The Art and Practice of Diagnosis in Chinese Medicine

by the same author

The Fundamentals of Acupuncture
Nigel Ching
Foreword by Charles Buck
ISBN 978 1 84819 313 0
eISBN 978 0 85701 266 1

of related interest

Acupuncture and Chinese Medicine
Roots of Modern Practice
Charles Buck
ISBN 978 1 84819 159 4
eISBN 978 0 85701 133 6

The Acupuncture Points Functions Colouring Book
Rainy Hutchinson
Forewords by Richard Blackwell, and Angela Hicks and John Hicks
ISBN 978 1 84819 266 9
eISBN 978 0 85701 214 2

The Spark in the Machine
How the Science of Acupuncture Explains the Mysteries of Western Medicine
Dr. Daniel Keown MBChB MCEM LicAc
ISBN 978 1 84819 196 9
eISBN 978 0 85701 154 1

The Acupuncturist's Guide to Conventional Medicine
Second Edition
Clare Stephenson
ISBN 978 1 84819 302 4
eISBN 978 0 85701 255 5

Intuitive Acupuncture
John Hamwee
ISBN 978 1 84819 273 7
eISBN 978 0 85701 220 3

The Art and Practice of Diagnosis in
CHINESE MEDICINE

NIGEL CHING
Foreword by Jeremy Halpin

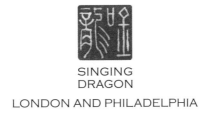

SINGING
DRAGON
LONDON AND PHILADELPHIA

English language edition first published in 2017
by Singing Dragon
an imprint of Jessica Kingsley Publishers
73 Collier Street
London N1 9BE, UK
and
400 Market Street, Suite 400
Philadelphia, PA 19106, USA

www.singingdragon.com

First published in Danish as *Kunsten at diagnosticere med Kinesisk medicin*
by Klitrose Publishers, Copenhagen, Denmark, 2009

Library of Congress Cataloging in Publication Data
Names: Ching, Nigel, 1962- author.
Title: The art and practice of diagnosis in Chinese medicine / Nigel Ching.
Description: London ; Philadelphia : Singing Dragon/Jessica Kingsley
    Publishers, 2017. | Includes bibliographical references.
Identifiers: LCCN 2016056990 (print) | LCCN 2016058175 (ebook) | ISBN
    9781848193147 (alk. paper) | ISBN 9780857012678 (ebook)
Subjects: | MESH: Medicine, Chinese Traditional--methods | Diagnostic
    Techniques and Procedures
Classification: LCC R601 (print) | LCC R601 (ebook) | NLM WB 55.C4 | DDC
    610--dc23
LC record available at https://lccn.loc.gov/2016056990

British Library Cataloguing in Publication Data
A CIP catalogue record for this book is available from the British Library

ISBN 978 1 84819 314 7
eISBN 978 0 85701 267 8

Printed and bound in Great Britain by Bell and Bain Ltd, Glasgow

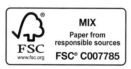

Dedicated to my granddaughter '5316', my parents and all the family and friends between them.

If a man will begin with certainties, he shall end in doubts; but if he will be content to begin with doubts, he shall end in certainties.

Francis Bacon 1561–1626

CONTENTS

FOREWORD

Another way of seeing things

One of the most important contributions that Chinese medical diagnosis has given to the collective medical knowledge is the unique way it comprehends and describes conditions of disease. Chinese medicine does not use polarised belligerent metaphors that try to identify internal and external 'enemies' that must be destroyed. Neither does it see the body as a dissociated and isolated island on which this 'war' is waged. Chinese medicine's focus is more on the constant adaptation to change.

To understand why this is so, it is necessary to understand the underlying medical model, or the logical principles that form the basis for this approach. To use a modern metaphor, the approach in this model focuses on 'software data flow' and not 'hardware', i.e. on what is happening inside and not on the physical structure.

The model is energy based; it is not an anatomical/physiological model. It does not involve the study of dead bodies or the deconstruction of the body into ever smaller components in an attempt to describe the whole. Chinese medicine always sees everything in the context of the whole.

The Dao that can be named is not the Dao[1]

The attentive reader will note that all the diagnostic models in this book describe the body's response to change and not separate and arbitrary disease symptoms as such. This is because the state of balance in the body is in a state of constant flux and a skilled therapist will be able to track the signals that the body is emitting. In this context, to name something is to fossilise it. People are not their 'diabetes' or 'migraine'. They are unique individuals whose conscious and unconscious responses have brought them to this place. The art of diagnosis is to identify these unique patterns of response in each individual. In other words, it is the patient who is diagnosed and not the disease.

An exchange of stories

So what is diagnosis? In the late 1800s the meeting between the patient and practitioner was called an 'exchange of stories'. This is where the patient presents their problem ('story') as best they can, based on their subjective experiences. They can also present their story in more subtle and non-conscious ways, for example their posture, movement and other factors that can be observed by the clinician.

Diagnosis, which is the subject of this detailed book, forms the therapist's story – the therapist's interpretation and response to the patient's history through the filter of their knowledge and experience. It will include aspects such as observation, palpation and the use of other senses, such as the sense of smell or noting the way the person's *shen* is manifesting, to expand the practitioner's perspective of the whole. All these factors are sorted in the diagnostic process through the various sub-models (the Eight Principles, Four Levels, Six Stages, etc.) to differentiate the possible diagnoses.

This does not, however, mean that the diagnosis ends here. For example, it is common to recheck the pulse diagnosis during the treatment to measure the response. In fact, treatment and diagnosis are never separated. They are constantly influencing each other and are two sides of the same coin.

When looking at new models such as this one, it is easy to drown in the volume of cultural references that permeate it. What Nigel Ching has achieved in this thorough and detailed study of traditional Chinese diagnosis is to outline and explain clearly both the methodology and, perhaps more importantly, the thinking behind it. It is especially this that I am convinced will prove to be indispensable to both students and interested readers.

Jeremy Halpin
Acupuncturist, Zen-shiatsu therapist and teacher
Stockholm, June 2008

ACKNOWLEDGEMENTS

I would like to express gratitude to the practitioners and scholars of Chinese medicine who have developed and documented this unique medical system. The world is a much better place to live in thanks to their knowledge, wisdom and efforts. I am deeply indebted to all of my teachers through the years, the authors of English language Chinese medicine textbooks and the doctors and practitioners who I have had the pleasure and honour of working with.

I would also like to thank the people directly involved in the genesis of the original Danish version of the book. Primarily my thanks go to Ole Bidsted from the Klitrose publishing house who published the original version of this and all my other books. Thank you for your tireless idealism and enthusiasm in publishing unprofitable but indispensable textbooks.

My gratitude and appreciation is also sent towards Singing Dragon for their support and belief in my books. A special thanks to Claire Wilson, Jane Evans and Victoria Peters.

Thanks to Aske Ching for tweaking the illustrations and making them presentable.

Thank you to the various students who have made valuable comments to the book, both when it was still only in the form of teaching handouts and later on after it was published in Denmark. There is a lot of proofreading talent gone to waste out there!

Thanks to friends and colleagues who have helped with their encouragement. I would particularly like to thank Wendy Norris for shelter, encouragement and support, both before and during the writing of the original version of the book.

PREFACE

An experienced Chinese medicine doctor can often diagnose a patient before the patient has even begun to tell the doctor what their disorder is. This may sound fantastic, as if the doctor has supernatural abilities, something that only a few people with special powers can do. This ability, though, depends on years of experience and a thorough understanding of the body's physiology and pathology. The doctor will have consciously and subconsciously picked up on a myriad of small and sometimes extremely subtle signs, such as the expression in the patient's eye, the facial complexion, the tone of the flesh, how the movement of the person is, how their posture is, the strength of their handshake and whether the hand feels clammy or dry, whether the hand is cold or hot and if it is warm whether it is the whole hand or only the palm that feels hot, how their attire is, the smell of their body, the sound of their voice, etc. All these individual small signs and signals will create an overall impression in the doctor's mind, enabling the doctor to identify the patterns of imbalance that the patient is presenting with.

Charlie Buck once said that this ability which experienced Chinese doctors possess is the same ability that a good ornithologist possesses. If a novice like me is going to be able to identify a bird in my garden, the bird must stand still and I must also have sufficient time to take note of the size of the bird's body, its wingspan, the colours in the plumage, the colour and length of the legs and beak, how it moves and so forth. Furthermore, I must then compare this information with the descriptions presented in an ornithology manual to see which bird it is that has precisely these colours and characteristics. However, an experienced ornithologist will immediately recognise which bird it is that is sitting on the bird table. An experienced ornithologist will not only recognise the bird when it sits on the bird table outside the window, but will also be able to identify the bird at a distance, even when it flies quickly past. Where others will barely have noticed the bird at all, just a few fleeting impressions will enable the experienced ornithologist to identify the bird with certainty. This ability is the result of many years of experience of studying the bird both through binoculars and with the naked eye, as well as having studied pictures and read descriptions of the bird in ornithological manuals. This will have resulted in an ability to recognise birds quickly from a minimum of signals.

This is also the case with an experienced Chinese medical doctor. The doctor will have gathered sufficient information before the patient talks of their problem to be reasonably certain of their diagnosis. The rest of the consultation is then used to confirm the diagnosis and to identify the aetiology and whether there are contributing patterns of imbalance.

This might give the impression that diagnosis goes from being analytical to being simply intuitive, but this is not so. Diagnostic intuition is nothing other than the rapid, subconscious analysis and interpretation of impressions and signals and relating these impressions to all the previous experiences of these signs. At the same time, these signs and impressions are subconsciously compared with the theoretical knowledge that has been gleaned from books and teachers. The subconscious is much quicker at analysing and sorting information than the conscious brain. Intuition is therefore not a supernatural ability but something that most of us are capable of. It just requires experience and a sound theoretical foundation.

What Chinese medical doctors have done over the centuries is to observe all the changes that occur in a person when a person's body is out of balance – both which symptoms there are and what other signals the body emits in these situations. They have been aware of the relationships between these symptoms and signs or the patterns that they constitute. Chinese medicine developed methods to collect and collate this information and these models systematically, and to classify and differentiate the symptoms and signs so that an accurate diagnosis can be determined, thereby creating a solid foundation for the treatment strategy.

The purpose of this book is to enable the practitioner to gather the necessary information from the patient to make an accurate and correct diagnosis through the use of traditional Chinese diagnostic methods.

The book is divided into two parts. The first part of the book is a summary of the four diagnostic approaches or diagnostic pillars. This part of the book covers the methods used to collect information from the patient – through observation and palpation and by listening to and smelling the patient – and the information that can be gathered through interviewing the patient. The clinical significance of what these signs represent in Chinese medicine is also detailed and explained.

The second part of the book examines the various diagnostic systems or diagnostic models used to classify and rationalise the information that has been collected through the four diagnostic pillars. It is only by making an accurate diagnosis that one is able to give the correct treatment to each individual patient.

As well as reviewing the various patterns of imbalance, this part of the book also gives suggestions for their treatment. It is important to remember that the acupuncture points and herbal formulas that are mentioned in the text are suggestions and not a rulebook. Excellent results will also be obtained using other relevant combinations of acupuncture or herbal formulas.

Furthermore, the acupuncture points suggested are just a starting point and only some of the points listed will be used. These points will often be combined with other points that are relevant to the individual symptoms or other imbalances that are to be addressed concurrently. The herbal formulas presented should also be modified in practice so that they are tailored to match the individual patient's presentation. It should also be noted that treatment with herbal prescriptions should only be administered by practitioners who have a relevant herbal medicine training. Acupuncture needles forgive mistakes, but herbal prescriptions can be merciless and one can easily worsen a patient's condition if the diagnosis and herbs do not match each other. Furthermore, there is a risk that even if the prescription is suited to the diagnosis, it can still create new imbalances in the body. Only when you have learned what signs you should be aware of do you know how to intervene and adjust the treatment in time.

It should also be made clear that this book is an analysis of Chinese medical diagnosis as a complete system. This means that some of the diagnostic categories are a reflection of life-threatening conditions that you will rarely meet in the clinic. Even if you work exclusively with Chinese medicine, it is important not to forget which signs and symptoms to be aware of in Western pathology and to know the limits of your competence and when to send a patient on to a Western medicine doctor for further examination or hospitalisation.

In keeping with *Fundamentals of Acupuncture* (Ching 2016), I have as far as possible used Chinese words, such as *qi, xue, xu, shi, shen*, instead of an English translation of these terms. The reason for this is that English words will usually either be too specific, representing only one of the multiple meanings or interpretations of the term, or they will not express the connotations that are present in the Chinese character. *Xue*, for example, is something other and more than blood is in the Western definition of the word. Furthermore, terms such as *shen* or *qi* cannot be adequately translated into a single English word. These Chinese words are therefore written in italics.

Furthermore, organ names, pathogens, pulse qualities, etc. are capitalised when the Chinese understanding of this term is inferred. This is done in order to emphasise that it is the Chinese medicine concept that is being referred to and that the word is not to be understood in the usual definition of the word in English.

I hope that this book can help the reader to develop a systematic approach to the diagnosis of their clients and that it gives the reader a thorough understanding of how and why pathological changes arise in the body. This book will never be able to replace practical instruction or teach the more tactile aspects of the diagnosis, but it is my hope that the book can be a guide to what needs to be felt, seen, smelt or heard and how these sensations are often experienced.

I am indebted as a practitioner, teacher and author to the Chinese doctors and scholars who have developed the theories and methods that are described in this book, as well as to the teachers and authors who have transferred this knowledge on to me.

My hope is that I can be a medium or pathway so that their knowledge can be of benefit to you and your patients.

Nigel Ching
Copenhagen

THE ART OF DIAGNOSIS OR HOW TO DIAGNOSE IN CHINESE MEDICINE

Before we even start to look at how to diagnose in Chinese medicine, it is appropriate to consider the following questions.

• Why do we diagnose at all?

• What is the aim of the diagnosis?

• In what way are we going to use the diagnosis?

We use the diagnosis as one of several steps that must be taken when we want to move from point A, which is a person who has some form of disorder or suffering, to point B, which is the same person who no longer has a disorder or is no longer suffering. Traditional Chinese Medicine (TCM)[2] has a logical and linear approach to enable the practitioner to get from point A to point B.

Patient with a problem ⟶ Diagnostic techniques to reveal the patient's symptoms and signs ⟶ Classification of these symptoms and signs into the various diagnostic models ⟶ Creation of an appropriate treatment strategy ⟶ Choice of relevant acupuncture points and needle techniques, appropriate herbal formulas and appropriate dietary and lifestyle advice ⟶ Patient without a problem

---

By diagnosing and identifying the underlying pattern or patterns of imbalance, we have not only a treatment strategy in relation to acupuncture and Chinese herbs, but we have also created a foundation from which we can give relevant advice to the client. This advice will often, but not always, have a direct relationship with the aetiology of their disorder. When we know which patterns of imbalance are present, we will also have an idea of the probable aetiology. These aetiological factors can often still be a part of the person's life. In this case, they are something that must be altered if the patient is to have a long-term benefit from the treatment. At the same time, when we know which other aetiological factors can negatively affect the imbalance, we can also give the client advice with regards to these factors.

Chinese medicine usually diagnoses on two levels at the same time: *bian bing lun zhi* (differentiation of symptoms and signs in relation to the disease category) and *bian zheng lun zhi* (differentiation of symptoms and signs in relation to the patterns of imbalance). *Bian bing lun zhi* is very similar to a Western medicine diagnosis in that it classifies the symptoms and signs with respect to a specific disease category, for example headache, menstrual cramps, vomiting, etc. Although the *bian bing* diagnosis is characterised by the name of a specific disorder, it is still important to remember that you must still think of this pathological process from a Chinese medical perspective. This means that we must understand the disorder through the pathomechanisms that have generated it. We must think of *qi*, *xue*, Phlegm, *zangfu*, etc. and not through the lens of lymphocytes, antibodies and hormone receptors. We do this even if the *bian bing* category has the same name as a Western disease category.

Dizziness, for example, is a disease category in both Chinese and Western medicine, yet the understanding of how and why dizziness arises is very different. In both Chinese and Western medicine there are several causative factors and various subcategories of dizziness. These pathomechanisms cannot simply be translated from one system into another. Dizziness can, for example, be diagnosed in Western medicine as being caused by a virus on the balance nerve. If we just translate this into Chinese medicine, we may think that we have to expel invasions of exogenous *xie* (pathogenic) *qi*. There will only be a few situations in which this would be a relevant treatment strategy. Dizziness in Chinese medicine can arise from many factors, such as internally generated Wind, *xue xu* or *yin xu*. Although the disease names and the underlying aetiology can sound similar, the treatment focus will often be decidedly different. This is because it is with the Chinese medical system that we will be treating the disorder. There is a linear progression in all medical systems from physiology, pathology and diagnosis through to treatment. Each stage is determined by the previous stage and these stages cannot be separated from each other.

The *bian zheng lun zhi* approach to diagnosis is radically different from Western medicine concepts. *Bian zheng lun zhi* is the classification of symptoms and signs in relation to the various patterns of imbalance, such as Liver *qi* stagnation, an invasion of Wind-Damp or *shaoyin* Stage Cold. Chinese medical diagnosis is not a choice between either *bian bing lun zhi* or *bian zheng lun zhi*. For the treatment to be truly effective, we must in reality use both differentiations. This can be illustrated with the following example. The acupuncture point GB 20 and the extra point *taiyang* (Ex-HN 5) are effective acupuncture points that can be used to treat headaches (*bian bing lun zhi* diagnosis). This is because these acupuncture points move and circulate *qi* and *xue*, as well as being able to drain *xie* (pathological) *qi* downwards from the head. GB 20 and *taiyang* are not, though, indicated in the treatment of nausea, which is a separate *bian bing lun zhi* diagnosis. The reason for this is precisely because the actions of these points is in the head. If the headache was the result of Phlegm (*bian zheng lun zhi* diagnosis), then St 40 and Sp 3 would be obvious points to combine with GB 20 and *taiyang*. This is because St 40 and Sp 3 can transform Phlegm, which in this case is underlying the headache. If, on the other hand, the headache had arisen from an invasion of Wind-Cold (*bian zheng lun zhi* diagnosis), then St 40 and Sp 3 would not be relevant, because they do not 'open to the exterior and expel invasions of *xie qi*'. St 40 and Sp 3 would, though, be relevant when treating nausea (*bian bing lun zhi* diagnosis) if the nausea is due to the presence of Phlegm (*bian zheng lun zhi* diagnosis). In this situation, these two points could be combined with Ren 12 and Pe 6, as these points are effective in regulating Stomach *qi* so that it descends. Ren 12 and Pe 6 are, however, not suitable for draining Phlegm down from the head. It is for this reason that an adage in Chinese medicine states, 'A single ailment can have many causes; a single cause can result in many ailments.'

Western medicine trains practitioners to distinguish symptoms separately and to understand them individually or as part of a particular disease or disorder. In Chinese medicine it is the opposite. Here one is trained to try to see patterns in the symptoms and signs and to see how these are related and what they can be an expression of.

A Dutch lecturer, whose name I have unfortunately forgotten, once gave a good illustration of the difference between the two systems' approaches to analysing a client. He said that the two systems both look at the same scene through a telescope. Western medicine views the body through the focus of the telescope, so when you look through it, you can, for example, see a hand. Western medicine can even see through the skin and can zoom in on the tendons, the muscles and bones in the hand and how these interact with each other. The telescope can zoom even closer in and see how the nerves affect the muscle fibres and how various neurotransmitters can activate the nerves. It can see into the cells themselves and see how the various components in the individual cells operate. Chinese medicine reverses the telescope. Chinese medicine sees the same hand, but it also sees what is going on at the same time. It observes that the hand is on an arm that belongs to a woman, who is waving to her husband, whilst a train is pulling out of a station. Both images are correct. To stop the hand moving, you could, for example, sever the muscles and tendons, break the bone or inject a chemical that disrupts the nerve signals. You could also, though, stop the train. Both approaches will result in the same result: the cessation of the hand waving.

In Western medicine, the focus is on the physical causes and effects. In Chinese medicine it is more the context and the relationship that are the most important, and not the individual components. For example, migraine headaches, menstrual pain, alternating diarrhoea and constipation, hypochondriac tension, a sensation of having a lump in the throat, the voice having a slight staccato quality and the pulse having a Wiry quality in the left middle (*guan*) position are not coherent symptoms in a Western medicine perspective and they will be seen as being expressions of several disparate disorders. Chinese medicine sees these symptoms and signs collectively as a clear indication that the person is presenting with Liver *qi* stagnation. Chinese medicine will therefore not treat these individual symptoms separately but instead treat them as a single pattern. Chinese medicine will also try to identify the underlying aetiology that has resulted in the development of Liver *qi* stagnation, because the pattern of imbalance itself must also be seen in a context. Imbalances do not arise by themselves.

The adage 'a single ailment can have many causes; a single cause can result in many ailments' means, therefore, that there are no standard treatments for specific diseases. There will, of course, be particular acupuncture points that are often used in the treatment of certain ailments, but there will also be utilised acupuncture points that treat the specific patterns of imbalance that have resulted in the disorder. In order to do this, one must be able to differentiate the individual patterns of imbalance from each other.

Patterns of imbalance can be differentiated according to various diagnostic models. These models can be used individually and they can be used together. They are, in fact, overlapping. Liver *xue xu* for example is both a diagnosis based on the Eight Principles and a *zangfu* diagnosis, as well as being a diagnosis according to *qi*, *xue* and *jinye*.

The *bian zheng lun zhi* diagnosis will not only identify the root cause of the disease manifestation, it will also identify where or at which level in the body the imbalance is. At the same time, it will give an indication of the relative strength of the body in relation to the imbalance. For example, the diagnosis 'invasion of the Wind-Cold' indicates that the imbalance is to be found in the *taiyang* aspect, which means that it is in the exterior aspect of the body, and implicit in this diagnosis is that there is a relatively strong pathogenic assault on the body – a *shi* or excess condition. Liver *xue xu* diagnosis, on the other hand, indicates that the imbalance is in the interior aspect of the body and that it is specifically the functioning of the Liver that is disturbed. Liver *xue xu* further implies that *xue* is deficient, and therefore the organ is weakened, so the Liver is *xu* or deficient.

A Chinese medicine diagnosis is the foundation of the treatment strategy, i.e. how to restore balance in the body. The treatment strategy is already indicated in the diagnosis. If there is an invasion of *xie qi, xie qi* must be expelled. If there is a *shi* condition, then that which is *shi* must be drained, spread or expelled. If there is a *xu* condition, then that which is *xu* should be tonified, nourished or strengthened.

By differentiating patterns of imbalance, the clinician is not only able to develop an appropriate treatment strategy and thus utilise relevant acupuncture points or herbal prescriptions, but also will have an idea of what the aetiology of the imbalance could be. It is vitally important to remember that patterns of imbalance are not the causes of the disease. Diseases are certainly manifestations of patterns of imbalance, but the real causes lie in the aetiological factors that result in the pattern of imbalance. This will be factors such as environmental influences, a person's diet, lifestyle or emotional influences.

Liver *qi* stagnation, for example, can manifest with the symptoms and signs described earlier. However Liver *qi* stagnation is not the cause of these symptoms and signs. Liver *qi* stagnation is, like all other patterns of imbalance, a related collection of signs and symptoms. The pattern of imbalance is exactly this – a 'pattern' the patient presents with. The underlying cause of the pattern in this case will often be related to a person's emotional situation. If we are able to recognise patterns, we can have a logical idea of the underlying aetiology. When we have an idea of the aetiology, we have an opportunity to give relevant advice to the client. This is in reality the most important part of the treatment. By administering herbs or inserting needles, we can rectify an imbalance and relieve its symptoms. By giving relevant advice, we can help a person to prevent the imbalance from arising again.

To be able to detect which patterns of imbalance are present requires a comprehensive and thorough diagnosis. This entails the gathering of large amounts of disparate information from the client. This information has to be gathered through several sensory organs at the same time. Gathering and processing so much information simultaneously can appear to be overwhelming, but Chinese medicine is very logical in its approach from having developed specific diagnostic models and, especially, from having a very systematic approach to the collection of this information.

This foundation for this systematic approach to the gathering of diagnostic information was laid 2000 years ago in the classical text *Nan Jing* (The Classic of Difficulties). This book initiated the diagnostic approach that we use to this day: the four diagnostic pillars. In the book it says that one must first see and observe the patient. Then you should listen to and smell the patient. Next you have to ask the patient questions. Finally, you should palpate the patient. This requires that you are systematic and logical, whilst being sensitive and aware. This is because much of the information that needs to be gathered and utilised is something you have to perceive through your fingers, nose, eyes and ears, rather than simply asking questions.

To observe and absorb this much information at the same time, you need to be centred and focused when the patient comes through the door and free from all mental distractions so that your senses are open and receptive. This is obviously easier said than done when you are already behind schedule with your clients. Nevertheless, it is important to try at all times to be as focused and present as much possible.

However, being sensitive and receptive is, in itself, not enough when diagnosing. You also need to have an intellectual understanding of the material. You need to learn which signs and symptoms you should be aware of and what these symptoms and signs mean. This can done by learning either the various signs and symptoms and what these are a manifestation of by heart, and what the pathomechanisms behind these signs and symptoms are – how these symptoms and signs arose. Organising and structuring our approach and the way we process this information means it becomes more manageable and easier to access the relevant information. This frees you up so you can be more intuitive. Intuition that is not based on a strong fundamental understanding of theory will always only be speculation and guesswork.

Diagnostic prerequisites

A strong theoretical foundation and understanding of Chinese medicine physiology and pathology

By having a solid understanding of both the Chinese medicine physiological and pathological models, you will be able to understand the pathomechanisms (the pathological dynamics) behind the various symptoms and signs.

Let us look at an example. The Stomach sends its *qi* downwards. When a person vomits, this will be due to a rebellious movement of Stomach *qi*, which has sent the contents of the Stomach upwards and out of the mouth. We do not yet know why the Stomach *qi* is rebellious, but we know that Stomach *qi* is moving in the opposite direction to the direction in which it should when the Stomach is in balance. We know this, because we have studied the Chinese medicine physiological model and we therefore know that the correct movement of Stomach *qi* is downwards. Having also studied Chinese medicine pathology, we will already have several ideas of how and why this disturbance of Stomach *qi* could have arisen. There could, for example, be something that is blocking the Stomach *qi* from descending (such as exogenous Cold, Phlegm, *qi* stagnation, *xue* stagnation or food stagnation). We also know that Stomach *qi* could be too weak to be able to send the food downwards (Stomach *qi xu*) or there may be Heat present, causing the Stomach *qi* to rise upwards (Stomach Fire or an invasion of exogenous *xie qi*). This means that we can start looking for relevant symptoms and signs that relate to these particular patterns of imbalance and we can ask the patient relevant questions: Is there anything that provokes the vomiting? Is there anything that ameliorates it? When and how did the vomiting start? And so on. All these things will give an idea of why the person's Stomach *qi* has become rebellious.

Observe and analyse deviations from the 'norm'

A concept that is central to the art of diagnosis is the norm. The norm is that which we expect to observe. It is that which we should observe when the body functions perfectly and is completely harmonious. This condition is also known as the utopian state!

If we constantly maintain a clear image in our minds of how the body should be, we can recognise signs which indicate that the body is not in balance. At this point, it is very important to be constantly aware of the crucial difference that there is between what is normal and what is common. It is common to have a pale tongue with teeth marks, a greasy yellow coating on the root and a red tip. This is seen in a lot of people, perhaps the majority of Northern Europeans, but it is not what a normal tongue should look like. A normal tongue should be pink, without tooth marks and with a thin, pale, even coating.

We must train ourselves to spot deviations from the norm, and to think about and determine what has caused the change.

There will often be nothing, or very little, to observe. The closer you are to the norm, whether this is the strength and speed of a person's voice, the colour of the tongue or something else, the fewer signs of imbalance there will be to observe.

By observing the deviations from the norm, and by understanding pathomechanisms behind these changes, you are in fact liberated from having to learn long lists of symptoms and signs, as well as having to remember what these signs and symptoms signify diagnostically. This is not the typical Chinese approach to learning how to diagnose: in China, it is more common to learn things by heart, which is also a valid way of learning the significance of the various signs and symptoms. I personally think, though, that it is easier to learn and remember the relevance of diagnostic signs and symptoms, by thinking of *qi* dynamics and pathomechanisms. This also has the advantage that you become more flexible in your thinking and comprehension of problems when they present themselves differently from the textbooks.

By learning to understand the pathomechanisms, you become accustomed to thinking: 'This is not as it should be. How and why is it not as it should be?' When you have done this, you can start to figure out why something has deviated from the norm.

As always, it is easiest to use an example. Normally, a person's respiration is gentle and rhythmic. If a person has difficulty breathing gently, quietly and rhythmically, and if their respiration is very shallow, this is a sign that the Lung[3] is not descending and spreading *qi* as it should. We must then try and determine why the Lung is not able to perform this function optimally. Is it because the Lung is *qi xu*? Is it because there is a stagnation of *qi* in the upper *jiao*? Is there exogenous *xie qi*, such as Wind-Cold, obstructing the Lung so it cannot spread and descend *qi*? Is there Phlegm in the Lung and the upper *jiao* that is blocking the *qi*? Has the person been exposed to a shock, and *qi* in the upper *jiao* has become chaotic? This way of thinking can be used with any symptom or sign. This approach also means that we then start to look for other relevant signs and symptoms that may confirm our hypothesis.

Study and become adept at using the various diagnostic techniques

In order to practise Chinese medical diagnosis, it is a prerequisite that you have learned the various diagnostic techniques – the observational skills required to be able to utilise the techniques involved in the four diagnostic pillars. This means that you must have learned to palpate the pulse, observe the tongue, palpate the channels and interview the client. This is something that is taught in basic training, but it requires constant practice to become adept at it. I often meet former students who ask me for advice about a client they are treating. Unfortunately, when I ask about the tongue and pulse diagnosis, it is not uncommon that the practitioner says that they have not checked the pulse. When I ask why, the answer is that they think it is difficult and they do not feel that they are competent enough to be able to utilise the pulse. Learning diagnostic skills is no different from learning to play the guitar or learning a foreign language. Some people have natural talents and they are adept right from the beginning. These people will only improve with time if they practise. Others, myself included, are less gifted. I could learn to play some simple chords on a guitar if somebody showed me where to put my fingers. However, I would never become a virtuoso who could play in a concert hall, although I might become competent enough to sit around a fire and entertain my friends. However, even this will take practice – a lot of practice! The same is true of pulse diagnosis, tongue diagnosis, observation techniques and palpation. Diagnostic techniques are something that must be practised every day or at least every time you have a patient. You may well feel that you are not feeling or observing anything, but it is important to keep on practising. It is often easier, when diagnosing, if you deconstruct the process and analyse each aspect separately.

If we take the pulse as an example, you might ask yourself, whilst your your fingers are palpating the patient's artery: Is the rate of the pulse fast or slow? Does the pulse feel strong or weak? Wide or narrow? Shallow or deep? Rhythmic or not? Has the pulse got qualities that could be perceived of as being 'Slippery', 'Choppy', 'Wiry' or 'Tight'? Are there variations between the individual pulse positions? You can also reverse the process. If you know which patterns of imbalance are present in a patient, you can search for the relevant pulse qualities and see if you can recognise them in the patient's pulse. When you have felt the same quality several times, you may start to recognise this same quality in a new patient's pulse.

Study the various patterns of imbalance

There are, unfortunately, no short cuts here. The various patterns of imbalance should be learnt by heart. You should be able to classify the various symptoms and signs you experience and categorise them into the various patterns of imbalance. However, there is the loophole that I described above: if you have a firm grasp of Chinese medicine physiology and understand the dynamics of the various forms of *xie qi* (pathological *qi*) and other disruptive factors, you will be able to assess which organs, substances or aspects of the body are affected and in what way. For example, if a person freezes, especially suddenly, and they cannot get warm even though they put on thick clothes and tuck themselves under a duvet, our thinking will be as follows. We know that it is *yang qi* that heats the body, so if they had *yang qi xu* – a condition where there is too little of the warming *yang qi* – the person ought to be able to keep warm by putting on sufficient clothing or by tucking themselves under a duvet. This is not the case here, so it is probably not a *yang xu* condition. If, on the other hand, the person has been invaded by exogenous Wind-Cold, which blocks the *wei qi* whose function it is to warm the skin, then even though they pack themselves into warm clothes and bedding, they would still feel cold. Therefore, this is probably a *shi* Cold condition – an invasion of exogenous *xie* Cold. Further confirmation that their *wei qi* is being blocked by exogenous *xie qi* will be found if the person does not sweat and has muscle aches. This is because all these signs either relate to the functions of *wei qi* (warming the skin and controlling the pores) or they are signs of a stagnation of *qi* in the exterior aspect of the body, where the *wei qi* circulates (muscle aches). We know that the *wei qi* can be blocked by exogenous *xie qi* and that Cold, due to its contracting dynamic, will cause the pores in the skin to close. Cold will also inhibit the free movement of *wei qi*.

The other option is, of course, to learn everything off by heart. You can memorise the various symptoms and signs that define the individual patterns of imbalance. By studying the textbooks, we know that all of the above symptoms and signs can be found in the diagnostic category 'invasion of Wind-Cold'. This is similar to how a computer works. The computer does not understand why the symptoms occur, but it can nevertheless recognise a pattern when it is presented with a particular group of symptoms and signs. This is because it has been programmed to recognise these symptoms and signs as being representative of this pattern of imbalance.

An alternative approach is to learn the importance of the individual symptoms and signs by heart. In the example above, when a person freezes, you can look at all the possible imbalances that manifest with a sensation of cold or an aversion to cold. You can then collect additional information to see whether the person has other symptoms and signs that can confirm the presence of one or more of these patterns of imbalance.

Experience

The main difference between an experienced practitioner and a novice with regards to diagnosis is simply a question of experience. An experienced practitioner has had more years to read books and study other practitioners' case histories. More importantly, the experienced practitioner has had more years of experience in visually observing, interviewing, listening to, palpating and smelling patients and subsequently comparing what they have read about in books with what they meet in practice. This means that the experienced practitioner knows what is probable in certain situations, but also has experienced situations where the opposite is the case.

An experienced practitioner has also learned to place more emphasis on certain symptoms and signs than others in particular situations. Moreover, the experienced practitioner, through practice and experience, just becomes better at recognising characteristic signs of an imbalance in certain people. They have, however, also become better at not latching onto, and sticking with, the first idea that comes to mind. They have become more flexible in their approach.

In general, an experienced practitioner is often quicker at diagnosing a patient than a novice. This is because the experienced practitioner does not need to think for as long about things. When observing a symptom or a sign, the experienced practitioner automatically know what questions they will subsequently ask or what signs they should observe in this situation. They do not need to think about it. Neither do they need to look things up in books or search the corners of their memory when they want to find out what the various symptoms, signs and observations signify. It is something that they just know.

Intuition

Another major difference between experienced and less experienced practitioners, is how much they trust their intuition and, especially, how trustworthy their intuition is. Intuition must be based on a solid theoretical understanding coupled with practical experience, otherwise it is nothing more than just guesswork.

Intuition is one of the most important skills an experienced practitioner possesses. Intuition, however, is nothing other than a person's ability to let their subconscious brain recognise and process the information that they, at some point, have had to collect consciously and think about. Their subconscious brain can more rapidly sort this information into useful conclusions than the conscious processes of the mind can.

Western diagnosis

There can be a tendency amongst some practitioners to use a Western medicine diagnosis as their starting point. A question that I often meet, both when I talk to other acupuncturists and when I read online discussions is: Which acupuncture points should you use to treat some Western named disorder? This raises several issues.

- **Western diagnoses can be incorrect.** There is a significant risk involved in relying on another person's diagnosis. It is not uncommon for a patient to receive different diagnoses from different doctors. This is not a critique of Western doctors, but a fact when different people subjectively analyse objective material. If you treat according to another doctor's diagnosis, there is a risk that you will administer an incorrect treatment if the initial diagnosis was wrong. This is only made worse by the fact that the Western medicine diagnosis is based on a completely different physiological and pathological model than that of the Chinese medicine diagnoses and treatments. I will expand on this below. However, it is not only the Western medicine diagnosis that we must be wary of. We should also be wary of Chinese medicine diagnoses made by other acupuncturists or herbalists. I regularly receive clients from other practitioners who want me to either treat their patient with herbs or continue their acupuncture treatment. It is not uncommon that my and the other acupuncturist's diagnoses do not match. If I prescribed herbs or inserted needles based on another acupuncturist's diagnosis, I would often be giving the patient the wrong treatment (assuming that my diagnosis is correct). Likewise, if I gave an acupuncture treatment on the basis of a Western doctor's diagnosis, I cannot be sure that the doctor's diagnosis was correct in the first place.

- **A Western medicine diagnosis is based on the Western medicine physiological and pathological model.** The acupuncture points that are recommended in Chinese medicine textbooks for the treatment of certain organs, bodily substances, pathological factors, etc. are usually selected based on an understanding of the actions that they have in Chinese medicine. It is not certain that they have the same effect when viewed from a Western medicine analysis of their physiological actions. A very obvious example of this is when a Western medicine diagnosis says that a person has a problem with their spleen. It is far from certain that a point such as Sp 3 will have any effect on the physical spleen in this situation. This is because the same pattern of symptoms and signs in a patient will often not be diagnosed as a Spleen pattern of imbalance in Chinese medicine. We need to translate diagnoses to our own diagnostic models. It is only in this way that the treatment will match the diagnosis perfectly. This also applies to other complementary medicine diagnostic methods, such as iris diagnosis or a homoeopathic diagnosis. In these cases, the diagnosis of organs and their functions will again be based on another physiological and pathological model. Treatments and the physiological and diagnostic foundation must match each other. We would not expect a Western medical doctor to treat a patient based on our diagnosis. They would immediately exclaim that what we are saying does not make sense in relation to their way of understanding the body. Likewise, we should not treat the body from a diagnosis based on a Western medicine understanding of the body but through a Chinese medicine interpretation of the symptoms and signs.

- **The same disorders can have many causes.** A Western diagnosis will always be a *bian bing lun zhi* diagnosis. The foundation of Chinese medicine is the differentiation of disorders both in relation to the disorder or disease and in relation to the patterns of imbalance. This means that even if we diagnose multiple patients with the same *bian bing lun zhi* diagnosis, we may well treat each of these patients differently, precisely because their patterns of imbalance or *bian zheng lun zhi* diagnosis are different.

In what way can we then use a Western medicine diagnosis?

As written above, a Western medicine diagnosis is basically a *bian bing lun zhi* diagnosis that is based on a Western medicine understanding of the body. This means that the Western diagnosis will often relate to aspects of the body that are not found in the Chinese medicine model, such as hormones, neurotransmitters or intestinal bacteria. We know that intestinal flora, for example, has many of the functions that we relate to Spleen *qi*, but we also know that Spleen *qi* is much more than just the functions performed by the intestinal flora. Similarly, the intestinal flora also have functions that do not relate to Spleen *qi*. When we are informed of a Western medicine diagnosis, we need to deconstruct this into its component symptoms and pathological processes. We should then reconstruct the individual symptoms and signs, as well as the pathological processes, into a Chinese medicine diagnosis using a Chinese medicine understanding of the body. Unfortunately, we cannot just say that oestrogen, for example, is equivalent to Kidney *yin* and thereby treat an oestrogen imbalance with the acupuncture point Kid 3. It may well be that the treatment will work, but not all of the functions of oestrogen in the body can necessarily be interpreted as being Kidney *yin*. There may well be individual processes that we will interpret differently, and if we are to treat these processes then there may be a greater physiological effect if we warm Kidney *yang* or move Liver *qi* or something else altogether. This is especially relevant if there are other symptoms and signs that also point in this direction. What we must find is a pattern – a relationship between the various symptoms and signs and how they relate to the Chinese medicine model of health and illness.

A Western medicine diagnosis will give us an idea of which direction we should look in. We can definitely examine the Western medicine diagnosis and try to analyse the symptoms and the pathological processes that lead to these symptoms from a Western medicine perspective, but we should always be thinking: How would I interpret this from a Chinese medicine perspective? Which organs or types of *qi* perform these functions? How could this process be disturbed, for example, by *qi* stagnation, Phlegm, Heat, etc.? We should also look at the individual patient and ask ourselves: Do they actually have these symptoms and signs? At the same time, we need to correlate these symptoms and signs with all the other symptoms and signs that the patient manifests. This is because Chinese medicine often places emphasis on signs and symptoms that are not viewed as being relevant in a Western medicine diagnosis of a disorder. This could, for example, be that the person talks rapidly and gesticulates a lot with their hands whilst they are talking, indicating the presence of Heat in the Heart.

The diagnostic process

As previously written, diagnosis is part of a process where we proceed from point A, where a patient has a problem, to point B, where the same patient does not have a problem any longer. This is most easily achieved by having a structured approach where you are aware of what the aim of each step is. This is especially true in the diagnostic part of the process.

The diagnostic process starts at the first contact

We start the diagnosis the moment we first see the patient or at the first moment of contact that we have with the patient. This process can actually start even before the patient enters the room, when we talk to them on the phone or read their email. From the moment we are in contact with them, and certainly from the moment they step into the room, we must constantly gather information from them and begin to form a diagnostic hypothesis. We will subsequently continue to verify and check this hypothesis in an attempt to confirm or refute our assumptions. We must then constantly investigate all the various diagnostic clues that reveal themselves. At times, it is something of a difficult balancing act. We must trust our first impressions. This is because the first impression can often be of great diagnostic importance, especially as it is at this moment that we are usually most intuitive and least rational in our thinking. We must, however, simultaneously have and maintain a flexibility in our thinking and our approach to the patient. We must not stubbornly cling to a diagnosis and thereby become blind to the diagnostic signs that point in other directions. We must be aware of the risk of interpreting symptoms and signs exclusively from the perspective of our first hypothesis. It's like being a detective. We must follow a hunch, but not become blind to other possibilities or exclude other suspects.

Have a structured approach

Having a structured approach is very important. Moving from the metaphorical point A (the patient has a problem) to point B (the patient no longer has a problem) is most easily achieved when taking deliberate steps, where you are conscious of what you want to achieve with each individual step. A structured approach is also important, because our clients often present us with many, varied and sometimes conflicting symptoms and signs. It is therefore essential that you constantly have a clear idea in your head of where you are going and what you want to know. You must not let yourself be driven around like driftwood in a sea of symptoms and signs. You must have a clear direction and deliberately paddle using your eyes, ears, mouth, nose and fingers as oars and your theoretical foundation as a rudder. This can be especially difficult when new pieces of information constantly keep emerging, each of which must be investigated. You will have to travel down each diagnostic track one at a time, but at the same time remember to come back and investigate the remaining tracks. In these situations, having a pen and a piece of paper is invaluable, so that you can jot down notes and key words whilst the patient is talking to make sure you do not forget to investigate everything thoroughly. A good intake sheet with boxes and rubrics that list various qualities is a diagnostic essential that enables you to investigate all relevant areas thoroughly.

Complex patients, where there are many signs and symptoms, will always be a challenge. Unfortunately, these clients are not uncommon. This is because many of the clients who seek Chinese medicine are clients who have chronic conditions that have not been helped in the conventional medical system. These conditions are called 'difficult to treat, knotty diseases' in China. In these cases, there will typically be many patterns of imbalances at the same time – at least six or seven – and often in excess of ten patterns. There will also be a tricky mixture of *xu* and *shi* and Hot and Cold imbalances. This means that there will be a myriad of symptoms and signs to discern and decipher. These signs and symptoms will often be contradictory, pointing in opposite directions at the same time.

There is a vast amount of information that we have to keep track of whilst we diagnose. At the same time, we must be open and attentive on several levels, both intellectually and intuitively. We need to listen to what the patient says and at the same time listen to how they are saying it, what qualities their voice has, how fast they talk and how structured their conversation is. We must observe their appearance, their movements and their body language while we ask them questions and mentally analyse their responses.

A structured approach is also important when interviewing clients who have a tendency to take over the interview. There are definitely some clients who are more difficult to interview than others. This is usually an important diagnostic sign in itself. As the practitioner, we should try to maintain control of the conversation. After all, it is us who is the therapist. When this control is challenged by the client, we can try and interpret diagnostically why and how they cause us to lose control. We must, of course, be conscious of our own patterns of imbalances and how these might be involved in us having difficulty in controlling the interview. If it is not our own patterns of imbalances that result in us losing control, then we can try to see how the patient makes us lose our footing. For example, some patients with Heart Fire will often be very garrulous and we will have difficulty getting succinct answers to our questions. Patients with Phlegm-Heat blocking and agitating *shen* will also often talk a lot and much of what they say may be completely irrelevant, because Phlegm is blocking their *shen*. Liver *qi* stagnation patients may have a tendency to want to control the situation and the conversation. Phlegm-Dampness patients may be slightly confused and have difficulty keeping their focus, and so on. It can also be difficult when patients have a lot of ideas about what is wrong and why they have a disorder. These people tell you a lot of things that to us are not necessarily relevant to the diagnosis. They could, though, have been treated by other acupuncturists or have read things on the internet or in an acupuncture textbook and believe that they know which Chinese medicine patterns of imbalances they are manifesting. It is important that it is us who interprets the information we gather and the information they tell us. What they conclude or what they have been told may not be correct. It is important that it is us who makes the diagnosis.

A structured approach is more than just a checklist

As written above, all the information that we need to collect and process simultaneously can be overwhelming and confusing, especially with a client who takes control of the conversation. A well-designed diagnostic journal or intake sheet is a massive help here. It ensures that we collect all the information that we need to use. A diagnostic journal must never become a checklist where you just tick boxes. I have often experienced in exam situations and school clinics that some students tend to ask a question – often a yes or no question – and then they just move on to the next question. Each and every answer we get is a springboard for further investigation. It is a door that we should walk through to see if there is more information inside that room. For each answer we get, or for each sign we observe, we must look for further signs or ask clarifying questions. This is both in order to understand the mechanism behind this sign or reply and to see if there are other symptoms and signs that these are connected to. We must see whether the sign or the answer is part of a pattern. An example could be that the patient has replied that yes, they do suffer from headaches. We then need to know: When do they have headaches? How would they describe the pain? Whereabouts in the head is the pain? What makes the headache better or worse? When did they begin to suffer from headaches and what happened in this period of time? We must ascertain what type of headache they have. If we have the impression that the headache is possibly a manifestation of, for example, ascending Liver Fire, we must then look for further signs of Liver Fire to confirm or refute our hypothesis. Furthermore, we also know that many patterns of imbalance may be a consequence of the other patterns of imbalance. We should therefore also investigate whether there are signs and symptoms of these patterns.

Use all four of the diagnostic pillars

If we have a structured approach, we should consciously utilise all four diagnostic pillars. A skilled diagnostician will also utilise as much information as possible from each pillar. A pillar is not just built from one or two blocks of stone, it also consists of sand and mortar. Palpation is more than just pulse diagnosis, and observation is more than just tongue diagnosis.

Furthermore, there can be a tendency to prioritise the diagnostic pillar of interviewing or questioning the client. This is often at the expense of the other three approaches. This is mainly due to the way we have been educated, since we started in primary school when we were children. This has resulted in the development of an intellectual bias. We feel secure and trust an intellectual approach based on questions and verbal responses. It is relatively easy to translate a verbal response to intellectual knowledge. This is something the education system trained us to do for more than a decade. There are, however, a lot of pitfalls in this diagnostic approach. We must be very conscious of what the questions are and how we ask them. We need to know what their response implies. We also know that patients do not always respond truthfully. It could well be because it is something that they are not conscious of. Also, clients sometimes, for various reasons, deliberately answer misleadingly or use words that you can interpret in a different way from them. More typically though, they comprehend the question in a different way from the practitioner. For example, if you ask a woman if she has regular menstrual periods, she may well answer yes, even if her menstrual cycle is only 21 days long or is 35 days long. Another woman might answer yes – it is regular, because it comes about once a month. The problem for us is that 'about once a month' is not regular in Chinese medicine if it's 25 days in one month and 33 days in the next month. Similarly, regular bowel movements can be interpreted by a client as being once every three days or four times each day. Some of these problems can be minimised by having a good interview technique with unambiguous questions and constantly ensuring that you have asked additional and clarifying questions and not let yourself be satisfied with simple yes and no answers.

The fact that we are so conditioned to be intellectual by the education system means that we actually have an intellectual handicap. We blindly trust our intellect at the expense of our other senses. We must learn to retrain and hone our observational abilities. This is also a challenge, because it is much easier to translate verbal responses to intellectual knowledge that can be analysed and categorised than it is to transform sensory information to something we can rationally analyse and intellectually classify.

Each of the four diagnostic pillars has their inherent strengths and their weaknesses. These will be investigated in Part 1.

Conflicting information

It is, unfortunately, not uncommon for there to be a conflict in the information, and thereby diagnostic conclusions, obtained from the different diagnostic approaches or within the same aspect of the diagnosis. It is quite common, for example, for the tongue to exhibit signs of certain imbalances, whilst the pulse manifests something else and the patient's voice and demeanour something else again. In reality, we must not think of these discrepancies as being conflicts but more as puzzles to be solved. These discrepant signals will usually just reflect different aspects of the diagnosis, i.e. different patterns of imbalance, all of which are present at the same time. We just need to understand how to separate them from each other and see whether they interact with each other or are independent of each other. We must also be aware of other factors that may have blurred these diagnostic signs, for example medicine, the fact that the patient just ran up the stairs or that they are angry.

Time constraints

A major problem we have is a lack of time. It can take a long time to gather all the information, especially when you are not experienced and therefore as quick to spot what is relevant and important in this situation. This means that you have to either allot an appropriate period of time to the diagnosis of clients or learn to prioritise information and make sure that you have control of the dialogue with the client.

Different processes, different strategies

Some teachers believe that you should only investigate the patterns of imbalance that are relevant to the specific disorder that you are asked to treat. This means that, for example, you do not start asking questions about signs of a Lung imbalance, if a person has chronic diarrhoea. Bob Flaws, an American author of numerous Chinese medicine textbooks, is an advocate of this approach and considers that you must learn all the relevant patterns of imbalance for the different *bian bing lun zhi* categories and only investigate these when diagnosing a *bian bing* condition. Personally, I do not agree with him. First, the relevant pattern of imbalances that can manifest with a specific disorder can in itself be the consequence of other patterns of imbalance. For example, Liver *qi* stagnation can be a consequence of Liver *xue xu*, which itself may be a consequence of Spleen *qi xu*. It is important to understand the dynamics involved in the genesis of the patterns of imbalance. I personally, therefore, do not think that it is enough only to investigate the patterns that are relevant to the specific *bian bing lun zhi* conditions.

Furthermore, the patterns of imbalance that are presently manifesting may be precursors to other patterns of imbalance. It may therefore be relevant to investigate whether these patterns of imbalance are evolving. Furthermore, it is not uncommon to uncover other disorders through the diagnostic process that are more serious than the disorder that the client has sought help for. It may be that the patient is not aware that you could also treat this problem but would actually want this problem addressed. For example, a patient may come to you because they want to have treatment for their weak immune system, but through your thorough and extended diagnosis you find out that they suffer from anxiety and insomnia, which is something that is a serious problem for them.

Diagnostic models

It is an advantage to memorise the various symptoms and signs of all the various *bian zheng lun zhi* categories, i.e. all the various pattern of imbalances. You can, of course, look these up in your textbooks or on the computer, but this is much more time consuming in the long run. Once you have learned the different diagnostic models and categories, you can quickly recognise patterns in the symptoms and signs that are in front you. The diagnostic models are templates that we can place on top of all the information we have collected. We can then see if the information we have gathered fits into a particular template.

Some diagnostic models are only used in specific situations, for example diagnosis according to the three *jiao* or the Four Levels; others are used constantly and in combination with other diagnostic models, for example diagnosis according to *zangfu* and diagnosis according to *qi*, *xue* and *jinye*.

One of the typical mistakes that I made when I started was that I believed that all the symptoms and signs that were listed as being representative of a specific pattern of imbalance should be present. Often, we diagnose a pattern of imbalance from the presence of as little as three or four key symptoms and signs. The trick is to learn which of the various symptoms and signs are important and essential and in which situations. Furthermore, I thought that the symptoms and signs that were listed in the textbook were the only signs and symptoms that were manifestations of this particular pattern. The signs and symptoms listed in textbooks are the most probable symptoms and signs of this pattern. There will often be other symptoms and signs that are not in the textbook but are created by this pattern's *qi* dynamic. When you suspect the presence of certain patterns of imbalance, you have to ask yourself whether all the things that you are observing can be interpreted as being manifestations of these patterns, even though they are not listed in the textbook. This is where you really benefit from the hours spent studying Chinese medicine physiology and pathology. These studies have, in reality, enabled you to determine for yourself what symptoms and signs can be manifestations of a particular imbalance. You are now capable of seeing a symptom or a sign in different context from that described in the textbook.

Another mistake that I made was to think that when diagnosing a particular disorder, the disorder was the result of either one or other of the imbalance patterns that were listed as being the root of the problem. In reality, a disorder is usually the consequence of multiple patterns simultaneously. For example, spontaneous bleeding will very often be the result of Spleen *qi xu*, *xue* stagnation and Heat simultaneously. Individually, these three patterns of imbalance may not have been sufficient to result in bleeding in this patient. This can also sometimes be the reason that a treatment has not succeeded. This is because you have not treated all the aspects of the problem. At other times there will only be the one underlying pattern of imbalance.

Treating complex patients with many patterns of imbalances

Keep it simple

When things seem complex and confusing, it is always a good idea to keep things simple and only diagnose and treat what you are certain is present. The diagnostic picture may well become clearer with time. The situation may seem daunting, because there are so many symptoms and signs all mixed in with each other. This is further complicated by the fact that some of these symptoms and signs are also contradictory. In these situations, the diagnostic model of the Eight Principles is a blessing. This is a solid rock that we can step back onto when we start to drown in a rough sea of multiple symptoms and signs. We can simplify the whole situation or the individual symptoms and signs momentarily and ask ourselves: Is this *xu* or *shi*? Cold or Hot? Interior or exterior? *Yin* or *yang*? This can then be used as a springboard to refine the diagnosis. If the diagnosis will not or cannot be further refined, we can always treat the patient from these principles alone. If we treat only from the Eight Principles, we can be reasonably confident that we will not harm the patient, but, on the contrary, we will probably benefit them. This is despite the fact that it would have been optimal to further refine the diagnosis.

Make inventory boxes and flowcharts

One technique that I utilised a lot in the beginning was to make inventory boxes and 'flowcharts' on a sheet of paper. I distributed all the symptoms and signs of the patient in various diagnostic boxes. The individual symptoms and signs could usually be listed in multiple boxes. Boxes that had many symptoms and signs in were probably relevant patterns of imbalances, whereas boxes with only one or two signs or symptoms were less probable, especially if these symptoms and signs could be seen and explained better in other boxes. However, it is important not to write off a pattern of imbalance simply because there are only one or two signs or symptoms in the box. This is because some signs and symptoms are definitive signs of particular patterns of imbalance or these signs are simply the only two signs that are manifesting at this point in time. When you have made these boxes, you can then see how the dynamic is in this patient – how these patterns of imbalance affect and create each other. You can also continue the exercise by including the aetiological factors.

Part 1

THE DIAGNOSTIC PILLARS

INTRODUCTION TO THE DIAGNOSTIC PILLARS

The first half of this book concerns itself with the so-called 'diagnostic pillars'. These pillars are all the information that can be gathered through visually observing, listening and smelling, palpating and interrogating the client. The pillars are the systematic approach that Chinese medicine has developed over the years to gather and analyse all the information from a patient that has diagnostic relevance. The four pillars enable the practitioner to construct as precise and solid a diagnosis as possible.

Through the use of the practitioner's eyes, hands, ears and nose, as well as their intellect, Chinese medicine has over the millennia developed a diagnostic system that is both coherent and logical. This is because any change in the physiology of the body will not only affect the functioning of the body, but it will also manifest with tangible signs that can be seen, felt, heard and smelt. By systematically organising the collection and categorisation of this knowledge, Chinese medicine has developed a very precise and scientific diagnostic system. While modern Western medicine has chosen to focus more and more on less and less, Chinese medicine historically chose a different approach. Chinese medicine has focused on collecting as much information as possible about a person. This includes not just the individual symptoms and signs themselves, but also information about the person as an individual and the world around them. By gathering as much information as possible, the picture becomes more defined and precise.

In the beginning, the sheer volume of the information that is presented in the following chapters can appear to be overwhelming and intimidating. The intention is not that you should slavishly follow the contents of each chapter section by section when diagnosing a client. Instead, you should train yourself to be aware of when and how a patient differs from what is normal or to be expected, i.e. the norm. There will always be an ideal norm – the norm being what we ought to see or hear, all things being equal, if the body is physiologically harmonious – and then there is the reality that is in front of us. This reality will be an aggregate of various deviations from the norm. Each of these deviations will usually be linear movements away from a midpoint. There will often be too little or too much of each individual variable. Each norm or midpoint is, of course, itself variable and is dependent on many factors, such as gender, age, season or time of day. It is, for example, normal to be wide awake at three o'clock in the afternoon but not at three o'clock in the morning.

Whenever there's a change in a person – a deviation from the norm in how they look or smell or the sounds they emit – it will be a manifestation of an imbalance in their physiology. Every sign and every change is significant. What Chinese medicine has done is to document the systematic observation of how imbalances manifest themselves and the diagnostic significance of these physiological changes.

We must therefore constantly ask ourselves the following questions every time we observe something in a patient.

- What should I expect to be seeing, hearing, smelling or feeling right now?

- In what way does this manifestation differ from the norm?

- Which mechanisms and dynamics could be the cause of this change?

- Which pathological process can be the cause of this dynamic?

- How can this be interpreted in Chinese medicine terms? What imbalance and which pathological processes could be the cause of this manifestation?

Something imperative that is important to be constantly aware of is the crucial difference between what is normal and what is common. Being common does not make something normal. This is evident, for example, when considering the tongue. Most of my clients present with tongues that are pale and swollen, with teeth marks on the sides, a red tip and a greasy coating. Is this therefore a normal tongue? No, this is a common tongue, manifesting signs of very common patterns of imbalance.

I have tried, wherever possible, to provide physiological explanations of how and why changes in the body arise in pathological conditions. This is because I, personally, think that it is easier to learn the diagnostic significance of these changes if you understand how and why they have arisen, rather than just learning the signs and symptoms by heart and blindly accepting that things are as they are. Furthermore, by developing a comprehension and understanding of how changes occur, you will be able to figure out why a body presents as it does without having to remember the importance of all the symptoms and signs by heart.

Some signs and symptoms are, of course, more important than others; some will be seen more frequently and others more rarely. However, I have chosen in this part of the book not to weight some signs and symptoms as being more important than others or as being 'key symptoms'. Even though the signs and symptoms are themselves objective, the diagnostic process itself is subjective. Some therapists weight certain signs as being more important than others. I know from my own experience that the signs and symptoms that I weight most now are somewhat different from the ones that I weighted ten years ago. Where ten years ago I relied much more on the interrogative approach to diagnosis, my focus is now much more on the visual and auditive signs that the patient is manifesting. On the other hand, a person trained in Japanese acupuncture will often place more emphasis on palpable signs, and a Five Element acupuncturist may well focus more on smelling and listening to the client. It is not because one area is more important than others. All information has a value and ought to be involved in the diagnostic process. There will, however, often be a personal and subjective weighting of which information is deemed to be most relevant or reliable. What is crucial is to keep an open mind whilst diagnosing. Even though there may be a clear sense of what the diagnosis is from the outset or during the initial stages of the diagnosis, one must consciously search for evidence that can confirm this thesis or assumption. It is also important not to focus blindly on this thesis. This is because most signs and symptoms can mean different things in different contexts. This is the core of Chinese medicine and oriental philosophy in general. It is the context that the object is observed in that provides the definition, not the object itself. A sign or symptom should be comprehended as a part of a whole and it is this whole we are trying to determine, not the individual components. This is the reason that the Chinese medicine diagnostic process is so comprehensive and the reason that each of the four pillars comprises of so many elements. It's also why you have to use all four pillars together and not neglect the use of any of them. A roof is only stable if there are four pillars supporting it. A diagnosis is no different; it relies on four pillars. There are also some aspects of these diagnostic approaches that are indispensable. They should not be forgotten or omitted. This is especially true of tongue and pulse diagnoses, which are such important cornerstones in their respective columns that the pillars, and therefore the diagnostic roof, would be unstable if they are not present.

THE DIAGNOSTIC PILLAR: VISUAL OBSERVATION

Introduction

Visual diagnosis is something that people constantly utilise without necessarily being aware of it. What you must learn, as a practitioner, is to refine this ability. When someone who is angry or distressed enters a room, you are usually in no doubt about their mood. Similarly, if a person is exhausted or has a heavy cold, you will usually also pick up on this, both by seeing them and when talking to them. This is because there is a multitude of signs and signals, some more subtle than others, that we pick up on. We perceive and mentally record these signs without even thinking about it. What we, as therapists, must do is refine this ability to observe relevant signs and see them as part of a pathological pattern.

The above examples are, of course, fairly obvious and the signs are easy to spot, but the difference between these examples and the signs that we encounter in the clinic when interviewing clients is only a matter of degree. The signals are always there. They're just not always as pronounced. The trick is to refine and train one's perception. This is an ability that virtually everyone possesses, but they are not accustomed to using it in such a refined way or, importantly, using it systematically as part of a structured diagnostic system.

Visual diagnosis in Chinese medicine has two prerequisites: you must learn what the different visual diagnostic signals are a manifestation of in a Chinese medical context, and you must train your observational skills – your visual attentiveness. The former is a matter of understanding and remembering how changes in the body's internal physiology will manifest on the exterior of the body. The latter requires honing your visual awareness and focus so you are able to perceive these signals.

Something that is also vital when utilising visual diagnosis is good lighting. This is especially relevant when observing the complexion in the face and the tongue. A great many details can be overlooked because the lighting conditions are poor or the signs can be misinterpreted because the light source causes the colours to have a different hue.

What are the signs and symptoms that we will be looking for in this diagnostic pillar? Which signals from the body should be observed and what is the diagnostic significance of these signs?

In the moment a client steps through the door, we immediately start to form an impression of the person. We do this based on their body shape, their posture, their way of moving, the colours in their face, the complexion of their skin, the expression in their eyes, their body language, how they sit down on the chair and much more.

During the diagnostic procedure, we actively observe specific areas of the body – including the tongue, the fingernails and the skin. This is because certain aspects of the body manifest a lot of relevant information that can give us vital information about the patient – information that can often determine the diagnosis.

In Chinese medicine visual diagnosis, this information is utilised in a structured manner. We consciously focus on and interpret the signals that are being radiated by the patient. We process the information and relate it to our understanding of the body's physiology. Within the first three to four minutes, an experienced Chinese doctor may well have determined the fundamental aspects of the diagnosis. The rest of the consultation is then used to confirm and further refine the diagnosis.

Having said that, it does not mean that you should blindly adhere to your initial diagnostic impression or solely approach the diagnosis using intuition. At times this becomes a difficult balancing act. We must learn to trust the first impression we have received. This is because this first impression can often be of great diagnostic importance, especially because it is in this moment that we are often most intuitive and least rational in our thought processes. However, we must simultaneously maintain a flexibility in our thinking and our approach to the patient. Our mind must not get stuck on a diagnosis and thereby become blind to the diagnostic signs pointing in other directions. We must be aware of the risk of interpreting symptoms and signs only from the perspective of our initial hunch. It's like being a detective. We must follow a lead, but not get stuck trying to pin the evidence on our initial suspect.

Intuition without a theoretical foundation is nothing other than guesswork. Intuition requires that you have a strong theoretical basis that you subconsciously utilise. Most of us, at least to begin with, have to look systematically and consciously for each visual sign. We must consciously ask ourselves questions whilst we observe the patient: How is their facial complexion? How are their body movements? How do they dress? And so on.

Later on you will begin to answer these questions subconsciously and just say to yourself when you see a client: 'Liver *qi* stagnation and Heart *yin xu*,' without having consciously thought about it.

Some diagnostic areas are more straightforward than others. Diagnosis of body movements is usually fairly straightforward and can be observed from a greater distance than, for example, the skin in the area around the eye. Several signs that have relevance must be consciously sought out, for example skin lesions that are covered by clothing. They will first be seen only when the relevant area is uncovered.

J. R. Worsley advises practitioners to set up their practices so that they can see their patients when they arrive in their car and walk towards the clinic. This means you will have time to see the client and their natural posture and body movements, etc. without the client being aware that they are being observed (Worsley 1990, p.77).

As stated, good lighting is crucially important in visual diagnosis. You should, whenever possible, take advantage of daylight. Unfortunately, this is often not an option because there is a building just opposite your window that blocks the light or your client has come in the early morning or evening.

It is therefore a good idea to decide on what form of artificial lighting you will be using in the clinic and then investigate how this source of light affects the various colour tones. This can be done by initially observing the skin, tongue or other aspect of the body in natural daylight and then observing the same area when it is illuminated by the artificial light source and mentally noting the difference.

Visual diagnosis

Relative strengths of visual diagnosis

- Observation, together with auditory diagnosis, is the cornerstone of the intuitive approach to diagnosis. Through these two approaches we can often determine a substantial part of the diagnosis. We must learn to trust this ability but at the same time not confuse intuition with guessing.
- When observing the client, we are not dependent on the client's subjective interpretation and presentation of their diagnostic signs.
- Visual diagnosis is central in the diagnosis of children.

Relative weaknesses of visual diagnosis

- Many of the visual signs are very subtle and thereby difficult to differentiate.
- There are almost too many signs, which can be overwhelming, making it difficult to maintain an overview.
- The facial signs can be concealed by make-up.

Diagnostic tips

- Remember to notice petechiae and nevi whilst palpating and locating acupuncture points.
- Remember to notice whether the skin is dry whilst palpating and locating acupuncture points.
- Skin that is red or ruddy is a sign that Heat is present, at least in the local area.
- Skin that is purple is a sign of *xue* stagnation in the area.
- Discharges and exudations that are yellow or greenish are always a sign of Heat.

Visual diagnosis of a person's *shen*

Observation of the *shen* is probably one of the most important aspects of diagnosis. Even though observation of the *shen* is something many people do without even thinking about it, it is a good idea to be aware of what you are doing and subsequently draw relevant conclusions from what you have observed.

We immediately start to form an impression of the patient's *shen* from the first point of contact. The state of a person's *shen* is critical in determining the prognosis.

This is because *shen* is formed from *jing, qi* and *xue.* These are the material basis for the more ethereal *shen.* For its part, *shen* is the exterior manifestation of these substances. This means that the person's *shen* will reflect the state of these vital substances and the condition of the body that generates them.

If the person is healthy and their *yin, yang, qi, jing, xue* and *zangfu* are strong, they will have a strong *shen.* If they are weak, or if *xie qi* (pathogenic *qi*) is virulent and injuring the vital substances, their *shen* will be weakened.

Shen can be observed in a person's eyes, face, hair, body movements, tongue and breathing, as well as the way they act, react and interact with their surroundings. Vitality is a key word here. When there is *shen,* there is vitality. If a person radiates a vitality, there will still be a good prognosis, even if their symptoms are serious. Contrarily, if the person lacks this radiance, the prognosis is poor. This is because a lack of *shen* is a sign that the vital substances are injured and/or that *xie qi* is virulent.

If *shen* is strong, healthy and harmonious, there will be a shine and a sparkle to the person's eyes. The eyes will be bright. Conversely, a person's eyes can seem dull and lifeless if their *shen* is weak or blocked. If the person's *shen* is agitated, their eyes can seem very intense or they will be restless, their gaze darting around the room.

Because *shen* manifests in the eyes, a person with a healthy *shen* will be able to look you directly in the eye and maintain prolonged eye contact. If the *shen* is out of balance, you can have the sensation that even though you are looking them directly in the eyes, there is no contact. They may have difficulty maintaining eye contact because their eyes are darting around in various directions or they may maintain eye contact but have dull and lifeless eyes. They may give the sensation that there is no-one there, there is no vision coming out through the eyes or you are not able to create a connection into them.

The skin of the face is another place where a person's *shen* can be observed. The skin in the face should have a faint glow. The facial skin should also be soft and elastic. It should not be grey, dry or lifeless. There should be a vitality in the skin. This is not dissimilar to the tongue. Both should appear fresh and have a vibrancy. There should be the same vitality that you see in a live fish, not a fish that has been lying on a fishmonger's slab for a few days.

As stated earlier, *shen* is the external manifestation of the internal organs and the vital substances. This means that a person's body and their muscles can also reflect the quality of their *shen.* A strong body with healthy muscle and strong bones will be a sign that there is a strong foundation for *shen,* i.e. that their *jing* and *xue* are strong and healthy. A person's movements should be light and agile and their reflexes sharp. This shows that *shen* is able to control the body, that the Emperor is in command of his realm.

There is a close relationship and cooperation between the Heart and the Lung. *Shen* can therefore also be observed in a person's breathing. The respiration should be calm, smooth and regular, indicating that the *shen* is in balance.

The concept of the *shen* encompasses both the concepts of the soul and the mind in Western terminology. Most people can recall having seen someone in the street or on a bus and instantly recognising that the person is mentally deranged. Their clothes, hair and body movements separate them from the crowd. If a person's *shen* is in balance, a person will have normal responses and behaviour in relation to their surroundings. A person whose *shen* is imbalanced will often dress oddly. The clothes may seem strange, unusual or disharmonious or just inappropriate for their surroundings or the season. Their hair can be eye-catching and eccentric, and they will act and behave in a way that arouses our attention. However, it is important to remember that even though a person's clothes and behaviour may seem odd or different to what most people think of as normal, it may just be something that is the norm within a certain subculture or ethnic group to which the person belongs or it may be a conscious choice by the person.

Observation of *shen*

	Strong *shen* that is in balance	*Shen* that is weak or imbalanced
Eyes	The eyes are bright and have a sparkle and a radiance	The eyes can seem either dull and lifeless or too intense
Eye contact	Good eye contact and the person is able to maintain this contact	Poor eye contact and the person has difficulty maintaining eye contact Their gaze can be too rigid and staring, their eyes can dart around the room or they may shyly look away, because it is too intimidating to maintain eye contact
Facial skin	The skin has radiance and is soft and supple	The skin is dull and lifeless, possibly grey or matt
The hair	The hair has shine and lustre	The hair is dull and lifeless
Muscles and flesh	Strong and solid body with good muscle tone	Weak and lax body with poor muscle tone
Body movements	Agile movements with good reflexes	Slow, uncertain movements with poor reflexes
Breathing	Calm and smooth breathing	Superficial, irregular or rapid breathing
Clothes and hair	Normal and harmonious clothing and hair	Outlandish or odd clothes and hair
Response to the environment	The person acts and reacts normally with their surroundings	The person is either very apathetic or agitated The person reacts inappropriately to their surroundings, saying and doing things that are odd or inappropriate

False shen

Something that can be seen in seriously ill patients is that they can go from a state where they are very exhausted and their *shen* appears to be extremely weak, possibly even lacking consciousness, to suddenly brightening up. They may suddenly start talking again and have a brightness in their eyes, their appetite returns and they get a rosier colour returning to their face. This is ostensibly a positive improvement, but it is actually the opposite. When a person is very weak and ill, recovery and returning to strength should occur gradually. What is being observed here is 'false *shen*' and is an indication that *zheng qi* is about to collapse and that *yin* and *yang* are separating. These apparently benign signs are in fact manifestations that *yang* has detached itself from *yin* and is no longer controlled, thereby rising upwards. This is a very serious and negative sign.

Visual diagnosis of the body shape and posture

General shape and posture

Everyone is born with a certain constitution. The shape and form of a person's body can give an indication of their constitutional foundation, as well as the balance between *yin* and *yang* in their body. A person with a strong and robust physical body will usually also have healthy organs and strong *qi*. When there are imbalances in this person's physiology, they will tend to be *shi* in nature. In contrast, a person with a weak and fragile body will tend more towards *xu* states of imbalance.

The body's posture also expresses the distribution of *qi* in the body and whether there are *shi* or *xu* conditions in certain organs. A person with too much *yang qi* will often appear to be slightly distended or pumped up in the upper part of the body with a barrel chest. Generally, it will look as if their muscles are slightly too tense. Their legs will seem to be relatively insubstantial in relation to the upper body. This will result in a V-shaped body. This is called a '*taiyang*' body type. It is more typically seen in men and people who are relatively *yang*, and the person will tend towards *yang shi* imbalances.

Conversely, a person with relatively too much *yin* or with too little *yang* will tend to become more pear-shaped. This is due to the accumulation of *yin* Dampness in the lower part of the body or because *yang* is not lifting the *qi* upwards in the body. This gives a more pear-shaped appearance. This body type is called a '*taiyin*' type. Where the *taiyang* body type's muscles will often appear to be slightly taut and tense, the *taiyin* type's muscles will appear to be more flaccid or doughy and the skin will be paler. This person's movements may well be slightly slower and more ponderous. *Taiyin* body types are more typical in women, and *taiyin* types will generally tend more towards *yang xu,* Dampness and Phlegm.

The '*shaoyang*' body type is mixture of the first two body types. In the *shaoyang* body type the proportions of the upper and lower parts are more even and the muscles will be neither too flaccid nor too tight. This is the healthiest body type because *yin* and *yang* are harmonious.

A fourth body type is the '*shaoyin*' body type. This person is very thin and sinewy. They can often be slightly nervous or restless in their body movements. These people tend to be *yin xu* and/or *xue xu*.

By observing the distribution of *qi* in the body, you can get an idea of how long-term influences have physically affected the body. When we see a person in front of us, we must ask ourselves: How is the *qi* distributed? Is there an impression of there being too much or too little *qi* in general? Are there areas of the body where there is relatively too much or too little *qi*? Are there areas where there appear to be signs that Dampness or Phlegm are accumulating? Are there signs that *yang qi* is ascending?

In general, a powerful body with strong muscles and bones is an indicator that a person has strong *jing* and *qi*. Because their *qi* is strong, they will be more likely to develop *shi* patterns of imbalance. A person with weak muscles and a more delicate bone structure whose posture is more slumped will probably be *qi xu* and possibly even *jing xu*. When these people get sick, their patterns of imbalance will tend to be *xu* in nature.

Qi xu and *yang xu* tend to result in a slumped posture. There is an impression that the *qi* is not lifting the body up and holding the person upright. The patient will typically sit slumped on a chair and their back will not be straight or erect. On the other hand, if a person is too rigid in their posture, it could indicate that they have Liver *qi* stagnation. Liver *qi* stagnation will result in muscles that are tense, their lack of flexibility on the mental and emotional level being reflected in their physique. Liver *qi* stagnation and ascending Liver *yang* can also be seen in shoulders that are raised and tense. This is due, not only to the ascending *yang qi* lifting the shoulders upwards, but also because the neck region is a 'bottleneck', and if there is ascending *yang qi*, the ascending *qi* will have difficulty passing through this narrow area and will accumulate, creating neck and shoulder tension. The tension is further exacerbated if there is already Liver *qi* stagnation creating a stagnancy of *qi* in the muscles.

A person with an excess of Damp-Phlegm can have a tendency to obesity or be overweight. In particular, the Dampness will accumulate around the hips, buttocks and the lower portion of the abdomen. This is due to the *yin* nature of Dampness, which results in it seeping downwards. The muscles and skin can be loose and flaccid.

If there is Lung *qi xu,* the person may be hollow chested or have poorly developed muscles in the thoracic region. An accumulation of Phlegm in the upper *jiao* will, on the other hand, result in a person being barrel-chested. This is due to the Phlegm blocking the movement of *qi* and causing *qi* to stagnate in the upper body.

A person with an excess of Heat in the body will have a more 'open' or 'splayed' posture. They will often sit with their legs and arms spread out to the sides. They will spread their limbs outwards in a subconscious attempt to create a larger surface area and thereby increase the dissipation of heat from the body.

A person who lacks physiological heat – a person who is *shi* Cold or *yang xu* – may sit with their arms crossed or even wrapped around themselves, in an attempt to reduce the loss of heat from the body. This posture is similar to, but slightly different from, a person who is emotionally blocked or suspicious (blocked *shen* due to Liver and Heart *qi* stagnation). They can also sit with a very 'closed' posture, with their arms folded in front of the chest. However, this is not an attempt to maintain body heat but is an external manifestation of their emotional rigidity.

Body shape and posture

Observation	Significance
Strong and sturdy body	Strong constitution and *qi*. Good *jing*. Tends towards *shi* imbalances
Weak and fragile body	Weak constitution and *qi*. Weak *jing*. Tends towards *xu* imbalances
Pear-shaped or '*taiyin*' type	*Yang xu*, Spleen *qi xu*, Damp-Phlegm
V-shaped or '*taiyang*' type	*Yang shi*
Thin and wiry or '*shaoyin*' type	*Yin xu, xue xu*
Even distribution between upper and lower parts of the body or '*shaoyang*' type	*Yin* and *yang* are in balance
Slouching posture	*Qi xu* or *yang xu*
Stiff and rigid posture	Liver *qi* stagnation
Overweight or plump	Phlegm-Dampness
Raised shoulders or tense shoulders	Ascending Liver *yang*, Liver *qi* stagnation
Sitting with arms and legs spread	Heat
Huddled around themselves	*Shi* Cold or *yang xu*
Arms folded and rigid body	Liver and Heart *qi* stagnation

Five Phase body shapes

Everyone is born with a constitutional body shape and form. This is the foundation of their subsequent development. There are five primary body shapes in Chinese medicine. These correspond to the Five Phases. However, it is rare that a person is exclusively one shape alone. People are combinations of all Five Phases simultaneously, but one or two phases may be dominant in relation to the others.

A person's experiences in life, their diet, the diseases they've suffered, their chronic patterns of imbalance, their environmental surroundings, etc. will all have had a fundamental influence on the way that their body has developed and changed through the years. This influence is particularly strong during childhood when the body is still developing and *qi* is less stable and more easily affected.

In the Five Element acupuncture system, people are diagnosed with regard to their constitutional types. The body's fundamental physical appearance is used to help to determine which phase is most dominant in the person's constitution. The Five Phase body differentiation can also be used to assess the seriousness of an imbalance. It is better to have an imbalance that is congruent with the dominant constitutional phase, rather than an imbalance that is characteristic of the controlling phase.

Huang Di Nei Jing – Ling Shu (The Yellow Emperor Classic – Spiritual Axis) chapter sixty-four lists the following characteristics of the five constitutional types.

Wood type

- Sinewy
- Greenish skin colour
- Small head
- Long face
- Broad back and shoulders
- Straight back
- Small torso
- Tall
- Small hands and feet
- Intelligent
- Not physically strong
- Persistent when they work
- Tendency to worry

Fire types

- Ruddy skin colour
- Small head
- Thin face
- Wide back
- Well-developed muscles in the shoulders, back, abdomen and buttocks
- Small hands and feet
- Curly hair
- Quick tempered
- Quick thinking
- Quick body movements
- Firm gait, and the body moves whilst they walk
- Can have a tendency to be anxious

Earth type

- Yellowish skin colour
- Rotund body shape
- Large head
- Round face
- Broad jaws
- Large abdomen
- Large thighs and calve muscles, strong legs
- Relatively small hands and feet
- Well-proportioned body
- Steady gait
- Raise feet slightly whilst walking
- Solid muscles
- Quiet and generous
- Not over-ambitious
- Easy to get on with

Metal type

- Pale skin colour
- Square face
- Small head
- Narrow shoulders and upper back
- Small abdomen
- Lean
- Small hands and feet
- Fine bone structure
- Powerful voice
- Thinks quickly
- Honest and reliable

- Quiet and calm, but solid

- Determined

- Good leader

- Quick, swift movements

Water type

- Dark complexion

- Wrinkled face

- Large head

- Angular jaw and chin

- Round and narrow shoulders

- Large abdomen

- Move the whole body when they walk

- Long spine

- Relaxed

- Loyal

- Attentive and sensitive

Visual diagnosis of a person's movements

A person's body movements are one of the first things, along with the shape of their body and their posture, that we notice when they enter the room. It is important to be aware of how they move, not only before they sit down in the chair, but also after they have seated themselves. We should observe how much movement there is in the body or whether there is a distinct lack of movement.

Heat and Cold will both have an influence on a person's movements. The more Heat there is, the greater the activity of *qi* and thereby the faster the movements and the greater the amount of movement. A person with Heat will not only move quickly, they will also tend to be more restless or just move their body more. A person with a lot of Heat – both *xu* Heat and *shi* Heat – will have difficulty sitting still because their *qi* is agitated. Their toes will tap, their arms and hands will constantly be in motion and they will keep moving about on the chair. This is usually noticeable in people with *yin xu* Heat. They will often be restless and nervous in their movements, having difficulty sitting still. The difference between *xu* and *shi* Heat can be seen in, amongst other things, the force of the movements. *Shi* Heat will manifest with more powerful movements, because there is simply more *qi*. *Yin xu* movements are typically more fidgety and nervous.

To gain an impression of how *yin xu* Heat movements can manifest, think about how small children are in the evening, especially when they are overtired. Their movements are not lethargic and slow, as would be expected when they are *qi xu*, due to them being tired and exhausted. Instead, their movements are frenetic and overexcited. The more tired they are, the more they run around and the more excitable they become.

The dynamic nature of Cold is to contract and constrict. This thereby restricts the movement of *qi*, leading to a lack of movement and slowness. The slowness is accentuated by a lack of physiological heat, which can activate the *qi* and thereby the body itself. There will be significant differences in the person's movements, depending on whether the Cold is *shi* or *xu* in nature. When there is *yang xu*, the movements will be slower and more lethargic. This reflects that there is a lack of the *yang qi* that creates activity. With *shi* Cold, the movements will also be slow, but the movements are not weary, weak and feeble, but stiff and inhibited. This is because the lack of movement is not due to a lack of *qi* but because *qi* is restricted in its movement by the Cold.

A localised invasion of Cold will affect the mobility of that area of the body. Invasions of Cold are typically seen in the joints of the limbs, the lumbar region or the shoulders and neck. These areas will be restricted in their movement and there will also be stiffness and physical pain.

Xue stagnation can also result in a joint's movements being inhibited and often painful. This will manifest with rigidity and a reduced mobility of the joint.

Elderly people's body movements are characterised by the decline in their *yin*, *yang*, *qi*, *xue* and *jing*. This will manifest in movements that are slow and weak. This, though, is not the only thing we see. Elderly people's movements are also stiff and inhibited. This is because there is an increasing stagnation of *xue* and Phlegm as people get older. Typically, their movements will be stiffest in the morning and after they have been sitting still for a while. They have difficulty getting up and moving again, due to the stagnation.

Liver *qi* ensures that *qi* in general can flow freely and the Liver thereby ensures the unimpeded flow of *qi* throughout the body and through all the muscles and tendons. If Liver *qi* is harmonious, the person will have smooth and fluent movements. If Liver *qi* has stagnated, the movements will be more uneven, clumsy and stiff. Liver *qi* stagnation may also result in stiffness and a noticeable rigidity to the body itself. The person may sit stiffly upright in the chair and there may be a conspicuous lack of movement in their body. This will particularly be seen in the hands and facial muscles, which will be noticeably immobile.

Qi xu and *yang xu* can result in a person's movements being limp and weak, the muscles lacking the energy to complete their movements. When the person enters the room, they may drag their feet slightly. Their movements will seem lethargic and will often be slow. Again, it can help to conjure a picture in your head. These are the movements that you will also see when someone is completely exhausted.

Dampness and Phlegm result in a heaviness in the body and this will be reflected in the movements of the body, which will be lumbering and ponderous. The Phlegm and Dampness can also block the joints in the limbs. The movements of these joints then become stiffer and inhibited due to *qi* being blocked in its movement by the Dampness and Phlegm. This will be more noticeable when the weather is damp or humid and when the joint has been inactive for a while.

Clumsiness can arise either because there is a stagnation of *qi*, so the movements of the body are uneven and rougher, or when there is Phlegm. Phlegm can block the *shen* so that there is a poorer coordination of the body's movements.

All of these movements are things that we should be picking up on as the patient enters the room and sits down in the chair. We should also be conscious of their movements whilst we interview them and again when they get up to walk over to the treatment couch. We should constantly ask ourselves: What are their movements like? Are they slow, quick or stiff? Do they drag their feet? How is the balance of *qi* and where is it in their body? Is there a lot of body movement in general or is there too little? Are the movements large or small, forceful or weak, rapid or slow, smooth or jerky, stiff, heavy and ponderous? How much do they use their hands when talking?

Do they sit too still and if so is it due to rigidity or lack of energy? Do they fidget and move about in the chair? If they are fidgety, is this due to nervousness or is it just excessive movement? We see this often in children, because children are generally warm and tend to be *yin xu*. This means an excess of movement will have more diagnostic significance in adults than it does in children, because the heat and relative lack of *yin* is the norm in children but not in adults.

We should also note whether there are changes in their movements when they talk about different subjects.

Body movements

Observation	Significance
Rapid	Heat
Quick and nervous	*Yin xu* Heat
Quick and forceful	*Shi* Heat
Restless	Heat
Slow and stiff	Cold
Lethargic, weak and slow	*Qi xu, yang xu*
Stiff and limited	Cold, *qi* stagnation, *xue* stagnation
Clumsiness	Liver *qi* stagnation, Phlegm
Heavy and ponderous	Dampness and Phlegm

Visual diagnosis of a person's clothing

A person's attire can relay useful information, but we must also pay attention to factors such as fashion and the identity statements of subcultures.

One of the first things that we can focus our attention on is how much clothing the person is wearing and how appropriate this is for the climate. This will give an indication of Heat and Cold, from an Eight Principles perspective.

A person with an excess of Heat will usually be more lightly clad than others, even if the weather is cold. This can be seen, for example, in alcoholics sitting on park benches. Even in the midst of winter, they will often only be wearing a t-shirt and a thin jacket, despite single-figure temperatures.

Conversely, a person with *yang xu* will often meet up in the clinic wearing a thick jacket or a sweater, even in the height of summer when everyone else is walking around in a t-shirt and shorts. You should always ask yourself: Is the clothing they are wearing appropriate for the climate? Are they wearing too much or too little clothing compared with other people? It is, of course, important that this judgement is made from an objective perspective and not from your own subjective feelings. If you yourself are *yang xu*, then you will also probably wear more clothes than others and only notice a discrepancy in people who are more scantily clad than yourself. It is therefore important to be conscious of your own patterns of imbalance.

Harmony

Our *shen* makes us conscious of what is normal and correct in any given situation. Our *shen* makes us aware of, and thereby helps us conform to, what is expected or normal in the society around us. When *shen* is disturbed, the person may have difficulty conforming to this norm. The person will often say and do things that other people find strange. This can be seen in their clothes. *Shen*-disturbed patients may have a lack of harmony in their clothing. People with an extremely disturbed *shen* – people who are mentally ill – can often be easily spotted on a bus or the street because their clothes are disharmonious and to others look a bit weird. This is typically exemplified in cartoons when depicting a person who is 'mad'. Focusing on extremes and looking at caricatures is useful training, as it helps us to tune our awareness so we can spot the more subtle cases. This is useful, as many of the patients we see are not 'over-the-edge wacko' cartoon characters, but their *shen* is still disturbed or disrupted in some way. These patients are definitely 'normal' in their own eyes, and often in the eyes of those around them, but their *shen* can still be disturbed from our point of view. They have deviated from the ideal 'norm'. It can just be subtle differences between what we expect and what we see, or it can be more extreme. We must ask ourselves: Is this voluntary, through choice, or are they unaware of their appearance? What we must be aware of is that many subcultures consciously choose to look weird or different or just adopt a rebellious way of dressing. These individuals' *shen* are usually harmonious, because they are just conforming to a subset of normality, rather than the normality of society. Often, they are more conformist in relation to the narrow rules of their social niche than other people whom they perceive as being normal and boring!

There is, of course, also a narrow line between genius and madman. It can often be difficult to see the difference in their appearance.

Colours

Another aspect of a person's clothing we can observe is colour. We can ask ourselves: Is a patient predominantly and/or repeatedly dressed in just one colour?

A preference for a certain colour can be a tenuous sign of imbalance, as it is more often fashion related and thereby of little diagnostic relevance. That said, *xu* and *shi* pattern imbalances may affect a person's relationship with certain colours. This is because colours have an energetic resonance. If there is a certain organ or phase that is *xu*, a person may have an attraction to the colour that is a manifestation of that phase's *qi*. A person with a Kidney *xu* condition, for example, may have a tendency or an attraction to wearing clothes that are predominantly black or dark blue. This is a subconscious attempt by the body to replenish its own deficiency of this particular resonance of *qi*. A person with a *shi* condition, on the other hand, may have an aversion to a certain colour because they already have too much of this type of *qi* in their body.

Drab colours and clothing

The brightness and vibrancy of a person's clothes can reflect the quality of their *shen* and *qi*. Young people often dress more brightly than older people, wearing more vibrant colours and patterns. These clothes will also suit them better than if somebody middle-aged wears the same clothes. This is because the clothes seem more harmonious with the person wearing them. They match their *qi*. Many people tend to dress more drably as they get older. They become more anonymous. This can reflect the imbalances and developments that are common as a person grows older. *Xue xu, qi xu, yin xu, yang xu, jing xu*, Phlegm and various stagnations will all mean that the *shen* shines less brightly because it is either undernourished or blocked. This reduced vibrancy can sometimes also be seen not just in their clothing, but also with reduced sparkle in their eyes. The vibrancy of their clothes and their eyes reflects the vibrancy of their *qi*. This, of course, is far from always the case. Some elderly people do wear bright clothes and look harmonious in them. However, this is usually a reflection of the quality of their *qi* and their *shen*.

Drabness can also be the complete opposite. It can be a manifestation of a *shen* in perfect balance – the apparel and physical appearance no longer being of any importance and clothing being just another ego attachment. That is why, like every other sign, it must be viewed as being part of a larger pattern.

We also see many people whose marital relationship or life has become stuck and non-giving become more and more drab or boring in their appearance. A person whose life, and thereby peace of mind, has fallen apart, for example a man whose wife has left him and who has emotionally imploded, may stop caring at all about his appearance and often start to look dishevelled. This is a reflection of emotional condition – the state of their *shen*. Even though this is common and understandable, it is not an expression of a *shen* in balance, i.e. the ideal 'norm' from a Chinese medicine perspective. Similarly, when some people stop caring about their appearance, it is a reflection of them no longer caring about themselves and lacking self-worth. This is, again, telling us something about their Heart and their *shen*.

A *shen* blocked by Phlegm and Dampness can sometimes manifest with confusion and muddle-headedness. This can be reflected in the appearance, for example shirts buttoned wrongly, different coloured socks, pockets hanging out or food stains on their shirt.

It is not just aberrations from the norm that are manifestations of a pattern of imbalance. Over-conformity can also be a relevant sign. The extreme tidiness and pristineness of some people reflects their controlling attitude to everything in their life and everything around them. This will often be seen in people with Liver imbalances.

The need to decorate themselves and conform to the latest fashion – the need to belong and conform – is for some people a sign of their imbalances. Like so many things in Chinese medicine, it is not the factor itself, for example the flavour, the climatic influence, the emotion or whatever, that is the problem. It is the amount, situation and context of the factor, in particular whether there is too little or too much. Too much control and conformity or too little are both signs of imbalance.

This means that when the patient comes through the door, we might take note of the clothing. Most often there is nothing to see or register. It is only when there is something that sticks out that we take note, and even then we can't necessarily use the information but occasionally we can. This is no different from many other signs. It is the aberrations that we look for and we only can use them when they appear part of a pattern, unless they are very extreme or are a unique manifestation of a certain pattern.

Finally, we must also take other factors into consideration when considering a person's attire. They may, for example, be on their way to or from work, where the clothing is specified, or be on their way to or from a social function.

Clothing

Observation	Significance
Wearing lots of clothes	Cold, *yang xu*
Wearing little clothing	Heat
Disharmonious clothing	*Shen* disturbed
Very pristine clothing	Liver *qi* stagnation
Predominance of a particular colour	Can be a sign of a *xu* condition in the *zang* organ that resonates with that colour, but usually it is fashion related
Aversion to a particular colour	Can be a manifestation of a *shi* condition in the *zang* organ, which resonates with that colour

Visual diagnosis of the face

When we visually diagnose the face, we must note changes and distribution in the colours on the face. We must also observe the moistness and the quality of the skin and whether there is radiance.

Visual diagnosis of the face is fairly straightforward, as the face is not usually covered by clothing. Furthermore, it is the face that we look at when we talk to the client.

It is important though to pay attention to the lighting conditions in the room and to take into account the fact that many women use make-up, which can shroud the true colours of the complexion. Both of these factors can complicate the diagnosis. Some therapists therefore ask their patients not to put on make-up before the consultation. Account must also be made for the natural difference in skin colours between various ethnic groups. A pale complexion, for example, will be darker in a person from Pakistan compared with a Norwegian. The facial colours that a person is born with are called their 'guiding colours'. The colours that the face can manifest because of changes in temperature, physical activity, mood swings, etc. are called 'visiting colours'.

The colours of the face

Facial colours in relation to the Five Phases

There are different diagnostic levels or models for analysing the colours of the face. Five Element acupuncturists place great emphasis on the client's facial colours, especially the area between eyes and temples. This can give an indication of which constitutional type the person is. Furthermore, changes in facial colours can reveal which element or phase is in imbalance.

The colours of faces in relation to the Five Phases

Observation	Significance
White	Metal constitution or imbalance in the Metal Phase
Blue/black	Water constitution or imbalance in the Water Phase
Red	Fire constitution or imbalance in the Fire Phase
Green	Wood constitution or imbalance in the Wood Phase
Yellow	Earth constitution or imbalance in the Earth Phase

Some colours are more favourable and some are more serious, depending on the phase that the colour represents. It is necessary to relate the colours to the *sheng* and *ke* cycles. If the person manifests a colour in the face that resonates with the 'mother' phase, it is called a conforming colour and this is a positive sign. If they manifest the colour that resonates with the 'son' phase, this is a slightly 'conflicting' colour and is seen as being a negative sign. This, though, is not as bad as if it is a 'contradictory' or very conflicting colour. A conflicting colour will be when the patient's face manifests the colour of the phase that should be controlled by the phase in the *ke* cycle. It is even worse when the patient manifests the colour of the phase that ought to be controlling the phase of the patient or the phase that resonates with their disorder.

Conforming and contradictory colours in relation to the Five Phases

	Earth	Metal	Water	Wood	Fire
Yellow		Conforming	Very contradictory	Contradictory	Slightly contradictory
White	Slightly contradictory		Conforming	Very contradictory	Contradictory
Black or dark	Contradictory	Slightly contradictory		Conforming	Very contradictory
Green or green/blue (*qing*)	Very contradictory	Contradictory	Slightly contradictory		Conforming
Red	Conforming	Very contradictory	Contradictory	Slightly contradictory	

Facial colours in relation to the Eight Principles

The observation of the facial colour is also an important tool in more classical Chinese medicine and TCM. The colours of the face can be used as an aid when differentiating the Eight Principles. The colours of the face can help to reveal whether there is an internal or external condition, whether the condition is *xu* or *shi* or whether it is Hot or Cold. The colour of the face can also give an indication of which types of *xie qi* are present.

The facial colour will normally match the underlying pattern of imbalance, for example if a person has a Hot condition, then the face will be red or reddish. If it is not, there can be various explanations. One of the most common reasons that the colours in the face do not correspond to a pattern of imbalance is that the patient is manifesting multiple patterns simultaneously, and not all the colours can manifest at the same time. For example, a patient with *shi* Heat, Spleen *qi xu* and Liver *qi* stagnation will not have all three colours simultaneously; most often, we only see one colour. When the colour of the face is not consistent with what we expect to see, this can be used as an aid to understanding the pathological dynamics that are taking place. If we expect to see a dark colour because the person is manifesting *xue* stagnation but their face has a pale colouration, this could tell us that the root of their *xue* stagnation is a *qi xu* or *xue xu* condition. This will then influence our approach to treatment and we may well utilise a different treatment strategy than we would if it were a purely *shi* stagnation. The facial colours can also be affected by things such as the person's occupation, for example if they work outdoors. The change in the colour could also be due to the weather, the season or the person's emotional state.

There may also be situations in which there are conflicting signs of Heat and Cold in the patient's facial colour, their symptoms and the tongue and the pulse. This can be seen when there is 'false' Heat or 'false' Cold. False Heat and Cold arise when the patient's *yin* and *yang* are in the process of separating. This is always an ominous sign.

It is not only the colour itself that has a diagnostic significance. The intensity of the colour, its depth and the radiance and moistness of the skin are also of relevance.

Intensity and depth of the colours

When diagnosing the face, we have to observe the qualities of the facial colours. The colours will be more superficial in an exterior condition. There will be an appearance of the colour almost floating on the surface of the skin without the colour having any 'root' or depth. Interior conditions usually manifest with more deeply rooted colours. These colours will have depth, appearing not to be lying on the surface of the skin. A *xu* condition will result in weaker or more dilute colours. These colours will not be as intense and concentrated as the colours in a *shi* condition, where the colours are more substantial.

In addition to the intensity and depth of colour, moistness must also be taken into account, as well as whether there is radiance or the colour seems dull, matt and lifeless.

Radiance

The facial complexion should have *shen* in the same way that the pulse and tongue do. This means that the complexion must have radiance. The presence of *shen* is always a good prognostic sign. Conversely, a lack of *shen* is always interpreted as a negative prognostic sign.

Moistness

In the same way that Stomach *qi* gives the pulse a smooth and slippery quality and the tongue a thin, rooted coating, Stomach *qi* ensures that the face and thereby the complexion has a slight moistness. If the complexion appears to be matt, dry and without lustre, it will be a sign that Stomach *qi* is injured and is not producing sufficient *jinye*.

Face colour in relation to the Eight Principles

Observation	Significance
Superficial hue	Exterior condition
Deep hue	Interior condition
Weak, diluted colours	*Xu* conditions
Strong, intense colours	*Shi* conditions
Red and ruddy hues	Heat
White, pale or blue hues	Cold
Clear, bright colours	*Yang* conditions
Matt and dull colours	*Yin* conditions

It is also necessary to note the distribution of the facial colourations. The individual areas of the face relate to the various *zangfu* organs.

Normal colours

The normal colour will, as stated previously, depend on the person's ethnicity. Northern Europeans' facial colour should be a mixture of white and a slightly red colour. Adjustments to this base colour should therefore be made for different ethnic groups. Despite differences in skin colours between the various ethnic groups, there will still be the same dynamics and the same variations in facial complexion.

A slightly red colour indicates that there is sufficient Heart *xue*. The facial colour should have lustre and radiance, indicating the presence of *shen*. The colour should be 'subdued'. This means that it should not be too obvious. *Huang Di Nei Jing – Su Wen* (The Yellow Emperor Classic – Simple Questions) chapter ten states that 'the colour should appear, as if it is being seen through a thin piece of silk'. This means that the colour should be seen through the skin, i.e. the skin itself should not have the colour and the colour should not appear to be lying on the surface of the skin.

The skin should be slightly moist and the colour should have a slight lustre

The normal colour will be seen in a person who is healthy and in balance. If these colours are seen in a person who is ill, this in itself will be a good prognostic sign. This means that the disease has arisen recently and has not taken root. It indicates that the disease has not injured *qi*, *xue*, *jinye* or *zangfu* yet.

Pathological colours

WHITE

The white colour is seen when there is *qi xu*, *yang xu*, *xue xu* and Cold. The white colour can be: dull and matt when there is *yang xu*; dull and pale or almost greyish when there is *qi xu*; a sallow, wan white that is slightly yellowish and without lustre when there is *xue xu* or sometimes Phlegm; an almost bluish white colour when Cold is present.

GREY

A greyish white, sallow complexion that is slightly dry can sometimes be seen in the face when there is Phlegm blocking *xue* from nourishing the skin.

QING[4] (GREEN/BLUE), GREEN

The green or green/blue colour is seen when there is pain, when there is a stagnation of *qi*, especially Liver *qi* stagnation, or when Cold creates stagnation. It can also sometimes be seen when there is Heart *xue* stagnation.

BLUE

The blue colour is often classified as being a shade of *qing*. It will usually be seen when Cold stagnates *xue*. It can also be seen in the area between the eyebrows of young children when there is Liver Wind. If the entire face of a pregnant woman is bluish, this is a sign of *xue* stagnation and *yang xu*. This is an adverse sign.

RED

The red colour will always indicate the presence of Heat. *Shi* Heat will cause the cheeks or the entire face to become red or ruddy, whereas *xu* Heat will result in the cheekbones and the region around them becoming red. The red colour in *yin xu* will also be thinner and look more like make-up brushed on to the surface of the skin. Heat can also result in the eyes becoming red.

BLACK

The black colour includes a very dark complexion, as well as black. The dark complexion will be a sign that there is Kidney *xu*, Cold, Damp-Phlegm or *xue* stagnation. When there is Kidney *yin xu*, the skin will be dark and dry. When there is Kidney *yang xu*, the skin will be dark and moist. Damp-Phlegm or Damp-Cold can result in the area around the eye becoming dark. If the colour is very dark, then there may be *xue* stagnation.

YELLOW

The yellow colour is seen when there is *xue xu*, Damp, Damp-Cold and Damp-Heat. *Xue xu* can result in the face being pale and wan with a slightly yellowish tinge. *Shen* accompanies *xue* as it circulates around the body. If there is *xue xu*, the face will therefore lack radiance and lustre.

   The yellow colour resonates with the Earth Phase. When there is Spleen *qi xu*, it can sometimes manifest with a yellowish hue in the facial complexion if there is Dampness at the same time. Damp-Heat imbalances will also manifest with a yellowish tinge to the face. Damp-Heat can arise when there are Spleen imbalances, but also in other organs, for example jaundice is often seen when there is Damp-Heat in the Liver and Gall Bladder. The yellow hue will often be seen in the facial complexion, as well as the sclera of the eyes. The more Heat that there is present, the brighter the yellow colour will be. If there is Damp-Cold, the complexion will be darker and more smoky. If the face is dry and yellowish without radiance, there may be pathological Heat in the Stomach or Spleen.

PURPLE

The purple colour is seen when there is extreme *xue* stagnation and poisoning. As with the tongue, the purple colour is differentiated according to whether the complexion is reddish-purple or bluish-purple. Heat can condense *xue* and thereby stagnate it. This will be seen with a reddish-purple complexion. Cold will congeal *xue*. In this case the facial complexion will be bluish-purple.

Facial colouration

Observation	Significance
Normal colour	No disease or a disease of shorter duration and with a good prognosis
White	*Qi xu*, *yang xu*, *xue xu* and Cold
Red	Heat
Blue/green	Pain, *qi* stagnation, Cold, Heart *xue* stagnation or Wind
Yellow	Damp, Damp-Heat, Damp-Cold or Spleen *qi xu*
Black	Kidney *yin xu*, Kidney *yang xu*, Damp-Cold, Damp-Phlegm or *xue* stagnation
Purple	*Xue* stagnation or poisoning
Greyish	Phlegm

Facial areas

In classical texts such as *Huang Di Nei Jing – Su Wen* and *Huang Di Nei Jing – Ling Shu* there are descriptions of the facial areas and the internal organs that these areas relate to. An imbalance in a *zangfu* can manifest with changes to the colours or the skin in these areas. There are significant discrepancies between these two texts, as well as between other sources, with regards to the diagnostic relationship of the various areas of the face and the internal organs. Figure 1.1 shows the positions of the *zangfu* organs in the face according to *Huang Di Nei Jing – Ling Shu* Difficulty forty-nine, but, as written, there are many different interpretations of the diagnostic significance of these areas.

Tics

Tics occur when there is internal Wind in the muscles. The Wind makes *qi* become chaotic in its movement and thereby lose control of the muscles. The Wind will be internally generated and will always be related to Liver imbalances. This also explains why tics can often develop or worsen when a person is stressed or emotionally affected.

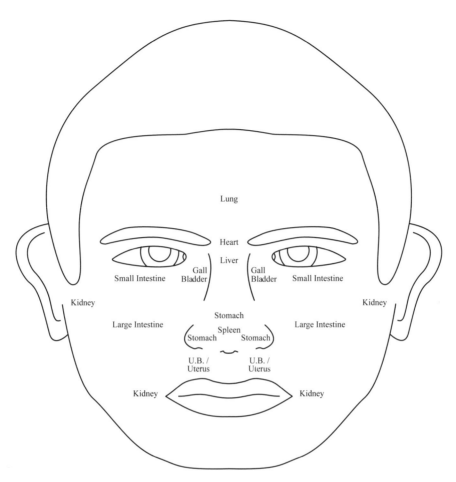

Figure 1.1 Positions of the *zangfu* organs in the face according to *Huang Di Nei Jing – Ling Shu* Difficulty forty-nine

Visual diagnosis of the eyes

Before discussing the eyes as a diagnostic tool, it is important to state that it is the Chinese medicine version of eye diagnosis that should be utilised in a Chinese medicine diagnosis. Whilst iris diagnosis is an effective and precise diagnostic tool, it should not be used as part of a Chinese medicine diagnosis. This is because iris diagnosis is based on the Western medicine anatomical and physiological model. This means an observation of an imbalance in the kidneys, for example, in iris diagnosis does not necessarily mean that the Kidneys, as understood in Chinese medicine, have an imbalance and need treatment. Conversely, one can imagine a situation in which there is an obvious pattern of Kidney *yin xu* or Kidney *yang xu* without this manifesting as a problem in the person's physical kidneys, and therefore this will not register with changes in the iris. It is important to keep the diagnostic tools from different physiological and pathological systems separate, otherwise there is a risk of formulating a treatment principle based on a false premise.

There are many different aspects and levels to ophthalmic diagnosis. Most of us have taken advantage of some of these, even before we started learning and practising Chinese medicine. Chinese medicine has just taught us to focus our attention on these signals and systematise the information that they give us.

Shen

One of the first things we determine, both consciously and subconsciously, on meeting a person is how much vitality and radiance there is in their eyes. From a Chinese medicine perspective, this will inform us about the person's *shen*. In the same way that we in the West say that the eyes are the windows of the soul, Chinese medicine states that *shen* can be observed in a person's eyes.

There are two definitions of *shen* that are relevant here: *shen* meaning vitality and radiance and *shen* meaning spirit/mind/consciousness.

A person who is in good health will have eyes that are bright and sparkling. It is possible to have direct eye contact with them and this will feel comfortable for both persons.

A person with Heart *qi xu* will have difficulty maintaining, or feel uncomfortable with, direct eye contact. This is because their *shen* is undernourished and they are therefore often very shy; direct eye contact can feel too intense for them. It can also seem as if there is just too little sparkle in their eyes; it can remind you of the eyes of a person who is exhausted. The *shen* is simply not shining brightly enough.

It can also be difficult to have eye contact with a person who has Heart and Liver *qi* stagnation, due to the lack of movement of their *hun* and *shen*. The difference between this and the former situation is that a person with Heart *qi xu* will have a tendency to look away and they will lower their gaze when you look directly into their eyes. In a person with Heart and Liver *qi* stagnation, it will seem as if they are staring inwards, are unable to look outwards and are locked within themselves. This is reflective of their mental condition. Their *hun*, which normally looks forwards and outwards, is inhibited in its movement by the stagnation, and the person can have difficulty in seeing a future for themselves.

An over-active Liver can in turn result in a person having very intense, rigid staring eyes. They stare at you and instinctively you want to look away from them because their gaze is too intense and piercing. In this case, the *hun* is over-active. It is very focused on a goal or its own individual vision of the future. This type of person is used to being in control and getting their own way.

When Heat agitates the *shen*, it becomes restless and the person can be manic. Their eyes will become restless and frenetic. This is because '*hun* follows *shen* in its entering and exiting'. When *shen* is agitated and thereby over-active, *hun* is forced to follows its movements. This results in eyes that are constantly shifting their point of focus in the room.

When *shen* is obscured and blocked by Phlegm, it can have difficulty radiating outwards, thereby creating a barrier in making contact with other people's *shen*.

The eyes will appear matt and blurry. The person will often have the feeling that they are not fully present and in touch with the outside world. It is as if they are sitting in a bell jar or there is a mist between their eyes and the outside world.

Observation of the eyes

Observation	Significance
Lack of eye contact	Heart *qi xu*
Staring and piercing eyes	Liver *shi* imbalances
Darting or restless eyes	Heat agitating the *shen*
Blurry or matt eyes	Phlegm blocking the *shen*
Lack of brightness	Liver and Heart *qi* stagnation, Heart *qi xu*

The zones in the eyes

The eyes can be divided into different zones, as with the ears, feet and other parts of the body. When there are colour changes in these areas of the eye, this can tell us something about the corresponding *zangfu* organ. It is important to remember, though, that the condition of other organs may also affect these areas. A condition of Heat, even though it is not in the Lung, will make the sclera in the eye redden and become bloodshot. Heat's *yang* nature means that it will always rise upwards and therefore all forms of Heat in the body can affect the sclera of the eyes.

The zones in the eyes

Zone	Significance
The pupil	The Kidneys
The iris	The Liver
The sclera	The Lung
The canthus	The Heart
Lower eyelid	The Stomach
Upper eyelid	The Spleen

The colours in the eyes

Various imbalances can affect the eyes. Although the eyes, when taken as a whole, relate to the Liver, the colours in the eyes can be affected by other organs and by *xie qi*.

Heat, especially *shi* Heat, will make the eyes red. Heat is *yang* in nature and therefore rises upwards. Systemic Heat, unless it is bound together with Dampness, will always rise up to the upper part of the body and to the head. This is why it is most often the head and not the lower part of the body that manifests symptoms and signs of Heat.

Heat manifesting with a redness of the eyes will often have its root in Liver Fire, Stomach Fire or an invasion of exogenous Wind-Heat. The Heat can be so intense that it affects the fluids in the eye. This will result in dryness as the body fluids evaporate from the area or in an inflammation when the Heat is so intense that it becomes 'Toxic-Heat'.

Yellowish eyes result from conditions of Damp-Heat. *Xue xu* and *xue* stagnation can also cause the eye to turn yellowish.

Less common, but still of relevance, are the colours green and blue. A bluish tinge to the eyes may be a sign of Cold and greenish tinge may indicate Liver Wind.

Colours in the eyes

Observation	Significance
Red	*Xu* and *shi* Heat
Yellow	Damp-Heat, *xue xu* or *xue* stagnation
Blue	Cold
Green	Liver Wind

Inflammation and styes

Inflammation and styes in the eye have two main root causes. They can result from an invasion of Wind-Heat or when Heat that has been generated internally rises up to the eye. Often the Heat will have ascended from the Stomach via its channel connection to the eyelid. The Heat can damage the fluids and be so intense that it generates Toxic-Heat.

Tears and mucous in the eyes

In theory, sleep and secretions of mucous in the eyes can be observed by the therapist, although this is not usually the case in practice because the person will often have removed it before you meet them. This means it is best to ask the patient about it instead.

In the same way that Phlegm can accumulate in the Lung or in the respiratory passages, it can also accumulate in the corners of the eyes. This is because the corner of the eye is a cavity in which there is a limited flow of *qi*. Fluids can stagnate in this cavity and turn into Phlegm. This can be seen in the morning after the eyelids have been closed for several hours, resulting in a lack of movement of *qi* in this area. A person with a tendency to have Phlegm may often experience small blobs of mucous in the eyes forming throughout the day.

Watering eyes can be due to the circulation of fluids in the area being disturbed by exogenous *xie qi* or a Liver imbalance causing the movement of fluids in the eyes to become chaotic. Liver imbalances that lead to the eyes watering can be both *xu* and *shi* in nature. The tears may be spontaneous, but they will often arise when the eyes are exposed to wind or draughts. This is consistent with the fact that the Liver, wind, the eyes and tears are all aspects of the Wood Phase in Chinese medicine.

Secretions and mucous in the eyes

Observation	Significance
Sleep and mucous in the eyes	Phlegm
Watering eyes	Liver imbalances, Wind-Cold or Wind-Heat
Styes and inflammation	Wind-Heat, Stomach Fire

Visual diagnosis of the area around the eyes

The area around the eyes includes both the eyelids and the area just below the eyes. Visible changes in the colour of the skin and in the moistness of these areas may be observed. Attention should also be paid to the presence of oedema or puffiness in the area around the eyes.

Colour

The colours most often observed in this area are black, green, blue/green, yellow, red and white. Changes in skin colour will most often be fairly subtle – often only a slight tinge.

Blackness of the skin around the eyes usually indicates a Kidney imbalance. The colour in this case must be seen in relation to the moistness of the skin in the area. If the skin is black and moist, then this can be a sign of Kidney *yang xu*. There may well also be puffiness as a result of a slight oedema in the area. This will be due to the inability of the Kidneys to transport body fluids away from the area. If the skin is dry, there may be Kidney *yin xu*. A black colour can be easily confused with the blue/green (*qing*) colour, therefore you should, as always, compare this characteristic with the other signs and symptoms.

A dark, dusky colour around the eyes can also arise when Phlegm or Dampness block the movement of *qi* and *xue* in the fine network of vessels in this area.

Blue/green and green around the eyes is usually a sign of Liver *qi* stagnation. The difference between these two colours is an indicator of the degree of the Liver *qi* stagnation that exists. Liver *qi* stagnation can result in *xue* not circulating in the fine network of vessels as it should. Because the skin around the eyes is very thin and almost transparent, it will be easier to see the stagnation of *xue* here than in other areas of the body. The stronger the *qi* stagnation, the more *xue* will stagnate. The blue/green colour indicates a stronger stagnation of *qi* than the green colour does.

A purple colour indicates *xue* stagnation.

Redness around the eyes is a sign of Heat, generally *xue* Heat. The redness can also be a sign of Damp-Heat. In this case, the skin will often weep or flake as is seen in fungal infections of the skin.

Whiteness can be shiny, pale or pallid. A shiny whiteness around the eyes can be seen in an invasion of Wind-Cold. Pale or pallid skin around the eyes is a sign of *xue xu*. The sallow complexion here can almost be yellowish.

As is the case with the lips and the face in general, the use of make-up can negate the diagnostic observation of these areas.

The colours around the eyes

Observation	Significance
Black and dry	Kidney *yin xu*
Black and moist	Kidney *yang xu*
Dark brown, dusky	Phlegm or Dampness
Blue/green *(qing)* or green	Liver *qi* stagnation
Redness	Heat
White and shining	Cold
White, dry and sallow	*Xue xu*
Purple	*Xue* stagnation

Puffiness (including 'bags' under the eyes)

The area around the eyes may be swollen and puffy due to the presence of accumulated fluids. In chronic cases it may result in 'bags' under the eyes. If the condition is acute, this will usually be due to an invasion of Wind-Cold or Wind-Heat. This *xie qi* can disturb the Lung's ability to spread and distribute the thin fluids, so these then accumulate in the Lung. At the same time, *xie qi* will block the Lung in its function of sending *qi* downwards. Lung *qi* can then become rebellious and rise upwards. The rebellious *qi* will carry the accumulated fluids upwards with it, resulting in puffiness in the face, especially in the area around the eyes where the flesh is very thin.

If the puffiness is a chronic condition, it will probably be a manifestation of Spleen or Kidney *yang xu*. Spleen and Kidney *yang* are responsible for transporting and transforming fluids. If there is *yang xu* in either of these organs, there will be an accumulation of fluids. The result will then be bags below the eyes. As it is a *xu* condition, the bags will be more noticeable and pronounced when the person is tired or has overstrained themselves.

Visual diagnosis of the forehead, the root of the nose and the area between the eyebrows

Observation of the forehead and the area above the bridge of the nose between the eyebrows is particularly useful in paediatric diagnosis, but these areas can also provide relevant information when diagnosing adults.

I will start by discussing the relevance of changes in these areas in children. The area between the eyebrows (above the root of the nose) has particular diagnostic significance in children who are below the age of four. If the root of the nose is greenish, there will often be digestive problems. A dark green colour can sometimes be seen when there is an excessive accumulation syndrome and a light green colour if the accumulation syndrome is due to a *xu* condition.

Green macules in this area are sometimes seen when there is diarrhoea. Blue veins in the region can be seen when there is abdominal pain.

The forehead of small children should also be observed. If there is a bluish colour here, it can indicate that the mother has been exposed to a strong shock during pregnancy that may have affected the foetus's Heart *qi*. Post-natal shock and Cold will also be capable of producing a blue colour in this area.

In adults we should observe the colour of the forehead and the bridge of the nose, as well as noting the amount and distribution of wrinkles or lines in the forehead and between the eyebrows.

If the skin of the forehead is red and dry, there can be Heat in the Urinary Bladder. Acne in this area, particularly if the spots are large, red and pus-filled, can be seen when there is Heat and Damp-Heat in the Stomach and Intestines. The skin of the forehead will often also be oily when there is Damp-Heat. Small red spots on the forehead can be indicative of Stomach Fire.

If there is a single deep, horizontal line on the forehead, it can indicate a chronic Small Intestine imbalance. Multiple horizontal wrinkles or lines in this area can be seen when there is Spleen *qi xu*.

A single vertical furrow between the eyebrows can be seen when there are chronic Stomach imbalances, whereas two vertical lines or wrinkles between the eyebrows are indicative of Liver *qi* stagnation.

Liver *xue* stagnation can result in the bridge of the nose being dark and yellowish, whereas Liver *xue xu* and Lung *qi xu* can result in this area being paler than normal.

Observation of the forehead and root of the nose

Observation	Significance
Single deep, horizontal furrow or wrinkle on the forehead	Chronic Small Intestine imbalance
Multiple horizontal furrows or wrinkles on the forehead	Spleen *qi xu*
Single vertical furrow or wrinkle between the eyebrows	Chronic Stomach imbalance
Two vertical furrows or wrinkles between the eyebrows	Liver *qi* stagnation
Dry, red forehead	Heat in the Urinary Bladder
Large, red, pus-filled spots on the forehead	Damp-Heat in the Stomach and Intestines
Small red spots on the forehead	Stomach Fire
Oily skin on the forehead	Damp-Heat
Dark and yellowish bridge of the nose	Liver *xue* stagnation
Pale bridge of the nose	Liver *xue xu* or Lung *qi xu*

Observation	Significance
Dark green between the eyebrows in small children	*Shi* accumulation syndrome
Light green between the eyebrows in small children	*Xu* accumulation syndrome
Green macules between the eyebrows in small children	Diarrhoea
Blue vein between the eyebrows in small children	Abdominal pain
Dark green between the eyebrows	Accumulation syndrome
Light green between the eyebrows in small children	*Xu* accumulation syndrome

Visual diagnosis of the nose

The nose is under the influence of the Lung and has a channel connection with the Large Intestine, *du mai*, Stomach and Urinary Bladder channels. Secretions from the nose are differentiated in the section 'Observation of secretions, excretions and exudations' (page 113). The colours on the nose have a diagnostic relevance, in relation to not only the Lung, but also the Stomach, Spleen, Liver, Heart and Gall Bladder.

A pale nose tip will be a manifestation of Stomach and Spleen *qi xu*. If the tip is pale and swollen, there may be an accumulation of Phlegm-Fluids.

If the bridge of the nose is pale, this will be a sign of Liver *xue xu* or Lung *qi xu*.

A yellowish nose can be seen when there is Damp and Damp-Heat. When there is Damp-Heat the yellow colour be more intense.

Liver *xue* stagnation can result in the bridge of the nose being dark and yellowish.

A red nose can be seen when there is Heat. If the upper part of the nose is red, the Heat is in the Lung. The middle part of the nose can be red when there is Heat in the Liver and the tip can be red if there is Heat in the Spleen or *xu* Heat. A red nose can also be seen when there is Wind-Heat.

If the nose is not red but reddish-purple in colour, this will be a sign that the Heat has stagnated *xue*.

Liver *xue* stagnation can result in the nose having a green/blue tinge.

Both Phlegm and Cold can create stagnation where the tip of the nose becomes bluish in colour when these are present.

Dark or an almost black nose can be seen when there is extreme Heat, *xue* stagnation or Kidney *xu* conditions.

When there is Lung Heat, the nostrils may 'flap' as the Lung tries to create a greater circulation of air around its sense organ and thereby dissipate the Heat.

Bleeding from the nose may occur when Spleen *qi* is weak and cannot hold *xue* inside the blood vessels or when Heat agitates *xue* and causes the walls of the blood vessels to burst due to the pressure.

Observation of the nose

Observation	Significance
Pale nose tip	Spleen *qi xu*
Pale and swollen nose tip	Phlegm
Pale bridge of the nose	Liver *xue xu* or Lung *qi xu*
Red nose	Heat
Reddish-purple nose	Stagnant *xue* due to Heat
Green/blue nose	Liver *xue* stagnation
Blue nose tip	Phlegm or Cold
Flaring nostrils	Lung Heat
Nose bleeds	Spleen *qi xu* or Heat

Visual diagnosis of the ears

In the same way that the eyes are an aspect of the Liver but are influenced by many other organs in the body, the ears are an aspect of the Kidneys. The Kidneys, especially Kidney *jing*, have a direct influence on the ears, but several other organs can also influence the ears via their channel connections. Each of the *yang* channels, for example, connects to the ears, either via the main channel or via their internal and sinew channels. The ears can be invaded by exogenous *xie qi* or disrupted by internally generated *xie qi*.

The shape of the ears

The ears are created from and nourished by Kidney *jing*. The shape, size and texture of the ear can therefore relay information to us about the person's constitution.

A small ear can be a sign of *jing xu*. If the ear appears shrunken, it can be a sign of *jinye xu* or *yin xu*.

If the ears are inflamed or swollen, this may well be a sign of Damp-Heat or Heat forcing body fluid up to the ears.

Pain in the ears can be a sign of Heat in the Liver and Gall Bladder or an invasion of exogenous *xie qi*. It can also be a sign of an imbalance in the body or body part that corresponds to a specific area of the ear.

Discharges from the ear

An increased production of wax in the ear can be a sign of Damp or Damp-Heat, in which case the increased exudation will be thick and sticky. More watery wax can indicate Spleen or Kidney *yang xu*, because *jinye* is not being transported optimally and collects in the ears.

Inflammation of the ear may arise when there is either an invasion of Wind-Heat or Damp-Heat in the Liver and Gall Bladder. Damp-Heat in the Liver and Gall Bladder can be both chronic and acute in nature. Wind-Heat will always be acute. In both cases, the discharge will be yellowish and sticky.

If the discharge from the ear is more watery and clear, it will be due to Spleen *qi xu* creating Dampness, which has then accumulated in the ear.

Kidney *yin xu* can also manifest with a thin, watery secretion from the ear.

As with other excretions, information about this will probably be gained by interviewing the client, rather than direct observation, because the client will probably have cleaned their ears due to these secretions.

Observation of the ears

Observation	Significance
Small ears	*Jing xu*
Shrunken ears	*Jing xu* or *yin xu*
Pain in the ear	Liver and/or Gall Bladder Heat
	An imbalance in the organ or part of the body that corresponds to that zone in the ear
Inflammation of the ear	Invasion of Wind-Heat, Liver/Gall Bladder Damp-Heat
Yellowish sticky earwax	Phlegm, Damp-Heat
Thin, watery earwax	Spleen *qi xu*

Visual diagnosis of the lips

In general, the lips are an aspect of the Stomach and the Spleen, but they will also give an indication of the condition of *xue* in general, and they can indicate the presence of Heat and Cold in the body. *Du mai, ren mai, chong mai*, and the Large Intestine, Liver, Stomach and Kidney channels all course around or connect to the lips. This means that the state of these channels can also be seen in this area.

Xue is almost directly visible in parts of the body such as the lips, where the skin is very thin and delicate. *Xue xu* can manifest with lips that are pale. This is because there will be too little *xue* to give the lips their characteristic rosy, red colour. The lips in these situations will also often be dry due to the lips not being moistened and nourished by *xue*. A tendency to *xue* stagnation can be seen when the lips are more purple in colour. This is because *xue* is moving slowly and is not replenished with fresh *xue*. This is similar to Western medicine, where the lips will be darker in colour when there is poor blood circulation and the blood lacks oxygenation and is saturated with carbon dioxide. The purple lip colour can be either reddish or bluish, depending on whether it is a condition of Cold or Heat, which is the cause of the *xue* stagnating.

Cold will result in the lips being more blue in colour. This is due to Cold stagnating the movement of the *xue*, as well as the *yin* nature of Cold. The *yin* dynamic of Cold will cause *xue* to contract inwards to the centre of the body. This will result in a reduced flow of *xue* in the superficial network of vessels found in the lips. This, again, corresponds to the Western medicine physiological explanation of how cold affects the body. When the body temperature is lowered or the body is cooled down, there is a reduced movement of the blood in the superficial blood vessels. This is the body's attempt to reduce the dissipation of heat to the external environment, thereby helping to keep the vital internal organs warm.

Very red and full lips will indicate a condition of Heat. This is due to Heat increasing the circulation of *xue* and sending *xue* outwards and upwards to the surface to cool it down (again, this is an expression of the intrinsic nature of *yin* and *yang,* where Heat is *yang* and thereby has an upward and outward, expansive dynamic).

A temporary state of Heat can be seen during sexual arousal. When a person experiences desire or arousal, *mingmen* blazes up. This generates physiological heat in the body and can be seen in places such as the lips and nails. For centuries women have imitated this signal by painting the lips, cheeks and nails red. If a woman is wearing lipstick during the consultation, it will, of course, hamper the visual diagnosis of the lips.

The lips can have a yellowish hue when there is Damp present in the body.

Dry lips will logically indicate that there is a state of Dryness. This can be a local condition, in which case it will not have particular diagnostic significance or it can be systemic Dryness. When the lips are dry, the colour of the lips will help differentiate the cause of the dryness. Red and dry lips are a sign of Heat, either *yin xu* Heat or *shi* Heat, the lips being dry as a result of the Heat damaging *yin* fluids. Pale lips are a sign of *xue xu*, the lips being dry because *yin xue* is not moistening them. If the lips are very dry, the surface of the skin can crack. Using lip balm will, of course, veil the dryness of the lips, but the fact that a person needs to use lip balm can in itself be a diagnostic sign of Dryness.

Very moist lips indicate that the transportation of fluids is disturbed as in an invasion of Wind-Cold or when there is *yang xu.*

Weeping sores, such as those seen in herpes simplex, can be a sign of Damp-Heat in the Liver and Gall Bladder, when Heat is the dominant pathogen. This is because the Heat will rise up along the Liver channel to the mouth. If Dampness was the dominant aspect of *xie qi*, it would be more likely that the symptoms would have manifested around the genitals. This is because the *yin* nature of Dampness means that it tends to sink downwards. The Damp-Heat could also have its source in the Stomach and Large Intestine channels or it could be due to an invasion of Toxic-Heat. *Yin xu* Heat may in some cases also result in sores around the mouth.

Fine wrinkles around the lips are a sign of *yin* and *xue xu*. This is typically seen in post-menopausal women. This is due to *ren mai* and *chong mai* drying out and no longer overflowing with *xue* and *yin*. *Ren mai* and *chong mai* both circle around the mouth, moistening and nourishing the skin here.

Observation of the lips

Observation	Significance
Pale	*Xue xu, yang xu*
Very red	Heat (both *xu* and *shi*)
Purple	*Xue* stagnation
Pale blue	*Yang xu,* Cold, *xue* stagnation
Bluish	Cold (both *xu* and *shi*)
Yellowish	Dampness
Dry	Heat (both *xu* and *shi*)
Cracked	Heat (both *xu* and *shi*)
Weeping sore	Damp-Heat in the Liver, Invasion of Wind-Heat or Toxic-Heat Stomach Fire, *yin xu* Heat
Wrinkles around the lips	*Ren mai* and *chong mai* are *xue xu* and *yin xu*

Visual diagnosis of the mouth

Sores around the mouth have been discussed above. Other signs that can have a diagnostic relevance are distortion of the mouth and saliva from the mouth.

If the mouth is skewed without there being a history of physical trauma in the region, the distorted shape may be due to an invasion of Wind-Cold blocking the movement of *qi* and *xue* in the local area or Wind-Phlegm creating a chaotic movement of *qi* and blocking *qi and xue* in the area.

If there is a history of physical trauma to the area, the distortion will be due to local stagnation of *qi* and *xue*.

If the person drools from the corners of their mouth, this can be due to Spleen and/or Lung *qi xu*. The *qi xu* results in *jinye* accumulating in the mouth and an over-production of saliva.

Internal Wind can cause paralysis of the muscles around the mouth. This means that the lips cannot hold the saliva in the mouth. In these situations, the saliva will usually only dribble from one side of the mouth. An invasion of Wind-Cold can also block the movement of *qi* in the area, resulting in a unilateral paralysis and subsequent dribbling from this side of the mouth.

Heat in the Stomach can drive fluids from the Stomach up to the mouth, so that there is an over-production of saliva. In small children, the pattern of Stomach Heat can be caused by the accumulation of parasites in the digestive system.

Observation of the mouth

Observation	Significance
Distortion of the mouth	Wind-Cold, Wind-Phlegm, *xue* stagnation
Dribbling from the mouth	Wind-Cold, internal Wind, Spleen and/or Lung *qi xu*, Stomach Heat, parasites

Visual diagnosis of the gums

Like the lips and the tongue, the state of the gums can be used to diagnose c̣
of Heat and *xue xu*. Furthermore, the gums are under the direct influence of th̦
and Stomach. This means that imbalances in these two organs can manifest ̦
in the gums. This is also logical when viewed from a Western medicine perspe ̣ve:
the oral cavity is part of the digestive tract and has evolved from the same tissue as the
stomach in the embryological stage. In practice, this means that a state of Stomach
Fire can manifest with very red, bleeding gums. Bleeding gums can also arise from a *xu*
condition. Stomach *yin xu* Heat can also manifest with bleeding gums, as can Spleen
qi xu. In both *yin xu* and *shi* Heat, the haemorrhaging will occur because *xue* has
become agitated by the Heat, rupturing the walls of the vessels. When there is Spleen
qi xu, the Spleen may be unable to hold *xue* within the blood vessels. There can, of
course, be situations where both of these aspects are present simultaneously. It could
be that the *xue* is agitated by the Heat and the Spleen is too weak to keep the agitated
xue inside of the blood vessels. The primary diagnostic difference in bleeding gums is
the colour of the gums. In conditions of Heat, the gums will be red. If there is Spleen
qi xu, the gums will be pale in colour. The gums can also be pale if there is *xue xu*, *yang
xu* or Cold resulting in a lack of *xue* in this area.

When there is *qi* and *xue xu*, the gums can begin to recede, exposing the roots
of the teeth.

Heat, on the other hand, can damage the tissue, resulting in ulcers in the gums.

Observation of the gums

Observation	Significance
Pale gums	Spleen *qi xu*
	Can also be *xue xu*, *yang xu* or Cold
Very red gums	Heat (both *xu* and *shi*)
Weeping ulcers	Damp-Heat, Stomach Fire
Receding gums	*Qi* and *xue xu*

Visual diagnosis of the tongue

Analysis of the tongue and pulse are some of the most important diagnostic tools
we have at our disposal. The analysis of these two aspects of the body will often be
used to determine a diagnosis, especially when doubt has arisen due to the symptom
picture being contradictory and confusing.

The tongue can provide us with a great deal of information. It provides an
insight into the state of an individual's *qi* and *xue* and the state of the various *zangfu*
organs, and it is an important tool for differentiating patterns in relation to the
Eight Principles.

Most people find tongue diagnosis easier to learn than pulse diagnosis. This is
because tongue diagnosis is less subjective; with the pulse it is easier to feel doubt.

You can be uncertain that what you are feeling under the tips of your fingers, and define as Wiry for example, is the same sensation that another person feels when they say that a pulse feels like a guitar string under the finger. The tongue is more objective. It is something you can see with your eyes. A pale tongue with a thick white coating is a pale tongue with a thick white coating. It is something that you can compare with a photograph in an atlas of tongue photographs. Pulse diagnosis requires repeated hands-on training together with an experienced practitioner, whereas tongue diagnosis can be learned by studying photographs of tongues, with an explanation of which signs are significant on each tongue.

There is also a greater consensus in textbooks and amongst practitioners about which organs the various areas of the tongue relate to in the body and the significance of the changes in these areas. The pulse positions and definitions are much more open to debate and interpretation between the various systems.

The great strength of the pulse is that it is very precise, but it is also easily influenced and affected by many factors, which may only have limited diagnostic relevance. If you run up the stairs, if you are momentarily very irritated or if you have not slept all night, the pulse qualities will be radically different than if you had been sitting calmly for half an hour and had had a good night's sleep. The tongue though, for all intents and purposes, would remain the same in these situations.

The tongue gives us a good insight into the general condition of the patient. This is especially true of the tongue body itself. Compared with the pulse, the tongue is slower to manifest changes. However, the pulse's ability to change immediately is also an advantage. For example, you can perceive immediate changes in the pulse when the body is invaded by Wind-Cold, but changes in the tongue are difficult to detect in this situation. The pulse can also be used to control and adjust the needles that have been inserted into the body; again, something that is not possible with the tongue.

For its part, the tongue is excellent at showing the overall condition of the body and the imbalances that have affected the body over a longer period of time.

There are also internal variations with regards to how quickly the different aspects of the tongue can alter characteristics. The colour of the tongue body will not change as fast as the coating, which can change by the hour during an invasion of the body by exogenous *xie qi*. The tongue body's shape changes more slowly than its colour. The coating will reflect which influences the body has been exposed to during the previous hours and days.

There are several reasons that the tongue is such an effective diagnostic tool. To start with, the tongue is a bodily structure that is simultaneously on both the inside and the outside of the body. Visually, it is something that can be observed from the exterior, but it is also a part of the digestive tract and thereby a part of the interior. The tongue surface consists of a different cell structure than the normal skin. Both of these factors make it possible to see clearly the quality of *xue* through the surface of the tongue. It is possible to observe fluids on and in the tongue body, and you can see clearly the influence of factors such as Heat and Cold.

Changes in the pulse and the tongue

Pulse	Can change immediately	Can indicate what is affecting the body here and now. It can, of course, also supply information about long-term influences and changes, because these are the foundation for what is happening right now
Tongue shape	Can change over the course of weeks and months	Indicates which aetiological factors and imbalances have affected the body over a longer period of time
Tongue colour	May change during the course of the day and from day to day	Indicates which imbalances and aetiological factors have affected the body in recent days. Again, as with the pulse, chronic imbalances will also be seen, as they are part of the current situation
Tongue coating	Can change by the hour	Can indicate whether the aetiological factors and imbalances are chronic or acute

The tongue is directly under the influence of the Heart. The tongue is supplied with *xue* and *qi* via the Heart *luo mai*. *Shen*, which has its residence in Heart *xue*, is conscious of everything that is happening and in all changes that take place in the body. The *shen* will therefore influence the tongue via Heart *xue*. Apart from the Heart *luo mai* vessel, most channels have a branch that connects to the tongue. The Kidney channel terminates in the root of the tongue. The Spleen channel has an internal branch that connects with the tongue. The Liver, Stomach, Urinary Bladder and *san jiao* all have divergent channel connections with the tongue. The only channels that do not directly connect to the tongue themselves are the Lung, Large Intestine, Small Intestine and Gall Bladder channels. They connect to the tongue through either their partner channel or deep, internal channel connections. This means that changes in *zangfu* organs and their channels can be seen in the tongue.

The tongue coating is created from the impure residue that is sent upwards by the Spleen along with *gu qi* after transformation processes have taken place in the Stomach. The tongue therefore clearly shows the condition of the Stomach *qi*.

Finally, there are various micro-systems on the exterior surface of the body, where one can both treat and diagnose imbalances in the body. These are places where the whole body is reflected in a small, distinct area. This is clearly seen, for example, in the ear. These micro-systems exist because everything in the universe has an energetic resonance; things will resonate and influence other objects that have the same energetic vibration. This is also true of the body. Specific areas within the body can therefore be affected by changes elsewhere in the body. This means, for example, that when the Liver has been energetically or physically influenced, it can be observed and palpated in many parts of the body that resonate with the Liver, including observable changes on the side of the tongue.

The topography of the tongue

The tongue, as with many other parts of the body, reflects the condition of the various internal organs. This is seen in both the tongue's general appearance and changes in specific areas of the tongue.

There are three basic models that depict what the various areas of the tongue represent. The models are not intrinsically contradictory but support and supplement each other.

In the first model, the tongue is divided into three zones. Each zone represents one of the three *jiao*. The upper *jiao* can be seen in the front third of the tongue, the posterior third of the tongue is the lower *jiao* and in between them is the middle *jiao*.

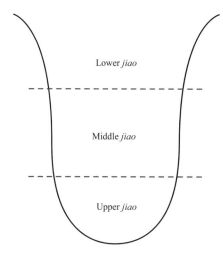

Figure 1.2 Positions of the three *jiao* on the tongue

In the second model, the front and the sides of the tongue are the areas that will manifest changes if there is an invasion of *xie qi* in the exterior. The areas that are inside of and behind these areas will reflect the body's interior. These areas will manifest changes if exogenous *xie qi* penetrates into the interior.

In the third model, the imbalances in the various *zangfu* organs manifest in specific areas of the tongue. It is important to remember that this model reflects an organ's physical location in the body and not its energetic or functional location. This means that the Liver, which physiologically belongs in the lower *jiao*, is to be found in the middle *jiao* area of the tongue (something that is also seen in its pulse position). This is in accordance with its anatomical location in the body. Some sources place the Liver on the left side of the tongue and the Gall Bladder on the right side; other sources assign both sides of the tongue to the Liver and Gall Bladder jointly. I personally utilise the latter in practice, as imbalances in the Gall Bladder channel are usually caused by Liver imbalances, and therefore both organs are involved and will be reflected on the tongue. Likewise, the very centre of the tongue is often assigned to the Stomach and the area around it to the Spleen, but the whole central area can also be seen as being representative of the Stomach and Spleen.

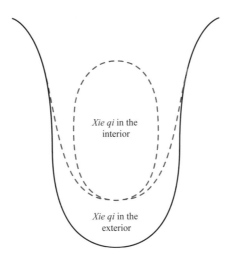

Xie qi in the
interior

Xie qi in the
exterior

Figure 1.3 Areas of the tongue that reflect how deep an invasion
of exogenous *xie qi* has penetrated into the body

Similarly, some sources divide the root of the tongue into four zones – Kidneys, Urinary Bladder, Small Intestine and Large Intestine – whilst other sources define the whole area as corresponding to all four organs at the same time. Again, I mostly utilise the latter interpretation. In clinical practice you must compare the tongue with the rest of the symptoms and signs. This will help to define which of these organs is manifesting on the root of the tongue. The Kidneys only have *xu* patterns of imbalance; conversely, the other three organs on the root tend towards *shi* patterns of imbalance. This means that if the root of the tongue, for example, has a greasy, yellow coating with raised papillae, it indicates that there is Damp-Heat present in the lower *jiao*. The Kidneys do not have a pattern of Damp-Heat, therefore it must be one of the other three organs that are manifesting Damp-Heat. If the person has a burning sensation when urinating, this will confirm that it is the Urinary Bladder and not the Intestines that is affected by Damp-Heat. On the other hand, if the person has diarrhoea, the Damp-Heat will not be in the Urinary Bladder but in the Intestines. If the root of the tongue is peeled and lacks coating, this indicates a *yin xu* condition. This will therefore be more indicative of a link to the Kidneys, rather than the Intestines or Urinary Bladder.

One must always remember that it is not only the *zangfu* organs, but also the three *jiao* that can be seen on the tongue. For example, a general condition of the Damp-Heat in the lower *jiao* could manifest on that area of the tongue.

The tip of the tongue reflects the Heart and the area behind the tip reflects the the Lung. The centre of the tongue manifests the Stomach and Spleen. The sides of the tongue reflects the condition of the Liver and Gall Bladder and the root the lower *jiao* organs – Kidney, Urinary Bladder and the Intestines.

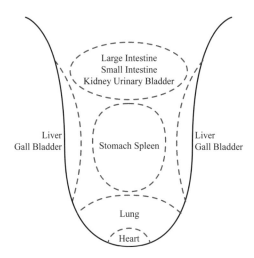

Figure 1.4 Areas of the tongue that reflect
the condition of the various *zangfu* organs

Tongue diagnosis according to the Eight Principles

Changes in the tongue can give a quick overview of diagnosis according to the Eight Principles.

The tongue and the Eight Principles

Significance	Observation
Exterior	No changes in the body of the tongue
	The coating can manifest change
Interior	The structure, form and colour of the tongue can have changed
	The coating will be affected in some way
Cold	Pale or bluish tongue body, white coating
Heat	Red tongue body, yellow coating or no coating
	Dry tongue
Xu	*Qi xu* – pale or swollen tongue body
	Yang xu – pale or bluish tongue body
	Xue xu – pale, thin tongue body and/or dry surface of the tongue
	Yin xu – red tongue body, cracked, dry, lacks coating
Shi	Thick coating

Optimal conditions for observing the tongue

There are various factors to take into consideration when observing the tongue that can influence its appearance.

- Consumption of various food and beverages can colour the coating on the tongue, leading to a false impression of how the coating looks. The following are typical examples of things that will affect the colour of the tongue: coffee, cigarettes, wine, liquorice, certain sweets, beetroot and Chinese herbal medicine, as well as spices such as turmeric, paprika, saffron, etc. It is therefore a good idea to ask the person whether they have ingested anything that could have affected the tongue colour, especially if the colour of the tongue is different to what you were expecting to see or when the colour is in contrast to the rest of the diagnostic picture.

- Many kinds of Western pharmaceutical medicine can affect the tongue. Whilst changes created by things that dye the tongue have no diagnostic relevance, as they will not have affected the physiology of the body, the changes created by medicines are relevant to the diagnosis. This is because medicine by its very nature affects the body's physiology, which creates a change in the tongue's appearance; therefore these changes in the tongue's appearance are diagnostically relevant. Antibiotics, for example, have a very cold energy and create Dampness in the body. When a person has been treated with antibiotics, they will often have a thick, white or a geographically peeled tongue coating. This is not a false sign and something that should be ignored when diagnosing the tongue; on the contrary, it tells us about the current situation, which will have relevance in the treatment of the patient. Likewise, some asthma sprays are hot and spreading in their dynamic. The long-term use of these sprays can result in a tongue whose front third is reddish and slightly peeled. Even though it is the medicine that is the cause of this change in the tongue's appearance, it is an indication that the medicine has injured the patient's Lung *yin*.

- It is increasingly common for people to brush their tongues. Removing the coating on the tongue makes the diagnosis more difficult and the conclusions more fraught with uncertainty. You should request that the patient does not brush their tongue in the days prior to a consultation, so that you can get a truer picture of their condition. It can sometimes be a diagnostic sign in itself that the person brushes their tongue. Dampness and Phlegm will often manifest with a thick, sticky tongue coating. This can result in an unpleasant sticky sensation in the mouth and the person may well brush their tongue to rid themselves of this unpleasant sensation.

- Lighting is important. The tongue should be well illuminated during inspection, preferably being viewed in natural light. Direct sunlight is optimal, but unfortunately most of us do not have clinics with panorama windows, and we do not live in the south of France but in countries with limited sunshine. Furthermore, many patients book appointments after work when it is dark. We must therefore view the tongue using sources of light other than sunlight. Halogen lighting is one of the best alternatives, but it is far from perfect. Energy-saving light bulbs and fluorescent lighting are, on the other hand, some of the worst alternatives, as they seriously affect the appearance of the colours. I normally observe the tongue in either the daylight that is available or illuminated by an ordinary light bulb and I then inspect the tongue using a torch with a halogen bulb. The advantage of using the torch is that I can focus the beam of light on specific areas of the tongue and on the root of the tongue, which is otherwise difficult to illuminate. It is a good idea to train yourself to look at various tongues, first in ordinary daylight and then with the light source that you will be using in your consulting room. This will give you an idea of how the tongue's colouration is affected by this particular light source.

- The tongue should be relaxed during inspection. It is better to get the patient to show you their tongue several times for a short duration (about 15 seconds each time) than to make them sit with their tongue hanging out for five minutes whilst you analyse everything you can see and consider the implications of any changes – it is both unpleasant and strenuous for the patient. It will also affect the colour and moistness of the tongue, thereby giving a false impression.

When analysing the tongue, it is important to remember that all aspects of tongue diagnosis are indispensable and that you should not see any aspect as being separate from the whole. This is because the various pieces of information must be seen in a context and as a part of a whole picture. This is particularly important, as most signs can have multiple interpretations depending on what other signs are present. A pale tongue body, for example, can be a sign that there is *yang xu*, *shi* Cold, *qi xu* or *xue xu*. Knowing that the tongue is pale therefore does not give enough information for us to be able to treat the patient. We must compare the tongue body's colour with other aspects of the tongue, especially the tongue body shape and the thickness, colour and distribution of the coating. In this example, the pattern of imbalance will be *shi* Cold if the pale tongue has a thick, white tongue coating. If there is *xue xu*, the tongue will not only be pale, but also thin and dry. *Yang xu* will manifest with a tongue that is pale, swollen and wet, whilst if there is *qi xu* in a specific *zang* organ, then the shape of that area of the tongue may be affected, as well as being pale.

All the information and signs that can be seen on the tongue can initially seem confusing and overwhelming. This will lessen if you proceed logically in your inspection and analysis. It is important that you are systematic, so that you are certain that you have observed all the relevant signs. I recommend having a checklist in the intake journal to ensure that you have observed and noted all relevant aspects of the tongue.

Remember to record the tongue body's colour, shape, size and structure, as well as variations between the various areas of the tongue body: the tongue coating's colour, thickness, distribution, moisture and quality; the movement and flexibility of the tongue; the tongue's vitality. Note each aspect separately and then compare the pieces of information with each other.

Something that is very important to remember is that the tongue reflects the body as a whole and can reflect several patterns of imbalance simultaneously. This means that even if there is a certain pattern of imbalance, if the tongue is manifesting another pattern of imbalance that veils these signs, it may not be very obvious. For example, the classic *xue xu* tongue should be thin, pale and dry, but if the condition of *xue xu* is due to Spleen *qi xu*, the tongue may well be pale, swollen and wet, thus negating the signs of dryness and thin tongue body.

The amount of information you need to take into account when you diagnose the tongue can seem overwhelming. Personally, I think that instead of laboriously learning by heart all the various colours, shapes, coatings, etc. and what each of these signs indicate, it is easier to try and think about how these changes will have arisen, i.e. what dynamic processes create these changes. For example, if the tongue is pale, instead of having to remember that a pale tongue is a sign of *qi xu, xue xu, yang xu* and *shi* Cold, you can think to yourself: Why does the tongue look pale? What could the dynamic be behind this change? The tongue can be pale because there is too little *xue* in the tissue of the tongue. This lack of *xue* in the tissue can be because there is too little *xue* in the body in general, i.e. a pattern of *xue xu*, or because something is either preventing the *xue* from reaching the tongue – *shi* Cold – or *xue* is not being lifted up to the tongue – *qi xu* or *yang xu*.

Shen

The first impression we get from the tongue is whether there is *shen*. *Shen* in this context means vitality and refers to the general appearance of the tongue. It is the same kind of *shen* that we talk about as being visible when the eyes or face have *shen*.

A tongue with *shen* radiates vitality, flexibility and is not limp or stiff. The tongue should radiate the same energy that a live fish has, not a fish that has been lying around for a couple of days on a fishmonger's slab.

Shen in this context is mainly used for prognosis. A tongue with *shen* means that although there may be many signs of a serious imbalance in the body, the patient's *zheng qi* is still strong and *xie qi* is not deeply rooted. This means that the imbalance can be rectified. The absence of *shen* in these situations, though, is serious and can indicate that the condition is deep rooted and therefore more difficult to rectify.

Tongue colour

The tongue colour refers to the colour of the tongue body itself and not the coating. If the coating is so thick that you cannot see the tongue body, the colours on the underside of the tongue may give an indication of the colour of the tongue's surface. The colour of the tongue can be used to diagnose conditions of Heat, Cold, *yin xu, yang xu, qi xu* and *xue xu*, as well as the state of the *zangfu* organs. The colour of the tongue can give an idea of how deep *xie qi* has penetrated into the body. The colour should always be seen in relation to the shape of the tongue. These two aspects cannot be seen separately from each other and they are the single most important aspect of tongue diagnosis. In cases where you are unsure of your tongue diagnosis because of conflicting information, it is the tongue's colour that should determine the diagnosis, because it is the most important aspect. This is because the colour of the tongue body reflects the long-term influences and the underlying patterns of imbalance.

Five pathological colours have traditionally been differentiated on the tongue: pale, red, dark red, purple and blue.

The overall colour of the tongue should be noted, as well as any colour changes in specific areas. The colour of the tongue as a whole will reflect the general condition of the body, and changes of colour in the specific areas of the tongue will relate to imbalances in these areas of the body, especially the *zangfu* organs that these areas pertain to.

Pale tongue

A tongue will be pale when there is not enough *xue* circulating in the it. This may be due to there being too little *xue* in the body in general – *xue xu* (and possibly *qi xu*), there being too little *qi* or *yang* to transport *xue* up to the tongue or there being something (Cold for example) that is blocking *xue* from reaching the tongue. It is necessary to compare the colour of the tongue with the shape of the tongue body, as well as the coating and the moistness of the tongue, in order to determine which pattern is involved. *Xue xu* will make the tongue not just pale, but also thin and dry. There is a rare situation in which *yang xu* can also result in a pale and dry tongue. This is when the *yang* is so weak that it is unable to transport fluids and *xue* up to the tongue and therefore the tongue is dry.

A *yang xu* tongue will not only be pale, but it will also be swollen and wet, as will a *qi xu* tongue. This means that you will have to compare the tongue with the patient's pulse and ask the patient relevant questions that can help to differentiate these patterns, such as whether they have an aversion to cold.

If there is *shi* Cold, the tongue can be pale with a thick, white and wet coating.

It is very common for the side of the tongue to be paler than the rest of the tongue. This is a manifestation of Liver *xue xu*. The sides of the tongue can also have a pale orange hue when there is Liver *xue xu*.

Red tongue

The presence of Heat can turn the tongue red. This is because the *yang* nature of Heat drives *xue* upwards to the surface of the body. In Western medicine physiology, the body opens and increases the flow of *xue* in the exterior aspects of the body when the temperature rises, enabling blood to dissipate some of the heat to the surroundings. This means that the tongue will be more red in colour. The opposite is the case when the body is too cold (*yang xu* Cold and *yin shi* Cold in Chinese medicine). In these situations, the tongue will be pale in colour due to the reduced amount of *xue* in the superficial blood vessels.

The whole of the tongue may be red, or it may only be specific areas of the tongue that are red. If an isolated area of the tongue is redder than its surroundings, it will indicate the presence of Heat in the organ that manifests in this area of the tongue.

The presence or lack of coating is diagnostically very important when diagnosing a red tongue. The presence or lack of coating will indicate whether to diagnose *shi* Heat or *yin xu* Heat: in *shi* Heat there will be a yellowish coating, whilst there will be a lack of coating on the tongue when there is *yin xu* Heat.

When there is Heat present, the tongue will usually be dry. There is, however, a situation where the tongue can be red and wet. This can occur if there is an acute condition of extreme Heat. In this case, the extreme Heat drives fluids in the body upwards and outwards. This will make the tongue temporarily wet. The person will probably also sweat profusely in this situation for the same reason.

Another scenario that can manifest with a red and wet tongue is the condition of Damp-Heat. Here, there is the presence of a *yin* and a *yang* pathogen simultaneously.

It is important to remember that *yin xu* can exist without resulting in Heat, in which case there will be a normal-coloured tongue that is dry and lacking in coating.

Red spots

Red spots and speckles always signify the presence of Heat. The size and height of the spots reflect the intensity of the Heat and how much stagnation the Heat has generated. The larger and more raised the spots, the more Heat there is present.

Sometimes you can see that the papillae on the tongue are raised without being red. This is also Heat, but the Heat is not as intense as when there are red spots although there is sufficient Heat to raise the papillae up from the surface of the tongue.

The distribution of the spots and speckles on the tongue's surface will indicate which organs are affected by Heat. Small speckles are mainly seen on the sides and tip of the tongue. Larger spots and raised papillae are usually seen on the rear of the tongue.

Purple

When *xue* stagnates, the tongue will become purple in colour. This reflects poor circulation, which in Western medicine will be a sign that the blood is not being optimally oxygenated. There may be a reddish-purple or bluish-purple colour. If the tongue is reddish-purple then it is Heat that has stagnated *xue*, resulting in *xue* becoming thick and sticky. *Xue* stagnation can in itself also generate Heat.

Cold can also stagnate *xue* by causing the vessels to contract, making it more difficult for *xue* to circulate through them. At the same time, Cold will block the *yang qi* that propels *xue* through the vessels. The tongue will be bluish-purple in colour when the stagnation is due to Cold.

The tongue can also have a slight mauve tinge, which the eye must be trained to perceive. This indicates Liver *qi* stagnation resulting in *xue* not circulating optimally.

There may also be purple spots in specific areas of the tongue. This will indicate that there is *xue* stagnation in the relevant area of the body. The sides of the tongue can be purple when there is Liver *xue* stagnation

Veins on the underside of the tongue

It is also important to observe veins on the underside of the tongue. These are often dark and purplish if there is *xue* stagnation. The veins in this case will usually also be swollen or knotted.

If the veins are pale and flat, it can indicate *xue xu* or *qi xu*. If the veins are milky in appearance, this can indicate the presence of Dampness and Phlegm.

The sub-lingual veins may also be longer than normal, which is a sign of Heat.

It is not only the two main sub-lingual veins that can change colour and shape. Small veins on the lower surface of the tongue changing colour and shape is a sign of *xue* stagnation. Similarly, small, purple spots appearing on the underside of the tongue is a sign of *xue* stagnation.

Tongue body colour

Observation	Significance
Pink	Normal
Pale and wet	*Yang xu* Cold or *shi* Cold patterns *Qi xu*
Pale and dry	*Xue xu* (in some cases *yang xu*)
Pale sides	Liver *xue xu*
Pale-orange sides	Liver *xue xu*
Red	*Shi* or *xu* Heat, depending on the coating The entire tongue can be red or only the area that relates to a specific area of the body or a specific organ
Red tip	Heat in the Heart
Red sides	Liver Heat
Red central area	Stomach Heat
Red spots	Heat, *xue* Heat and/or *xue* stagnation, depending on size The location of the spots gives an indication of where the Heat is in the body
Red and wet	Short-term Heat or Damp-Heat (in rare but very serious situations, this is a sign of true Cold/false Heat)
Red, swollen	*Xie* Heat in the interior Heart Fire

Purple or purple spots	*Xue* stagnation
	The whole tongue or just specific areas that relate to the organs involved, can be purple
	The purple colour will be either bluish purple (Cold stagnating *xue*) or reddish purple (Heat stagnating *xue* or the stagnant *xue* generating Heat)
Purple veins on the underside of the tongue	*Xue* stagnation
Pale veins on the underside of the tongue	*Xue xu* or *qi xu*
Milky veins on the underside of the tongue	Damp-Phlegm
Extended veins on the underside of the tongue	Heat
Purple spots on the underside of the tongue	*Xue* stagnation

Tongue body shape

The shape of the tongue includes the tongue's size, physical shape, whether there are cracks on the surface and the length and mobility of the tongue.

The tongue's shape will mainly reflect whether there is a *xu* or *shi* condition. The tongue shape will give an impression of the condition of *qi* and *xue*, as well as whether Wind and Dampness are present.

The shape of the tongue will also reflect the severity and duration of the imbalance.

A pale, wet tongue that has arisen due to *yang xu* is less serious and indicates a shorter duration than if the tongue is pale, wet and swollen. The swelling of the tongue indicates that the *yang* is chronically weak and therefore not performing its function of transforming and transporting fluids in the body. Similarly, *yin xu* that manifests with a tongue that is red and without coating is not as serious and chronic as *yin xu* that manifests with a tongue that is red, thin, lacking in coating and with cracks in the surface of the tongue. The latter shows that the *yin xu* is so deep rooted and chronic that it is starting to damage the body's tissues.

Even though the shape of the tongue is highly significant, it is still the tongue colour that is the single most important aspect in tongue diagnosis.

Thin tongue body

A 'thin tongue' refers to the thickness and not the breadth of the tongue. A tongue becomes thin when there is too little fluid and too little *xue* to 'fill' the tongue, i.e. there is too little *yin* in the tongue. This will be due to there being too little *yin* and/ or *xue* in general or there being something that has damaged these *yin* aspects, which will be some form of Heat. The colour of the tongue will be the determining factor.

A red tongue indicates that there is Heat damaging the *yin* aspects and a pale tongue that there is too little *xue*.

A thin tongue is not seen as often as might be expected. Many clients are *xue xu* and *yin xu*, but because they also have Dampness and Phlegm, this results in their tongues being swollen. This means that a tongue that would otherwise have been thin due to *xue xu* or *yin xu* can be swollen due to the presence of Dampness and Phlegm.

Swollen tongue body

It is necessary to distinguish between a tongue that is completely swollen and a tongue where only certain areas are swollen.

A swollen tongue will be the result of too much fluid accumulating in the tongue, i.e. Dampness, Phlegm or accumulation of fluids, which is the opposite of the previous situation where the tongue was too thin due to a lack of fluids. The accumulation of Dampness, Phlegm or fluids in the body is in itself a *shi* condition. *Shi* conditions will often, though not always, have their root in a *xu* condition. Heat, for example, can force fluids upwards to the tongue or condense them so that they transform into Phlegm.

As with the colour of the tongue, the swelling can encompass the entire tongue body or just be limited to a certain area that corresponds to specific organs or areas of the body.

Partially swollen tongue body

Whilst an entirely swollen tongue will be due to a *shi* condition of Dampness, Phlegm or accumulated fluids, a partially swollen tongue can be a sign of a *xu* or a *shi* condition. *Qi xu*, *qi* stagnation and Heat can all result in the swelling of certain areas of the tongue. The areas of the tongue that most often swell up are the tip, the central area and the edges of the tongue.

If the sides are swollen, it is important to differentiate between whether it is the whole side of the tongue that is swollen (a Liver imbalance) or just the sides in the central area of the tongue (Spleen *qi xu*). If the swollen sides are also red, this indicates Liver Heat. If they are normal in colour, there will be Liver *qi* stagnation.

The reason that Spleen *qi xu* can result in swelling of the sides of the tongue, which is an area normally associated with the Liver and Gall Bladder area, is that when the Spleen area in the middle of the tongue swells, this forces the side of the tongue outwards in this area. Spleen *qi xu* swelling will usually result in there being teeth marks on the side of the tongue.

If there is Phlegm-Dampness or *qi xu* in the Lung, there will be swelling of either the whole of the front third of the tongue or just the sides of this area.

The tip of the tongue can swell when there are Heart imbalances. This will typically be seen if the mental-emotional aspect of the Heart, the *shen*, is not in balance; the tip will usually also be red in these situations.

Sunken areas

Some areas of the tongue can appear to have sunk downwards. This indicates a condition of *qi xu* in the organ that is reflected in this area of the tongue. The depression in the tongue's surface can sometimes only be seen immediately after the person has presented their tongue, and then the area 'fills' up and the depression is no longer visible. It is sometimes necessary to get the patient to extend their tongue a couple of times to be sure that you have observed the depression correctly. On the other hand, an area of the tongue may only 'collapse' after the tongue has been extended for a while. In both cases, this will most typically be seen in the area corresponding to the Lung or the Spleen and Stomach, and is indicative of *qi xu* in these organs. If the root of the tongue is sunken, this can be a sign of Kidney *jing xu*.

Uncontrolled movement and stiffness

There should be flexibility and movement in the tongue. If the tongue movements are involuntary, this may be interior Wind causing *qi* to move chaotically or the Spleen failing to control the muscles. When the Spleen does not control the muscles in the tongue, the tongue can quiver. Sometimes the tongue will begin to quiver after the person has had their tongue extended for a few seconds. It is as if the Spleen is no longer capable of keeping the tongue still.

In the same way that a light wind will cause a flag to wave from side to side, high winds will make the cloth of the flag hard and stiff. The same applies to the tongue. Interior Wind can make the tongue sway from side to side or result in a tongue that is rigid and inflexible.

If the tongue deviates to one side, this can be due to the channels on one side of the body being *shi* (Wind or Phlegm) or the channels on the other side of the body being *xu*.

A flaccid tongue, especially if it is swollen, indicates *qi xu* or Phlegm.

Flaccidity

If the tongue seems limp and lifeless, this may be due to a lack of fluids or *xue*, causing the tongue to wilt. There may therefore be *qi xu* or *xue xu*. Alternatively, Heat may have damaged the fluids. The colour of the tongue will determine whether it is *xue xu* and/or a *qi xu* condition, on the one hand, or *yin xu* or Heat, on the other. In the first two cases the tongue will be pale, and in the latter two cases the tongue will be red.

Length

The *yang* nature of Heat is expansive. This can cause the tongue to become longer.

At the same time, Heat damages fluids and this can therefore cause the tongue to shrink, resulting in a short tongue.

Cold has a *yin* dynamic that makes things contract. Cold can therefore also result in a tongue that is shorter than normal.

The difference between a tongue that is short due to Cold and one that is short due to Heat will be seen in the colour of the tongue. Heat will result in a short tongue that is red, whereas Cold will manifest with a pale and short tongue.

Cracks

Cracks are often, but not exclusively, a manifestation of *yin xu*. Body fluids nourish and moisten the tongue, in the same way that rain moistens the soil. If there is too little rain, the surface of the earth cracks, and if there is too little body fluid, the tongue surface cracks.

The shape and distribution of the cracks will depend on the type of *yin xu* involved. The depth and size of the cracks will say something about how serious the situation is and how long it has existed. Deep, long and multiple cracks signify a more deep-seated imbalance than single, short, shallow cracks.

A very swollen tongue may look as if it is cracked, but this is because the tongue is 'wrinkled' and 'creased'. The patient can be asked to pull the sides of the tongue outwards. If the cracks disappear, the tongue is just swollen and not cracked. By pulling on the side of the tongue you can also get an idea of the depth and thus the severity of the cracks.

A short crack in the middle of the tongue indicates a *xu* condition in the Stomach or Spleen. If the crack and the area around it is red and lacks coating, this is a sign of Stomach *yin xu*. If the area is normal or pale coloured and has coating, it will not be *yin xu*, but Spleen and Stomach *qi xu*. If the crack is deeper or wider with a sticky, yellowish coating (it may look as if the crack is furry), it is a sign of Stomach Fire or Phlegm-Heat in the Stomach.

If there are more irregular or transverse cracks in the central area of the tongue, it will be a manifestation of Stomach *yin xu*. If the cracks are more extensive and cover the entire tongue, this indicates Stomach and Kidney *yin xu*. Likewise, a longitudinal crack along the middle of the tongue with several transverse cracks extending out from it, reflects Stomach and Kidney *yin xu*.

A crack that runs all the way down the centre of the tongue and out to the tip shows that there is a constitutional weakness and the person can have a tendency to develop Heart imbalances.

Two diagonal cracks on the front third of the tongue behind the tip is a sign of Lung *yin xu*. The cracks may be the remnants of an old condition, such as a severe respiratory disease in early childhood that damaged the Lung at the time.

Short transverse cracks on the sides of the tongue are a sign of Spleen *qi* and *yin xu*.

Veins on the underside of the tongue

If the veins on the underside are swollen or knotted, it indicates that there is *xue* stagnation.

If the veins are very flat and pale, there may well be *xue xu* or *qi xu*.

Tongue body shape

Observation	Significance
Neither swollen nor thin, the same shape all over, flexible but static No cracks	Normal
Thin	*Yin xu*, *xue xu* or lack of fluids (Dryness)
Pale, large, swollen, tooth marked	*Qi* and *yang xu* Damp-Phlegm
Normal coloured, swollen	Dampness or Phlegm
Red, swollen	Stomach and Heart Heat, Damp-Heat
Purple, swollen	Poisoning
Partly swollen	Depends on the colour and the area: Sides – Liver/Gall Bladder Fire if the sides are red or Liver *qi* stagnation if the sides are normal coloured Middle of the sides or teeth marks – Spleen *qi xu* Tip – Heart, usually Phlegm or Heat Front third – Lung usually Phlegm, but can also be *qi xu*
Sunken areas	Depends on the area: Middle – Stomach and/or Spleen *qi xu* Front – Lung *qi xu* At the rear – Kidney *jing xu*
Quivering	Wind or Spleen *qi xu*
Stiff	Interior Wind If the tongue is red, this is due to extreme Heat
Flaccid and pale	Spleen and Heart *qi* and *xue xu*
Flaccid and red	Heat
Flaccid, red and dry	Kidney *yin xu*
Long	Heart Fire
Short	If the tongue is red – Heat If the tongue is pale – Cold
Swollen veins on the underside of the tongue	*Qi* and/or *xue* stagnation
Very flat and pale veins on the underside of the tongue	*Qi xu* or *xue xu*

Observation	Significance
Cracks	A short crack in the centre, the area is pale and with coating – Stomach or Spleen *qi xu*
	A short crack in the centre, the area is red and lacks coating – Stomach *yin xu*
	The crack in the middle is deeper or wider with a sticky, yellowish coating – Stomach Fire or Phlegm-Heat in the Stomach
	Irregular or transverse cracks in the central part of the tongue – Stomach *yin xu* or Stomach and Kidney *yin xu*
	Long crack along the central area with several transverse cracks spreading outwards – Stomach and Kidney *yin xu*
	Crack all the way down the middle of the tongue and out to the tip – constitutional weakness with a tendency to Heart imbalances
	Two diagonal cracks behind the tongue tip – Lung *yin xu*
	Short transverse cracks on the sides of the tongue – Spleen *qi* and *yin xu*

Tongue coating

The tongue coating is a natural consequence of transformation of the ingested food and liquids in the Stomach. It is some of the 'dirty' residue rising upwards along with the pure *qi* that has been separated from the impure dross.

The tongue coating should be thin enough to enable the tongue itself to be seen through the coating. The tongue should look like a wheat field in the spring when the wheat has sprouted and is just beginning to push its way up through the soil. The soil can still be clearly seen, but the field has a green hue and when you look closer you can distinguish the individual wheat sprouts. Similarly, you should be able to see the body of the tongue through the coating and the coating should look like small individual dots on the tongue.

The coating will be thickest in the middle and at the rear. This is because these areas of the tongue correspond to the Stomach and Intestine, which are the organs that receive and transport the impure residue that is left behind after the transformation of the pure *qi*. This is reflected in these areas having a thicker and dirtier coating than the rest of the tongue. An alternative explanation for why the coating is naturally thicker on the rear of the tongue is that some of the impure residue from the transformation process rises from the Stomach and ascends towards the mouth. This impure residue settles on the back of the tongue, as it is this part of the tongue that it hits first. This is likened to when steam rises upwards from a kettle and condenses on the bottom of a windowpane, but the upper part of the glass is still transparent and dry.

The coating on the tongue does not usually extend to or cover the sides or the tip.

The tongue coating primarily reflects whether a condition is *shi* or *xu* in nature, whether the condition is Hot or Cold, and the condition of the *fu* organs. The coating is not necessarily directly associated with the tongue colour and shape and therefore can be viewed separately in certain situations.

The tongue coating can be used to rapidly differentiate the Eight Principles.

The tongue coating in relation to the Eight Principles

Significance		Observation
Interior/exterior		The distribution of the coating on the tongue will reflect whether *xie qi* is in the interior or the exterior
Hot/Cold	Heat	Yellow and dry coating
	Cold	White and wet coating
Shi/xu	*Shi*	Thick coating
	Xu	*Yin xu* – very thin or peeled coating
		Qi xu – coating lacks root
Yin/yang	*Yin xu*	Very thin or peeled coating
	Yin shi	Thick, white and moist coating
	Yang xu	White and wet coating
	Yang shi	Thick, yellow, dry coating

Observation of the tongue coating is particularly relevant in acute conditions. This is because the coating is the aspect of the tongue that is quickest to change; it can change by the hour. In an acute invasion of *xie qi*, it is sometimes possible to observe changes in the coating in the front third of the tongue, especially the outer edge of this area. If *xie qi* penetrates deeper into the body, the coating will change by becoming thicker in the central areas of the tongue and possibly also changing colour and consistency.

It is not only exogenous invasions that can produce rapid changes in the tongue coating. Food stagnation will also manifest with changes in the tongue coating relatively quickly.

A general rule of thumb is: the thicker the coating, the stronger the *xie qi*.

If an organ is *yin xu* the tongue may manifest with a lack of coating in the area of the tongue that corresponds to that organ.

A healthy coating should have root, be evenly distributed and be slightly moist. Having root means that the coating should appear to be growing out of the tongue and not just lying on top of the tongue. If we go back to the metaphor of a wheat field, the wheat should appear to be growing up through the soil and not lying uprooted on the top of the earth like mown grass.

When a coating lacks root it can be easily scraped off. This is because the Stomach, Spleen and Kidney are not functioning as they should and a new, healthy coating is not being formed to replenish the existing coating from below. The old coating eventually loses its connection to its root and starts to fall off.

A rootless coating is always indicative of a *xu* condition. There may be a rootless coating in the early morning upon waking. This is because the Stomach and Spleen are inactive at night and have therefore not created a new coating on the tongue whilst the person slept.

The coating also gives an impression of the development of a pathological condition. The coating suddenly disappearing in a disease is a negative sign, even if the coating was excessively thick. Intuitively, a thick coating disappearing might seem to be a positive development, but it is only positive if the change is gradual and not sudden. If the change is sudden, it is probably due to *yin* or *qi* being damaged by the *xie qi*.

A coating that suddenly becomes thick is usually seen when Dampness blocks the middle *jiao*.

When exogenous *xie qi* invades the body, the changes in the coating will usually only be seen in the front third of the tongue and the sides of this area. If the coating begins to thicken further towards the centre of the tongue and if the coating changes colour from white to yellow and starts to dry out, this indicates that *xie qi* has started to penetrate the interior and begun to generate Heat. This process can often be quite rapid.

In interior pathological conditions, the distribution of the coating will indicate where the imbalance is in the body and which organs are most likely to be affected. The colour and texture of the coating will give an indication of what type of imbalance is probable.

One should therefore observe whether the coating is thicker or thinner in certain areas of the tongue and whether there is a difference in the condition of the coating in these areas.

Colour of the coating

The coating is naturally a pale, white colour. It will also be white if there is pathogenic Cold present, but the coating will be thicker and moister.

When there is Heat, the coating turns yellow. The more Heat there is, the darker the coating becomes. The coating will usually be drier, unless there is Damp-Heat or Phlegm-Heat, in which case the coating can be sticky, greasy or oily.

In some situations, the coating is black or almost black. This may be a sign of extreme Heat or of Damp-Cold, depending on how moist the coating is and what colour the tongue body has. When there is extreme Heat, the Heat will have damaged fluids in the body; therefore the black coating will also be dry. If the black coating is a manifestation of Damp-Cold, the coating will instead be wet, because Cold can block the transportation and transformation of fluids, which then accumulate on the surface of the tongue.

There may well be differences in the colour of the coating from one area of the tongue to another. This can be a reflection of Heat in a certain area of the body or in an organ. Typically, the coating at the rear of the tongue is more yellow than at the front of the tongue. This is because Damp-Heat tends to accumulate in the lower *jiao*.

Heat in the Stomach will turn the coating yellow in the centre of the tongue or in a crack in the centre of the tongue.

If the coating on the sides of the tongue is yellow, it is important to observe how the colour is on the rest of the tongue. If there is a yellow coating on the sides and the rest of the tongue coating is white, this indicates that there is an invasion of Wind-Heat or Heat in the Intestines. If the rest of the coating is also yellow but the sides are even more yellowish, this usually indicates that there is Heat in the Liver and Gall Bladder. Finally, if one side of the tongue has a yellow coating and the other side is white, this can be a sign that exogenous *xie qi* is locked in the *shaoyang* aspect or that there is Heat in the Liver and Gall Bladder.

Moistness

Moistness refers to both the general moistness of the tongue and the moistness of the tongue's coating. Both the tongue and the coating should be slightly moist but not wet.

Pathogenic Heat will dry and damage fluids and *xue*.

Yin xu is characterised by a lack of fluids, therefore the tongue will also be dry.

Fluids and *xue* are closely linked to each other and *xue* helps to moisten the body. A dry tongue can therefore also be seen when there is *xue xu*.

Yang xu and Cold can mean that body fluids are not transformed and transported optimally and these will therefore accumulate on the tongue, causing the tongue coating to become wet.

Greasy and sticky coatings

Greasy coatings arise when *qi* does not transform fluids, causing Dampness and Phlegm to arise.

Greasy and sticky coatings are very similar in appearance and cause. Maciocia describes the papillae on the tongue in a greasy coating as looking like the bristles on a toothbrush that are covered in butter. You can still see each individual bristle, but they are thicker and have a greasy coating. In a sticky coating, the individual papillae are no longer distinguishable from each other and the coating will look more oily (Maciocia 2004, p.224).

A greasy or sticky coating always indicates the presence of Dampness or Phlegm.

Mouldy coating

A mouldy coating, is also called a 'tofu coating' in Chinese, because it seems as if there are small pieces of tofu on the tongue. In English this could translate as a cottage cheese coating, because it will look as if the person has just eaten cottage cheese. The mouldy coating is seen when there is Stomach Fire or Toxic-Fire in the throat.

Tongue coating

Observation	Significance
Thin, white, rooted, normal moistness	Normal
Rootless coating	Stomach *qi xu* or *yin xu*
White, thin, slippery	Damp-Cold disrupting *wei qi*
White, thick, slippery	Internal Damp-Cold, food stagnation of short duration
Thick, white	Food stagnation, *shi* Cold
Dry, white	Cold that is in the process of transforming into Heat. Fluids are being injured
Greasy, white	Internal Dampness or external Cold or Dampness. Spleen *yang xu*
Dry, yellow	Internal Heat is starting to damage *yin*
Thin, yellow	Wind-Heat
Thick, yellow	Food stagnation turning into Heat, *shi* Heat
Greasy, yellow	Internal Damp-Heat or Phlegm-Heat
Yellow stripes on the sides of the tongue and the rest of the coating is white	Exterior pathogen invading inwards. Heat in the Stomach and Intestines
Dark yellow stripes on the sides of the tongue and the rest of the coating is yellow	Heat in the Liver and Gall Bladder
Yellow on one side and white on the other	Heat in Liver and Gall Bladder. *Shaoyang* syndrome
Damp, grey-black/brown	Cold-Damp
Dry, grey-black/brown	Extreme Heat
Mouldy	Stomach Fire, Toxic-Fire
No coating	*Yin xu*
Dry tongue	Heat, *xue xu* or *yin xu*
Wet tongue	*Yang xu* or Cold

Visual diagnosis of the hair

This section deals mainly with observation of the head hair. Pubic and body hair will be discussed in the following section.

Head hair

Diagnosis of the hair on the head encompasses the volume of the hair, whether the hair is dry or greasy, the colour of the hair and the quality of the scalp.

In a healthy state, there should be an even distribution of hair, covering the entire scalp. The hair should be neither too dry nor too oily. It should have a sheen and be soft. Similarly, the scalp should be smooth and without dandruff.

A healthy head of hair that has lustre, shine and volume indicates that the person has sufficient *jing* and *xue* to nourish the hair.

The hair can also give an indication of the state of a person's *shen*. A person whose *shen* is disturbed can often have a slightly odd or eccentric appearance, the person's *shen* lacking the ability to conform to what is normal. This may manifest in the fact that their hair is either chaotic or looks slightly odd. This is sometimes seen, for example, in people who are mentally ill. An unusual hairstyle can, of course, be a conscious intention, especially in younger people. In this case, the appearance of the hair loses its diagnostic significance.

Hair loss

It is not only *jing* that has a direct impact on the head hair. The hair is created by *jing* in the same way that grass seed creates the grass on a lawn: seed alone is not enough, as the grass must be nourished and watered. The hair on the head is nourished and moistened by *jinye* and *xue*. This means that the quality and amount of head hair can be affected negatively if either or both of these are *xu*. The fact that *jing xu* is not the only cause of hair loss is seen in post-partum women who are *xue xu*. If the hair loss was only due to the loss of *jing* through pregnancy and birth, the condition would be more permanent and not improve with the improvement of their *xue*. Furthermore, Fire and Damp-Heat can scorch the roots of the hair, resulting in hair loss. *Xue* stagnation can prevent fresh, nourishing *xue* from reaching areas of the scalp, resulting in the roots of the hair not being nourished.

Dryness

If the body is in balance, the hair on the head has a healthy shine and is soft. This indicates that it is well nourished by *xue* and *yin*.

Dry hair will therefore be seen, when there is a condition of *yin xu* or *xue xu*. *Shi* Heat conditions such as Fire can also injure *yin* or *xue*, resulting in dry hair.

Greasy hair is usually an indication of Damp-Heat or Phlegm-Dampness.

It is, of course, important to take into account the use of various hair products that can give the hair an oily or greasy appearance, as well as hair treatments such as bleaching and perming that can desiccate the hair. In these situations, the dryness or greasiness is caused by factors that do not have a diagnostic significance.

Colour

If the hair turns grey or white, this is usually a sign that *jing* is weakened and is no longer strong enough to produce normal-coloured hair. This is a natural part of the ageing process, manifesting the decline of *jing*.

If the person loses their hair colour prematurely, this may well be a sign of *jing xu*. It can also be the result of a powerful shock injuring the Kidney and Heart or from Liver and/or Heart Fire damaging the hair. Some people lose their hair at an early age without this having diagnostic relevance. In these cases, the people will be otherwise healthy and strong, without any further signs of *jing xu*.

The scalp

The scalp is affected by the same factors as the rest of the skin. The scalp is nourished and moistened by *xue* and *jinye*. The most typical manifestation of an imbalance that can be seen in the scalp is dandruff. Dandruff can be dry, in which case it is usually due to *xue xu* or *yin xu* not nourishing the scalp. The dandruff can also be oily in appearance, in which case the cause will probably be the presence of Damp-Heat or Phlegm-Dampness. Damp-Heat will usually also result in the scalp being itchy at the same time.

Observation of the head hair

Observation	Significance
Hair loss	*Jing xu*, *xue xu*, Fire, Damp-Heat or *xue* stagnation
Greasy hair	Damp-Heat, Damp-Phlegm
Dry hair	*Yin xu*, *jinye xu*, *xue xu*, Fire or *shi* Heat
Grey or white hair	*Jing xu*
Dandruff	*Yin xu*, *jinye xu*, *xue xu* or Damp-Heat
Chaotic or odd hairstyle	*Shen* disturbance

Visual diagnosis of the body hair

The body hair is under the influence of the Lung and *wei qi*, but it is also nourished by *xue*. If there is a lack of body hair, it may indicate that there is Lung *qi xu* or *xue xu*. If the body hair is fragile, breaks easily or falls out, this is usually a sign of *qi xu* and/or *xue xu* resulting in the hair not being nourished.

Body hair is used to control and regulate the body temperature, especially when the person is exposed to cold. This is one of the functions carried out by *wei qi*. When the body is exposed to Wind-Cold, *wei qi* raises the body hair and closes the pores of the skin to keep the invading *xie qi* out.

The pubic hair should appear at the start of adolescence. This is a manifestation of the transition from the second to the third *jing* cycle. A lack of pubic hair can therefore be a sign of *jing xu*. It is important, however, to remember that as with the hair on the head, a lack of pubic hair can also be a sign of *xue xu* if the roots of the hair are not receiving sufficient nourishment.

An excessive growth of pubic hair, for example down the thighs or upwards towards the navel, can be seen when *chong mai* is disrupted by Phlegm or *xue* stagnation.

Observation of the body hair

Observation	Significance
Lack of body hair	Lung *qi xu* or *xue xu*
Fragile body hair that breaks easily	*Qi xu* or *xue xu*
Lack of pubic hair	*Yin xu* or *xue xu*
Excessive growth of pubic hair	Phlegm or *xue* stagnation in *chong mai*

Visual diagnosis of the throat

The pharynx

Observation of the pharynx is mainly relevant when there are invasions of exogenous *xie qi*. Invasions of Wind-Heat can manifest with redness and swelling in this area. If the Heat is so intense that it has created Toxic-Fire, there can also be ulceration and white exudate in the throat.

The throat can also become red and swollen when there is Stomach Fire that flames upwards, scorching the throat.

Swollen tonsils that are pale are an indication of Phlegm, Phlegm-Dampness or a retained pathogen.

If the tonsils are swollen and the throat is red, there will be an invasion of Wind-Heat.

The outside of the throat

The two most common diagnostic signs that can be observed on the outside of the throat are a swollen thyroid gland and redness of the skin on the throat and neck.

A swollen thyroid gland can be a sign of Phlegm. The Phlegm can be an independent pattern or it can be seen in combination with the following patterns: Liver *qi* stagnation, *xue* stagnation, Liver Fire, Heart *yin xu* or Liver *yin xu*.

Red skin on the neck is a sign of Heat. It will usually be seen when Heat ascends from the Lung or the Heart.

Observation of the throat

Observation	Significance
Red pharynx	Wind-Heat, Stomach Fire
Very red throat with ulcers or exudation	Toxic-Fire
Swollen tonsils	Invasion of Wind-Heat, Phlegm-Dampness or retained pathogen
Red skin on the outside of the neck	Heart or Lung Heat
Swollen thyroid gland	Phlegm

Visual diagnosis of the chest and the back

Observation of the thorax

The thorax is especially influenced by *zong qi* and the Lung and also the Heart. *Ren mai, chong mai*, Liver and Gall Bladder channels all also influence the area. Stagnation or accumulation of *qi, xue* or Phlegm in the area will create distension of the chest. This can give the appearance of being barrel-chested.

A lack of *zong qi* can cause the chest area to be hollow or sunken. *Jing xu* can also manifest with a sunken chest.

Observation of the chest

Observation	Significance
Distended	*Qi, xue*, or Phlegm stagnation
Hollow and sunken	*Zong qi xu, jing xu*

Visual diagnosis of the back

The Kidneys have a determining influence on the lumbar area, but the back is also affected by the channels that traverse the spinal column and the muscles alongside the spine. Furthermore, the muscles in general are affected by the Liver and the Spleen, so Liver *qi* stagnation, Spleen *qi xu* and Dampness and Damp-Heat can all affect the muscles of the back.

Abnormal curving of the spine

An abnormal curvature of the spine, such as scoliosis, lordosis or kyphosis, can be a manifestation of *jing xu* that has resulted in improper development of the body's structure, or it can be due to *du mai* imbalances. If there is only a slight distortion, this may be caused by muscle tension. The muscle tension may arise from Liver *qi* stagnation, *xue* stagnation, an invasion of exogenous Cold or Spleen *qi xu*.

Muscle tone

If the muscles along the spine appear to be tense and tight, it will be a sign of stagnation of *qi* in the area. The stagnation may be due to a local blockage of *qi* from an invasion of Cold or *xue* stagnation. It is often the consequence of a more general Liver *qi* stagnation that has caused the muscles to tense up.

A *shi* condition in one or more of the *zangfu* organs can manifest with the area around their back-*shu* point becoming tense and tight.

The muscles along the spine and in the back can be weak, lacking in tone or slightly sunken. This can be unilateral or bilateral. Weak muscle tone will indicate *qi* and *xue xu*. If the weakness of muscle tone is more local, this may be due to a disturbance of *qi* in the Urinary Bladder channel or it may be a sign of a *xu* condition in the organ, whose back-*shu* point lies adjacent to the area.

Observation of the back

Observation	Significance
Abnormal curvature of the spine	*Jing xu*, *du mai* imbalances, Liver *qi* stagnation, *xue* stagnation, an invasion of exogenous Cold or Spleen *qi xu*
Tight and distended muscles	*Qi* stagnation If the tightness and distension is localised to specific back-*shu* points, there can be a *shi* condition in these organs
Weak, soft and sunken muscles	*Qi xu* If the weakness and hollowness of the muscles is localised to specific back-*shu* points, there can be a *xu* condition in these organs

Visual diagnosis of the limbs

Visual diagnosis of the limbs includes observation of the size and quality of the muscles, whether there is oedema, observation of the skin and blood vessels and whether there are spasms, tremors or muscle cramps. Observation of the limbs has relevance in both acute and chronic patterns.

Stomach and Spleen *qi* is reflected in both the quality and mass of the muscles in the arms and legs. If there is Stomach and Spleen *qi xu*, there will be an inadequate production of *qi* and *xue*. This will mean that the muscles lack nourishment. A sign of Stomach and Spleen *qi xu* and *xue xu* can therefore be muscle atrophy or underdeveloped muscles. This can, of course, also be a sign of *jing xu*, especially in children, as well as Kidney and Liver *yin* and *xue xu* in older people.

Muscles that are flaccid and weak, but without a loss of mass, can be seen in acute conditions when Heat injures *jinye*.

Chronic conditions of weak and soft muscles are seen when Stomach and Spleen *qi xu* results in *xue* and *ying qi* not nourishing the muscles. Kidney and Liver *yin xu* can also result in muscles not receiving adequate nourishment. Dampness and Phlegm can block *qi* and *xue* from nourishing the muscles.

Very stiff and inflexible arms and legs usually indicate an invasion of exogenous Wind in acute cases or internally generated Wind in chronic cases.

The arms and legs can be rigid and stiff because joints are inflexible. This inflexibility can be due to Phlegm resulting in changes and deformity of the joint. It can also be due to *xue* stagnation or oedema on the muscles around the joint. Oedema around the joint arises when there is Damp *bi* or when there is Spleen and Kidney *yang xu*.

Liver and Kidney *yin xu* can result in the joint being too dry and becoming stiff.

Liver *xue xu* can mean that the tendons and sinews lack nourishment and thus become stiff.

Tremors, spasms and cramping of the muscles in the limbs will always be caused by Wind. There are, though, differences in how the Wind has arisen. It can be due to invasions of exogenous *xie qi* penetrating deeper into the body and generating Heat, resulting in the arousal of internal Wind. This is seen, for example, when there are febrile convulsions. Internal Wind can also arise when there is ascending Liver *yang*, Liver *yin xu* and Liver *xue xu*.

Acute oedema of the hands may occur during an invasion of Wind-Cold that interferes with the Lung's ability to spread *jinye*. If the oedema is chronic, and especially if it is pitting, it will probably be due to Kidney and/or Spleen *yang xu*. Oedema that is not pitting is more typical of *qi* stagnation.

Xue stagnation can manifest with small, but visible, purple thread veins or 'spider naevi'. This is typically observed on the ankle area in geriatric patients.

Varicose veins are a sign of Spleen *qi xu* that is failing to maintain the structure of the blood vessels and/or *xue* stagnation.

Observation of the limbs

Observation	Significance
Muscle atrophy or underdeveloped muscles	Stomach and Spleen *qi xu*, *qi* and *xue xu*, *jing xu*
Muscle weakness or laxity	Stomach and Spleen *qi xu*, Heat, Damp-Heat, Liver and Kidney *yin xu*
Rigid and inflexible arms and leg muscles	*Xue* stagnation, *qi* stagnation, Dampness, Phlegm, Wind, Kidney and Liver *yin xu*, Liver *xue xu*
Paralysis of the arms or legs	Wind (internal and external), Phlegm, Dampness, *xue* stagnation or Liver and Kidney *yin xu*
Tremors, spasms and muscle cramps	Wind (internal and external)
Oedema	Invasion of Wind-Cold, Kidney and/or Spleen *yang xu* or *qi* stagnation
Spider naevi	*Xue* stagnation
Varicose veins	Spleen *qi xu*, *xue* stagnation

Visual diagnosis of the joints

Visual observation of joints is imperative in the diagnosis of joint pain, including in *bi* syndrome.

Visual diagnosis can elicit useful information that can indicate the presence of Heat, Dampness, Phlegm or *xue* stagnation.

If there is Heat in the area, the skin will often be red and the area can be swollen due to the underlying stagnation of *qi* and thereby *jinye* that is creating the Heat. The skin will also feel warm on palpation.

If there is an accumulation of Dampness or *jinye* in the joint and surrounding tissue, the area will be swollen and spongy.

If the *bi* syndrome becomes chronic, the stagnation of *jinye* and Heat can result in the formation of Phlegm in the joint. This will result in the joint becoming deformed and gnarled. This will clearly be visible with the naked eye.

Xue stagnation in the joint can prevent the flow of fresh *xue* to skin above the joint. This means the skin will lack nourishment and moisture and can therefore be dry and flaky.

Observation of the joints

Observation	Significance
Redness and swelling	Heat
Swelling	Dampness, accumulation of *jinye*
Deformity	Phlegm stagnation
Dry flaky skin	*Xue* stagnation

Visual diagnosis of the hands

Visual diagnosis of the hands includes the observation of colour, shape and moistness of the hands and fingers, as well as the observation of the fingernails.

Colour

The normal colour of the hands in white Europeans should be pinkish red, indicating that the hands are being supplied with sufficient *xue* and *yang qi*. Account should be taken of the colouration of the skin in other ethnic groups.

If there is Heat, the hands can be more red in colour. If the Heat is *shi* in nature, this will be seen on both sides of the hand. If the Heat is *xu*, it will only be the palm that is red.

Pale hands are a sign of *yang xu* and *xue xu*.

Shape of the fingers

Thickened or swollen fingers can be caused by Phlegm or Dampness. They may also be due to oedema, but this will usually be periodic and sporadic.

Phlegm-Dampness can often manifest with 'chubby' fingers. Other causes of swollen fingers can be Cold or Damp *bi*. If there is Cold or Damp *bi*, there will also be pain in the fingers that is affected negatively by cold weather.

Fingers that are spoon-shaped (thicker at the tips) are usually an indication of a chronic Lung imbalance. It may be Phlegm-Cold, Phlegm-Heat or Lung and Kidney *yin xu*.

Very thin fingers may indicate Stomach and Spleen *qi xu*. The fingers will be thin because the muscles are malnourished and withered.

The joints in the fingers can change shape or become swollen or gnarled when there is a chronic *bi* syndrome if the stagnation has led to the formation of Phlegm in the joint.

Moistness

The skin in the hands, especially the palms, can become dry and even cracked. The dryness can be due to either Heat injuring *jinye* or a lack of nourishment and moisture due to *xue xu* and/or *yin xu*. If the dryness is due to Heat, the skin will be red. If the dryness is due to *xue xu*, the skin will be pale in colour.

Palms that are moist and sweaty can be seen when there is Heart *yin xu*, Heart *qi xu* or Heart Fire. In some cases this can be due to Lung *qi xu* or Lung Heat. Both of these organs' channels connect to the hands, and both organs have a direct influence on sweating. Sweaty palms after the insertion of acupuncture needles may be due to the person being nervous (a Heart imbalance) or to the needles causing the Lung and the Heart to lose their control of the pores temporarily, resulting in spontaneous perspiration along the course of the channel.

Account should be taken of the use of hand creams and other lubricants and moisturisers. It can be a good idea to ask whether the patient uses a hand cream and if so ask why. The need to use a moisturising cream can in itself be a diagnostic sign.

Tremors

Shaking of the hands can be a consequence of internally generated Wind. Internal Wind can arise from Liver imbalances – both *xu* and *shi* imbalances.

Veins

Veins on the hands and forearms that are very prominent, both in adults and children, are usually an indication of Heat.

In small children, observation of the vein on the side of the index finger is an important part of the diagnosis. The diagnostic significance of this vein is explained in the appendix to this section, where the visual diagnosis of children is discussed. This diagnostic sign does not have relevance when diagnosing adults.

Fingernails

Fingernails are viewed as being a tendon in Chinese medicine and therefore as being nourished by Liver *xue*.

The Liver, especially its *xue* aspect, has a determining influence on the condition of the nails. Attention should be paid to the nails' shape and quality, including their colour and strength.

There is a whole nail diagnosis system in which the various organs and areas of the body are reflected in the fingernails. For further information on this system see *Chinese Medical Palmistry* (Xiao and Liscum 1995) or *Diagnosis in Chinese Medicine* (Maciocia 2004).

The colour of the nail

The colours described in the table below are, with the exception of white spots, the colour of the nail bed that is seen through the surface of the nail.

The colour of the nail bed

Observation	Significance
Purple	*Xue* stagnation
Red	Heat
White	*Xue xu*, *qi xu* or *yang xu*
Yellow	Damp-Heat
Dark	*Xue* stagnation, Kidney *yin* or *yang xu*
Green nails in young children	Spleen *qi xu* and internally generated Wind
Blue	*Xue xu*
White spots	*Qi xu*

Fingernail shape

Nails that are ridged or have small indentations are a manifestation of Liver *xue xu* and sometimes of Liver *yin xu*. The ridging and unevenness will be due to the nails lacking nourishment. These nails will often appear to be dry.

Nails that are thicker than normal are due to Dampness, Damp-Heat, Phlegm, *xue* stagnation or Liver Fire, depending on the colour.

If the nails itself bends down or upwards, it can indicate that there is *qi xu* or *xue xu* combined with *xue* stagnation.

Very thin nails that lack strength are a sign of Liver *xue xu*, Liver *yin xu* or *jing xu*.

Nails that flake and break easily may be a sign of Liver *xue xu* or Liver *yin xu*. If they are also thickened and grey, this is a manifestation of Spleen *qi xu* combined with Dampness or Damp-Heat.

Nails that are ragged and frayed are also the result of Liver *xue xu*, Liver *yin xu* or Kidney *yin xu*.

Nails that are very dry are an indication of Liver *xue xu* or Liver *yin xu*.

It is important to be aware that the long-term use of nail varnish and nail varnish removers, as well as the glue used in nail extensions, can weaken the structure of the nail. They can also dry the nail out.

The form of the fingernail

Observation	Significance
Ridged or indented nails	Liver *xue xu* or Liver *yin xu*
Thick nails	Dampness, Damp-Heat, *xue* stagnation or Liver Fire
Thin, weak nails	Liver *xue xu* or Liver *yin xu*, *jing xu*
Broken nails	Liver *xue xu* or Liver *yin xu*, *jing xu*
Thick grey but weak nails	Spleen *qi xu* with Dampness or Damp-Heat
Nail that bends upward or downward	*Qi* and *xue xu* with *xue* stagnation

Visual diagnosis of the skin

The skin as a whole is under the influence of the Lung. This is because the skin is a respiratory organ[5] and also because the Lung controls *wei qi*, which circulates under the skin, and it is *wei qi* that warms and moistens the skin. There are, however, other organs and body substances that also have a direct influence on the skin.

Many of the changes that occur in the skin arise due to *xue* imbalances. This is because *xue* nourishes and moistens the skin. The Liver also has great influence on the skin. This is because the Liver is a reservoir for *xue*, and Liver *qi* ensures the free flow of *xue*.

The Heart controls *xue* and the vessels, therefore Heart imbalances can also manifest in the skin.

The Stomach and Spleen create *xue*. This means that *xue xu* imbalances manifesting in the skin can have their origin in Spleen and Stomach *qi xu* imbalance. Stomach and Spleen imbalances can also give rise to Damp-Heat, which can manifest as skin diseases. Furthermore, Damp-Heat can cause the skin to become greasy or spotty.

The Kidney is the root of *yin* and *yang* in the body. Kidney imbalances can affect the moistness of the skin.

All the channels course under the skin. This means that changes in the skin may also be caused by imbalances in the channels passing through the area. It is particularly the small *luo*-connecting vessels that affect the skin. These *luo*-connecting vessels are the most superficial aspect of the channel system and are similar in structure and function to the capillary network system in Western medicine anatomy.

There are two levels to visual diagnosis of the skin. One level is the general impression given by the skin. What colour is it? How intense or deep are these colours? How is the moistness? Is the skin greasy? Is the skin dry and flaky? How is the skin elasticity?

The second level is the diagnosis of specific skin disorders, such as eczema, psoriasis, acne and so on. The appearance of the affected skin is of vital importance in Chinese medicine dermatology.

Skin colour

When we observe the skin colour, it is often the facial colour that we notice first. This is because the face is the body area that is most often visible at first glance. This is also where much of our attention is focused when we are talking to the patient. It's not just in the face, though, that we look for variances in skin colour. In *bi* syndrome, it is important to see whether there are changes in the skin colour around the joint, and in the diagnosis of skin diseases, changes in skin colour are a determining diagnostic sign.

When diagnosing the colours of the face, it is important to pay attention to the use of make-up. Furthermore, one must, of course, take into account the ethnicity of the person. A pale colour in a person who originates from North Africa will still be much darker than the skin tone of a person who originates from Scandinavia; likewise, a yellow hue will be more diagnostically significant in this person than someone who is originally from East Asia. Changes in skin colour have the same diagnostic significance in all ethnic groups, but the starting point for the colour variations will be different.

The dynamics behind the changes in skin colour also correlate to the Western medicine physiological model. The skin colour is influenced by the amount and movement of blood in the superficial blood vessels. When blood does not flow optimally and stagnates, either in or outside of the vessels, for example when there is bruising after a physical trauma, the skin becomes purple or bluish-green. This is because blood is not being oxygenated optimally. When the body is too hot, it tries to dissipate heat by increasing the circulation of blood in the superficial capillary network just below the skin. The increased flow in these vessels will cause the skin to appear to be more red than normal. Conversely, when the body temperature is reduced, blood is drawn inwards to reduce temperature loss and keep the internal organs warm. This means that the skin will look more pale. This complements the Chinese medicine model, where the *yang* dynamic of Heat and the *yin* dynamic of Cold cause *xue* to be driven upwards to the surface of the body and the skin or to contract inwards away from the surface.

The following section discusses diagnosis of skin colour in general. Facial diagnosis is discussed in a separate section. It is important to note not only the colour of the skin, but also the depth of the colour. The colouration can appear to be relatively shallow, as if it is almost lying on the surface of the skin, or the colours can be more deep rooted.

When the colours appear to be more superficial, this may well be a consequence of an exterior imbalance, whereas interior imbalances tend to result in more deep-rooted colour changes. *Xu* conditions tend to manifest with weaker colours that are not as concentrated and as intense as those seen in *shi* conditions.

Pale

Pale skin arises when there is too little *xue* in the superficial vessels located below the surface of the skin. This can be due to there being *qi xu*. *Qi xu* can result in there being too little *xue* because there is a poor production of the post-heaven *qi* needed to create *xue*, but also because *qi* is not strong enough to propel *xue* to the exterior aspects of the body. *Yang xu* will likewise also mean that there is a reduced dissemination of *xue* in the exterior aspects of the body. Pale-coloured skin is differentiated from sallow or wan coloured skin, which is seen in *xue xu* conditions.

Wan

When there is *xue xu*, it is not only the quantity but also the quality of *xue* that is deficient. This means that the skin does not receive sufficient nourishment. The skin will therefore not only be pale, but also dry, matt and lifeless.

Phlegm can also result in the skin being sallow and lacking lustre. This is because Phlegm can block *xue* so that it cannot nourish the skin.

Yellow

A yellow skin colour can be due to Dampness or, if it is very dry, a chronic *qi* and *xue xu* condition. A more powerful or even shiny yellow colour will be a sign of Damp-Heat.

Black

Kidney imbalances, which will always be *xu* in nature, can result in a black hue on the skin. This can also be seen when there is *xue* stagnation. When there is *xue* stagnation, the skin will be more matt. This is because the stagnant *xue* will prevent the circulation of fresh and nutritious *xue* reaching the skin.

Purple

Purple skin will be seen locally after a physical trauma and is due to stagnation of *xue* in the area.

Blue

When Cold invades the body, it will block the movement of *qi* and *xue* due to its contracting nature. This will result in the skin having a bluish colour, because *xue* is less oxygenated.

Green

A greenish tinge of the skin is an indication of *qi* and *xue* stagnation. It is most often seen in the area around the eyes, on the bridge of the nose and on the abdominal cavity.

A useful technique for measuring the extent of *xue* stagnation in the superficial aspects of the body is to depress the skin with your fingers and observe how long it takes for the colour to return to where the fingers pressed the skin. The more stagnation there is, the more time it will take before the white fingerprints disappear from the skin.

Observation of skin colour

Observation	Significance
Red skin colour	Heat, both *xu* and *shi*
	Wind-Heat
Pale skin colour	*Yang xu* or *qi xu*
Sallow and wan	*Xue xu* or Phlegm
Yellow skin colour	Damp or Damp-Heat
Black skin colour	Kidney *xu* or *xue* stagnation
Purple skin colour	*Xue* stagnation
Green skin colour	*Qi* and *xue* stagnation
Blue skin colour	*Shi* Cold
White fingerprints that remain after palpation	*Xue* stagnation in the skin or muscles

The moistness of the skin

The skin is moistened and nourished by *jinye* and *xue*. If *xue*, *yin* or *jinye* are *xu*, the skin will not be moistened and will become dry.

If the skin is excessively damp or oily, there is probably Damp, Damp-Heat or Phlegm conditions. Dampness and Phlegm are forms of *xie qi* and therefore do not have nourishing qualities. They will, in fact, prevent the circulation of *qi*, *xue* and *jinye*. This will mean that the skin can be both oily and undernourished at the same time.

Yang qi xu can mean that there is not enough *qi* to keep the pores in the skin closed. The spreading dynamic of exogenous Wind can also force open the pores. Both of these situations will result in spontaneous sweating. Heat can also drive fluids upwards and outwards, causing the person to sweat. People who are anxious will also sweat spontaneously when they are nervous. This can be experienced before and during an acupuncture treatment. This is a sign that their *shen* is unsettled and the Heart therefore can no longer control sweat.

There may be certain areas of the skin that are not being nourished as they should. This will result in the skin in these areas becoming dry and flaky. This indicates that there is a *xue* stagnation deeper down, blocking fresh, nutritious *xue* and *jinye* from reaching the area, resulting in the skin lacking nourishment.

It is, of course, important to be attentive to the use of moisturisers and creams that will confuse or obscure the diagnosis.

Observation of the moistness of the skin

Observation	Significance
Dry skin	*Xue xu, jinye xu, yin xu, xue* stagnation
Oily or greasy	Damp, Damp-Heat or Phlegm
Wet (sweaty)	Lung *qi xu*, Spleen *qi xu*, *yang xu*, Heart *qi xu*, *shi* Heat, *xu* Heat, invasion of Wind

Visual diagnosis of the skin's elasticity

The skin should be soft, elastic and smooth, which reflects that the Lung and the Spleen are healthy.

If the skin is thickened or hard, this can be a manifestation of *xue* stagnation or Dampness.

Phlegm can cause the skin and connective tissue to become 'doughy'. The skin will usually also lack *shen*. This is due to Phlegm blocking the small spaces in the tissue (*cou li*) and preventing the circulation of *xue*.

Wrinkles or loose skin are an indication that the skin is not nourished optimally. This will usually be an indication of *yin xu* or *xue xu*. Sometimes the wrinkles are localised to specific locations and can indicate a *xu* condition in the channel or channels that traverse the area. An example of this is the fine wrinkles that can be seen around the mouth in post-menopausal women. This is because *ren mai* and *chong mai* have dried out.

Observation of the elasticity of the skin

Observation	Significance
Elastic and soft skin	Normal skin
Loose or wrinkled skin	*Xue xu* or *yin xu*
Doughy skin without lustre	Phlegm
Thickened skin	*Xue* stagnation or Dampness

Visual diagnosis of veins

Small, purple blood vessels that are visible in or below the surface of the skin, as well as spider naevi, are an indication of *xue* stagnation. These vessels can be a sign of a local stagnation, such as those seen on the lower back when the back pain is the result of *xue* stagnation. The vessels may also be indicative of a general *xue* stagnation. Many older people with *xue* stagnation have, for example, many visible, small purple veins in the area on the inside of the ankles.

Visual diagnosis of skin lesions

Skin lesions are mainly used in the diagnosis of skin diseases. In dermatology the diagnosis of the lesions is the primary diagnostic tool and is even more important than the tongue and the pulse.

Skin lesions are divided into primary and secondary lesions. The primary lesions are the lesions that arose originally. Secondary lesions occur as a result of the primary lesion.

Primary lesions

Macules

Macules are flat. They are neither raised nor sunken and they cannot be felt when palpating the area with a finger. They can only be observed visually. Macules can have various sizes[6] and colours, depending on the cause.

- Red macules will always be a sign of Heat. The redder they are, the more Heat there is. Red macules are often seen in febrile diseases. In these situations, their appearance will be a serious sign. When they are observed, it is an indication that *xie qi* has penetrated to the *xue* or *ying* level in 'Diagnosis according to the Four Levels' (see page 669). Red macules can also be seen in chronic skin diseases, but this is still a sign of Heat.

- White macules can arise when the skin is not nourished by *qi* and *xue*. This lack of nourishment can be due to *qi xu*, *xue xu* or a stagnation of *qi*.

- Brown macules arise when the skin is not nourished by *qi* and *xue*. This lack of nourishment can be due to *qi xu*, *xue xu* or a stagnation of *qi*.

- Purple or black macules are due to *xue* Heat creating *xue* stagnation. The difference between the purple and black macules is the intensity of the Heat, black being the most extreme of the two.

In general, the presence of macules indicates that the Heat is at a deeper level than in the presence of papules does.

Papules

Papules are elevated lesions that can be felt when running your fingers over the skin. They may be pointed or flat on top. Papules are less than five millimetres in diameter. If they are larger than five millimetres, slightly raised and flat, they are defined as being a plaque, but the diagnosis will be the same as the diagnosis of a papule. If they are larger than five millimetres and elevated, they are called a nodule (see below).

A papule is often red and is always a sign of Heat.

If the papule is the same colour as the rest of the skin, it will be a virus-induced wart.

- Red papules. If the papules are hard and itchy, they will be due to an invasion of Wind-Heat. If, at the same time, there are red macules, bleeding or scabbing, this will be due to *xue* Heat. If there is exudation, the cause will be Damp-Heat.

- Purple papules are due to *xue* stagnation generating Heat or the *xue* stagnation itself.

Weals

When larger areas of the skin swell up temporarily, these are called weals. The swellings are caused by localised oedema.

- White weals are due to Wind, Wind-Cold, or *yang xu*.

- Red weals can arise from Wind-Heat or *yin xu*. Red weals that arise after scratching are a sign that *xue* Heat is generating Wind.

Nodules

A nodule is raised and larger than five millimetres in diameter. There will always be an underlying stagnation, either of *qi* and *xue* or Dampness and Phlegm.

Vesicles

Vesicles, like papules, are elevated and less than five millimetres in diameter. The difference between the two is that vesicles contain clear fluids (which can become murky over time). Vesicles may be due to Damp-Heat or Toxic-Fire. The more Heat there is, the redder the vesicle is around the edge.

Bulla

If a vesicle is greater than five millimetres it is called a bulla. The diagnostic significance is the same as for vesicles. The more Heat there is, the redder the bulla is around the edge.

Pustules

Pustules are elevated and contain pus. They will always indicate the presence of Toxic-Fire. There is a difference in the presentation if Toxic-Fire is internally generated or caused by an invasion of *xie qi*. If the pustule has a thin wall and a red border, it will be due to exogenous Wind-Heat. If the wall of the pustule is thicker, the Heat will have been internally generated.

Secondary lesions

Dandruff

Flaky patches of skin are almost always a sign that there is some form of Wind. Differentiation is made between dry and greasy flakes.

- Dry and white flakes are seen in extreme Heat or when *xue xu* generates Wind.

- Oily and yellowish flakes are seen when there is Wind, Damp-Heat or Toxic-Fire.

Erosion

Erosion arises when the outermost layer of the skin is partially disintegrated, but it does not leave a scar when the skin heals again. This is usually seen as a consequence of vesicle or blister. It is a sign of Damp-Heat.

Ulcers

With an ulcer, the outermost aspect of the skin is eroded and there is scarring after the skin has healed. Ulcers are seen when there is Damp-Heat and Toxic-Fire.

Crusts

Crusting can be seen when there has been a bloody or watery exudate from a lesion. Crusts are a sign of Damp-Heat, *xue* Heat or Toxic-Fire.

Excoriation

These are scratch marks or superficial lacerations in the skin that are caused by the person scratching themselves. Excoriation is seen when there is Wind or *xue* Heat.

Cracking

Cracks in the skin are seen when there is Dryness. Dryness can be caused by Cold, *xue* Dryness or Heat.

Lichenification

Lichenification is thickening of the skin, possibly with visible wrinkles in the thickened skin. It can be seen when there is *xue xu* or *xue* stagnation.

Thin skin

The skin can be thin and almost transparent, enabling the blood vessels to be visible through skin. The skin is fragile and there will be easy bruising. This is a sign of *qi xu, xue xu* or *yin xu.*

Pigmentation

If the skin becomes darker or lighter, it is a sign that there is *xue* stagnation or malnutrition of the skin. Malnutrition occurs as a consequence of *xue xu* or Kidney *xu*.

Visual diagnosis of acupuncture points and channels

Observation of the channels

Imbalances in the channels can result in changes in the skin or muscles around the channel.

Changes in the skin's colouration and skin lesions are particularly important. Observation of changes in the skin along a channel will give an indication of which channel is out of balance and what type of imbalance it is. This is particularly helpful when utilising 'Diagnosis According to the 12 Regular Channels' and 'Diagnosis According to the Eight Extraordinary Vessels' (see Sections 10 and 11).

- Stagnation of *qi* in the channel can result in the skin above the channel becoming greenish in colour.

- Heat in the channel can turn the skin above the channel red.

- Cold in the channel can manifest with bluish skin above the channel.

- Dampness in the channel can be observed when there is yellow skin along the path of the channel.

- Purple skin or the presence of small purple veins along the path of the channel is seen when there is *xue* stagnation in the channel.

- Pale skin along the path of the channel will be observed when there is *qi xu* and *yang xu* in the channel.

There may also be skin lesions along the path of the channel.

- Red macules indicate the presence of Heat in the channel.

- Green macules indicate a stagnation in the channel.

- Bluish macules are seen when there is pain and *xue* stagnation in the channel.

- *Xue* stagnation in the channel can also manifest with purple macules.

- Papules along the path of the channel indicate the presence of Heat in the channel.

- Vesicles along the path of the channel indicate the presence of Dampness or Damp-Heat.

- Pustules along the path of the channel indicate the presence of Toxic-Fire.

Observation of yuan-source points

Changes can be observed in the skin and the flesh above and around the *yuan*-source points when there is an imbalance in the associated organ. Typical changes around the point include the area being sunken or swollen. There can also be changes in skin colour or visible veins.

Visual diagnosis according to micro-systems such as ear acupuncture

There are a vast number of various so-called micro-systems around the body. The most famous are ear acupuncture, the reflexology zones on the feet, abdominal acupuncture and ECIWO (Embryo Contains Information of the Whole Organism).[7] It is beyond the scope of this book to include a detailed explanation of the many and varied micro-systems. A common feature of many of these systems is that the points or zones that relate to specific areas of the body or organs become reactive when there is an imbalance or physiological change in this part of the body. This means that you will often be able to observe skin changes in these points or zones when the corresponding area or the organ is out of balance.

Observation of secretions, excretions and exudations

Excretions, secretions and exudations in this context will be discharges from the bodily openings that can be observed with the naked eye. It was previously a part of a doctor's diagnostic approach in Western medicine hospitals to observe the patient's stool and to see, smell and sometimes taste the urine. This elicited useful information for the doctor. Nowadays, microscopic and biochemical analysis of excretions from the body is utilised instead. Nevertheless, the physical appearance of an excretion will reveal important diagnostic information about a person. The excretions that will typically be seen in the clinic do not include excretions from the lower orifices. In fact, the observation of excretions from the body in general will be limited. This is because the exudations from the body will usually have been removed by the patient prior to visiting the clinic. The physical appearance of these exudations is therefore something we usually have to ask about.

The diagnostic guidelines are the same for all types of discharge from body openings. Generally speaking, discharges that are clear and watery are caused by Cold, *qi xu* or *yang xu*.

When discharges become thicker, sticky or yellowish, this is an indication that there is Heat that is condensing the fluids. Extreme Heat can result in the presence of blood in the excretion.

If the excretion is not just yellow but is also decidedly greenish, then there is Toxic-Fire.

Dampness makes excretions turbid and cloudy.

In addition to the general guidelines presented above, there are some more specific observations that are relevant to the specific orifices.

Exudations from the ears

Excessive earwax is a sign of Phlegm or Dampness.

Yellowish or greenish exudation is a sign of Toxic-Fire or Damp-Heat in the *shaoyang* channels.

Exudations from the eyes

A person with Phlegm will tend to have blobs of slime in the eyes, not only in the morning but also during the day.

Eyes that water can be a sign of an invasion of exogenous Wind and also of the internal Liver imbalances.

Secretions and exudations from the mouth

Saliva dribbling from the corners of the mouth can be a sign of Spleen *qi xu* and Dampness, but can also occur when the muscles around the mouth are blocked by Wind-Phlegm or when the channels in the local area are blocked by Wind-Cold.

Exudations from the nose

Watery mucus in the nose or a runny nose will be seen when there is Wind-Cold and Damp-Phlegm.

Yellowish and thickened mucus in the nose is due to Wind-Heat, Phlegm-Heat or Toxic-Fire if the mucus is decidedly greenish.

Spontaneous bleeding from the nose can be a sign of Heat and also of Spleen *qi xu* if the Spleen is not able to keep *xue* inside the vessels.

Secretions and exudations

Sweat also falls within the category of 'excretions'. If we observe that the patient sweats a lot, without the weather being particularly hot or humid, this will in itself be a diagnostic sign. If the person has just cycled or has been running, the heat that this activity has generated will have driven fluids upwards and outwards from the interior of the body to the surface as sweat. This is a natural consequence of physical activity. If the person has perspired due to less strenuous activity, such as walking up the stairs, or they just sweat spontaneously, it will be a sign of *qi xu*, *yang xu*, Heat or Damp-Heat.

There are two mechanisms in *qi xu* and *yang xu* that can make a person sweat during light exercise. The first mechanism is that even the heat that the light physical activity generates will be enough to make the person sweat. This is because the dynamic nature of heat will always force fluids up to the surface of the skin. Because there is a lack of *qi*, particularly *yang qi*, the pores will not be able to restrain the sweat. The physical activity itself will simultaneously consume *yang* and *qi*, resulting in there being less *yang qi* to control the pores.

Both *xu* and *shi* Heat drive fluids upwards and outwards resulting in increased pressure against the pores. If there is Damp-Heat, the sweat will usually be more sticky and yellowish.

Sweat is an important diagnostic sign in invasions of exogenous *xie qi*. The differentiation of the sweating can be used to locate which level or stage *xie qi* has penetrated to. When there is an invasion of Wind-Cold in the *taiyang* aspect, there will not be any sweating unless the person is *wei qi xu*. This is because the exogenous Cold is blocking the pores and preventing them from opening. When exogenous *xie qi* penetrates to the *yangming* aspect or *qi* level, there will be profuse sweating without any relief of the symptoms. This is because the extreme Heat is driving the fluids upwards and outwards. If sweating ceases during the day and is only seen at night, this will be because the invasion of *xie qi* has entered the *ying* level or *shaoyin* or *jueyin* aspects. It reflects that *yin* has been damaged by the *xie* Heat.

Yellowish, oily sweat beads can be seen on the forehead when *yang* collapses.

Vaginal discharge

A watery or whitish discharge from the vagina is due to Cold or Spleen and Kidney *yang xu*. The blockage by Cold or the lack of *yang qi* results in fluids not being transported away from the area, whilst the lower orifices lose the ability to hold the fluids in the body, either because there is a lack of *yang qi* or because *yang qi* is blocked by the Cold.

Yellowish and sticky discharge from the vagina is seen when there is Damp-Heat. The Heat condenses the fluids, turning them yellow.

Greenish discharge is seen when there is Toxic-Fire.

Urine

Dark and scanty urine is seen when Heat condenses the urine.

Yang xu Cold will give rise to copious amounts of clear urine. This is because a deficiency of *yang qi* means that fluids are poorly transformed and transported. These fluids then seep down to the Urinary Bladder in the lower *jiao*.

Dampness causes the urine to become cloudy or murky.

If analysis of the urine reveals the presence of blood in the urine, the cause can be Heat, *xue* stagnation or Spleen *qi xu*.

Stools

Watery stools that contain undigested food are seen when there is Kidney and Spleen *yang xu*. This is due to the inability of *yang* to transform the ingested food.

Sticky stools are a sign of Damp-Heat. The Heat condenses the fluid aspect of the stool so they become sticky.

Blood in the stool can be caused by Heat, *xue* stagnation or Spleen *qi xu*, which can all result in the walls of the blood vessels rupturing.

If the stool is very dry, there will be either Heat, *yin xu* or *xue xu*. The Heat injuring fluids or *yin xu* and *xue xu* result in a lack of fluids.

Stools that are small, hard and pebble-like, similar to goat droppings, are due to Liver *qi* stagnation, especially if the stagnation has generated Heat.

Long and thin stools, can be seen when there is Spleen *qi xu*. If the stools contain mucus, this is usually a sign of Phlegm-Dampness.

Observation of excretions and discharges

Observation	Significance
Watery and clear excretions	Cold, *qi* or *yang xu*
Yellow, sticky or thick discharges and excretions	Heat, Damp-Heat
Greenish discharges	Toxic-Fire
Cloudy and murky discharges	Dampness
Bloody discharges	Heat (but can also be Spleen *qi xu* or *xue* stagnation)
Copious earwax	Phlegm or Dampness
Eyes that water	Invasion of Wind, Liver imbalances
Saliva dribbling from the mouth	Spleen *qi xu*, Dampness, Wind-Phlegm, Wind-Cold
Clear, watery mucus in the nose	Wind-Cold, Damp-Phlegm
Nose or sinuses that are blocked with yellow or green mucus	Wind-Heat, Phlegm-Heat, Toxic-Fire
Spontaneous sweating or sweating on light activity	*Qi* and *yang xu*, Heat or Damp-Heat
Yellow or sticky sweat	Heat, Damp-Heat
Watery or whitish vaginal discharge	Cold or Spleen and Kidney *yang xu*
Yellow, sticky vaginal discharge	Damp-Heat
Greenish vaginal discharge	Toxic-Fire
Dark urine	Heat
Clear urine	*Yang xu*
Cloudy or murky urine	Dampness
Blood in the urine	Heat, *xue* stagnation or Spleen *qi xu*
Watery stools containing undigested food remnants	Spleen and Kidney *yang xu*
Sticky stools	Damp-Heat
Blood in the stools	Spleen *qi xu*, *xue* stagnation or Heat
Dry stools	Heat, *yin xu* or *xue xu*
Pebble-like stools	Liver *qi* stagnation
Long, thin stools	Spleen *qi xu*
Stools that contain slime and mucus	Phlegm-Dampness

VISUAL DIAGNOSIS OF CHILDREN

Observation is a significant aspect of Chinese medicine paediatric diagnosis, particularly when diagnosing babies and small children. Diagnostic information can be obtained by asking the parents and the child, but an essential part of diagnosis is also carried out by observing the child. The most important aspect of paediatric diagnosis is to assess whether it is a *shi* or *xu* condition and whether there is Heat present. The differentiation of these conditions is highly dependent on visual diagnosis.

Observation of the child

Radiance

One of the first things to observe is whether there is *shen*. *Shen* is seen in the radiance that there is in the skin of the face, especially in the child's eyes. Ideally, there should be a soft glow in the skin of the face, and the eyes should be bright and clear. This will show that *zheng qi* is strong and that *xie qi*, if it is present, has not penetrated very deeply.

If the eyes are dull and without lustre, and the skin of the face lacks radiance, this is a sign that *zheng qi* is weakened and *xie qi* is strong or that there is a significant *xu* condition.

If there is *shen*, there will also be good eye contact. The child should appear alert and take an interest in their surroundings. Something that can blur the picture is that children are often nervous when meeting a stranger, especially if that stranger is an acupuncturist. This is not such a problem with babies, but the parents' nervousness and fear that the needles will hurt the baby can affect the baby and make it nervous. This will affect the radiance from the eyes.

Movement

Children's movements are faster and more restless than adults. This is because children are relatively more *yang* and do not have as much *yin* in their body yet. Constitutionally, they tend to have an excess of *yang* and have too much Heat. Their *yin* is not strong and has difficulty controlling *yang* Heat. This is seen especially in the evening when the child is tired. Children will often have difficulty rooting their *yang*, and the more tired they are, the more their *yang* is active. An overtired child can become hyperactive in the evening. If the child is like this during the day, and is very restless, fidgety and has difficulty sitting still during the consultation, this is an indication of Heat. Heat will also result in rapid movements. A child with Heat will kick off their bedclothes when they sleep as they try to dissipate some of their Heat.

If the child seems very quiet and there is a lack of movement, this is a sign of a *xu* condition or Cold. In *xu* conditions the child will seem limp, whereas Cold will mean that they sit or lie huddled up. When they sleep, they may well lie curled up with a duvet pulled up over them to retain body heat. As stated earlier, this quietness and lack of movement can also be due to the child being shy. In an adult, this shyness would itself have diagnostic significance, but it is to be expected in small children, as their Heart *qi* is not stable.

Muscle spasms and cramps will rarely be seen in the clinic, but if they are, it will be a sign of Liver Wind.

Muscle tone

The muscles and posture should not be too lax, but at the same time they should not appear to be rigid. Flaccidity will be seen in a *xu* condition and muscle tenseness in a *shi* condition.

Sudden tenseness and cramping of the muscles, with rigid neck muscles, means there is internally generated Wind. A milder form of internally generated Wind is seen when there are spasms, convulsions, tics and muscle trembling.

The skin should be supple, elastic and not too loose.

Observation of children's movements and muscle tone

Observation	Significance
Restless or fast movements	Heat
Sitting or lying huddled up	Cold
Tense muscles	*Shi* condition
Lax muscles	*Xu* condition
Muscle spasms, convulsions, tics and muscle tremors	Liver Wind
Stiff muscles	Liver Wind

Observation of skin colours

The diagnostic significance of the colours in the skin in general, and especially in the face, is the same as it is for adults. In *xu* conditions, the colours will be paler, and they will be more intense in a *shi* condition.

Red colours are seen when there is Heat. A white or pale face is seen when there is *qi xu* and *yang xu*.

Cold and shock are capable of producing a blue colour. If the mother has been exposed to a strong shock during pregnancy, it may affect the foetus's Heart *qi*. This can be observed as a bluish colour on the forehead.

Pain and the internal Wind can manifest with a green hue to the face.

A yellowish hue in the facial complexion is a sign of Stomach and Spleen imbalances.

A blue or blue/green (*qing*) colour on the bridge of the nose between the eyebrows is a sign of Liver Wind and can be seen when there are muscle cramps.

Observation of facial skin tones in children

Observation	Significance
Red	Heat
Blue	Cold or shock
White or pale	*Yang* or *qi xu*

Yellow	Spleen and Stomach imbalances
Green	Pain or Wind
Paleness	*Xu* conditions
Strong, intense colours	*Shi* conditions

Visual diagnosis of the index finger vein

Something that is unique in the diagnosis of children under three years is the observation of the vein along the Large Intestine channel on the index finger.

The radial aspect of the finger should be rubbed lightly and then observed to see the length, colour, depth and distinctness of the vein.

The index finger is divided into three zones. The borders of these zones are the three creases in the joints of the finger. These creases are called 'gates'. The proximal finger joint, i.e. the metacarpo-phalangeal joint, is called the Wind Gate, the middle joint of the finger is called the *qi* Gate and the distal joint of the finger is called the Life Gate.

If the vein is only visible just beyond the Wind Gate, the disease is mild and *xie qi* has not penetrated deeper than the exterior aspects of the body and is located in the small *luo* vessels. If *xie qi* has penetrated deeper down to the channels, the vein will also be visible beyond the *qi* Gate. A visible vein beyond the Life Gate is a serious sign indicating that *xie qi* is virulent, has penetrated into the interior and has reached the *zangfu* organs. It is even more serious if the vein reaches all the way to the nail bed of the index finger.

A thin and pale vein will be seen if it is a *xu* condition, whilst a thicker and more deeply coloured vein will be seen in *shi* conditions, in particular when there is a stagnation in the Intestines.

Veins that disappear when massaged with your fingers are seen in *xu* conditions. If the vein does not disappear, even with strong massage, it is a *shi* condition.

If the vein is very superficial and clearly visible just under the skin, then *xie qi* is in the exterior. Conversely, if the vein appears to be deeper lying and is almost hidden, the *xie qi* is in the interior. The colours here will also be more intense.

Vein colour

Ideally, the vein should have a reddish, yellow colour. The vein will become bright red when there is an invasion of exogenous *xie qi* in the exterior.

If the vein is a purple/red, this is a sign of Heat, whilst a green/blue-coloured vein can be seen when there is internally generated Wind, pain or food stagnation. If the vein is more black/purple, this is more serious and that indicates Phlegm and stagnation Heat are blocking the vessels.

If the vein is thick and seems to pulsate, this is a *shi* condition, which is seen when there is food stagnation, Phlegm and *qi* stagnation.

Visual diagnosis of the eyes in children

The eyes can become red when there are invasions of Wind-Heat and when internally generated Heat ascends upwards to the head.

Yellow sclera can be seen when there is Dampness, particularly Damp-Heat.

Liver Wind can manifest with the sclera having a greenish blue tinge.

Red and fissured skin along the canthus is a sign of Damp-Heat or accumulation syndrome (food stagnating in the Stomach and Intestines).

Inflammation of the eyes with pus indicates the presence of Toxic-Fire. Toxic-Fire can arise from *shi* Heat conditions, in either the channels or their associated organs, ascending to the eyes. It can also arise from invasions of Wind-Heat.

Visual diagnosis of the ears in children

One of the most important diagnostic signs that relate to the ears in children is the size of the ears.

The ears are created from Kidney *jing*. This means that small, crumpled ears can be a sign of *jing xu*.

Red ears can be a sign of Heat in the Liver. Red ears are also seen when there are invasions of Wind-Heat or Toxic-Fire in the ears.

If there is yellowish/greenish discharge leaking out of the ears, Toxic-Fire is present.

Visual diagnosis of the tongue in children

Tongue diagnosis is basically the same in children as in adults. It can, however, be difficult to get to see the tongue in very young children. It can require patience and coaxing, but even then it is not always possible. For this reason, I often rely on observing the colouration, moistness and sometimes the size of the lips to provide me with some of the information that the tongue normally elicits. The relevance of the diagnostic signs on the tongue are no different from those in adults.

Visual diagnosis of the lips in children

The lips are under the influence of the Spleen and Stomach, but are nourished by *xue*.

Red lips can therefore indicate both *xue* Heat or Stomach Heat.

Pale lips can be a sign of Spleen *qi xu* or *xue xu*.

The lips can become dry when *yin* has been injured. This will be seen after or during a febrile disease.

The Liver channel is one of the channels that encircles the lips. Liver Wind, Cold in the Liver channel or abdominal pain due to Liver *qi* stagnation can manifest with a greenish colour around the mouth.

Visual diagnosis of the throat in children

Changes in the throat are mainly seen when there are invasions of *xie qi* or Phlegm or when there are Lung, Stomach and Intestinal imbalances.

A red and sore throat, where the condition is of short duration, will be seen in invasions of Wind-Heat.

If the redness and soreness are chronic, the Heat is more likely to come from the Lung, Stomach or Intestines.

If the throat is swollen and red and there is ulceration, this indicates the presence of Toxic-Fire. This is usually seen after or during an invasion of Wind-Heat. If the tonsils are swollen and red, the Wind-Heat has generated Toxic-Fire. The Fire can also have its origin in the Stomach or the Intestines, especially if the condition is chronic.

If whitish or yellowish exudation is observed in the throat or on the tonsils, it is a further confirmation of Toxic-Fire.

If the tonsils are swollen but have a normal colour, this indicates Phlegm and *qi xu*.

This can be seen when *xie qi* is retained in the body and has not been expelled or drained out of the body.

Visual diagnosis of the gums in children

The oral cavity is under the influence of the Stomach and Spleen. This means that pathological changes in the gums are usually due to Stomach imbalances.

If the gums are red and swollen, this can be a sign of Heat in the Stomach, food stagnation or parasites in the Intestines.

The gums can be red and swollen when a child is teething. This can be treated as Heat in the Stomach with good effect.

Visual diagnosis of the nose in children

The nose is under the direct influence of the Lung and is connected to the Large Intestine channel. This means that imbalances in the Lung will often manifest in the nose. Nasal discharges have particular diagnostic relevance.

Phlegm and Damp-Phlegm will often manifest with increased mucus in the nose.

A nose that is running with clear and watery mucus will be seen when there are invasions of Wind-Cold and when there is Lung *qi xu*.

If the mucus is whitish or yellowish, it is a sign of Wind-Heat.

If the nose is blocked with thick, sticky mucus, it will be Damp-Phlegm or Phlegm-Heat.

If the mucus is yellowish or greenish, it indicates the presence of Heat.

If there is a lot of Heat present in the Lung, the nostrils can 'flare'.

Visual diagnosis of the root of the nose in children

The root of the nose (the area between the eyebrows) can be used in the diagnosis of children who are below the age of four years old.

If the root of the nose is greenish, there will often be digestive problems.

A dark green colour can sometimes be seen when there is accumulation syndrome that is an excess condition and a light green colour can be seen if accumulation syndrome is due to a *xu* condition.

Green macules in this area are sometimes seen when there is diarrhoea.

Blue veins in the region can be seen when there is abdominal pain.

Visual diagnosis of the eyes, ears, nose, throat, lips and gums in children

Observation	Significance
Red sclera	Wind-Heat or internally generated Heat
Blue/green sclera	Liver Wind
Yellow sclera	Damp, Damp-Heat
Red and cracked skin around the canthus	Damp-Heat, accumulation syndrome
Small, crumpled ears	*Jing xu*
Red ears	Liver Fire, invasions of Wind-Heat or Toxic-Fire
Yellow or green discharge from the ears	Toxic-Fire
Red lips	*Xue* Heat, Stomach Heat
Pale Lips	Spleen *qi xu*, *xue xu*
Dry lips	*Yin* is injured
Green colour around the mouth	Liver Wind, pain, Liver *qi* stagnation affecting the abdomen or Cold
Red throat	Wind-Heat, Toxic-Fire, Lung Heat, Stomach Heat or Intestinal Heat
Red, swollen throat	Wind-Heat, Toxic-Fire, Stomach Fire
Swollen tonsils	Phlegm
Red and swollen tonsils	Toxic-Fire, Heat in the Stomach or Intestines
Red, swollen tonsil with exudate	Toxic-Fire
Red gums	Stomach Heat, accumulation syndrome or parasites
Runny nose with clear, watery mucus	Wind-Cold
Runny nose with yellow, sticky mucus	Wind-Heat
Blocked nose	Damp-Phlegm, Phlegm-Heat
Flapping or flaring nostrils	Lung Heat
Dark green between the eyebrows	Accumulation syndrome
Light green between the eyebrows	*Xu* accumulation syndrome
Green macules between the eyebrows	Diarrhoea
Blue vein between the eyebrows	Abdominal pain

Visual diagnosis of the sleeping position in children

This is usually something that we must ask about.

A child who sleeps curled up and packs themselves into the duvet has a Cold condition.

A child with Heat will toss and turn, kicking off the bedding, and will often sleep with the arms and legs splayed to the sides.

Visual diagnosis of the faeces and urine in children

The stools and urine are usually not observed in a clinical context. We are therefore again reliant on the parents' observations. The diagnostic significance of these signs is the same as for adults and is described on page 115.

THE DIAGNOSTIC PILLAR: LISTENING AND SMELLING

Introduction

The diagnostic pillar 'To Listen and to Smell' may seem to be a strange combination, because these are two separate senses that do not seem to be related. In Chinese, the same character, *wen zhen*, represents both of these words. Both of these senses are often used whilst carrying out other parts of the diagnosis. The diagnostic signs in this pillar can often be very subtle and hard to detect unless you are very attentive. We can gather olfactory information whilst we are in close physical contact with the client, for example whilst we are palpating them or when we are inserting needles. Sometimes, the subtle odours that a client emits are more pronounced when the needles are being removed. We will also have ample opportunity to listen to the patient's voice and breathing whilst they are relating their symptoms and medical history to us. We constantly utilise the first aspect of the pillar to listen, all the time, without necessarily thinking about it and without having structured it into a system. Even before we have met a client, when we have only talked to them on the phone, we have often formed an impression of who they are just by hearing their voice. The great strength of Chinese medicine is that it has systematised and categorised the impressions we get from a person in a diagnostic context.

Unfortunately, some practitioners prioritise listening and smelling less, for various reasons. This is a pity, because by listening to the client, you can gain vital information. It is important to listen to the various sounds emanating from the abdomen and chest, as well as to the sound of the patient's voice. Here it is important to be observant of not only the classical sound qualities in the voice that are described in Chinese medicine textbooks, such as laughing, crying, shouting etc., but also of how they are talking, the words they use, how they express themselves, how they converse and, very significantly, how easy it is to engage them in a conversation and how communicative they are.

Furthermore, many of the signs described in this section and the previous section on visual diagnosis, are not necessarily things that you will see or hear that often. What is important is to be sufficiently vigilant to spot the signs when they are there. Physiological harmony is characterised by an absence of pathological symptoms and signs. It is when things digress from the norm, from what is expected, that we prick up our ears and open our eyes. When we see or hear these signs, we must ask ourselves: What does this mean? How do I interpret this from a Chinese medicine perspective?

Olfactory and auditory diagnosis

Relative strengths of olfactory and auditory diagnosis

- Auditory diagnosis is, together with visual observation, the cornerstone of the intuitive approach to diagnosis. Through these two approaches we can often determine a substantial part of the diagnosis. We must learn to trust this ability but at the same time not confuse intuition with guessing.

- Listening to the client means we are not dependent on their subjective interpretation and presentation of their diagnostic signs.

- Many patterns of imbalance manifest with changes in how the person communicates and changes in the quality of their voice.

- We can hear the sounds emanating from the client, even when we do not interview them (for example, in the waiting room, on the phone or whilst we are needling them).

- Auditory diagnosis is very important in the diagnosis of children.

Relative weaknesses of olfactory and auditory diagnosis

- There is a limited amount of literature that you can use as reference material.

- Olfactory diagnosis is difficult because people frequently wash themselves, wash their clothes regularly and use creams, deodorants, perfumes, etc.

- Both diagnostic approaches are very subjective and you can be uncertain about whether what you hear or smell is the same as what is written in the textbook. This is particularly relevant in olfactory diagnosis.

- Some things, such as the patient's stools, urine or vaginal discharge, are not things that we smell ourselves. We are therefore dependent on the patient's subjective reporting of these signs.

- Many of the olfactory and auditory signs are very subtle and thereby difficult to differentiate.

Diagnostic tips

- Ask the client how the various excretions from the body smell and possibly taste (for example, mucus from the sinuses and nose).

- Things that have a strong smell or taste are usually a sign of pathological Heat.

- Ask some questions for which the answer is not important. This gives you the opportunity to listen to how the patient talks instead of having to focus on what they are saying.

- Ask the patient to put a t-shirt, vest or pillow case that they have been using in a plastic bag, which they then tie and bring to the clinic. This will make the odours more prominent.

Auditory diagnosis

There are two main focus areas in auditory diagnosis. When we are together with a client, we must be diagnostically aware of the sounds emanating involuntarily from their body, such as coughs, abdominal rumbles or respiration. At the same time, we must listen to the sound of their voice. We may well have already heard the sound of their voice on the telephone and answerphone. We may also have heard them talking outside our door whilst they were in the waiting room. This will have started to create an impression of who they are from a Chinese medicine perspective. A resonant or loud voice will usually indicate that the person has a *shi* condition, whereas a weak voice will tell you that their imbalances are probably more *xu* in nature. A gravelly voice will indicate Phlegm, whilst a staccato or clipped voice will point us in the direction of Liver *qi* stagnation. The patient can continue to provide us with auditory information before we see them. The way they press the doorbell, the sound of their steps in the hallway, the strength of their voice while talking on a mobile phone in the waiting room and their coughs and sniffles, etc. can all potentially elicit relevant information about the client and their patterns of imbalance.

When we initiate the verbal interview, we should be simultaneously gleaning information on two levels. We should be listening not just to their answers to our questions and their descriptions of their condition, but also to how they are communicating.

When they sit opposite us during the diagnostic interview and whilst they lay on the couch, we should pay attention to their breathing. If they have a cough, it is a great help to be able to hear the sound of them coughing, rather than them giving you a description of how it sounds. It is, unfortunately, necessary to ask about several aspects of this diagnostic pillar, rather than actually experiencing them. It is probably more likely that you are going to have to ask a woman with morning sickness about how her vomiting is, rather than actually hearing her vomit.

Auditory diagnosis of the person's voice

The voice is something we will hear during the consultation and we may well have already heard their voice on the phone or in the waiting room. This may even be the only auditory sign from the patient that we pick up. The voice will nearly always give us relevant diagnostic information about the patient, and this can be vital.

The voice is affected directly and indirectly by various organs and vital substances, the emotions and *xie qi*, particularly Heat. Listening to the patient's voice will give us an impression of more than one aspect of the client's imbalances.

It is the Heart that enables a person to communicate with others. The Heart gives a person the ability to express themselves and open up to others. A person literally tells other people what is in their heart or on their mind. It is therefore said that speech is controlled by the Heart.

When the Heart is in balance, a person has a desire and a need to communicate with others. At the same time, the Heart should also be able to close when appropriate and have a sense of *li* or propriety. When the Heart is imbalanced, a person can have a tendency to either over- or under-communicate – to talk too much or too little and give out too much, too little or inappropriate information. The Heart has a very close relationship with the tongue. The tongue is the sense organ that relates to the Fire Phase and to the Heart organ. Whereas the other sense organs are hollow and therefore can receive and absorb impressions, the tongue is solid. This is relevant to the Heart, which needs to be empty and not filled so it can receive and manifest the *dao*. Where the other *zang* organs receive stimulation and impressions via their sense organs, the Heart can empty itself through the use of the tongue. The tongue communicates a person's thoughts, ideas and emotions via speech. The more activity and movement that there is in the Heart and *shen*, the more the tongue will be active.

A person with Heart *qi xu* or Heart *qi* stagnation will tend to be reserved, and thus they will talk less and you will have the sensation of having to draw each word out of them. There is, though, a difference in their taciturnity. A person who is Heart *qi xu* will be more shy and timid, whereas a person with Heart *qi* stagnation will be more terse and uncommunicative. If there is Heat agitating the Heart, on the other hand, the person will often have a tendency to over-communicate, i.e. they will be loquacious.

The speed of the voice is also affected by how much Heat there is in the Heart. A person with Heart Fire will tend to talk more quickly. This is because Heat accelerates processes, including speech, but also because Heat will agitate the *shen* and thereby increase mental activity. At the same time, Heat in the Heart will often result in a person 'opening' too much and over-communicating. An extreme example of this is someone who is manic.

The voice should have vitality. This is not dissimilar to the tongue, pulse and skin, which should all have *shen* – a quality of vitality. The same is true of the voice, but it does not have the same connotations. When there are *xu* conditions or stagnations in the Heart and the *shen* is either blocked or malnourished, the voice will lack a certain quality. This quality isn't volume and it isn't necessarily joy, it is more movement. The voice should vary and change as they talk, especially as the subject area that they are talking about changes. This reflects the natural movement of the *shen*. The voice should not be stuck in a certain gear. Where the pulse with *shen* is firm, solid and rhythmic in its beating, the voice should have an even flow and not be stuttering or confused. It should also have the sound of joy and happiness in it. If there is no joy – if Heart *qi* and *shen* are either blocked or undernourished – there will be a flatness and maybe even a tone of sadness in the voice. On the other hand, if there is too much Heat in the Heart, there can be too much of the quality of joy and happiness. The voice can be unnaturally glad. This is the 'life and soul of the party' voice. Here, the voice will often be voluble and accompanied by too much laughter. Also, there will frequently be too many and inappropriate jokes. All this indicates too much Heat in the Heart. The Heart *yin xu* Heat voice won't, of course, be voluble, and the laughter accompanying the voice is more a nervous laughter, often at the end of the sentence like an inappropriate punctuation mark.

It is not only the Heart and Heat that affect the voice, *zong qi* is also used to create the voice. This means that the Lung will give the voice resonance and force.

It is said that the Lung controls the voice. A person with Lung *qi xu* will have a weak or quiet voice.

The Liver ensures that the flow of *qi* is free and uninhibited throughout the body. This means that even though *zong qi* gives the voice its strength, it is Liver *qi* that ensures that the voice flows freely and evenly. When there is Liver *qi* stagnation the voice can have a hardness and become staccato, sounding a bit like a machine gun firing.

The vocal cords, which create the sound of the voice, depend on being moistened and nourished. This moisture and nourishment is provided by *xue* and *jinye*. This means that *xue xu*, *yin xu* and *shi* Heat can all affect the sound of the voice. The vocal cords can also be coated and thereby blocked by Phlegm.

Strength and quality of the voice

The strength of a person's voice will give us an immediate indication of the quality of a person's *qi* – of whether it is an overall *xu* or *shi* condition. A *shi* condition, particularly Heat, will make a person's voice become louder and more resonant. These are the people whose voices travel through doors and walls into the next room. This is the voice that is heard on the streets on a Saturday night when people have consumed large amounts of alcohol. The alcohol creates *shi* Heat in the Liver, their voices become loud and they no longer talk quietly and softly with each other; their voices have volume and resonance. When you speak to these people on the phone you instinctively move the earpiece further away from the ear, and you lean backwards slightly when sitting next to them. The opposite is the case with people whose voice is so quiet and soft that you have to strain your ears and sometimes even physically move closer to them to hear them. These people will usually have a *qi xu* condition. They will lack the *zong qi* necessary to give the voice volume.

Listening to the strength and volume of the voice is something most people already do subconsciously. We must consciously observe this and place the impression in a diagnostic context.

We must also pay attention to the quality of the voice. Whether the voice sounds dry or gravelly and whether the person sounds hoarse or nasal. Furthermore, the tone of the voice can also impart important diagnostic information. Besides listening to the overall tone and strength of the voice, we should observe how the voice is influenced by what they are talking about. If the quality of their voice changes when talking about a particular subject, situation or person, this may be an aetiological factor that is relevant to their imbalance. If a person's voice, for example, becomes harder and more staccato when they talk about their job, it could indicate that their job or work environment is detrimentally affecting their Liver *qi*. Conversely, if this person talks about something else and their voice becomes gentler and more mellow, this may be something that can help to alleviate their imbalance.

It is particularly important to notice how much and how fast they speak. The more Heat there is, the more verbose they are and the quicker they talk.

Normal voice

The normal voice is neither too loud nor too soft and should sound harmonious. 'Harmonious' here means that the tone of the voice naturally goes up and down and the tone is appropriate to what is being talked about. A discordant voice, for example, could be when a person has joy in their voice when they talk about something worrying or sounding sad or unenthusiastic when they talk about a happy event. On the other hand, the voice will be harmonious if there is joy in the voice when they are happy.

The volume and depth of the voice will, of course, depend on the person's gender, age and build. I don't expect a loud, resonant voice in an 80-year-old woman or three-year-old child, in the same way that I don't expect a timid, weak voice in a 30-year-old builder. If the voice is incongruous, we must immediately ask ourselves why. What is the possible or probable cause of this difference between what I expect and what I hear?

The Five Phases in the voice

Each of the Five Phases imparts a specific quality in the voice. All five qualities should be present. There should be neither too much nor too little of these qualities. These qualities should also vary and be appropriate to the situation. For example, it is natural that the voice is harder, louder and angrier if a person is exposed to an injustice. A lack of anger in the voice in this situation is as much a sign of an imbalance as there being too much of this quality in other situations. If the voice is dominated by or lacking a certain quality, this indicates an imbalance in the relevant phase or its related organ.

Five Element acupuncture utilises the quality of the voice when determining which constitutional type a person is. Furthermore, in Five Element acupuncture, it is a more serious sign when a person's voice has a vocal quality from a different phase than their constitutional type. It is less serious if they manifest with a powerful vocal quality from their own phase.

As stated above, it is a sign of imbalance when there is too much and too little of any of the vocal qualities that relate to the Five Phases and their associated organs. When we are talking to the client we must therefore listen to whether a certain vocal quality is lacking or dominant in their voice.

Fire – joy and laughter

Fire gives the voice a quality of joy and happiness. It's the voice you hear when someone tells you about a happy event. The voice will have vitality. The Heart is nourished by and manifests with joy. In Heart *xu* imbalances or Heart stagnation conditions, the voice will often lack this quality. There will be a flatness and sadness to their voice. Too much joy and laughter in the voice is usually an indication of some form of Heat in the Heart. Heart *yin xu* Heat will affect the voice, so there will be nervous laughter. This nervous laugh will often end the sentences, almost like an inappropriate punctuation mark. Heart Fire will be more of the 'life and soul of the party' voice. This person is exaggeratedly jovial. There can often be an actual laugh, rather than a nervous giggle, in the middle of sentences. The voice must be appropriate to what they're talking about. A person whose voice is cheerful and lively, or who laughs while talking about something sad, will undoubtedly indicate a Heart imbalance; the question is which one. It could easily be nervousness or embarrassment (which in themselves are manifestations of Heart imbalances). Similarly, a Heart imbalance could be manifested by a person who talks about a happy event but has a noticeably sad and flat voice.

Earth – singing

The Earth Phase manifests with a singing voice. This is a voice that is varied in its tone. The tone fluctuates up and down. It is the voice that you would use when reading a story out loud. A voice that has either too much or too little of this quality indicates a Spleen or Earth Phase imbalance.

Metal – crying

The emotion of the Metal Phase is sorrow. Grief can also be heard in a person's voice when there are Lung or Metal Phase imbalances. There may be a slight choking of the words. The voice will sound as if the person is on the verge of tears. An extreme version of this voice is when a child is telling you something just after they have been crying. In Lung imbalances the voice may be lacking in strength and the sentences can have a tendency to ebb out before they are completely finished. This is because *zong qi* is often weak in many Lung imbalances and there will not be enough strength to complete the sentence.

Water – complaining and moaning

This voice is heard when the Kidneys or the Water Phase are out of balance. It is a very flat voice, lacking in tonal variation. The voice also sounds like it is about to break into tears. It is the opposite of the Fire Phase voice, which is full of joy and laughter.

Wood – shouting

The voice of the Wood Phase is a hard voice. When the Liver and the Wood Phase are in balance, the voice is neither too hard nor too soft. The voice should be resonant without shouting. If there is imbalance, the person's voice can acquire a very hard tone. It will have a shouting quality. The voice will sound sharp and have force and direction. It is a voice that has no problem being heard and is not hesitant. It is the tone that is heard when someone is angry.

If a person's Liver *qi* stagnates, the words will be clipped and the voice will become staccato.

These Five Phase qualities can be seen as balancing qualities when you place the Five Phases in the Cosmological Five Phase sequence – North, South, East, West with Earth located in the centre. The Water Phase's flatness is the *yin/yang* antithesis of the Fire Phase's joyful voice. They are opposites and they therefore balance each other. Too much of one will mean that there is, as a consequence, too little of the other. The more happiness there is in the voice, the less flatness there will be and vice versa. This is fundamental *yin/yang* principles and dynamics. The more *yin* there is, the less *yang*. They are opposites that consume each other. If we look at the other axis, the Metal Phase voice has a tendency to be strangled by sorrow, and both the words and sentences have a tendency to ebb out before they are finished. There is less definition, especially at the ends of words and sentences. This is the opposite of the Wood Phase voice, which is hard and clear cut and the words don't drag out before ebbing away but are instead sharply clipped and well defined. Where the Metal Phase voice lacks strength due to *zong qi* being affected, the Wood Phase voice is expansive. It can travel through walls and doors when it is in excess. It is difficult to be aggressive and sorrowful at the same time; you have to alternate between the two. This then leaves the Earth Phase. Here, the voice is described as singing – a voice where the tone is variable and going up and down. This makes sense, as the Earth is the centre – the axle that everything revolves around and passes through. The other phases' voice qualities are constantly moving backwards and forwards, up and down through the Earth centre giving the voice a singing quality.

Five Phase vocal qualities

Phase	Significance
Fire	Laughter, joy
Earth	Singing
Metal	Crying
Water	Complaining and moaning
Wood	Shouting

Emotions and the voice

The five emotions are similar to, but not exactly the same as, the five vocal qualities. Sometimes there are certain emotions that are prevalent, not only in the vocal quality, but also in the conversation itself. This can be heard in the answers and explanations that the patient gives and in the questions they ask. Some patients with Kidney or Water imbalances, for example, will be excessively fearful. You can hear in the way that they describe their life and their symptoms how there is an undertone of fear and anxiety. There are many things that they are scared of, not just the disorder they suffer from. They will often wonder whether: the treatment is safe or dangerous; you think that their condition is life threatening, even though the doctor has told them it isn't and that there is nothing to worry about; there is a danger of the needles puncturing an organ; the needles are sterile. They will also be scared that you have forgotten to take all the needles out again. You will hear, repeatedly, how fear dominates their life. A person with Liver or Wood imbalances may, on the other hand, tell you about all of the frustrations and problems that they have in their life and all the dissatisfaction and frustration that they have had when visiting other therapists. It is not that emotions themselves are imbalances but they should be appropriate to the situation and, importantly, neither too dominant nor too weak. This means that we must be listening to how and what they are communicating. Do they, for example, constantly apologise, even though it is not necessary – sorry for coming early, sorry for having chewing gum in their mouth, sorry for not taking their clothes off quickly enough, sorry for the state of their clothes? Do they constantly or excessively compliment and praise you and others? Do they express excessive gratitude? As with so many things, there is no hard-and-fast definition of any of these things, it depends on the underlying emotion, the tone of the voice and the emotional motivation. If we look at apologising, for example, it can be an expression of constant worrying, it can be fear, it can be lack of self-worth and it can be a combination of all three. We therefore have to see this in the context of the other symptoms and signs.

The emotion in the voice should also be appropriate to the subject being talked about. We listen subconsciously to the tone of the voice as much, if not more than, what is being said. The same sentence can have a multitude of meanings, depending on the tone of the voice and where the stress in the sentence is placed. It is also important that the tone of the voice changes in relation to what they are talking about.

Sometimes an imbalance that can be heard in the voice only becomes obvious when they talk about a subject that generates a certain emotion, such as anger, fear or sorrow.

Five Phase emotional qualities

Observation	Significance
Fear and anxiety	Kidney *xu* or Water imbalances
Worry and speculation	Spleen *qi xu*, Dampness or Earth imbalances
Sorrow and grief	Lung or Metal imbalances
Anger and frustration	Liver or Wood imbalances
Excessive merriment or sadness	Heart or Fire imbalances

How easy is it to engage the patient in conversation?

When we are sitting in front of a patient, we are listening to what they are saying and the quality and volume of their voice. We must, though, also have a focus on the conversation itself – not only how quickly and how structured their conversation is, which will be discussed below, but also how effortless the conversation is between you and them. How easy is it to create contact with them? Are they open and communicative? If not, in what way are they not? Is it shyness, which will usually indicate a Heart *xu* condition, or is it because they are closed, uncommunicative and difficult to engage? As always, things must be seen in a context of the other signs and body language. These will be significantly different between a person who is difficult to engage because they are shy and reticent and a person who is stubborn and dour due to stagnation of their Heart and Liver *qi*.

If the Heart is harmonious, the person will be easy to engage and they will open themselves but with a degree of restraint. The Heart not only has the ability to open up and communicate with others, it is also responsible for 'closing' and not communicating when this is appropriate. A person who has Heat in their Heart can be over-communicative. They can initially be very easy to engage, quickly opening up and creating a connection, but if there is a lot of Heat, they can have a tendency to be too communicative, too open and lose the sense of *li* or propriety that is an aspect of *shen*. These people will not only start talking to anyone and everyone, they will also 'open up' too much, even when it is not appropriate or relevant. This is the person who, whilst sitting in the waiting room, tells the person sitting next to them all sorts of personal details about their life, family, neighbours, illness and journey into the clinic. The Heat opens the Heart so much that it is unable to close when appropriate and is therefore open and communicating all the time.

These people are very easy to engage, but in this case it is an expression of imbalance rather than harmony. As with everything in Chinese medicine, both too little and too much of something is a sign of imbalance and a lack of harmony. What is too much and too little will, as always, be dependent on the situation, and a person should be able to adjust to the various situations and contexts.

How easy is it to engage the client?

Observation	Significance
Easy to engage in conversation and communicate with	Normal or Heat in the Heart
Shy, reserved and reticent	Heart *qi xu*
Closed, uncommunicative and terse	Liver and Heart *qi* stagnation
Opens excessively, no boundaries	Heart Fire, Phlegm-Fire

Flow and structure of their speech

The flow of the voice will reflect the condition of the patient's *shen*. This is obvious when we experience fright, start to stutter and become 'tongue-tied'. This is one of several manifestations indicating that Heart *qi* has been spread and has become unstable due to the fright. We will probably also be sweating in the armpit and in the palms of our hands, and our heart will be thumping, beating rapidly and possibly slightly irregularly.

When the Heart and the *shen* are affected, the flow of the voice can also be affected in other ways. These changes in the speech pattern reflect what it is that is affecting *shen*. If *shen* is agitated by Heat, the structure of their speech and their replies to your questions can become disrupted. The mind can start rushing – moving faster than the words can keep pace with – so the conversation loses some of its structure. Heat, by agitating *shen*, will result in the person not always finishing describing or explaining what they were talking about before they start veering off in other directions because new thoughts have overtaken the ones that they were elaborating on.

When Phlegm is blocking *shen*, there will also be a disruption in the structure of the conversation. The speed of the voice can be slower due to Phlegm slowing the ability to formulate what is in their mind, but at the same time the blockage of *shen* will also mean that the person has difficulty thinking clearly. They will be more easily confused and they may even lose the thread of their thoughts when talking. The flow of the conversation can pause whilst they mentally search for a word or something that they were going to say but somehow just can't recall. Their conversation can also change tack almost without them being aware of it themselves. If there is a lot of blockage, their responses can also be inappropriate and confused. This is because *shen* ensures that our reactions and responses are appropriate to the stimulation we have received. When Phlegm is blocking the Heart's orifices, the patient may also have difficulty clearly understanding what you are asking them and therefore have difficulty answering precisely. This is something most of us can recognise, either from when we have a heavy head cold where it feels as if your head is full of cotton wool or when we have a hangover. For people with a lot of Damp-Phlegm, this is a chronic sensation that they may not even be conscious of any more, as it has become normal. It will often be worst in the morning when the person has been lying flat all night and this *yin xie qi* has seeped down to the head and the Heart, thereby blocking the 'orifices of the Heart'. It will also be aggravated when the person consumes Phlegm- and Damp-producing foods.

In general, a person with Phlegm blocking the *shen* will tend to meander verbally back and forth, going round in circles, jumping from subject to subject, losing their thread or completely wandering off the path in irrelevant and inappropriate directions. This is different from the person with Heat agitating the *shen*. The structure of their conversation can be disrupted by an over-eagerness and a surfeit of ideas and things they want to tell you. They lose their thread because they keep changing subject before the last subject area is finished. A person with Heat in the Heart will lack the necessary composure to maintain the structure of a conversation.

If *shen* is undernourished, as it is, for example, when there is Heart *xue xu*, the structure of the conversation can be affected by forgetfulness. They will also have difficulty finding words or remembering what they were talking about, but this is more due to absentmindedness than confusion or over-exuberance.

When there is *yang xu* and *qi xu*, the conversation will retain its structure, but the speed of delivery and the volume can be affected. The conversation is less animated. It may seem as if it is an effort to talk. People who are *yang xu*, in particular, will tend to speak slower and more lethargically. The other person in the conversation sometimes wants to finish the sentences for them, because they get impatient. This is something we must try to be consciously aware of. Whilst interviewing the client, we have to constantly ask ourselves: How does their voice and the way they talk affect me? How am I reacting to them? Do I feel stressed, annoyed or bored? If so, why? Am I dominating or are they dominating the conversation? It is very important to be aware of your own patterns of imbalance – we can feel that they are dominating the conversation because they are preventing us from doing so when we normally would, or they can dominate the conversation because we are too passive and taciturn. We may be tired and *qi xu*. If we are annoyed by them, is it because they talk too much or too little or is it their subject matter or their aggressiveness? There are definitely some patients in whom you quickly pick up on a latent aggressiveness. You can feel them almost looking for something to pick a fight over. It is not against you personally, and it isn't something that they are conscious of, but in situations outside of the clinic – such as at home or at work – it probably is a problem; a problem they may not be aware of. They are often people who have a lot of conflict in their relationships. This is a problem because it is often caused by Liver *qi* stagnation, and the conflicts their persona provokes will in themselves become causes of Liver *qi* stagnation.

It is, as stated, important to be aware of your own patterns of imbalance. These will affect how you react to other people. If you have Heat, you will more easily become impatient with someone who speaks slowly and laboriously but possibly enjoy the snappiness of talking to someone who also has Heat. The opposite can also be the case. If you are yourself verbose and loquacious, it can be frustrating when someone else dominates the conversation. If you have Heart *qi xu* or Heart and Liver *xue xu*, you may well find many people intimidating and find that you quickly feel overwhelmed by others when you are talking to them. Likewise, if you are *yang xu*, you may well think of people who talk slowly and methodically as being an example of how everyone should speak.

Our imbalances can often mean that we either over-diagnose our own patterns of imbalance – we easily recognise these signs and symptoms because we know what they are – or under-diagnose these patterns of imbalance – we are blind to them because we subconsciously or consciously think that these signs and symptoms are normal.

Structure and flow of the conversation

Observation	Significance
Loquacious and verbose	Heart Fire, Phlegm Fire
Taciturn, silent	Heart *qi* stagnation, Phlegm, Heart *qi xu*, *zong qi xu*

Observation	Significance
Talks quickly	Heat
Talks slowly	*Yang xu*, Phlegm-Dampness
Confusion, delirium	Phlegm, Heat in the Pericardium
Incoherent speech	Phlegm blocking the Heart's orifices
Difficulty finding words or maintaining their thread	Heart *xue xu*, Phlegm
Talking to themselves	Phlegm blocking the Heart's orifices
Laughing excessively or inappropriately	Heart imbalances
Stuttering	Heart *xue xu*, Heart Fire
Talking in their sleep	*Shi* Heat, Heart *xue xu*
Sudden shouting	Liver *qi* stagnation, Liver Fire, Heart Fire

Quality of the voice

Apart from observing the emotional qualities, the volume and the flow of the conversation, we should also note other qualities in the voice. These will again reflect patterns of imbalance that have affected the voice and made it deviate from the norm. We should, as always, be thinking: What should I expect to be hearing and how does what I am actually hearing differ from this? What is the pathomechanism that could create this aberration?

Gravelly voice

Phlegm, especially Phlegm-Heat in the Lung, will manifest with a gravelly voice. This is the typical barfly and heavy smoker's voice. If it is extreme, there will also be a rattling sound in the throat and a sticky cough. Cigarettes are drying and heating. They will damage Lung *yin* and generate Lung Phlegm-Heat. Alcohol will create Phlegm and Heat that can rise up to the Lung and the throat, affecting the vocal cords.

Hoarse or husky voice

Invasions of Wind-Heat, as well as chronic Heat and *yin xu* conditions, will mean that the throat and the vocal cords lack moisture and lubrication. Again, alcohol and tobacco are often contributing or causative factors.

Dry voice

A person with *yin xu* or *xue xu* will lack *yin* and *xue*'s moistening qualities. This can be heard in the voice, even though it is a very subtle quality (or lack thereof). Often, elderly patients' voices have this quality.

Nasal voice

The voice should be clear and ring like a bell. If the bell is smothered, as when the sinuses are filled with varying amounts and consistencies of Phlegm, the voice becomes more or less nasal. This can be both acute and chronic, depending on the underlying imbalance.

Staccato voice

Some people have a staccato voice. Their voice sounds like a machine gun when they talk. They do not necessarily talk quickly, but their words are clipped and the voice is hard, sometimes even aggressive. This relates to the Liver *qi* and its function of helping the *qi* and thereby the voice to flow freely and unhindered. Liver *qi* stagnation will also result in a tendency to be irritable, which one will often hear in the voice.

Aggressive voice

Again, Liver imbalances can give an aggressiveness or anger to the voice. It may be a general tone or only heard when patients talk about certain subjects.

Slurred voice

Phlegm can slur the voice. This is heard when people are drunk and the intense Heat and Dampness of the alcohol results in Phlegm. It can, though, be a more chronic condition. An extreme example is after a stroke where Wind-Phlegm has resulted in Phlegm blocking the orifices and the person has difficulty speaking, their voice being heavily slurred.

Very soft voice

Liver *xu* imbalances can manifest with a voice that lacks resonance and the hard qualities that the Liver gives to the voice. The voice will be too soft and will lack authority.

Sleep talking, talking to themselves and delirious speech

There are also some situations where various forms of *xie qi* have affected the speech, but we are unlikely to experience these in the clinic. *Shi* Heat can agitate the *shen* at night when it should be calmly resting in the Heart. This can result in the person talking in their sleep. *Shen* can also become active when it is not rooted by Heart *xue*, i.e. Heart *xue xu*. In this case, the voice will be more quiet and tranquil.

In some febrile diseases where Heat has invaded the Pericardium, the Heat can agitate the *shen* so much that the person's speech is delirious and incomprehensible.

Another sign in the voice that usually isn't heard in the clinic is people talking to themselves when Phlegm has blocked the orifices of the Heart and they are locked in their own world. This can be observed in people who are mentally ill and hold conversations with themselves, the content of which can sometimes be meaningless to outsiders.

Sudden shouting is seen in some types of Tourette's syndrome. This is usually a sign of Heat in the Liver and Heart.

The sound of the person's voice

Observation	Significance
Loud, resonant voice	*Shi* condition
Quiet, soft voice	*Xu* condition
Hoarse voice	Invasion of Wind-Heat or Wind-Dryness, Liver or Lung *qi* stagnation, Phlegm, Heat, *xue* stagnation, Kidney *yin xu* or Lung *yin xu*
Staccato voice	Liver *qi* stagnation
Aggressive voice	Liver *shi* condition
Shouting voice	Liver *shi* condition
Dry voice	*Yin xu*
Gravelly voice	Phlegm
Slurred voice	Phlegm
Nasal voice	Phlegm, Dampness

Auditory diagnosis of other sounds coming from the mouth, nose and chest

As well as all these verbal impressions, we also have the classical diagnosis of sounds. We can ask the client about these, but they should also be things that we keep our ears open for when we are interviewing the client. We should, for example, listen to the patient's breathing, both whilst interviewing them and whilst they are lying on the couch.

Yawning and sighing

When there is Liver *qi* stagnation, the body will instinctively try to set *qi* in motion again. One of the ways of doing this is to sigh or yawn. When we sigh or yawn, we inhale a larger amount of air. This increases *zong qi*, which then helps to force the blocked *qi* into circulating again. The patient may well be unaware that they sigh frequently, especially as the sighs can be quite subtle. This means that they might well answer negatively, when you ask about sighing. These more subtle sighs can often be heard when the patient talks about a particular subject area or about things that frustrate or annoy them. This is important in that it not only can help to reveal a pattern of imbalance, probably Liver *qi* stagnation, but also, importantly, it can help to reveal the aetiology, i.e. one of the contributing causes of the client's Liver *qi* stagnation.

Yawning can be a way of moving stagnant *qi* and a way of increasing *qi*. When a person is *qi xu*, from, for example, a lack of sleep, the body will try to compensate by increasing the production of *qi*. The quickest way to do this is to increase the production of *zong qi* by inhaling a larger amount of air.

Moaning, complaining, gasping, screaming and crying

These sounds are often heard as a response to pain. This may be a pain on movement or palpation or a constant pain. It indicates that there is a stagnation of *qi* and/or *xue* with accompanying pain.[8] The strength of the sound will often reflect the degree of stagnation.

Snoring

You will not hear snoring during the consultation, but you may hear it when the patient is lying on the couch. Otherwise, snoring is something you will have to ask the patient about. Snoring occurs most frequently when there is Phlegm blocking the nasal passages. The strength of the sound will tell you whether it is an exclusively *shi* or a *xu/shi* condition.

Respiration

Listening to the respiration can elicit vital information, especially about the condition of the Lung. The breathing should be calm, relaxed and deep.

Weak and shallow breathing shows that the Lung is not descending and spreading *qi* optimally. The weakness of the breath indicates that it is a *xu* condition.

The breathing can be laboured and shallow if Lung *qi* is blocked by *xie qi*, Phlegm or *qi* stagnation.

The Kidneys grasp the *qi* that the Lung sends downwards to the lower *jiao*. This means that Kidney *qi xu* can also affect the respiration, causing the person to become breathless.

Heat accelerates physiological processes. This can cause the person to breathe more rapidly.

The presence of Phlegm can be heard when there are sounds accompanying the respiration. This could be a wheezing or rattling sound when the person breathes.

Sounds from the person's mouth, nose or chest

Observation	Significance
Calm, relaxed and deep breathing	Normal
Weak and shallow breathing or breathlessness	Lung *xu* conditions, Kidney *qi xu*
Laboured and shallow breathing or breathlessness	*Xie qi* blocking Lung *qi*, *qi* stagnation, Phlegm
Rapid breathing	Heat
Wheezing	Phlegm
Rattling sound during breathing	Phlegm
Snoring	Phlegm
Moaning, complaining, gasping, screaming and crying	Stagnation of *qi* and/or *xue*
Sighing and yawning	Liver *qi* stagnation

Coughs, sneezes and sniffles

You may hear coughing during the consultation or whilst the patient is waiting outside the treatment room, and this is often something you ask about (see page 226). If you do not hear the cough during the consultation, you can ask them to cough in order to gain an impression of it, although it is best if you can hear an involuntary cough, as this will give a more accurate impression.

Fundamentally, a cough is nothing other than rebellious Lung *qi*. The stronger and more explosive the sound of the cough, the more *qi* there is rebelling. An explosive and loud cough will therefore be a sign of a *shi* condition.

Heat in the Lung will manifest with a barking cough. The Heat will make the sputum in the Lung stickier and more difficult to expectorate. This means that the person will often cough vigorously several times until the sputum disengages.

The sputum will be looser and more watery if there is Phlegm-Dampness or an invasion of Wind-Cold. The cough will sound wetter and it will require less effort to expectorate the sputum.

If the person is Lung *yin xu*, the cough will be very dry. If there is sputum, it will be rubbery and dry. It will require a greater effort to expel the sputum. The cough will not be as loud as when there is Phlegm-Heat and Lung Heat but will instead be a dry, 'ticklish' cough. You can almost hear how it tickles the throat and the Lung.

An invasion of Wind-Cold disrupting the Lung's ability to spread *jinye* or the presence of Damp-Phlegm in the Lung can lead to the accumulation of thin, watery mucus in the nose, causing the person to sniff repeatedly.

The sound of the cough and sniffles

Observation	Significance
Loud cough with the sound of loose sputum	Wind-Cold, Damp-Phlegm
Loud cough with sputum that is difficult to expectorate	Lung Heat, Phlegm-Heat
Barking cough	Lung Heat, Phlegm-Heat
Loud and explosive cough	*Shi* condition
Dry or ticklish cough	Lung *yin xu*
Weak cough	*Xu* condition
Sniffles	Wind-Cold or Damp-Phlegm

Diagnosis of sounds from the abdominal cavity

Borborygmi and other sounds

Sounds emanating from the abdominal cavity can sometimes be heard whilst talking to the client. More often though, they will be heard whilst the client is lying on the couch. This is mainly due to the change in posture as gases and liquids move from where they were to a new position in the gastrointestinal tract. The sounds can be anything from a rumble to the sound of liquid sloshing around. Rumbling sounds will usually be heard when there is Spleen *qi xu* and *qi* stagnation in the Intestines. A sloshing sound of fluid in the Intestines will be heard when there is *yang xu* or *shi* Cold in the Small Intestine or Large Intestine.

Hiccup

Hiccupping occurs when Stomach *qi* becomes rebellious and starts to ascend. This may indicate that there is a *shi* condition such as Stomach Heat, Stomach Cold or Liver *qi* invading the Stomach, in which case the sound of hiccups will be loud. The Stomach can also be too weak to send its *qi* downwards, i.e. Stomach *qi xu* or Stomach *yin xu*. In these cases, the sound of the hiccup will be weaker and more subdued.

Vomiting

It is unlikely that we will experience the sound of vomiting in the clinic and this will therefore be information that we are reliant on the client reporting to us. Vomiting that is loud and explosive is heard in *shi* conditions, particularly when there is Heat, the *qi* being forcibly propelled upwards and out of the body. In *xu* conditions there is not enough *qi* to transform the food and liquid consumed nor to send them downwards into the Small Intestine. The accumulation of food and liquid will eventually force *qi* upwards, but the sound and the force of the vomiting will not be strong.

Flatulence and belching

Flatulence is usually a sign of stagnation of *qi* in the Intestines, food stagnation or Damp-Heat in the Intestines. The louder the flatulence, the more *shi* the imbalance is.

Like vomiting, belching is a sign of rebellious Stomach *qi*. Again, it can be due to both *shi* and *xu* conditions, depending on the volume of the belching – the louder the eructation, the more *shi* the condition.

Sounds emanating from the abdominal cavity

Observation	Significance
Hiccup	Rebellious Stomach *qi*, may be due to Stomach Fire, Stomach Cold, Stomach *yin xu*, Stomach *qi xu* or Liver *qi* invading the Stomach
Rumbling sounds from the Intestines	Spleen *qi xu*, *qi* stagnation
Borborygmi	Fluid accumulation due to *shi* Cold or *yang xu*

Diagnosis of the sounds of the person in the clinic

Auditory diagnosis is not limited to the sounds emanating from the client's body, such as their voice, cough and respiration. All the sounds they create can have a diagnostic relevance. Imbalances affect the body's physiology – the way the body moves and reacts and the way the person interacts with their environment. This means that different patterns of imbalance can, in certain circumstances, manifest as audible sounds created by the person.

One of the first things we hear is the client ringing the doorbell. Often there is nothing to note, and at best it is a very tenuous sign, but when there is something to note, it can say a lot about certain people. The most obvious example of this is someone who has Heat in their Liver. The person is often extremely goal oriented and impatient. They tend to press the doorbell repeatedly and for a long time. More importantly, they will often not wait very long before re-ringing the bell if you do not buzz them in immediately. A person with Liver and Heart *xue xu* is more likely to wait longer before ringing again, as they do not want to be a bother to you.

The time it takes for them to come from the street door to the clinic door can also have relevance if you have stairs. Someone who is *qi xu* or *yang xu* will usually take longer than someone who has *shi* Heat. This is, of course, a very small sign, and there may be other explanations, for example if the person is talking on their phone.

If you have a door that they knock on, the sound of their knocks will be more revealing than an electric bell. Sometimes the knock can give an impression of the person. Again, this is an extremely tenuous sign that must be seen in the context of all the other signs and symptoms. A person who is *shi* will tend to knock harder and more times than a person with a *xu* condition. A shy person, for example a person with Heart and Gall Bladder *qi xu*, will tend to be more hesitant and will not knock so many times, if they knock on the door at all. As a rule, they will wait until you come out to them. A person with Heat in the Liver is more likely to knock on the door even though they have arrived ahead of schedule. In extreme cases, they will not even wait for you to open the door before entering the room.

A more dependable auditory sign is the sound of their steps in the hallway or waiting area. Quick steps can indicate Heat and heavy steps a *shi* condition. The sound of shuffling or dragging feet can indicate *yang xu*, *qi xu* or Damp-Phlegm conditions. Other factors, though, such as the person being late or heavy winter boots, must also be taken into account.

Other audible signs from the waiting area could be the sound of them repeatedly getting up and sitting down again or walking backwards and forwards. This could again indicate Heat agitating the *shen*, creating restlessness and impatience. It could, though, also be due to pain and discomfort or nervousness. We must, as ever, place these small impressions into a bigger picture before we can allot any significance to them.

Another sound that can have relevance in some patients is the need to rush to the toilet to urinate immediately on arrival. This, of course, does not have to mean anything, but some clients urinate both on arrival before lying on the couch and immediately after the treatment. This will tell you that they have frequent urination without you having to ask them.

We can also hear the sound of the patient's voice whilst they are sitting in the waiting area if they are talking on the phone or speaking to their family members or other clients. Is the voice so loud and resonant that we can hear it through our door? Is the voice so soft and quiet that we cannot really hear it, even though there is only a curtain and a short distance between us and them? Are they a person who immediately starts talking to complete strangers in the waiting area? Do they constantly make jokes and try to be funny? Do they start revealing very personal information to people they don't know?

The diagnostic significance of the voice itself was discussed earlier. What we hear can also reveal something of their relationships with other people. We may hear a lot of bickering or arguing, for example, something that could be an aetiological factor or something that we should at least consider when feeling their pulse, as this will have affected the pulse quality.

Olfactory diagnosis

The second aspect of the diagnostic pillar 'Listening and Smelling' is the impressions we receive from the client via the nose. Unfortunately, these impressions are more difficult to use in modern times in the developed world. This is because many people bathe daily and wash their clothes frequently, as well as using deodorants, creams, perfumes, etc. This means that we often cannot smell their natural odour, because they have washed it off their body and out of their clothes and masked it with various fragrances. A trick can be to get the patient to put a t-shirt, vest or pillow case that they have been using in a plastic bag, which they then tie and then bring into the clinic, making the odours more prominent. In general, the odours that have a diagnostic significance can be difficult to smell. It is usually only when there is a very dominant smell that it is noticeable. If we do pick up a certain odour, it usually has diagnostic significance. In these situations, it is often a very important diagnostic sign.

There are two aspects to olfactory diagnosis. First, the person's body odour, which can provide information that can help to determine a person's constitutional type or their imbalance in Five Element acupuncture diagnosis. Second, the diagnostic significance of the various discharges and excretions from the body.

Olfactory diagnosis of the body odour

Olfactory diagnosis plays a central role in the Five Element acupuncture system, founded by J. R. Worsley. Worsley and the schools inspired by him place great emphasis on training their students to be able to distinguish between the odours that resonate with the Five Phases. It is considered a serious sign of imbalance if a person does not manifest the odour that is characteristic for their own constitutional types but instead has the smell of one of the other phase's odours.

The following descriptions of the odours are mainly based on *Five Element Constitutional Acupuncture* by John Hicks, Angela Hicks and Peter Mole (2004) and J. R. Worsley's book *Traditional Acupuncture Volume II – Traditional Diagnosis* (Worsley 1990).

- **Water Phase – Rotten and putrid:** The Chinese character *fu* can be translated into English as 'putrid'. The character is built up of two components. The first has the meaning of a building or shed and the second component means to dry meat that is tied together. This gives the character a sense of the odour you would expect to smell in a shed that is used to dry meat. The difference between this odour and the odour of the Metal Phase is that the *fu* odour is more tart and caustic.

- **Wood Phase – Rancid:** *Sao*, as this smell is called in Chinese, is the smell that animals or urine can have. This is rancid, as in rancid butter or rancid fats, but even sharper. Hicks *et al.* describe this smell as newly mown grass but without that smell being pleasant (2004, p.57).

- **Fire Phase – Burnt:** This odour is called *zhuo* in Chinese. The smell can be described as being similar to toast that has been burnt, clothes that have just come out of a tumble dryer, a shirt that has been burnt with an iron or vegetables burning dry in a saucepan. In the same way that the smell varies depending on what it is that is burning, the burnt smell can vary from person to person. The aroma may be noticed when a person has a high fever.

- **Earth Phase – Sweet and aromatic:** The Chinese word *xiang* means aromatic. It is a word that is used in the name of many aromatic herbs for example. This can be misleading, as the odour referred to here has a heavy, sticky, almost nauseating aroma.

- **Metal Phase – Rotten:** Rotten is *lan* in Chinese. This is the rotten odour that is smelt when meat, fish or vegetables rot. This odour can be smelt in old dustbins or garbage trucks.

Odour

Phase	Significance
Water	Putrid
Wood	Rancid
Fire	Burnt
Earth	Sweet and aromatic
Metal	Rotten

Some imbalances can have specific smells that can be difficult to describe but are immediately recognisable when you notice them on another patient with the same pattern of imbalance. Phlegm patients, for example, often have a very heavy, sticky odour. It smells a bit like a wet leather jacket, but it lingers in the room long after the person has left. Sometimes you can go into the treatment room an hour after they have gone and the smell still lingers in the air.

Olfactory diagnosis of the body's excretions
We are usually dependent on the patient's reporting of how the various discharges and excretions from the body smell. Very few clients bring an example of their stools, urine or vaginal discharge for inspection in the clinic. We can, though, still smell things like their sweat and their breath during the consultation.

A general rule of thumb is that strong-smelling excretions and discharges are a sign of Heat. If there is no significant odour to the discharge, this will not be pathological unless there is a change in the volume, consistency or frequency of the discharge. These aspects are dealt with in Sections 1 and 4 on visual diagnosis and interviewing.

Olfactory diagnosis of the urine and stools
Urine and stools that have a strong odour will most often be a sign of *shi* Heat, usually Damp-Heat.

If the stool or urine does not smell, the lack of smell will only be relevant if there are other disturbances in the frequency and consistency of the stool or the volume and frequency of the urine, in which case the lack of odour can contribute to a diagnosis of *shi* Cold or *yang xu* Cold.

Stools that smells like sewage will be a symptom of food stagnation.

Olfactory diagnosis of sweat

A strong body odour from sweating is a manifestation of Damp-Heat. As explained in the introduction, this will probably be something that you have to ask the patient about because the strong body odour means they will have used deodorants and antiperspirants. Sometimes, though, you can still smell the sweat because the odour is very strong or your nose is close to their body whilst treating them with needles.

Olfactory diagnosis of the breath

A person's breath can sometimes be smelt whilst conducting visual diagnosis of the tongue or needling points in the face; otherwise it will be something you have to ask about.

Malodorous breath can result from imbalances in the Stomach, Spleen and Large Intestine. Heat from Stomach Fire or food stagnation can rise up to the mouth and be smelt on the breath. Heat in the Stomach and Large Intestine channels can result in paradentosis, rotten teeth, etc., which can give bad breath.

Olfactory diagnosis of nasal and pulmonary mucus

This will more likely be something the client can taste, but sometimes it is so powerful that the therapist also can smell it. If sputum in the Lung is infected, it may smell slightly of fish. This will be experienced when there is Toxic-Fire in the Lung. Strongly smelling mucus in the nose will be a sign of Lung Heat.

Olfactory diagnosis of menstrual blood and vaginal discharge

Menstrual blood and vaginal discharge that have a strong, pungent odour is a sign of Damp-Heat. If the vaginal discharge has a fishy odour, it is a sign of Damp-Cold.

Olfactory diagnosis of flatulence

An increased amount of intestinal gas that smells strongly is a sign of Damp-Heat or, in extreme cases, Toxic-Fire in the Large Intestine. An increased amount of intestinal gas that does not smell is a sign of Spleen *qi xu*.

The smell of excretions and discharges

Observation	Significance
Strong-smelling urine	*Shi* Heat, Damp-Heat
The urine does not smell, but there is increased volume and frequency of urination	*Shi* and *xu* cold
Strong-smelling stools	*Shi* Heat, Damp-Heat
The stool smells of sewage	Food stagnation
Strong-smelling sweat	Damp-Heat
Bad breath	Stomach Fire, Heat in the Stomach or Large Intestine channel
Nasal mucus that smells or tastes strongly	Lung Phlegm-Heat
Pulmonary sputum that smells strongly or has a significant flavour	Lung Phlegm-Heat or Toxic-Fire in Lung
Strong-smelling menstrual blood	Damp-Heat
Strong-smelling vaginal discharge	Damp-Heat
Vaginal discharge that smells of fish	Damp-Cold
Strong-smelling flatulence	Damp-Heat
Flatulence without odour	Spleen *qi xu*

THE DIAGNOSTIC PILLAR: PALPATION

Introduction

The diagnostic pillar 'palpation' includes all the information that can be acquired by palpating the patient. In addition to feeling the pulse, this also includes the palpation of the channels, acupuncture points, skin and various areas of the body.

Some aspects of this diagnostic pillar can seem daunting and difficult to learn. This can be the case with pulse diagnosis and its 28 qualities, 12 positions and three depths. At the same time, we need to train our abilities that we are not accustomed to using intellectually. We are well trained in translating verbal information into intellectual knowledge so the interviewing approach to diagnosis feels more reliable and trustworthy. Visual diagnosis also appears to be more accessible, because we can look at pictures in a manual and compare them with what we can see in front of us. However, we are not used to using our fingertips to provide information that we can utilise intellectually. Furthermore, it is more difficult to compare and contrast what we feel with our fingers with the descriptions presented in a textbook. What we experience will be a subjective assessment, and we can be in doubt about whether what we are feeling is the same as what's described in the book or whether it is, in reality, something else. Nevertheless, palpation is a vital and indispensable part of the diagnostic process and should not be neglected. Diagnosis is like a roof supported by four separate diagnostic pillars. If one of the pillars is missing or incomplete, the diagnosis will be unstable and unreliable.

Pulse diagnosis is particularly important in the differentiation of the Eight Principles, in *zangfu* diagnosis, *qi* and *xue* diagnoses and diagnosis according to *xie qi*. You will not be able to make a reliable diagnosis without having first palpated the pulse.

One of the great advantages of palpation is that it can be used to monitor and adjust treatments. There should be qualitative changes in the pulse, the abdomen or the skin and muscles in general after the needles have been inserted and stimulated. By feeling the pulse or the abdomen, one can see if the treatment has had an affect. Because the pulse can change instantly, it can reveal the state of a person's *qi* right now.

The pulse will also be able to give an indication of changes in the body's *qi* and vital substances, and it can reveal the presence of *xie qi* before actual symptoms have started to manifest.

The diagnostic techniques in this pillar require participation in practical training with an experienced teacher. Hands-on training will help to refine and clarify the details of these diagnostic methods and techniques. That said, a lot can be achieved by following the descriptions of these methods presented in various textbooks, especially if you use a logical and systematic approach, consciously ensuring that you have examined all the relevant aspects and compared the findings with those that are presented in the textbooks.

One way to become familiar with the various pulse categories when you are not with a teacher who can monitor your approach and conclusions is to systematically feel the pulse of each and every patient you come into contact with. When you have a patient with a very clear and definite diagnosis (using the other three diagnostic pillars), you should ask yourself: What should I be experiencing right now? You should then compare this with the sensations that you are experiencing in your fingertips. For example, if you have a patient with an obvious pattern of Liver *qi* stagnation, you would expect the pulse to have a Wiry quality in the left *guan* or middle position. You can then compare what you are feeling beneath your fingertips with the description in the textbook and see if you can recognise the qualities described in the book. By constantly repeating this procedure, you will eventually learn with certainty how, for example, a Wiry pulse feels. The more you practise, the faster you learn to diagnose with your fingers.

Palpation

Relative strengths of palpation

- It is indispensable when diagnosing muscular and skeletal problems.
- We are not dependent on the patient's interpretation and presentation of their diagnostic signs.

Relative weaknesses of palpation

- It is a subjective diagnosis. It can be difficult in the beginning to determine whether you are actually feeling what you are supposed to be feeling.

Diagnostic tips

- Always remember to palpate muscles and joints when a person has physical pain and impaired movement.
- Everything that feels hot is a sign of Heat, at least in the local area.
- Consciously investigate the skin temperature whilst palpating and whilst you are locating acupuncture points.
- Consciously investigate the skin moisture whilst palpating and whilst you are locating acupuncture points.
- Consciously investigate the skin elasticity whilst palpating and whilst you are locating acupuncture points.
- Consciously investigate the muscle tone whilst palpating and whilst you are locating acupuncture points.
- A rapid pulse is always a sign of Heat.

~~d~~iagnosis

~~Introd~~uction

~~Pulse d~~iagnosis is regarded by some as a precise but at the same time esoteric diagnosis tool. Some acupuncturists have shied away from it because they have not had teachers and textbooks that have presented it as an accessible tool that is indispensable in practice. Despite its reputation, pulse diagnosis is not difficult to learn and, even with very little practice, it can provide vital diagnostic information to the novice. With practice and hands-on instruction the novice can soon develop their skills and gain a deeper insight into their patient's physiological condition.

At first, seeing a list of 28 pulse descriptions with 12 separate pulse positions can be daunting and confusing. Furthermore, people are astounded when they hear stories of Chinese doctors who can relay to the patient their entire medical history just by feeling their pulse. This gives pulse diagnosis a veil of mysterious complexity and unattainability. It is important not to be deterred. There are many different levels of competence in pulse diagnosis. An expert in pulse diagnosis may get a lot of incredibly detailed information from the pulse, but you can learn in ten minutes to take the pulse to a degree where you will always be able to gain a quick and accurate overview of the client imbalances. You can gain vital information just by quickly feeling the pulse. It does not take long to feel whether a pulse is weak or replete, fast or slow, deep or superficial. These six characteristics of the pulse are relatively easily perceived. It's something anyone can do. The differentiation of these six parameters will help to define at least six out of the Eight Principles (*xu/shi*, Heat/Cold, interior/exterior). This can be essential, as we often need to determine whether a diagnosis is one or the other of these – whether it's a *shi* or *xu* condition for example.

Most patients we see present with complex conditions consisting of several conflicting patterns of imbalance at the same time. This creates the need for a bird's-eye perspective. Pulse diagnosis can be used both to refine and to simplify a diagnosis. We can use it to get a deeper insight and thereby a more accurate diagnosis. An example of this could be a client who suffers from fatigue and shortness of breath. Their pulse is weak, so we know that it is a *xu* condition. By feeling whether the pulse is weakest in the front or the rear position on the right wrist, we can determine if there is Lung *qi xu* or Kidney *qi xu*. But we can also move in the opposite direction and use the pulse to take a step back and clarify a situation. If the symptom picture is complex and messy with conflicting symptoms, you can quickly feel the pulse to answer questions like: Is there Heat or Cold? Is it a *shi* or *xu* condition? Is it *yin* or *yang*?

Pulse diagnosis has the strength to be utilised on its own. Where other changes in the body's physiology need to be compared with other symptoms and signs, or to be corroborated by asking supplementary questions, the pulse can be used alone. A deep and weak pulse in the rear or *chi* position is a sign of a Kidney *xu* condition; a rapid pulse is a sign of Heat. Tongue diagnosis and Hara (abdominal) diagnosis can in certain instances be used unaccompanied, but not to the same extent as the pulse.

Learning to take the pulse is not dissimilar to learning to play a musical instrument. It is reasonably easy to learn the most basic aspects, especially with a good teacher, but it takes years of practice to attain a high level of skill. As with learning a musical instrument, some people have natural talents and rapidly achieve a high level of proficiency, the rest of us have to work harder to achieve these skills. Everyone, though, whether they are natural prodigies or have more mediocre talents, will need to practise to become more adept. The only way to do this is to place your fingers on the radial artery of the wrist a great many times.

As well as constant practice, you must also study and commit to memory the diagnostic interpretations of the various pulse qualities, for example that a Full,[9] i.e. replete, pulse signifies that it is a *shi* condition.

History

Pulse diagnosis has been discussed in Chinese medical texts ever since *Huang Di Nei Jing – Su Wen* (The Yellow Emperor's Classic – Simple Questions). The book describes how the pulse is felt at nine locations on the body. The positions are directly related not only to the specific channels, but also to the five *zang*[10] organs and to specific areas of the body.

In the *Nan Jing* (The Classic of Difficulties), we can recognise the pulse diagnosis that we use today, with three positions on each wrist and three depths. The three positions reflect the three *jiao*, and specific organs are attributed to the different positions. There have been varying definitions over the following centuries of what the different positions relate to, but there has always been a general consensus on their relationship to the three *jiao*.

Physiology

The pulse that we feel under our fingertips is *xue* that is being circulated by *qi*. *Xue* can be more easily felt than *qi*, because it is more *yin*, i.e. more physical. *Qi* and *xue* have a close relationship: *qi* is the commander of *xue* and *xue* is the mother of *qi*. This means that we can perceive *qi* via *xue*.

We can perceive changes in how the artery feels when there is a *qi* imbalance. This is because changes in *qi* will affect the way *xue* moves through the vessels. Furthermore, *xue* is created from *gu qi* and *yuan qi*, driven by *zong qi* and guided by Heart *qi*, whilst the Liver ensures that *qi* flows freely and unhindered throughout the body. This means that imbalances in the Stomach, Spleen, Kidney, Lung, Liver, Heart and *san jiao* will be felt directly in the pulse quality and strength.

The structure of the pulse

Something that can initially create confusion and frustration is the diagnostic relevance attributed to the depths and positions of the pulse positions in the various pulse diagnosis texts.

The pulse was originally palpated in nine different locations on the body. The nine sites were specifically related to the various *zang* organs and to the three *jiao* in general. The pulse was felt in three locations in the head and neck, three places on the torso and three places on the legs. These three areas of the body in themselves related to the continuum of Heaven, Man and Earth. The same was therefore also true of each of these three pulse positions in these areas of the body. When the pulse was later felt only on the radial artery, this division into nine positions on each wrist was maintained as: three positions in the superficial level, three positions deeper down and three positions in the level between the superficial and deep levels.

The pulse can be comprehended as a two-dimensional structure. On the horizontal plane there are three positions along the length of the artery – *cun*, *guan* and *chi*. The vertical plane has three depths – deep, middle and superficial. In reality, it is a three-dimensional structure because the width of the pulse has also significance. Furthermore, some pulse diagnosis systems operate with positions lateral to the *cun*, *guan* and *chi* positions.[11]

Some people have a very rigid definition of the pulse positions and their relation to the organs or channels. In this approach, the deep level of the pulse relates to the *zang* organs or channels and the superficial level to the *fu* organs or channels. Personally, I prefer a more dynamic approach to the pulse, with changes in the pulse being seen in the context of changes in the body's *qi* and how these changes will have affected the pulse.

In most situations I view the organ pairs as an organic whole, the different levels reflecting both organs simultaneously. An example of this is when there is ascendant Liver *yang*, the pulse will manifest with a Full, Wiry and Superficial pulse in the left-hand side *guan* position, whereas Stomach *qi xu* will often manifest with a relatively deeper, Weak pulse in the right *guan* position. This is because *yang* rises upwards and outwards and therefore the pulse in the left *guan* position becomes tenser and more superficial than it otherwise would be. *Qi xu*, on the other hand, will mean that the pulse is weaker and there is not enough *qi* to lift the pulse up to the superficial level.

The three levels

There are three levels or depths in the pulse. The superficial level is felt with a very light touch, being located just below the skin. The deep level is felt with the exertion of greater pressure by the fingers. It is not so deep, though, that you are pressing into the muscle below. The middle level is located between the superficial and deep level.

The different levels represent different aspects of the body. It may seem paradoxical that the same level can reflect several aspects simultaneously. What is important to bear in mind is that the different levels reflect where *qi* is, or is not, in the body. A pulse that is only felt in the deep level, for example, will indicate that there is *yang xu* – that there is not enough *yang* to be able to raise the pulse up to the superficial level. At the same time, a pulse that is only present in the deep level can also indicate that there is a stagnation of *shi* Cold in the interior, the Cold blocking *yang qi* and thereby preventing *yang* from lifting the pulse upwards. There will, though, be significant differences in the qualities of these two pulses, even though they are both felt only in the deepest level. In this instance, the *yang xu* pulse will be not only deep, but also lacking in strength, whereas the pulse when there is a stagnation of Cold in the interior will feel tight and hard. There will also, importantly, be differences in the other symptoms and signs that the patient is presenting with.

The superficial level of the pulse represents both *qi* and *yang*, as well as the *yang* organs and channels. At the same time, the superficial level can also indicate whether an imbalance is located in the exterior (which is the *yang* aspect of the body) from an Eight Principles perspective.

There are only contradictions when you do not see the pulse in a greater context. If there is a Tight, Superficial pulse and the person freezes and has an aversion to Cold, a stiff neck and sore muscles, the Superficial pulse will indicate that the imbalance is located in the exterior. This does not contradict the other aspect of the Superficial pulse, which is that the Superficial pulse represents *qi* and *yang*. When there is an invasion in the exterior, it is the *yang wei qi* that is activated and the struggle takes place in the outermost aspect of the body, just below the skin. Conversely, a pulse that is only present in the superficial level, but feels thin and weak, could be a sign that there is *yin xu* and *xue xu*. In this case the *yin* and *xue* are no longer capable of anchoring *qi*, which therefore drifts up to the surface.

According to Ming dynasty doctor and author Li Shi Zhen, the condition of the various *zang* organs can be felt in the different levels. This model sees the three levels as a reflection of the three *jiao*. Again, this analysis does not in reality contradict the other perceptions of levels, but is in fact complementary. The superficial level relates to the Heart and the Lung. The Lung governs *qi* and *wei qi*. This means the exterior imbalances will directly and indirectly affect the Lung through its relation to *wei qi*. The Lung and the Heart have a close relationship, with *zong qi* driving *xue* from the Heart through the vessels.

The middle level reflects the quality of *xue*. Because *xue* is produced by the Stomach and Spleen and because the Stomach and Spleen are both in the middle *jiao*, their status also affects the pulse of the middle level.

The deepest level reflects *yin*, i.e. the *yin* organs and *yin qi*. When an imbalance is in the interior, it will be felt in the deepest level of the pulse. Furthermore, *yin* imbalances from an Eight Principle perspective will create changes here. When there is *yang xu*, the upward momentum of *yang* will be too weak to push the pulse up to the superficial level.

Kidney and Liver *yin* are the deepest level of *yin* in the body. This means that weaknesses of Kidney and Liver *yin* will be felt, not just in their respective organ positions, but also in the deepest level of the pulse in general.

Level	Type of *qi*	Level	Organs according to Li Shi Zhen
Superficial	*Qi* and *yang* (as well as *yang* organs)	Exterior	*Yang* (Lung and Heart)
Middle	*Xue*	Stomach and Spleen	Stomach and Spleen
Deep	*Yin* (as well as *yin* organs)	Interior	*Yin* (Liver and Kidney)

The three positions

The pulse is felt in three positions on each wrist. The distances between the positions depend on the size of the patient's body, so one must align the fingers in a way that is relative to the patient's anatomy. In small children it may be necessary to use only one or two fingers to feel the pulse. The three positions are named *cun*, *guan* and *chi* in Chinese, which translate as 'inch', 'gate' and 'foot' respectively. Their names are derived from their locations: inch and foot being units of measurement and a gate connecting these two positions.

The middle or *guan* position is located on the radial artery medial adjacent to the styloid process. The front or *cun* position will be nine fen (9/10 of a *cun*) distal to the *guan* position, proximal to the crease in the wrist at the base of the thenar eminence. The rear or *chi* position is 1 *cun* proximal to the *guan* position. This means that if you place the middle finger on the artery next to the Lu 8 and the index finger on the *cun* position proximal to the wrist, the ring finger will be placed proximally in almost the same distance from the *guan* position (it will be 1/10 of a *cun* further away).

Chinese name	English names
Cun	Inch
Guan	Bar or gate
Chi	Foot

It is important not to have a rigid idea of a pulse position's significance. The pulse reflects changes throughout the body in the organs, the channels and *qi* and *xue*. This means that changes occurring in the same pulse position will have different connotations when seen in different contexts. Like so much of Chinese medicine, it is the context that is the defining factor, for example other symptoms and signs that are present and the prehistory leading up to the situation. When one understands the pulse positions as being a reflection of the three *jiao*, instead of being a template of the organs' and channels' locations, it's easier to reconcile the different models. If the pulse is, for example, Superficial and Tight in the right *cun* position and the patient has a shoulder pain, the pulse will be reflecting a disturbance of the Large Intestine channel and therefore treatment of the Large Intestine channel would be relevant. If the pulse has the same quality and the person has been exposed to Wind and Cold, they have an aversion to cold and feel tired and have sore muscles, the pulse will tell you that there is an invasion of Wind-Cold blocking *wei qi*, which is a *yang* aspect of the Lung. The same pulse could also be seen when there is toothache, headache, tightness of the chest or something else.

Initially, it can be difficult and confusing to remember all the different divisions of the pulse. Some people start by just learning one of the pulse models. It is important, though, to remember that there are other models. If the pulse is not consistent with what one expects to feel, it may well be because the pulse is reflecting another aspect of the body's physiology.

The three horizontal pulse positions can also be seen as a reflection of *yin*, *yang* and *xue* in the same way as the three levels, where changes in *yang* and *yin* will affect the *cun* and *chi* positions respectively and changes in *xue* will affect the *guan* positions.

Pulse position	Type of *qi*	*Jiao*
Cun	*Qi* (*yang*)	Upper
Guan	*Xue*	Middle
Chi	*Yin*	Lower

The following are four of the best known representations of pulse positions from different historical textbooks.

Nan Jing (The Classic of Difficulties) ca. 100 CE

The pulse positions are defined by the channel pairs in relation to the Five Phase *sheng* cycle.

	Level	Left	Right
Cun	Superficial	Hand *taiyang* (Small Intestine)	Hand *yangming* (Large Intestine)
	Deep	Hand *shaoyin* (Heart)	Hand *taiyin* (Lung)
Guan	Superficial	Foot *shaoyang* (Gall Bladder)	Foot *yangming* (Stomach)
	Deep	Foot *jueyin* (Liver)	Foot *taiyin* (Spleen)
Chi	Superficial	Foot *taiyang* (Urinary Bladder)	Hand *shaoyang* (*san jiao*)
	Deep	Foot *shaoyin* (Kidney)	Hand *jueyin* (Pericardium)

Mai Jing (The Pulse Classic) – Wang Shu He, 280 CE

The pulse positions are also distributed in relation to the Five Phases. In this model the organs rather than the channels are evaluated. This is because this book focuses more on interpreting the pulse in relation to treating the patient with herbs rather than needles, so the internal organs are more relevant than the channels.

	Level	Left	Right
Cun	Superficial	Small Intestine	Large Intestine
	Deep	Heart	Lung
Guan	Superficial	Gall Bladder	Stomach
	Deep	Liver	Spleen
Chi	Superficial	Urinary Bladder	*San jiao*
	Deep	Kidney	Pericardium

Bin Hu Mai Xue (The Study of the Pulse by the Bin Hu Lake Master) – Li Shi Zhen, 1564 CE

In this model there is no distinction between the superficial and deep levels and it is mainly the *zang* organs that are being diagnosed.

	Left	**Right**
Cun	Heart	Lung
Guan	Liver	Stomach/Spleen
Chi	Kidney	Kidney

Jing Yue Quan Shu (Jing Yue Complete Book) – Zhang Jie-Bin 1624 CE

Here it is not necessarily the *zang* organ that is deepest or the *fu* organ that is most superficial.

This is the model that is mainly utilised in TCM-style Chinese medicine, i.e. the model utilised in mainland China today and also in much of the Western world.

	Left	**Right**
Cun	Heart and chest	Lung and chest
Guan	Liver and Gall Bladder	Stomach and Spleen
Chi	Kidney, Urinary Bladder and Small Intestine	Kidney and Large Intestine

The right *chi* position is perceived as representing Kidney *yang*, whereas the left *chi* position is seen as reflecting the condition of Kidney *yin*.

Although all these different models can appear to be confusing and contradictory, there is logic in the different systems. Common to them all is the fact that three pulse positions represent the upper, middle and lower aspects of the body. There is generally consensus with regards to most of the organs' and channels' positions. As written earlier, some people initially choose only to utilise one model, for example the model used in modern China, and learn these positions by heart, whilst keeping in mind that there are other models that could also be relevant.

How to take the pulse

There are various factors to take into consideration and preparations to be made before you take the pulse.

The client should sit or lie in a comfortable position. The therapist should also sit or stand in a position that is relaxed. This is because diagnosing the pulse can take a long time and if the patient is tense and uncomfortable this will affect the pulse. If you are not positioned comfortably with a relaxed arm, this will affect your concentration.

The patient's wrist should be level with or lower than their heart.

Place the middle finger on the radial artery next to Lu 8, the front finger proximal to the crease in the wrist at the base of the thenar eminence and the rear finger at a similar distance proximal to Lu 8. The distance between the positions depends upon the person's build. In children, it may be necessary to use only two fingers and afterwards palpate the different positions separately with one finger.

It is important to align the length of the three fingers. The middle finger is longer than the ring and index fingers and therefore it must be slightly bent. If the middle finger is not bent it will press harder against artery than the other two fingers, and this will give a false impression of the *guan* position's strength.

Start by noting the impression received from all three positions as a whole. This will give you a general idea of the pulse's overall quality. It can be a good idea to write down the first impression you get from the pulse, as this is often the truest. Take note of whether the pulse corresponds to the expectations that you have with regards to the person's body type, gender, age and so on.

Afterwards, you can lift two fingers so that only one position is being felt. Focus on the sensation below the tip of the finger and not the side of the finger. It is important to be aware that a strong pulse in a neighbouring position can pulsate on the side of the finger and give the impression of a pulse position below the fingertip that is stronger than it really is.

Roll the fingers back and forth and from side to side. This is to measure the breadth and width of the pulse and to feel qualities such as slipperiness and wiriness.

Press your fingers downwards and gently release the pressure again to get an impression of the depth. It is important to be conscious of the sensation in the fingertips, while both pressing and releasing the pressure. It is often whilst releasing the pressure that you get the clearest impression of the Superficial pulse and the Wiry pulse. In general, the clearest impression of depth is obtained by repeatedly pressing and releasing the finger pressure.

Let your fingers rest gently on the pulse, so you can feel the speed and rhythm of the pulse.

Count the beats.

Allow ample time to feel the pulse. Repeat the above procedures more than once. The pulse can be volatile and some of the qualities can change whilst you are feeling the pulse. This in itself can be a diagnostic sign.

Note the various qualities you have felt and the differences between the various positions and depths.

The following should be noted:

- whether the pulse has *shen*, Stomach and root

- the depth of the pulse

- the width of the pulse

- the strength of the pulse

- the rate of the pulse

- the rhythm of the pulse

- other qualities

- the *cun*, *guan* and *chi* positions.

It is a good idea to have these parameters printed in the journal or intake sheet, so you do not forget to take note of all of the qualities.

Take into account different factors that may have an effect on the pulse: the person's physical build, gender, age and profession, whether the person is tired, has just eaten, is stressed and in a rush, has just drunk coffee, etc.

The normal or healthy pulse

A healthy pulse is called *ping mai* in Chinese. For a pulse to be healthy, it must have certain qualities. It must have *shen*, Stomach and root. A pulse that lacks these qualities is called a sick pulse or *bing mai*.

Having *shen* means that the pulse has vitality, is soft and yet has strength and is regular in its beating. The pulse gets the *shen* quality from the Heart. This is similar to the quality that should be seen in the tongue and the eyes. If a pulse has *shen*, the Heart is harmonious and the prognosis is good.

Having Stomach means that the pulse is relatively slow (60–66 beats per minute), is calm and is soft. The Stomach quality comes from the Stomach and Spleen's transformation of body fluids during digestion. This is similar to the tongue, where the coating on the tongue is generated by the transformation processes in the middle *jiao*. Just as the tongue should have a thin coating indicating health, the pulse should have a smoothness and softness. Too much of these qualities on the tongue and in the pulse indicate Dampness, reflecting that there is too much impure *qi* being sent upwards with the pure *qi*.

Having root means that the pulse can be felt at the deepest level and in the *chi* positions. It is the Kidneys that give the pulse 'root'. If the pulse has root, it indicates that the Kidneys are strong and can anchor *qi*.

These three qualities represent the three treasures: *shen*, *qi* and *jing*. All three qualities must be present and in adequate amounts for the body to be harmonious. Even though the pulse can have many different qualities and even if the person is ill, a *ping mai* or healthy pulse, will indicate a good prognosis.

Disturbing factors and natural differences

There are several factors that must be taken into account when diagnosing the pulse. This is because these factors can alter the quality of the pulse. Some factors are natural differences caused by, for example, the changes in the seasons or the person's gender or age. Other things can be artificial factors, such as medicine or coffee.

The best time of day to take the pulse is early in the morning, just after the person has woken up and before they have become physically and mentally active. At this time the pulse will give the truest impression of the person. This is obviously unrealistic in a normal clinic and only something you would be able to do if you worked with in-patients.

If a person has just walked briskly, cycled or run up the stairs or is stressed, heat will have been generated in the body and the pulse rate will be faster and stronger than normal. The pulse is not giving a false impression of the body's physiology; on the contrary, it is giving a very accurate impression of the body's condition right now. The pulse is showing that there is a state of *shi* Heat caused by the physical activity. Their face will probably also be slightly redder and their skin warmer than normal. It is therefore important that the client is calm and relaxed when taking the pulse. I usually delay taking the pulse until the end of interviewing of the client. This is because I want the patient to be as relaxed as possible after their arrival at the clinic and because new patients may be nervous if it is the first time that they have been treated with acupuncture or Chinese herbs and this could affect the pulse. By waiting, one can hope that they will relax as they gain confidence in the therapist and become comfortable with the situation.

The position of the patient's arm is important. If the arm is raised above the heart itself, gravity will cause the blood to flow downwards and away from the wrist. This will make the pulse felt weaker than it really is.

Pay close attention to whereabouts on the fingertip you are feeling the pulse. If a pulse position is weak and thin, and the position next to it is strong and replete, you can risk misinterpreting the sensation in the fingertip. This is similar to the way that a loud radio can drown out the sounds coming out of a radio closer by that is turned down low.

Remember to ask the patient if they are taking medication for blood pressure, heart medications, blood thinners, anti-depressives, etc., because these will corrupt the pulse image.

Factors that can interfere with the pulse diagnosis

Factor	Effect
The person is stressed, just ran, cycled or walked quickly	Generates heat and makes the pulse rate increase in speed and strength
Stress	Can stagnate Liver *qi* and produce a Wiry pulse Stress can also generate Heat
Nervousness	Unsettles the *shen* and spreads Heart *qi*
Medication	Blurs and complicates the pulse image
The arm is higher than the heart	The pulse will be weaker

Several other factors must also be taken into account. These factors are natural differences or changes that are normal and to be expected. It is only when the person's pulse differs from what we expect to feel that it is defined as being pathological.

The pulse, like many other things, manifests the fluctuation of *yin* and *yang* throughout the year. Summer is the most *yang* time of year, so the pulse should be more *yang* in nature. It will be more superficial and overflowing. The *yang* heat of summer can increase the pulse rate so it is faster. Winter is the most *yin* time of the year when everything is drawn inwards and becomes quieter. The pulse in winter should therefore be deeper. Spring is young *yang*; it is the Wood phase. This can be felt in the pulse, which should gain a slight Wiry quality in the spring. In the autumn the pulse should become softer, because *yang* is decreasing and *yin* is increasing. This means that if a pulse is Superficial and Flooding in the winter, it is a more serious sign than if this sensation is felt in the pulse in the summer.

Men generally have stronger and more replete pulses, whilst women's are generally weaker. Because men are *yang* in nature and the left side of the body is perceived of as being *yang*,[12] their left pulse should be stronger than their right pulse, and their *cun* pulse should be stronger than their *chi* pulse. Conversely, because women are *yin*, their right pulse and their *chi* positions should be strongest. This means a deficient pulse in the left *cun* position is diagnostically more significant in a man than in a woman.

People whose occupation involves hard physical work should have a stronger pulse than someone who works in an office. Therefore, it will be a more serious sign if a man who works as a builder has a deficient pulse than it would in a woman who works as a secretary.

People who regularly play a lot of sport, physically train or work out will often have a slower pulse. Children have faster pulses and the pulse rate decreases with age. It will therefore be a more significant sign of Heat when a 50-year-old marathon runner has a pulse rate of 80 beats per minute than if it is a ten-year-old child. However, it is not necessarily a healthy sign if a person who is very physically active with a hard training programme has a slow resting pulse. The physical exertion of training and sport can damage their *yang qi*, which is why their pulse rate is slow.

The person's body build will also have an influence. An obese person's pulse will be deeper than a thin person's, whose pulse will be more superficial.

In the week before menstruation the pulse has more of the Slippery quality and in the week after menstruation the pulse is weaker, because the woman is relatively *xue xu* at this time.

The pulse is more Slippery during pregnancy. If the pulse becomes Choppy during the pregnancy, this is a negative sign and may indicate the threat of a miscarriage.

If the person is tired or has not slept properly, the pulse will be weaker.

If the person has just eaten, the pulse can be affected in two ways. The pulse may be fuller and Slippery in the right *guan* position, because there is an accumulation of food and *qi* in the Stomach. Or it may be weaker in this position, because Spleen *qi* is burdened by having to transform the meal.

The *qi*-producing organs' pulses are felt on the right wrist. The left-hand pulse includes the organs that are the root of *xue* and that store and govern *xue*. This means that the right-hand pulse will reflect the condition of *qi* and the left the state of *xue*.

Natural variations in pulse

Factor	Variation
The seasons	Spring – more Wiry
	Summer – more Superficial and Flooding
	Autumn – softer
	Winter – deeper
Gender	Men – stronger pulse than women's, stronger in the left and *cun* positions
	Women – weaker pluse than men's, stronger in the right positions and in the *chi* positions
The person's profession	Physical work – stronger pulse
	Sedentary work – weaker pulse
Individuals who physically train a lot	Slower pulse
Age and speed	Age Beats per minute
	1–4 90+
	4–10 84
	10–16 78/80
	16–35 76
	35–50 72/70
	50+ 68
Body build	Heavy set or obese – the pulse is generally deeper
	Thin body – the pulse is generally more superficial
Menstruation	The week up to menstruation – the pulse is more Slippery
	The week after menstruation – the pulse is weaker
Pregnancy	The pulse becomes more Slippery during the pregnancy
Fatigue or lack of sleep	The pulse will be weaker
The person has just eaten	The pulse can be stronger and Slippery or weaker

Diagnostic parameters

When you see the list of all the 28 different pulse qualities, it can seem overwhelming and complicated. This does not need to be the case if you utilise the correct methodology and are systematic and logical in your approach.

When you feel the pulse, you must ask yourself the following questions.

- Is the pulse superficial or deep?

- Is the pulse wide or narrow?

- Is the pulse deficient or replete?

- Is the pulse fast or slow?

- Is the pulse rhythmic?

- What other qualities are there?

Each of the questions is fairly simple, and the points are easy to differentiate individually, which is what you have to do. You must consciously investigate and answer each of these questions one by one, noting down the answers on a piece of paper. When you have the answers to these questions, you can, from the following descriptions, see which type of pulse the patient has. This is because the majority of the 28 pulse images are just different combinations of the parameters listed above.

It is easier to remember the pulse images if you divide them into categories. Seven of the pulses are superficial, four are deep and three are irregular. As a result, just determining that the pulse is superficial, for example, limits the possibilities to only seven definitions. Many pulse images can be divided into pairs, either as opposites of each other or as developments of each other. A hidden pulse, for example, has the same qualities as a weak pulse; it's just more extreme. This approach means that the 28 images quickly become much less overwhelming and more applicable in practice.

You can choose to learn the list by heart, meaning that you would be able to identify a pulse automatically when you feel it in a client.

If you cannot learn the 28 qualities by heart, you can make a copy of the table with the 28 pulse images, which you can keep close at hand. You can then compare the answers to the questions written above with the descriptions of the various pulse images.

Pulse qualities

It is important to remember that the various parameters can be combined with other qualities such as speed and strength. For example, a pulse can be both Deep and Rapid, or it could be Superficial and Tight.

The pulse depth

Learning to judge the depth of a pulse is best achieved through hands-on training with a teacher, because the differences in the depths is quite subtle. That said, learning to feel the depth of a pulse is something that can be learnt quite quickly.

The pulse should be palpable in the area just below the skin and you should be able to feel the pulse continuously while increasing the pressure and pushing deeper with the fingers. About two thirds of the way down to the bone, the sensation from the pulse will cease. The pulse should, therefore, not be felt all the way down to the bone. You should press the fingers slowly downwards and then release the pressure again slowly several times. This is because we often do not notice certain qualities as the pressure increases, but these qualities become evident on releasing the pressure, as the fingers return to the surface again.

Account must be taken of a person's body size. A thin person's pulse will generally feel more superficial than a corpulent person's. The corpulent person's pulse will feel deeper than that of a person who is thin and slender.

A healthy pulse can be felt equally clearly in all three levels. It will, though, be slightly deeper in the *chi* positions and slightly more superficial in the *cun* positions.

A Superficial pulse will be palpable with very little pressure. If the pulse is very superficial, it will be felt with no pressure at all. The Superficial pulse will either disappear completely when you push deeper or its strength will diminish as you press downwards.

The Superficial pulse is sometimes described as feeling like a piece of wood floating in water. When you push it down it disappears, but when you release the pressure, the wood floats back up again. This means that if you push your fingers down to the deepest level of the pulse and then release the pressure again, so that the fingers return to the superficial level, the sensation from the pulse increases as your fingers release the pressure.

The pulse is often only superficial in the *cun* position. The more positions the pulse is superficial in, the more serious or dominant the imbalance is.

The Deep pulse is either only palpable with pressure or its strength decreases as the pressure is released and the fingers return to the surface of the skin – the Deep pulse is felt most clearly in the middle and deepest levels and is weakest or is not present in the superficial level.

It is important to combine the pulse's depth with other factors such as speed and strength.

The pulse rate

Chinese doctors traditionally measured the speed of the pulse by counting the number of pulses in relation to their own respiration. This was before the invention of watches with a second hand. A simpler and more reliable method of counting the number of beats per minute is to count the number of beats in a period of 15 seconds and multiply this number by four. It is a good idea to repeat this measurement a couple of times, as the rate can vary. If there is a variation, this will in itself have diagnostic significance.

It is important to note that the speed of the pulse diminishes with age. The average speed of the pulse in various age groups is as follows.

Age	Beats per minute
1–4	90+
4–10	84
10–16	80
16–35	76
35–50	70
50+	68

A Rapid pulse is defined as a pulse where the beats per minute exceeds the pulse rate that you would expect for someone of that age. This means that a pulse rate of 84 beats per minute is normal for a child under the age of 10, but fast for a woman of 60. The faster the pulse, the more Heat there is. If the pulse is slower than the average, it can indicate Cold or a lack of *yang*.

People who work out and train hard physically usually have a slow pulse. This is considered by many people to be normal, so if these individuals have a normal speed pulse, it is in reality a Rapid pulse. Others, myself included, disagree with this point of view. The slow pulse rate in people who train and play a lot of sport or work out may well reflect that they have damaged their *yang* through excessive physical exertion and that their languid pulse is in fact a true reflection of their physiology.

The strength of the pulse will determine whether it is a *shi* or *xu* condition.

Situations in which the pulse is not fast, even though there is Heat present

- The person trains hard or is very physically active
- The person takes medicine
- Old age
- Damp-Heat
- Damp-Phlegm
- Mixed patterns where there is both Heat and Cold simultaneously or where there is also *qi xu* or *yang xu*
- The person has both Kidney *yin xu* and Kidney *yang xu*
- True Cold, false Heat

The pulse strength

In order to determine whether a pulse is Weak or Full, you must judge how much strength the pulse has. The strength of the pulse is determined by how much it pounds against the fingers.

A pulse without strength will only be felt faintly beneath the fingers and will disappear with pressure. There are several types of pulse that lack strength, such as an 'Empty' pulse, a 'Weak' pulse and a 'Faint' pulse. You therefore have to be careful when you use these terms, because they define specific pulse images, each with its own diagnostic significance. This is why I have capitalised the names of specific pulse qualities. If a pulse feels weak and is not very palpable, it is better to say that the pulse lacks power or strength.

It is important to distinguish between the size of the pulse, i.e. the width and depth, and how replete it is. A pulse can quite easily be large without being replete. Conversely, you could feel a pulse that is superficial and thin, yet has strength. This pulse will only be felt strongly in the superficial level and will feel weaker or non-existent when you push downwards with the fingers.

A pulse with strength can feel hard, full, tense and long. It strikes back against the finger and does not yield when pressed. It lacks softness and pliancy. It is important to be aware of where in the fingertip the sensation is felt. It should be felt just below the fingertip. If a pulse position is Weak, while the position next to it is Full, the strong pulse position can drown out the weaker one. The pressure from the Full position will be felt on the side of the fingertip, which can therefore give the impression that the pulse position that is Weak also feels as if it is Full.

A pulse that has too much strength or is Full generally indicates a *shi* condition. This reflects that there is too much *qi* present. If a Full pulse is felt in a client who has an acute illness, this is a good sign – the strength of the pulse indicating that the person has strong *zheng qi*, which is combating the *xie qi*.

The width of the pulse

Divergences in the width of the pulse result in the pulse being described as being either wide or thin. The width of the pulse can be determined by slowly rolling the fingertips laterally back and forth around the artery. A wide pulse feels broader than a thin pulse.

The pulse's width is independent of its strength and depth.

The length of the pulse

The pulse's length is determined by rolling the tips of the fingers backwards and forwards along the length of the artery. The length of the pulse is defined by how far up the arm the pulse is felt or, in the case of a Short pulse, how little it fills out the three pulse positions.

A Long pulse can be felt further up the arm towards the elbow beyond the *chi* position. The Long pulse can be a sign of Heat or rebellious Liver *qi* (Liver *qi* stagnation or ascending Liver *yang*). If the pulse is normal in its rate and strength, this is a normal pulse and it will not be given any diagnostic significance.

A Short pulse will not fill out all three pulse positions, i.e. it is not as long as a normal pulse, or it will feel as if the pulse cannot be felt fully in each of the individual pulse positions, i.e. the pulse positions themselves seem shorter than normal.

The rhythm and regularity of the pulse

The pulse should be rhythmic in its beating. It should not skip any beats and the speed, strength and other qualities should remain constant whilst you feel it. Some pulses are rhythmic in their beating but irregular in terms of strength and speed. Other pulses skip beats. When a pulse skips beats, it is important to determine whether it is the same beat that it skips, for example every fifth beat, or whether the breaks in the rhythm are random. The speed of the pulse has diagnostic significance in an irregular pulse.

Other qualities of the pulse

The other qualities will be discussed under the individual pulse categories.

Diagnostic pulse images

The easiest way to learn the various pulse images is to learn them as groups.

- Seven superficial pulses: Superficial, Drumskin, Hollow, Empty, Flooding, Soggy and Scattered.

- Four deep pulses: Deep, Weak, Hidden and Confined.

- Three irregular pulses: Knotted, Intermittent and Skipping.

- Other pulse images: Long, Short, Wiry, Tight, Choppy, Slippery, Stirring, Rapid, Very Rapid, Slow, Full, Large, Fine and Faint.

I have included the Chinese names of the pulse images because they are often translated differently from book to book. The Chinese name can be used as a reference point when reading other books.

Superficial pulse

There are several types of pulse that are classified as being superficial. It is important to note which other qualities the pulse has to distinguish the different pulses from each other. Many of the pulses are very similar to each other and their diagnostic significance is often also very similar. The main differentiating factor amongst the superficial pulses is their strength. It is important, therefore, to ask yourself whether the pulse feels strong or deficient.

A Superficial pulse will be a consequence of the presence of *xie qi* in the exterior or an interior *xu* condition. In an internal *xu* condition, the pulse will feel weaker or absent when you press down to the deep level. When there is an invasion of exogenous *xie qi*, the pulse will generally be powerful, but even more so in the superficial level. It is also important to note whether the pulse is Rapid or Slow, in order to determine if there is Heat or Cold.

The seven superficial pulses are: Superficial, Drumskin, Hollow, Empty, Flooding, Soggy and Scattered.

SUPERFICIAL PULSE (*FU MAI*)

The Superficial pulse is a pulse that is superficial and is not felt in the deep and/ or middle levels or the strength of the pulse decreases when you press your fingers downwards and increases again when the pressure is released again.

The Superficial pulse reflects that there is more *qi* and *yang* in the exterior aspects of the body. There will be a relative excess of *qi* and *yang* in the exterior aspects, either because there is a lack of *yin* to anchor *yang* or because *xue* is very weak and cannot hold *qi* down. In these cases, the pulse will be both superficial and without strength. *Yang* and *qi* may also be relatively strong in the exterior, because there is an invasion of exogenous *xie qi*. In this case, the pulse will be more replete, because there is a struggle between *wei qi* and *xie qi*. An exception, though, is if there is an invasion of exogenous *xie qi* whilst there is *wei qi xu*. In this situation, the pulse will be superficial and without strength. If there is Heat present, the pulse will be Rapid. The presence of *shi* Cold will result in a pulse that is Tight.

Extreme *yang xu* can also manifest with a Superficial pulse. This is a very serious sign and signifies that *yin* and *yang* are in the process of separating and the remaining *yang* is now drifting upwards.

Superficial pulse
Patterns of imbalance: *Xie qi* in the exterior, *yin xu*, *xue xu*, severe *qi xu* (in extreme cases *yang xu*).

Typical combinations

Superficial and Tight	Wind-Cold
Superficial and Rapid	Wind-Heat
Superficial and Slow	Invasion of exogenous Wind
Superficial and without strength	*Wei qi xu*
Superficial and empty in the middle and/or deepest level	Interior *xu* condition

DRUMSKIN (GE MAI)

Ge mai is often translated as a 'drumskin', 'leather', 'tympanic' or 'hard' pulse. This type of superficial pulse is wider than a normal pulse and it feels hard. It will provide the fingertips with resistance when you press downwards, but when you reach the middle level the resistance disappears. The width of the pulse will be felt when rolling the fingers laterally back and forth. The Drumskin pulse will be felt more laterally than the Empty and Soggy pulses. It is called a Drumskin pulse, because the pulse feels hard and wide in the same way that a drum skin does. It will also feel empty beneath the hard surface like a drum skin. The Drumskin pulse is not something that you will ordinarily encounter in a normal practice; it arises when there is a significant loss of blood. In Chinese medicine, the heavy blood loss will result in an extreme *xue xu* and/or *yin xu*. This will result in an abundance of *yang qi* ascending up to the surface. *Yang* is expansive in its dynamic; the pulse will therefore be superficial, hard and wide, but because there is an extreme deficiency of *yin* and *xue*, it will feel empty further down. Extreme *jing xu* can also manifest with this type of pulse.

Drumskin pulse
Patterns of imbalance: *Xue xu, yin xu.*

EMPTY PULSE (*XU MAI*)

This pulse is also translated as 'vacuous' and 'deficient'. Similar to the Drumskin pulse, the Empty pulse is superficial and wide, but the difference between the two is that the Empty pulse is not hard and the pulse is without force. The Empty pulse's weakness is reflective of a *xu* condition. If the pulse is also Rapid, it will be a manifestation of *yin xu* Heat. This pulse can also be seen when there is *jing xu* or *qi xu* or if a person has been invaded by exogenous Summer Heat that has injured *jinye* and *yin*. If there is an invasion of Summer-Heat, the pulse will be Rapid.

Empty pulse
Patterns of imbalance: *Yin xu, xue xu, qi xu* and *jing xu*.

Typical combinations

Empty and Rapid pulse	*Yin xu* Heat or Summer-Heat

HOLLOW PULSE (*KOU MAI*)

This pulse is often translated as a 'scallion stalk' pulse. This pulse, like the Empty pulse, is superficial and without strength. The difference between the two is that when you push down to the middle level, the Hollow pulse disappears completely. There is disagreement in the texts about what happens if you push further down to the deep level. Some books write that you will feel the pulse again at the deepest level, others that you will not. Some also state that the edges of the pulse can be felt clearly when you roll your fingers back and forth across the pulse.

The reason that the pulse is called a 'scallion stalk' is that it feels like the stem of a spring onion. If you put your fingertips on a scallion stalk, it will feel round and wide but also frail and without strength. There is nothing in the centre of it and a void will be felt when you press harder on the scallion stalk.

The middle level of the pulse reflects the condition of *xue* and the Stomach and Spleen. An emptiness in this middle level will therefore be interpreted as more a severe *xu* condition than if there was an 'Empty' pulse that was not empty in the middle level.

Hollow pulse
Patterns of imbalance: *Yin xu, xue xu, qi xu* and *jing xu*.

Typical combinations

Hollow and Rapid pulse	*Yin xu* Heat or Summer-Heat

SCATTERED PULSE (SAN MAI)

This pulse is superficial, wide and without strength and disappears on pressure. The difference between this and a Hollow pulse is that the Hollow pulse has clearly defined boundaries when the fingers are rolled back and forth. This is not the case with the Scattered pulse. The edges of the vessel are not defined, making them difficult to perceive. The pulse is so feeble that it disappears with the slightest touch. Maciocia describes the sensation as being like a lot of small dots below the fingertip instead of a wave. (Maciocia 2004, p.484)

The Scattered pulse arises in the same situations as the Drumskin pulse. The difference between them is that in the Scattered pulse the loss of *qi* means that the walls of the vessel lack *qi* and this can be felt by the lack of clear definition. The diagnostic significance of the two pulses is therefore almost identical, but with the difference that in a 'Scattered' pulse the loss of *qi* is greater.

Scattered pulse
Patterns of imbalance: *Yin xu, xue xu, qi xu* and *jing xu*.

SOGGY PULSE (RU MAI)

Some sources term this pulse 'soft'. This pulse image is described in *Huang Di Nei Jing – Su Wen* as being like a piece of silk thread lying on the surface of water. This description is very apt. The pulse will be felt superficially; it is without strength and feels narrow when rolling the tips of the fingers back and forth. The pulse will disappear when you press your fingertips downwards. The Soggy pulse can be felt when there is *qi xu* and *xue xu* and when there is Dampness. The Dampness will 'smother' the pulse as if it is wrapped in cotton wool. The *qi xu* and *xue xu* will mean that the pulse does not have the strength to be 'heard' through the Dampness.

Soggy pulse
Patterns of imbalance: Dampness, *qi xu* and *xue xu*.

Typical combinations

Soggy and Rapid	Damp-Heat
Soggy and Slow	Damp-Cold

FLOODING PULSE (HONG MAI)

This pulse is also translated as 'overflowing' and 'surging'. This pulse is felt when there is extreme Heat. The pulse's name alludes to the sensation it creates. It is large, replete, wide and superficial. It is like a flood wave that overflows or a tidal wave. The pulse rises powerfully from the deep level and hits the fingers with force in the superficial level.

The Flooding pulse will often be experienced when exogenous *xie qi* has penetrated down to the *qi* level or the *yangming* aspect. At this point there will usually be a fierce struggle between *zheng qi* and *xie qi*. This struggle will manifest with a very replete pulse. At the same time, the exuberant Heat that the struggle generates will increase the speed of the pulse so that it is quite fast. The Heat is so intense that it forces *qi* and *jinye* to the surface and this can be felt in the pulse.

The Flooding pulse can start as a deep or normal pulse in the *chi* position and increase in strength and width, rising upwards so that when it reaches the *cun* position, it is superficial, wide and replete.

Maciocia writes that the Overflowing pulse will sometimes only be felt in one position (Maciocia 2004, p.487). In this case, this pulse position will feel very strong and full in the superficial aspect relative to the other pulse positions. This is a sign that there is Heat in the organ or organs related to this pulse position.

If the pulse is generally weak, but is relatively full and superficial in a single position, it will be a manifestation of *yin xu* Heat in this organ or organs.

Flooding pulse
Patterns of imbalance: *Shi* Heat, *yin xu* Heat.

Deep pulses

The clinical significance of the deep pulses is that the imbalance is in the interior. The imbalance can be both *xu* or *shi* in nature. The pulse can be deep because it lacks *yang* and *qi* to lift it up to the surface or there may be *xie qi*, which inhibits *qi*, *xue* and *yang* from lifting the pulse upwards. The difference between a *xu* condition and a stagnation will be felt by the pulse being either without strength or being forceful, respectively.

The four deep pulses are: Deep, Weak, Hidden and Confined.

DEEP PULSE (*CHEN MAI*)

The Deep pulse will be felt when you have pressed down from the superficial level (and will only be felt in the middle and/or the deepest levels) or when the strength of the pulse increases as you press down and decreases again upon releasing the pressure of your fingers.

That the pulse is Deep is not enough information in itself and it must be coupled with other qualities before it can be used diagnostically.

If the pulse lacks strength, it will be because there is not enough *qi* or *yang* to 'raise' the pulse upwards.

If it is forceful, it is because *qi* and *yang* are blocked by Cold, food stagnation, *qi* stagnation, *xue* stagnation or a stagnation of fluids. The speed of the pulse will also determine whether it is a Hot or Cold condition.

Deep pulse
Patterns of imbalance: The imbalance is in the interior, *yang xu*, *qi xu*, *qi* stagnation food stagnation, Phlegm, Dampness, *xue* stagnation, Cold.

Typical combinations

Deep and Slow	Internal Cold
Deep and Rapid	Internal Heat
Deep and forceful	Internal *shi* condition
Deep and without strength	Internal *xu* condition
Deep and Tight	Internal stagnation
Deep and Slippery	Phlegm
Deep and Fine	Dampness or *qi* and *xue xu*

WEAK PULSE (*RUO MAI*)

The Weak pulse is felt only in the deepest level or the pulse feels weak in depth and decreases even more when pressure is released by the fingers. The Weak pulse lacks force and when the tips of the finger are rolled back and forth it feels narrow. This is because there is either not enough *yuan qi* and *xue* to fill the vessel or because *yang* is so weak that it cannot push outward and upwards.

Weak pulse
Patterns of imbalance: *Qi xu*, *xue xu* and *yang xu*.

Typical combinations

Weak and Slow	*Yang xu* Cold
Weak and Choppy	*Xue* and *qi xu*

HIDDEN PULSE (*FU MAI*)

The Hidden pulse is a more extreme version of the Deep pulse. The Hidden or 'deep-lying' pulse will only be felt near the bone and only when the fingers are pressed down firmly, so it is much deeper than the Deep pulse. You have to press very deeply and be very attentive to your fingertips before you can feel it. It is, again, important to differentiate between a feeble and a forceful pulse. The diagnostic significance of the Hidden pulse is the same as for the Deep pulse but more extreme and more serious.

Hidden pulse
Patterns of imbalance: Stagnation or extreme *yang xu*.

Typical combinations

Hidden and without strength	Severe *yang xu* or *qi xu*
Hidden and forceful	Severe stagnation in the interior
Hidden and Rapid	Internal Heat
Hidden and Slow	Internal Cold

CONFINED PULSE (*LAO MAI*)

The Confined pulse, which is also sometimes called a 'firm' pulse, is a deep, long, forceful and hard pulse. It provides resistance when you press down on it and it lacks softness. The difference between this pulse and the Full pulse is that the Full pulse is felt clearly in all three levels, whereas the Confined pulse is only felt in the deepest level. When you feel a pulse that is deep and hard, it will be because there is something that is stagnating *qi* and *xue* in the vessel. This could be Cold, food stagnation, *qi* stagnation, Dampness, Phlegm or *xue* stagnation.

> **Confined pulse**
> Patterns of imbalance: Cold, *qi* stagnation, *xue* stagnation or food stagnation.

Typical combinations

Confined and Slow	Internal *shi* Cold
Confined and Choppy	*Xue* stagnation

Irregular pulses

The three irregular pulses are the Knotted, Intermittent and Skipping. All three of these pulses miss beats. The difference between the three lies in their overall speed and whether they are irregular or regular in which beats they skip. When the pulse is very irregular, it can be difficult to assess how rapid the pulse really is. This is because if the pulse skips a lot of beats, it is difficult to estimate how many beats per minute there otherwise would have been.

An irregular pulse is always indicative of a Heart imbalance, both in the Western medicine and Chinese medicine sense.

KNOTTED PULSE (*JIE MAI*)

This is sometimes also translated as a 'bound' pulse. The Knotted pulse is slow and irregular in its rhythm. It randomly misses beats. The reason for it missing beats and its slowness is because there is something (Phlegm, Cold, *xue* stagnation or food stagnation for example) inhibiting the Heart from circulating *xue* through the channel and vessels, or because Heart *qi* or Heart *yang* are too weak to perform their functions.

In the former, the pulse will also be forceful, whereas it will lack strength in a *xu* condition.

Knotted pulse
Patterns of imbalance: *Qi* stagnation, *xue* stagnation, Phlegm stagnation, food stagnation, Heart *qi xu* or Heart *yang xu.*

Typical combinations

Knotted and forceful	*Qi* stagnation, *xue* stagnation, Phlegm or food stagnation
Knotted and without strength	Heart *qi xu* or Heart *yang xu*

INTERMITTENT PULSE (*DAI MAI*)

Unlike the Knotted pulse, the Intermittent or 'regularly interrupted' pulse is regular in terms of which beats it skips. After it has skipped a beat, it will feel like the pulse waits momentarily before it starts beating again. This is because *qi* is so weak that it is unable to keep *xue* in motion and the body must gain strength before it can move *xue* again. It may be necessary to feel the pulse for a long time before it skips a beat – perhaps as many as 50 beats. The Intermittent pulse arises in *xu* conditions of the Heart and in one or more of the other *zang* organs.

Intermittent pulse
Patterns of imbalance: *Zang* organ *xu.*

SKIPPING PULSE (*CU MAI*)

The Skipping pulse is also termed 'hasty' in some books. This pulse is rapid and irregular. It randomly skips beats. The Skipping pulse can arise when internal Heat over-activates the Heart. It is as if the Heart beats so fast that the pulse cannot keep pace. *Yang qi* has become more powerful than *yin* can control and harmonise. This means that *qi* separates from *xue* and 'races' ahead. The Heat can also create stagnations of *xue* or Phlegm, which then block the flow of *xue* in the vessels.

The Heat is usually *shi* in nature and will be due to factors such as *xie qi*, stagnations of *qi*, *xue*, Phlegm or food, or Heat from other organs. This pulse image can also arise in extreme and severe conditions where *yin* and *yang* are beginning to separate from each other. In this case, the pulse will be very frail.

Skipping pulse
Patterns of imbalance: Heat.

Typical combinations

Skipping and forceful	*Shi* Heat
Skipping and without strength	Extreme *yin xu*

Other pulse qualities

WIRY PULSE (*XIAN MAI*)

This pulse is also translated as 'bow string' or 'taut'. This is a very common pulse quality, and when you have felt it a few times, you are never in doubt about it again. It is thin and hard and pushes into the fingers like a guitar string. This will be especially noticeable when you release the pressure and let your fingers move upwards from the deep level to the surface – it is as if the pulse is in a hurry to get back to the surface after it has been pressed down.

The Wiry pulse will most often be seen when there is a Liver imbalance, usually Liver *qi* stagnation or ascending Liver *yang*, and also when there is Liver Wind or Liver Fire.

The Wiry pulse can also arise when there is pain or *xue* stagnation and in Phlegm conditions.

> **Wiry pulse**
> Patterns of imbalance: Liver imbalances *xue* stagnation, Phlegm, pain.

Typical combinations

Wiry and Rapid	*Qi* or Phlegm stagnation that generate Heat
Wiry and Slow	Cold stagnation in the Liver channel
Wiry and Slippery	Phlegm

TIGHT PULSE (*JIN MAI*)

This is also a 'hard' pulse like the Wiry pulse, but here the pulse is wider and less springy. It feels like a rope that has been twisted and tightened, such as a tightrope. The Tight pulse is seen when there is Cold. The Cold can be both in the exterior and in the interior. The depth of the pulse will be decisive.

The Tight pulse can also be experienced when there is pain.

> **Tight pulse**
> Patterns of imbalance: Cold, pain.

Typical combinations

Tight and Slow	Cold
Tight and Superficial	Invasion of Wind-Cold
Tight and Deep	Internal *shi* Cold
Tight and Slippery	Cold and Phlegm stagnation

SLIPPERY PULSE (*HUA MAI*)

The Slippery pulse feels very smooth, like 'glass beads rolling in a bowl' or the sensation that is felt when you squeeze an almond that has been boiled and the skin slips off. It has also been described as water droplets on a duck's back. Like the Wiry pulse, this pulse will be easily recognised once you have felt it a few times.

Women who are in the later stages of pregnancy should have a Slippery pulse, so this may present an opportunity to experience this pulse in practice.

A normal pulse or *ping mai* should feel slightly slippery. This is due to the movement of *xue* through channels and vessels giving the pulse this quality. It is part of the pulse's 'Stomach' quality. It indicates that there is sufficient *xue*, *qi* and *jinye* and that *xue* is flowing freely through the vessel system. The pulse should have an aspect of the slippery quality in the same way that the tongue should have a thin coating. A small amount is a healthy sign, but too much coating on the tongue or slipperiness in the pulse is a pathological sign.

Heat can agitate *xue*. This will cause *xue* to flow faster through the vessels. The increased movement of *xue* will give the pulse a more slippery quality. In this case, the pulse will be Slippery and Rapid.

The Slippery pulse is often an indication that there is Dampness and Phlegm in the body. Dampness and Phlegm will mean that there is extra lubrication in the vessels, so *xue* flows more smoothly than usual.

Food stagnation can also lead to the creation of Dampness, Phlegm and Heat, thereby making the pulse Slippery.

Slippery pulse
Patterns of imbalance: Phlegm, Dampness, food stagnation, Heat, pregnancy.

Typical combinations

Slippery and Superficial	Wind-Damp or Wind-Phlegm
Slippery and Deep	Food stagnation, Phlegm or Dampness in the interior
Slippery and Rapid	Phlegm-Heat or Damp-Heat
Slippery and Slow	Damp-Cold or Phlegm-Cold
Slippery and Large	Phlegm-Heat
Slippery and without strength	Dampness or Phlegm due to *qi xu*

CHOPPY PULSE (*SE MAI*)

This pulse is often also translated as a 'rough' or 'hesitant' pulse. A Choppy pulse can be experienced in various ways. The pulse can feel coarse and rough like sandpaper beneath your fingers. The pulse feels a bit 'dry'. Another quality the pulse can have is that the strength and rhythm may vary whilst you are feeling it. It is therefore also called a 3/5 pulse in Chinese, because sometimes there are three beats to each breath and sometimes there are five beats for each breath. Even though the rhythm can vary, the pulse does not skip any beats, it just accelerates and decreases in speed and/or strength.

One of the classical images used to describe this pulse is that it feels like a knife being scraped along a piece of bamboo. This conjures up two images. First, there is a roughness in the fingers as the knife scrapes along the bamboo. Second, the knots in the bamboo are unevenly distributed and are different sizes. This means that there will be an unevenness in the frequency and the size of the bumps as the knife passes over them. Another classical image that demonstrates how the Choppy pulse feels is fine rain falling in sand. This again conjures up a slightly abrasive sensation in the mind. In comparison, the normal pulse feels like rain running off a smooth jade stone.

The reason why this pulse has these rough and choppy qualities is that *qi* and *xue* are not flowing freely. The pulse has therefore lost some of its smoothness. The Choppy pulse will almost always arise due to there being too little *xue* in the vessels, meaning that *xue* cannot flow unhindered and smoothly through the vessels. This is like a stream that is starting to dry out. The pulse will be relatively weak. If the pulse is replete and Choppy, it is because there is a *shi* pattern of *xue* stagnation, and the stagnant *xue* is preventing *xue* from flowing freely through the vessels.

Apart from *xue* stagnation and *xue xu*, the Choppy pulse can also be seen when there is *jinye xu* and *jing xu*.

Where the Slippery pulse is normal and signifies positive qualities in pregnancy, the Choppy pulse is a very negative sign if it suddenly appears in a pregnancy, as it may indicate a possible miscarriage.

Choppy pulse
Patterns of imbalance: *Xue xu*, *xue* stagnation, *jinye xu*, *jing xu*.

Typical combinations

Choppy and Wiry	*Qi* and *xue xu*
Choppy and replete	*Xue* stagnation
Choppy and Weak	*Qi* and *xue xu*
Choppy and Soggy	*Qi* and *xue xu* with Dampness
Choppy and Deep	*Qi* and *xue xu*
Choppy and Knotted	*Xue* stagnation due to *shi* or *xu* Cold

S<small>TIRRING PULSE</small> (*DONG MAI*)

This pulse is also called a 'moving' or 'shaking' pulse. The Stirring pulse will be seen when a person is in shock or acute pain. It is as if the pulse does not travel in a wave but remains in the individual positions and vibrates. The pulse is described as being like a bean that spins around on its own axle. The pulse is fast, smooth and strong. Pain results in the pulse contracting and becoming Wiry; shock causes *qi* to become chaotic. *Qi* and *xue* separate from each other and *qi* races ahead without *xue* being able to follow.

> **Stirring pulse**
> Patterns of imbalance: Shock, acute pain.

S<small>LOW PULSE</small> (*CHI MAI*)

As described earlier, what is defined as a Slow pulse will be different from person to person. A rule of thumb is that a pulse that is slower than 64 beats per minute is a Slow pulse. The Slow pulse arises when there is Cold. *Xu* Cold can be seen when there is *yang xu*, in which case the pulse will be Weak and Slow. *Shi* Cold blocks *yang* and inhibits *xue* in its movement by contracting the vessels together. When there is *shi* Cold, the pulse will feel Tight or Confined. The depth of the pulse will give an indication of which aspect of the body the Cold is located in.

> **Slow pulse**
> Patterns of imbalance: Cold.

Typical combinations

Slow and Weak	*Yang xu*
Slow and Full, Tight or Confined	*Shi* Cold
Slow and Superficial	Invasion of exogenous Cold
Slow and Deep	Internal Cold
Slow and Slippery	Slim or Damp-Cold

R<small>APID PULSE</small> (*SHU MAI*)

The Rapid pulse is usually a pulse where there are more than 80 beats per minute. What defines a rapid pulse will depend on the person's age. The Rapid pulse is always a sign of Heat. Heat agitates the Heart accelerating its circulation of *xue*. The strength of the pulse will determine if it is *yin xu* Heat or *shi* Heat; the depth of the pulse will determine in which aspect of the body the Heat is located.

Even though a fast pulse always indicates the presence of Heat, the opposite is not always the case. There are several situations in which the pulse is not rapid even though there is Heat. In some of these situations the lack of speed in the pulse has diagnostic relevance; in others it does not.

Some of the reasons that the pulse is not rapid, despite the presence of Heat are:

- the person plays a lot of sport or is very physically active
- the person takes medication
- old age
- Damp-Heat
- Phlegm
- the Heat is chronic and has weakened *qi*
- mixed patterns where there is both Heat and Cold
- concurrent Kidney *yin xu* and Kidney *yang xu*
- true Cold, false Heat.

There are also situations where the pulse is Rapid, even though the person does not have a Heat imbalance. This will usually be due to the temporary presence of Heat in the body, for example, because the person has just run up the stairs, which will have generated warmth in the body. The person's face will be red, they will sweat and their pulse will be faster than normal. These are all Heat signs, indicating that the person has Heat in the body right now. This is, however, a temporary condition with no diagnostic relevance.

Other conditions that can cause the pulse to temporarily accelerate are:

- mental stress
- irritability and anger
- shock
- overexertion in a patient who is *qi* and *xue xu*
- nervousness.

> **Rapid pulse**
> Patterns of imbalance: Heat.

Typical combinations

Rapid and without strength	*Yin xu* Heat
Rapid and forceful	*Shi* Heat
Rapid and Superficial	Invasion of exogenous Heat
Rapid and Deep	Internal Heat
Rapid and Slippery	Phlegm-Heat or Damp-Heat

VERY RAPID PULSE (*JI MAI*)

This pulse is the same as a Rapid pulse but even faster. The dynamics of the pulse are the same. The Heat is so powerful here that *yin* is being injured.

> **Very Rapid pulse**
> Patterns of imbalance: Extreme Heat.

Typical combinations

Very Rapid and without strength	*Yin xu* Heat
Very Rapid and replete	*Shi* Heat
Very Rapid and Superficial	Invasion of exogenous Heat
Very Rapid and Deep	Internal Heat
Very Rapid and Slippery	Phlegm-Heat or Damp-Heat

SHORT PULSE (*DUAN MAI*)

The Short pulse does not occupy all the positions. It will often be in the *cun* position that the pulse is not fully present. The pulse reflects that *yang qi* cannot ascend all the way up to the upper *jiao*. This may be because there is something blocking it, probably food stagnation, or because there is a severe *qi xu*.

> **Short pulse**
> Patterns of imbalance: *qi* stagnation, food stagnation, *qi xu*.

Typical combinations

Short and without strength	*Qi xu*
Short and forceful	Stagnation
Short, forceful and Rapid	Stagnation condition that is generating Heat
Short and Slippery	Phlegm stagnation

LONG PULSE (*CHANG MAI*)

The Long pulse can be felt further up the arm proximal to the *chi* position. Most people have a Long pulse and therefore the Long pulse is a *ping mai* (healthy pulse) unless there are other qualities present. If there are other qualities present, the Long pulse will usually indicate that there is Heat or rebellious Liver *qi*. A long pulse can also be defined as a pulse that extends further than an individual position itself, i.e. a pulse that is felt when rolling the individual fingertip distally and proximally along the pulse.

> **Long pulse**
> Patterns of imbalance: Heat, rebellious Liver *qi*.

Typical combinations

Long and Rapid	Heat
Long and Wiry	Rebellious Liver *qi*

LARGE PULSE (*DA MAI*)

The Large pulse is a pulse that is broad and replete. It is rarely used as a separate pulse image, but is usually used as an aspect of other pulse images. The expansive dynamic of Heat is the mechanism behind this pulse image.

> **Large pulse**
> Patterns of imbalance: Heat.

FINE PULSE (*XI MAI*)

The Fine pulse is also translated as 'thin' and 'thready'. The Fine pulse is thin, weak and soft. It will feel like a piece of silk thread, but, unlike the Soggy pulse, the Fine pulse is not superficial. The Fine pulse arises when there is too little *xue*, *yin* or *qi* to fill the vessel or when Damp 'smothers' the vessels.

> **Fine pulse**
> Patterns of imbalance: *Xue xu, yin xu, qi xu*, Damp.

Typical combinations

Fine and Rapid	*Yin xu* Heat
Fine and Slow	*Qi* and *xue xu* plus Cold
Fine and Choppy	*Xue xu*
Fine and Slippery	Dampness

FAINT PULSE (*WEI MAI*)

The Weak pulse is also called a 'minute' pulse.

The Weak pulse is a more extreme version of the Fine pulse, as it is even thinner, weaker and softer. The pulse can be difficult to palpate because it is so weak and thin. The diagnostic significance and the dynamics are the same as those for the Fine pulse. The Faint pulse is seen when there is extreme *qi xu*, *xue xu* and *yin xu*. It will always be a chronic condition.

> **Faint pulse**
> Patterns of imbalance: Extreme *qi xu*, extreme *yin xu*, extreme *xue xu.*

Typical combinations

Faint and Rapid	Extreme *yin xu* Heat
Faint and Slow	Extreme *qi* and *xue xu* plus Cold
Faint and Choppy	Extreme *xue xu*

FULL PULSE (*SHI MAI*)

The Full pulse is also known as an 'excessive' or 'replete' pulse. The Full pulse feels strong, long and hard to the touch. It is felt on all three levels. The Full pulse will arise from *shi* patterns of imbalance. This is because when there is *xie qi* present, there will be more *qi* present in the body than normal. This results in the pulse feeling 'fuller'.

The speed of the pulse will determine if there is *shi* Heat or *shi* Cold.

> **Full pulse**
> Patterns of imbalance: *Shi* conditions.

Typical combinations

Full and Slow	*Shi* Cold
Full and Rapid	*Shi* Heat
Full and Tight	*Shi* Cold
Full and Slippery	Phlegm

Overview of the 28 pulse qualities

English name	Pinyin name	Significance	Quality
Superficial	*Fu mai*	*Xie qi* in the exterior, *yin xu*, *xue xu*, severe *qi xu* (in extreme cases *yang xu*)	Superficial, lacks strength in depth
Drumskin	*Ge mai*	*Xue/yin* loss, extreme *jing xu*	Superficial, wide, hard
Flooding	*Hong mai*	Heat	Superficial in *cun* position, but not in the *chi* position Forceful, superficial, wide
Empty	*Xu mai*	*Xue xu*, *yin xu*, *qi xu*, *jing xu* and Summer-Heat	Superficial, without strength
Hollow	*Kou mai*	*Xue xu*, *yin xu*	Superficial, wide, without strength, empty in the middle

English name	Pinyin name	Significance	Quality
Scattered	*San mai*	*Xue*, *yin* or *qi* loss	Superficial, wide, without strength, no edges, empty upon pressure
Soggy	*Ru mai*	*Qi xu*, *xue xu*, Dampness	Superficial, thin without force
Deep	*Chen mai*	*Yang xu*, *qi xu*, *xie qi* in the interior or stagnation	Deep
Weak	*Ruo mai*	*Yang xu*, *xue xu*, *yuan qi xu*	Deep, thin, no strength
Hidden	*Fu mai*	Stagnation or extreme *yang xu*	Very deep
Confined	*Lao mai*	Stagnation of Cold, food, *qi*, *xue* or Dampness	Deep, wide, long, hard
Knotted	*Jie mai*	*Qi* stagnation, Phlegm, *xue* stagnation, food stagnation, *shi* Cold, *yang xu*, Heart *qi xu*, *yuan qi xu*, *jing xu*	Slow, irregular
Intermittent	*Dai mai*	Organ *qi xu*	Regular disturbance in the rhythm
Skipping	*Cu mai*	*Shi* Heat or *yin* and *yang* are separating	Rapid, irregular
Wiry	*Xian mai*	Liver imbalances, pain, Phlegm	Thin, hard, feels like a guitar string
Tight	*Jin mai*	Cold, pain	Wide, hard
Slippery	*Hua mai*	Dampness, Phlegm, food stagnation, Heat, pregnancy	Feels slippery, like small beads in oil
Choppy	*Se mai*	*Xue xu*, *xue* stagnation	Variable strength and speed or rough feeling
Stirring	*Dong mai*	Shock, pain	Slippery, rapid, forceful, vibrating
Slow	*Chi mai*	Cold	Less than 60 beats per minute
Rapid	*Shu mai*	Heat	More than 80 beats per minute
Very Rapid	*Ji mai*	Extreme heat	More than 110 beats per minute
Short	*Duan mai*	Extreme *qi* or *xue xu*, food stagnation	Does not completely occupy all the positions
Long	*Chang mai*	Heat or rebellious Liver *qi* (can also be normal, if there are no other pathological changes in the pulse)	Longer than normal
Large	*Da mai*	Heat	Wide, overflows its boundaries, is forceful
Fine	*Xi mai*	*Yin xu*, *xue xu*, Dampness with *qi xu*	Soft, weak, thin
Faint	*Wei mai*	Extreme *xue xu*, *qi xu* or *yin xu*	Very weak, very thin
Full	*Shi mai*	*Shi* condition in which there is *xie qi* at the same time as strong *zheng qi*	Wide, forceful in all levels

Palpation of the abdomen, including Hara diagnosis

Palpation of the abdomen includes observing the general sensation and warmth of the abdominal region. Palpation of the abdomen also encompasses palpation of the channels, *mu*-collecting points and the so-called Hara diagnosis. In Hara diagnosis the abdominal area is divided into various zones that relate to the internal organs. Changes in these zones will indicate that there is an imbalance in the organ.

Palpation of the abdomen

Varying amounts of pressure should be applied whilst palpating the abdomen. Start by gently placing the hand lightly on the skin and slowly draw your fingers over the skin. This allows you to get a sense of the temperature, smoothness and moistness of the skin. Next, slowly apply pressure to the different areas of the abdomen with the fingers. Start with a light, superficial touch to get a sense of the elasticity of the skin and resistance in the superficial tissue. Then, gently press deeper to gauge the resistance further down. Take note of how hard and elastic the area feels and whether there are any lumps. The abdomen should be relatively soft and elastic in the surface aspect, but there should be an increasing resistance the deeper one presses.

Whilst palpating, be aware of any noises from the patient. The noises can be the patient's verbal responses, indicating discomfort, pain or pleasure, or involuntary sounds from the body, such as sloshing or bubbling sounds in the intestines.

A woman's abdomen should generally be softer than a man's. This means that if you feel a very soft and flaccid abdomen in a man, it has greater diagnostic significance than if you feel the same quality in a woman. Conversely, a very tense and hard abdomen is a more negative sign in a woman than it is in a man.

Temperature

It is important that the entire abdomen has a uniform temperature. Hotter skin in one area will indicate the presence of Heat, whereas cold skin will tell you that there is Cold or *yang xu* present. It is, of course, important to take clothing into account. If the person has just come in from outside and is wearing clothes that only partly cover the abdomen or are very thin, this area of the abdomen will probably feel colder. In children, palpable heat in the abdomen will usually be an indication of food stagnation, the Heat from the food stagnation emanating through the abdominal skin.

Tension and hardness

When the abdomen feels hard and tense, it indicates that there is a *shi* condition.

Qi stagnation will manifest with abdominal distension. The abdomen may be visibly bloated or the area may just feel hard and tense but also elastic. It will feel a bit like a trampoline. The patient will usually experience discomfort being palpated. This is because the pressure from the fingers increases the amount of *qi* in an area that already has an excess of *qi*.

If there is food or *xue* stagnation the abdomen will also feel hard and tense, but there will not be the same elasticity in the abdomen as when there is *qi* stagnation. A sharp pain on palpation is a further indicator of *xue* stagnation. Food stagnation can elicit a distended sensation in the abdomen. Dampness can also give a similar sensation.

The area below the costal region can become tense and hard when there are Liver and Gall Bladder imbalances or when there is *xie qi* locked in the *shaoyang* aspect.

Tightness in the epigastric area, inferior to the sternum, will indicate a stagnation in either the Stomach or the Heart.

Tension in the central area of the lower portion of the abdomen above the pubic bone is felt when there is a *shi* condition of the Urinary Bladder or the Small Intestine.

If the areas lateral and inferior to the umbilicus are tight, this indicates a *chong mai* stagnation or a stagnation in the Intestines. Stagnation of *qi* or *xue* in the *chong mai* can also manifest with tightness around the umbilicus. If this area is flaccid and loose, it can indicate that there is a *xu* condition in the Kidneys, *ren mai* or *chong mai*.

An abdomen that has an overall flaccid and soft sensation is felt when there is a *xu* condition. Spleen and Stomach *qi xu* will manifest with softness in the upper part of the abdomen whilst Spleen and Kidney *qi xu* can manifest with a lack of tension in the lower part of the abdomen.

Palpation of the abdominal flesh is indispensable in paediatric diagnosis.

Pain

When there are *shi* patterns of imbalance, pain and discomfort can be experienced by the patient during palpation. A sharp, severe pain is a more serious diagnostic sign than a deep tenderness or soreness. If there is a pain or discomfort that is alleviated by pressure, or if the palpation feels pleasurable, the imbalance will be *xu* in nature. On the other hand, a pain that is aggravated by palpation indicates a *shi* condition.

Lumps

If lumps are felt during palpation, it will be a manifestation of a *shi* imbalance. This is because the physical masses arise when there is an accumulation of *qi*, *xue* and/or Phlegm.

Differentiation is made between lumps that are localised and do not move and lumps that can change position when you press them.

Physical accumulations that are not fixed will be palpable sometimes and not at other times. *Qi* stagnation can create temporary accumulations, because *qi* is more volatile than *xue* and Phlegm. This means that accumulations that arise from a stagnation of *qi* will move around the area and will sometimes vanish. *Xue* stagnation and Phlegm stagnation lumps will be fixed in location and will not be movable.

Xue stagnation accumulations will feel harder than Phlegm accumulations and will have more defined edges. *Xue* stagnation lumps are also characterised by being more painful.

Damp-Heat can also create lumps in the lower *jiao*. These will be very sore and painful on palpation.

Physical accumulations can also be palpated in the area of the intestines. These may be stools in the intestines, which do not have diagnostic significance.

Physical accumulations can also be used prognostically. If the lump is reduced in size after the treatment, this is sign of progress and a good prognosis.

Patients with physical accumulations should always be referred for further examination by a Western medical doctor.

Sounds

Water retention due to Cold or *yang xu* can result in sloshing sounds as if there is liquid that is swishing around the Intestines or the Stomach.

Palpation of the abdomen

Observation	Significance
Warm skin	Heat conditions, food stagnation in young children
Cold skin	*Yang xu* or an invasion of Cold
Hard and tense abdomen	*Qi* stagnation, food stagnation, *xue* stagnation or Dampness
Soft and flaccid abdomen	Spleen and Stomach *qi xu* (upper abdomen) or Spleen and Kidney *qi xu* (lower abdomen)
Pain and tenderness	Cold, Heat, *xue* stagnation, Damp-Heat, *qi* stagnation, food stagnation or Dampness
Lumps	*Xue* stagnation, *qi* stagnation, Damp-Heat or Phlegm
Sloshing sounds in the abdomen	Accumulation of fluids in the Intestines due to Cold or *yang xu*
Tension in the hypochondriac region	Liver and Gall Bladder imbalances, *xie qi* in the *shaoyang* aspect
Tension in the epigastric region	Stomach and Heart stagnation
Tension around the umbilicus	*Chong mai* stagnation
Tension in the lower region of the abdomen	*Chong mai* stagnation, *shi* imbalance in the Urinary Bladder, Small Intestine or Large Intestine
Flaccid upper abdomen	Stomach and Spleen *qi xu*
Flaccid lower abdomen	Kidney and Spleen *qi xu*
Flaccid around the umbilicus	Kidney *qi xu*, *ren mai xu* imbalances or *chong mai xu* imbalances

Hara diagnosis

Hara diagnosis is a diagnostic technique utilised in some forms of Japanese acupuncture and shiatsu. Hara diagnosis differs from conventional abdominal palpation in that the abdomen is divided into different areas that relate to specific internal organs based on the descriptions from the *Nan Jing*. This is especially useful when utilising a Five Phase diagnosis. By palpating the abdomen, one can determine whether an organ is out of balance. When an organ is out of balance, there will be palpable changes in the area upon palpation. There are several different diagnostic models and accompanying techniques. The following approach is mainly based upon the writings of Kiiko Matsumoto and Stephen Birch in their book *Five Elements and Ten Stems* (Matsumoto and Birch 1983).

Start by holding the hand just above the abdomen without touching the skin. Let the hand pass slowly through the air above the various zones. Notice whether you can sense any variations in the perceived temperature or if there are changes in the sensation experienced in the palm of your hand. Some people sense or describe feeling a slight breeze on the hand. This is not as mysterious as it sounds: it's just a refined sense of *qi*. You do not have to feel anything. If you feel something, it is a sign of an imbalance, whereas the absence of a sensation may just be a sign that there is harmony and balance. Next, palpate the abdomen to ascertain whether there are areas that are tense and hard or soft and flaccid. Differences in the temperature in the various areas should be compared with the rest of the abdomen and between the abdomen and the rest of the body. Tenseness, tightness and resistance in an area is an indication that there is a *shi* condition. An area that feels flaccid, soft and weak will conversely be experienced when there are *xu* conditions. Areas that feel hot or cold will also indicate *shi* and *xu* conditions. Strong pulsing sensations can also be felt in *shi* conditions.

In addition to physically palpating the abdomen, visual observation should also be conducted to see if there are any changes in the skin, such as colour changes, visible blood vessels and increased moistness or dryness.

Diagnosis and treatment will typically merge into each other. When an aberration is felt in a specific area, this will dictate which needles are inserted. Once the needle has been inserted, the area is palpated again to see if the needle has engendered qualitative changes in the area. If there is no change in the area, the therapist will either adjust the manipulation of the needle or insert another needle. The area is then palpated again and the process is repeated until there is a perceptible improvement in the abdomen. It is important that the practitioner releases the physical pressure on the site each time before palpating again, thereby allowing a change to take place.

Diagnostic areas

The diagnostic areas described below are based on the areas outlined in the *Nan Jing*. It is important to take into account the various channels that traverse the abdomen. Palpable changes in the abdomen can also reflect imbalances in the channels themselves. Furthermore, imbalances such as *qi* stagnation and *xue* stagnation in the Stomach and the Intestines can also be felt when palpating the abdomen. It is also important to note that the following is just one interpretation of the abdominal areas and there are also other diagnostic interpretations of the abdominal zones.

LUNG AREA

The Lung area is located between the acupuncture points St 25 and St 27 on the right hand side of the umbilicus (the patient's right-hand side).

SPLEEN AREA

The Spleen area circumscribes the umbilicus in a circle that is one *cun* in diameter and in a line from Sp 14 to Sp 15.

LIVER AREA

The area below the patient's right costal region relates to the Liver. Furthermore, palpable lumps in the area to the left of and below the patient's navel in a line running St 25 to St 27 can be seen when there is Liver *xue* stagnation.

HEART AREA

The Heart area is located in the area around Ren 14 and Ren 15.

KIDNEY AREA

The Kidney area extends from Ren 4 to Ren 6 between the two Stomach channels.

Palpation of the Ren channel

Whilst palpating the abdomen, the various channels that traverse through the area should be palpated. Special attention should be paid to palpating along *ren mai*, especially the points Ren 6, Ren 12 and Ren 15. Ideally, there should not be any feelings of heat, cold, lumps, hardness or weakness, but there should be qualitative differences in how the three areas feel. Ren 6 should feel tighter and more elastic than Ren 12, and Ren 12 should feel tighter and more elastic than Ren 15, i.e. there should be an increasing resilience from Ren 15 to Ren 6. Aberrations in the form of increased tightness, softness, cold or heat in these areas will be an indication of imbalance in the respective *jiao*.

Palpation of the thorax

The thorax is mainly influenced by *zong qi* and the organs that are in the area – the Lung, Pericardium and Heart. The Liver will also have an influence on the area, as will the channels that traverse the area. The patient should be asked whether they experience pain, tenderness, discomfort or relief whilst being palpated

Tenderness in the area around Ren 17 can be experienced when there are stagnations in the Heart. Lung *shi* conditions can manifest with pain and tenderness in the entire area around the sternum and the ribs will often be sore. If there are *xu* conditions in the Heart or Lung, palpation will relieve the soreness and tenderness.

Liver and Gall Bladder imbalances can manifest pain, tenderness and tension below the ribs and on the side of the chest.

Palpation of the thorax

Observation	Significance
Pain and tenderness around Ren 17	Heart *shi* conditions
Pain and tenderness in the central area of the chest	Lung *shi* conditions
Pain and tenderness on the sides of the thorax	Liver and Gall Bladder imbalances
Tension in the hypochondriac region	Liver and Gall Bladder imbalances *Shaoyang* stage imbalances

Palpation of the skin

Palpation of the skin includes the inspection of the skin's temperature, humidity and elasticity, as well as palpating the tissue below the skin.

Palpation of the skin is especially important in the diagnosis of *bi* syndrome and in dermatological disorders.

Skin temperature

Gauging the temperature of the skin can give an indication of whether there is pathological Heat or Cold in the body. Investigation of the skin temperature is vital when diagnosing invasions of *xie qi*, particularly when there are *bi* syndromes.

Hot skin

If the skin feels hot when you place your hand on it, this will be a sign that there is Heat. The Heat can be both *xu* and *shi* in nature.

If it is only a limited area of skin that feels hot, for example the elbow, this will indicate that there is a localised condition of Heat, which is likely to be due to a stagnation in the area. Localised accumulations of Heat can also be seen when there is Toxic-Fire.

Cold skin

Cold skin can be experienced when there is both *shi* Cold and *yang xu*. Again, it can be the skin in general that feels cold or a limited area. Localised areas of Cold arise from invasions of exogenous Cold.

Skin temperature

Observation	Significance
Hot	*Shi* heat or *yin xu* Heat
Cold	*Shi* Cold or *yang xu*

Note: If the person is wearing a lot of clothes or has just run or cycled, their skin will feel hotter. Likewise, exposed areas of skin will feel colder than areas that are covered.

Humidity

Dry skin

The skin is moistened and nourished by *jinye* and *xue*. Skin can feel dry due to a lack of moisture if *xue*, *yin* or *jinye* are *xu*, injured by Heat or prevented from flowing to the area. The latter is important, as both Phlegm and *xue* stagnation can inhibit the circulation of *yin*, *xue* and *jinye*.

Sticky or oily skin

The skin can feel oily, sticky, greasy or moist when there is Damp-Heat or Phlegm.

Moist skin

Yang xu, *qi xu* or invasions of exogenous Wind can result in the pores in the skin not closing and sweat seeping out. Heat can also drive fluids upwards and outwards, causing the person to sweat. In all these cases, the skin will feel wet.

People who are very anxious will often sweat spontaneously when they are nervous. This can be experienced before and during an acupuncture treatment.

Rough or flaky skin

Certain areas of the skin can become dry or flaky when they are not nourished by *xue* or *jinye*. If the skin in general is dry and flaking this indicates *xue xu* or *yin xu*. Localised areas of dry, flaking skin can also arise due to *xue* stagnation blocking the flow of *xue* and *jinye* to the area.

It is, of course, important to take into account the use of creams and moisturisers, which can confuse or veil the diagnosis.

Humidity of the skin

Observation	Significance
Dry	*Xue xu, jinye xu, yin xu, xue* stagnation
Greasy or sticky	Dampness, Damp-Heat or Phlegm
Moist (sweaty)	Invasion of Wind, Lung *qi xu*, Spleen *qi xu, yang xu*, Heart *qi xu, shi* Heat, *xu* Heat
Rough or flaking	*Xue xu, xue* stagnation

Note: The use of creams and moisturisers will obscure the diagnosis.

Suppleness of the skin

The skin should be soft, elastic and smooth. This reflects that the Lung and Spleen are harmonious. It shows that there is sufficient *xue* and *jinye* to nourish and moisten the skin. The flesh below the skin should also feel firm but not hard. This indicates that *qi* and *xue* are nourishing the tissue and that fluids are being transported away from the tissue again.

Stagnations of Phlegm and/or *xue* will block the flow of fresh, nutritious *xue* and *jinye*. This will result in the skin feeling hard and thickened.

Loose skin is an indication that the skin is not being nourished, usually an indication of *yin xu* or *xue xu*.

The connective tissue and the muscles beneath the skin can feel hard and tense when there is a stagnation.

If the Lung, Kidneys or Spleen do not perform their task of spreading, transporting and transforming the fluids, either because there is an invasion of *xie qi* blocking their functioning or because they are *qi xu*, an accumulation of fluids in the tissue can arise.

Palpation of the hands and feet

The first handshake can give an indication of which patterns of imbalance may be present. The strength of the handshake, the temperature and the humidity of the hand will all reveal information that can be utilised in the diagnosis.

A person who is extremely *qi xu* will often have a limp handshake. This is not a hard and fast rule, especially as some people deliberately try to send signals to other people via their handshake, for example that they are strong (crushing handshake) or that they are trustworthy (firm handshake).

A person who is nervous will often sweat in the palms of their hands. This is because the Heart controls sweating. The other area where people sweat when they are nervous is under the arms. Both these places are located at the ends of the Heart channel. A person with Heart *qi xu* will often be slightly more nervous than others, which can manifest with sweaty palms. *Shi* Heat, especially Damp-Heat, can also manifest with sweaty palms. When there is Damp-Heat, the palm will usually also feel hotter. Invasions of *xie qi* can also make a person sweat, but the sweat in these cases will not be localised on the hand.

Hands and feet that feel hot are a sign of Heat. If the hands feel warm or hot, it is important to ascertain whether it is the whole hand or only the palm that feels hot. The whole hand will feel hot if the Heat is *shi* in nature, whereas *yin xu* Heat manifests with only the palms feeling hot.

Damp-Heat can manifest with hot and sweaty feet.

Cold hands and feet can be experienced when there is *yang xu* and *xue xu*, as well as Liver *qi* stagnation. If there is *yang xu*, usually the hands and arms are cold. The further away from the torso, the colder the sensation will be. This is because *yang* warmth is too weak to expand and extend away from the centre, but also because warmth is retained in the interior so the internal organs can utilise the transforming power of *yang*.

Xue and *qi* travel together. This means that if there is *xue xu*, there can be a lack of warming *qi* in the extremities with cold hands and feet as a consequence.

A very common cause of cold hands and feet is when there is Liver *qi* stagnation. The body itself will feel warm enough, but because *qi* is stagnated, the warmth remains trapped in the torso and is not distributed to the extremities. Because their hands and feet are cold, these people will often report that they have an aversion to cold when asked about their perception of temperature, leading to an incorrect diagnosis of Cold. Often it is not only the hands and feet that are cold, but all the extremities such as the tip of the nose and the buttocks.

Phlegm can block *qi* and in some situations manifest with cold extremities.

Palpation of the hands and feet

Observation	Significance
Weak and limp handshake	*Qi xu*
Sweaty palms	Heart *qi xu*, invasion of *xie qi*, Heat
Sweaty feet	Damp-Heat
The entire hand is hot	*Shi* Heat
Only the palm is hot	*Xu* Heat
Cold hands and feet	*Yang xu*, *xue xu*, Liver *qi* stagnation or Phlegm

Palpation of acupuncture points, channels and micro-systems

Palpation of acupuncture points

Palpating acupuncture points is an important, but unfortunately sometimes overlooked, area of diagnosis. Specific groups of points, for example *mu*-collecting and back-*shu* points, can be palpated to diagnose imbalances in their associated *zangfu* organs. Palpation of channel and a-*shi* points is especially relevant in relation to channel diagnosis. Palpation of acupuncture points is also useful when determining which points to use therapeutically and to judge the depth of insertion.

When palpating points, it is best to run your finger lightly over the skin where the point is to sense the point and its location. Next, press gently downwards into the point, paying attention to the sensations in the fingertip and at the same time registering any responses in the patient's reactions.

Tightness, stiffness, weakness, flaccidity, sponginess, granulations, lumps, skin changes, heat or cold can all be experienced when palpating in and around an acupuncture point. The area at the point can be raised or sunken. It is also possible to observe ruptured capillaries and spider naevi in the area. The patient can experience pain, discomfort, soreness, tingling or relief whilst the point is palpated.

Palpation of channel points and *a-shi* points

Channel points can be palpated both as part of the diagnostic process itself and of the point selection process. Palpation of the point can also give an indication of how deeply *qi* is located in the point and thereby determine the depth of the needle insertion.

Points that are sore, tight and tender can indicate that there is a stagnation of *qi* in the channel in this area. Tenderness and soreness arise because of the accumulation of *qi*. Pressure on the point will increase the amount of *qi* in the area, causing the point to feel painful on palpation. Furthermore, sensations of cold, heat and sponginess in and around the point can respectively indicate the presence of Cold, Heat or Dampness. The points will often lie on the channel itself, but they can also lie outside of the channels. These points are called *a-shi* points.

Tingling sensations are felt when stagnated *qi* is activated by the pressure from the finger.

If the patient experiences a pleasant sensation or relief upon point palpation or if the area in and around the point feels flaccid and soft, this indicates a *xu* condition. This is because there is too little *qi* present in the point, resulting in a lack of tension in the area. Pressing the point will increase the amount of *qi* in the point so it will feel pleasurable.

Palpation of acupuncture points can be a significant aid to determining which points to utilise in a treatment. It is not uncommon, when formulating a treatment protocol, to have a choice of several acupuncture points that have similar actions. By palpating the various acupuncture points, you get a sense of which points are the most reactive or dynamic and can then select these points.

By pressing slowly and gently into a point, one can sense how deep you have to press before there will be a response from the patient or a feeling of *qi* in the finger. The depth in which one experiences the response is the depth that *qi* is located, and this is the correct depth for needle insertion (whilst of course paying regard to the underlying anatomy).

Palpation of acupuncture points

Observation	Significance
Sore, painful and tight	*Shi* conditions
Soft and flaccid	*Xu* conditions
The sensation in the point feels worse with pressure	*Shi* conditions
The sensation in the point feels better with the pressure	*Xu* conditions
Heat	Heat
Cold	Cold
Sponginess	Dampness

Two categories of points that are very important, both therapeutically and diagnostically, are *mu*-collecting and back-*shu* points. They are important because the points in both of these categories are directly in contact with their associated organs. This means that these points may well be reactive when there are imbalances in these organs. The diagnostic significance of sensations felt in these points is the same as those described above.

Palpation of the channels

Palpation of the channels is indispensable in the diagnosis of *bi* syndromes and channel disorders. The information from channel palpation can also provide significant and relevant information in the diagnosis of internal imbalances, such as *zangfu* imbalances. This is because the organs and channels are directly connected to each other and the channels are, in reality, a manifestation of the organ itself. Unfortunately, channel diagnosis has been less emphasised in TCM acupuncture training in China and here in the West. I will give a very brief overview of channel diagnosis below. For a deeper elaboration of the techniques and diagnostic interpretations of channel diagnosis, the reader is referred to Professor Wang Ju-Yi and Jason D. Robertson's excellent book *Applied Channel Theory in Chinese Medicine* (Wang and Robertson 2008).

All 12 channels should be palpated from the tips of the fingers and toes to the elbows and knees respectively. The side of the thumb is slid along the path of the channel three or four times, first superficially and then deeper each time. The aim is to find changes not in the texture of specific acupuncture points but in the tissue in and around the channels themselves. This is because imbalances in the internal organs and in the channel as a whole can manifest with changes along the path of the channel. Changes in the tissue can be the presence of nodules, graininess in the tissue, sponginess, tightness and hardness, and softness and weakness. There can also be changes in the temperature of the skin along the channel.

The size, depth and hardness of any changes along the path of the channel are also important diagnostic factors.

Tightness, hardness and tension are usually indicative of a *shi* condition in the channel or its associated organ. The more superficial the hardness, the more acute the condition is likely to be.

Softness and weakness in the tissue along the path of the channel is a sign of a *xu* condition in the channel or its associated organ. If there is a *xu* condition, the palpation will feel more pleasant for the patient than if there is a *shi* condition.

Deep hardness and tightness will often be seen when there are interior and chronic imbalances.

Cold and *xue* stagnation can manifest with nodules that are hard and immobile with clearly defined edges, whereas Phlegm and Dampness nodules will tend to be smoother and slippery with less clearly defined edges. Phlegm and Damp nodules will be easily moved when palpated.

Longer, stick-like nodules can also be felt along the path of the channel. If the stick-like nodules are very bumpy and lie along the channel, this is a sign that it is a chronic condition that can be difficult to treat. Stick-like nodules that can be felt across the path of the channel are more typically acute or are due to stagnations of *qi* and are thereby easier to treat.

If the patient reports sensations of numbness whilst an area is being palpated, this can be due to Phlegm blocking the channel.

Palpation of the channels

Observation	Significance
Tenderness, tightness and tension along the channel	*Shi* condition in the channel or its associated organ
Softness and weakness along the channel	*Xu* condition in the channel or its associated organ
The sensation in the channel feels worse with pressure	*Shi* condition in the channel or its associated organ
The sensation in the channel feels better with pressure	*Xu* condition in the channel or its associated organ
The channel feels warm	Heat in the channel or its associated organ
The channel feels cold	Cold in the channel or its associated organ
Superficial hardness or nodules just below the surface of the skin	Acute conditions
Deep hardness, graininess or nodules	Chronic conditions
Hard, clearly defined nodules	Cold or *xue* stagnation
Hard, defined nodules that are slippery and smooth	Phlegm, Dampness
Hard, bumpy, longitudinal 'stick-like' lines	Chronic condition
Hard, transverse 'stick-like' lines	Acute condition, stagnation of *qi*
Numbness	Phlegm

Palpation of micro-systems, including ear acupuncture

There is a vast number of different so-called micro-systems around the body, the most famous being ear acupuncture. It is beyond the scope of this book to give a detailed description of these various zones in the body. The reader is therefore referred to relevant literature, for example Terry Oleson's *Auriculotherapy Manual* (Oleson 2014). Common to most of these systems is that the points and the areas that relate to different areas of the body and the organs are reactive when there is an imbalance or a change in these areas of the body. This means that palpation of these points or zones can help to identify where in the body an imbalance is and what its character is.

Section 4

THE DIAGNOSTIC PILLAR: INTERVIEWING

Introduction

This diagnostic pillar ostensibly appears to be more accessible than the other three diagnostic approaches. This is because interviewing the client is not dependent on the subjective perception and interpretation of the signals that are being received through the fingertips, nose and ears. You do not, for example, have to judge how much a certain hue in the complexion is an aberration from what you ought to be seeing right now in the complexion. In general, we are better at intellectually interpreting verbal responses than we are at intellectually interpreting visual, olfactory, auditory or palpable signals. Nevertheless, this pillar contains the most pitfalls. This is because the same verbal response can have multiple diagnostic interpretations. The person's responses can also be misleading, since the client may not understand the question in the same way as you do. They may not remember correctly what you are asking them about or they may not even be consciously aware of what you have asked them about. They may, for example, believe that they do not sweat at night, but if you asked their wife, she would say that they do indeed sweat at night. They may also be imprecise in their answers. For example, a woman may not place any significance in her menstrual cycle being 26 days long or 30 days long. This for her is a regular cycle, because her menstruation arrives once a month. Even though her cycle can vary in length by up to four days, it is still regular in her eyes, because it comes once a month. Even if you ask her to elaborate with a supplementary question about the number of days in the cycle, she might reply that it is 28 days long, because for her there is no significant difference between a 26-, 28- or 30-day cycle, but for us as a diagnostician, there is. Even if you get precise and detailed answers, they will still not be definitive in relation to the diagnosis. They will just be pieces of a jigsaw puzzle, because in Chinese medicine everything must always be seen in a context. Night sweats can, for example, be a manifestation of *yin xu* and Damp-Heat. You will need to compare each answer you get with all the other symptoms and signs, as well as comparing the individual answers with the answers to all the other questions. This is a major difference between Chinese medicine and Western medicine. In Western medicine, A is often equal to B. In Chinese medicine, A will only be equal to B if D, G and R are present, whereas A will be equal to C, if D, F, J and W are present. It is therefore important that the questions you ask are very precise and comprehensive. For example, when you ask someone how their stools are and they say that they are regular, you need to find out what they really mean by this? Daily? Three times a day? Once a week? Furthermore, if they have constipation, it is important to know

195

what the stools are like – whether they are dry, pebble-like or long and thin like a pencil, whether there is pain and whether they are exhausted or relieved after they have passed the stools. Each answer you get will usually result in having to ask a further elaborative question, and each response to these questions must be seen in the context of the other answers and in the context of all the other signs and symptoms that you have observed.

Interviewing techniques

When we listen to the patient, we should not only listen to what they are saying, but also to the sound of their voice and its tone, speed and strength. We should also observe their body language, posture and eyes, the speed and strength of their body movements and so on. These things are not an aspect of this diagnostic pillar, but interviewing the client gives us ample opportunity to observe the person. It does, though, require a degree of 'multi-tasking' to focus intellectually on the conversation and the information that is being given, whilst trying to observe visually and listen to the more subtle diagnostic signs emanating from the client.

As written above, interviewing the client is perhaps the most accessible of the four diagnostic approaches, but it can also be the most difficult, because it is not always easy to get the information you need from the client. This may be because the client is not particularly aware of their bodily functions. They may consciously or subconsciously not want to answer all the questions that we ask. The opposite is often also the case: the patient tells you too much. These patients can start to take control of the conversation or they relay to you too many details and a surfeit of information that has no relevance to what you are asking them about. This is a problem because you only have a limited amount of time set aside for each patient and because it can be very exhausting as a therapist to spend so much energy staying focused and trying to steer the conversation back to the topic. Patients with Heat in the Heart are especially problematic in this way. Heat in the Heart means that they are over-communicative. Their *shen* can have difficulty distinguishing between what is relevant and irrelevant, and it cannot control how much they open up to others. What they say may have relevance for the diagnosis, but often they begin to talk about something other than what you asked them about. It is, of course, an important diagnostic sign in itself that they are talking and telling you so much. It is, perhaps, only this and a red tip on the tongue that tell you that they have some form of Heat in the Heart. Once you have established this, it is important that you gain control of the interview again. It is important to learn how to cut people off in a polite and courteous manner. This can be difficult because they might feel that what they are telling us is relevant to their situation or that they are paying you to listen to them. It may also be that what they are telling us has a great deal of relevance to their imbalances, but that we do not possess the relevant therapeutic skills to help them as a counsellor. This could, for example, be a woman who says that she has been subjected to incest or rape. This will be an extremely important aetiological factor, but after we have listened and sensed how it affects and has affected her, it's not our job as an acupuncturist or herbalist to provide her with psychological counselling. We are not qualified to do this. We can offer empathy and we can give her the space to talk about it, but we must also be conscious of where our therapeutic tools and skills start and stop. In these situations, we must refer the client to others who possess these skills. We can, importantly, help her on the energetic level, and people who have undergone several years of counselling often experience a therapeutic breakthrough as a result of acupuncture. This, though, is through the actions of the needles and herbs and the space we create, not through our abilities as amateur psychotherapists.

Respect, sensitivity and being non-judgemental are keywords when interviewing clients. The patient must always feel that you have respect for them, that they can trust you and that you do not judge them. The latter is something most clients are excellent at doing themselves and they do not need any additional help! It is a great leap for some people to contact an acupuncturist or herbalist, as this is something that they may perceive of as being 'alternative' or even 'mystic'. It is important that they understand why we ask so many questions that can seem irrelevant and even strange. They may well have thought that it was enough to say that they suffer from migraines – that you would then stick some needles in the headache point and that would be all. It is therefore a good idea to explain how in Chinese medicine we are constantly looking for patterns and relationships, rather than isolated symptoms. You should explain to them how ostensibly disparate symptoms and signs can relate to a specific organ's functioning. For example, that the soreness in their knees and their tinnitus can relate to the Kidneys and that these signs therefore have relevance in the treatment of their night sweats – something that they have been told is hormonal. It is also important to inform the client of the difference between the Western medicine and Chinese medicine concepts of the internal organs. For example, when we say that there is an imbalance that relates to their Liver or Heart, this does not mean that they have cirrhosis or that they are about to have a cardiac arrest. We must explain to them that organs in Chinese medicine are more about functional relationships than physical structures.

Tact and respect are needed when you are enquiring into areas that may be sensitive or private. Some people may find it embarrassing to talk about certain aspects of the body. For example, a 15-year-old girl may not be completely comfortable talking to a 50-year-old man about her vaginal discharge. For others, it could be certain emotional aspects that they are sensitive about. It is therefore important that we win the client's trust in us as therapists and help them to understand why our questions are relevant.

It's also a good idea to rephrase questions so the person can relate to them or comprehend them. It is important to remember that the patient is not trained in Chinese medicine. It is, for example, unlikely that they will know what 'plumstone qi' is. This can, of course, easily be rephrased to asking them whether they have a sensation that there is a lump in the throat, as if there is something that they cannot swallow. Other questions that are ostensibly straightforward should sometimes be reformulated, such as asking them whether they have a sensation of heat in the evening. The difference in temperature may be too subtle for them to register it as a sensation of heat or fever, but if you ask them whether they remove their jersey or are less sensitive to cold in the evening, they may answer yes.

There are various strategies that can be employed when interviewing the client. It is definitely important to gather as much information as possible that is relevant to the diagnosis. However, Bob Flaws believes that you should be systematic and only ask questions that are relevant to the imbalance patterns that may be manifesting in the specific disorder that the patient has sought help for. His view is that you should only investigate the patterns of imbalance that are relevant in the treatment of this disorder. His strategy is to look for confirmation or rejection of the patterns of imbalance that manifest in this disorder. Once you have received enough information to confirm or reject a pattern, you do not have to investigate further. He believes it is a sign of sloppiness when you ask haphazard questions and lack focus.

The second strategy is to investigate all the available avenues. In this way, it is possible to identify patterns of imbalance that may not initially seem relevant but are subsequently found to be significant in relation to the disorder that the patient presents with. The information obtained can also reveal symptoms and imbalances that the patient has not sought treatment for but that may well be more important to address in the treatment. They may, for example, have sought treatment for allergic rhinitis, but through the diagnostic investigation you discover that they suffer from insomnia, stress, palpations and cardiac pain. In these situations, you must make the patient aware that Chinese medicine can treat these disorders or the imbalance. They may well decide that they still only want treatment of their rhinitis, but now they can make a conscious choice.

The two approaches are, of course, not mutually exclusive. In both scenarios it is important to follow a thread when interviewing a person and not just ask them random questions. You should thoroughly investigate a certain topic before moving on to another area of questioning. My personal opinion is that the more information that you can gather from a patient and the more detailed a picture you can paint, the more accurate the diagnosis will be. In both strategies, it is important that you do not just leap to the next question when a patient has given you an answer. You must ask yourself whether their response generates a new question or whether the answer needs elaboration or more specific details. For example, if when asking about their bowel movements, they respond that they have loose stools, you need to find out: what the consistency of the stools are; whether the stools are watery containing undigested food particles; whether the stools are sticky; whether the stools have a strong odour; whether there is a burning sensation in the anus during or after defecation; whether there is pain or if they feel bloated in the abdomen before they have bowel movements; whether the stools and their movements are influenced by certain foods or stress and so on

Interrogating the client is an integral part of the consultation and treatment. We must, though, be conscious from the outset and during the interview of precisely what information we are trying to gain. We must also be aware of how much time we have available to achieve these goals. If we have set aside an hour to diagnose and treat the client, we cannot sit talking to the client for three-quarters of an hour, as apart from treating the client, we must also receive payment and book a new appointment and they must dress and undress. This means that we, not the client, must be the one who controls the structure and direction of the interview.

The 10 questions

There are some classic questions or areas of verbal investigation. Classically, between 8 and 10 questions or areas of interrogation have been described. The list below is slightly longer, as I have expanded some of the areas of interrogation. Most of the 10 questions are also more categories of questions, rather than individual questions. The areas that I investigate when interviewing a client are:

- general questions, including: age, occupation, family situation, medical history and medication

- specific questions relating to the disorder or symptom that they are seeking treatment for, including the history and specific details of the disorder

- questions relating to body temperature and their relationship to heat and cold

- energy levels

- sweating

- thirst, appetite, taste, nausea and vomiting

- defecation and urination

- questions relating to the Heart

- questions relating to the Lung

- dizziness

- questions relating to the skin and hair

- questions relating to the ears, eyes, vision and hearing

- sleep

- pain, including headaches

- questions that are specific to women, for example questions about menstruation and childbirth

- questions that are specific to men

- emotions

- lifestyle and diet.

This list is not comprehensive and there are other areas that can be investigated verbally, but these are some of the most traditional focus areas.

The order of questions is not important. The questions will often be determined by the responses and in relation to the disorder that the patient has sought treatment for. What is important is to ensure that all relevant issues are investigated during the consultation. A well-designed journal is of great help here.

General questions

Age/gender

Knowing the age and gender of a person already gives us an idea of what imbalances are probable and thereby which signs and symptoms we should look for. This is because there are specific physiological factors that affect the respective genders and people of different ages. There are also certain lifestyle and emotional influences that are more relevant to specific genders and age groups. These are, of course, only probabilities and are definitely not certainties. This is because even though a person's age and gender will predispose them to certain imbalances, there are a great many other factors that will also have had an influence that may have resulted in completely different imbalances.

Women lose blood when they menstruate and when they give birth. This means that they have a tendency to develop not just *xue xu*, but also Spleen *qi xu*, because the Spleen will have to generate *gu qi* constantly to help replenish the *xue* that has been lost. This constant demand on their Spleen will also lead to their *mingmen* becoming weaker, especially when they are 35 and enter the fifth *jing* cycle, where there is a natural decline in strength of the *mingmen*. This will manifest with an increased tendency to Dampness and Phlegm. This is the reason many women's bodies become more pear-shaped at this age. When a woman is 49 years old, her *yin* and *xue* will be so depleted that she will enter menopause. This means that patterns of *xue xu* and *yin xu* Heat are more probable from this age onwards in women. As stated, it is very important to be observant of other possible patterns. Women's tendency to *xue xu* means that women may also manifest with Liver *qi* stagnation. This is because *xue* helps to moisten the Liver and make it flexible. Furthermore, women's position in society and the expectations placed on modern women, in terms of having a career whilst being a good mother, looking after the home, trying to look good and having an active social life, can all help to create a sense of frustration that will stagnate her Liver *qi*.

Young men tend more towards *shi* Heat, especially in the Liver and Stomach, because young men are more *yang* in general, but also due to their lifestyle, where a higher intake of alcohol is more likely than in women and older men. As written, these examples are only broad generalisations and many people do not necessarily fit into these descriptions.

Teenagers tend to develop *shi* Heat. The reason for this is that their *mingmen* flares up during this period. This creates Heat in various organs. Heat in the Stomach can manifest in their appetites – most people have experienced a 16-year-old boy's insatiable appetite – and in their skin, where the Heat in the Stomach and Damp-Heat will mean that they are prone to acne. The increased heat from *mingmen* will also affect their mood. This is because the Heat will agitate the Liver and Heart making them more hot-tempered and moody. Their libido is also relatively high, due to the increased Heat from the *mingmen.*

Babies and small infants tend to develop food stagnation. This is because their Stomach and Spleen are not fully developed yet. The Stomach and Spleen are first fully developed from about the age of seven. This means that babies find it difficult to transform and process the food that they consume. One must therefore be careful of what they are given to eat; how much they are fed at a time and how often they are fed. This also, of course, applies to older children, but it is especially relevant for infants. Many disorders that affect babies and toddlers will relate to their tendency to develop what is known as accumulation disorder and the patterns of imbalance that this can engender.

Because children's *yin* is not strong, they tend to generate pathological Heat, especially when they get ill. When they are affected by *xie qi*, they will quickly develop a high fever, because their *yin* is not capable of controlling the Heat. This is also seen in the evening when they are tired. When their *yin* cannot control *yang* in the evening, they become overexcited and restless, and their cheeks become red and flushed.

The older people get, the more they become both *yin xu* and *yang xu*. This is because their Kidney *jing* becomes continuously weaker and the Kidneys are the root of all *yin* and *yang* in the body. However, this is not the whole story. It is because Kidney *yin xu* and *yang xu* will undermine other organs and these organs' production of the vital substances, resulting in a tendency to *qi xu* and *xue xu*. At the same time, there is also an increasing tendency to develop stagnations of *qi*, *xue* and Phlegm the older one gets. This can be clearly seen in the body movements of older people. There is not only a lack of strength, but also a lot of stiffness in their movements. Their skin will often manifest signs of *xue* stagnation, with many spider naevi, visible purple blood vessels and 'liver spots'.

Some Chinese medicine doctors also believe that there is an increasing accumulation of *xie* Heat retained inside the body as people get older. This is because each time there has been a pathological invasion of *xie qi*, there will remain a residue of the *xie qi* in the body. These residues of *xie qi* will accumulate, creating Heat and stagnating the vital substances. This is one of the theories behind the development of age-related cancer.

Employment

Some jobs or occupations will predispose people to particular imbalances. People who work in environments where there is a pronounced or constant climatic influence can be invaded or weakened by these exogenous influences. This could, for example, be a person who works on a trawler or in a cold storage unit. All day long they will be exposed to dampness and cold. Steel mill workers are, on the other hand, constantly exposed to heat, whilst laundry workers and kitchen staff are often affected by dampness and heat. Clerical staff can also be affected by climate. This could, for example, be due to dryness, resulting from a poor indoor climate in concrete buildings, even though Dryness is not usually a form of exogenous *xie qi* that is often seen in Western and Northern Europe. They could also sit in a draught.

Repetitive or excessive strain and poor posture can also be an aspect of some people's jobs and this can damage the muscles and channels and weaken certain organs. Lifting heavy objects weakens Kidney *yang*. Standing for long periods of time also weakens the Kidneys, whereas sitting excessively can weaken Spleen *qi*, as well as stagnating Liver *qi* and *qi* in the Intestines. Lung *qi* is weakened by sitting with the shoulders slumped forwards.

One must also listen to the person's voice and observe their eyes whilst they talk about their employment. Do they sound happy or frustrated and sad? How do they talk about their work? Does it sound as if there are conflicts and friction? Does it sound as if their work gives them inspiration and joy? Their work can be a part of their aetiology, but it can also be something that contributes positively to their lives.

Habitation

The standard of housing used to be a major aetiological factor here in Northern Europe, and it still is in many other parts of the world. This is because the home is a place we spend a lot of time. To live in an abode that is cold, damp or draughty would have been a major aetiological factor in the past. The standard of living has generally increased over the last 50 years, but the person's housing can still be a relevant factor. Some people still live in damp and cold buildings, while others who live in modern concrete constructions can have the opposite problem, i.e. that the indoor air is too dry. Others are affected by there being fungus, for example dry rot, in the building where they live or work. This fungus will often give the person the same symptoms and signs that are seen in Dampness. It is important to find out whether a person's symptoms improve when they are not at home or at work in this building.

Family situation

Enquiring about the person's family situation – whether they are married or have a partner, whether they have children and whether they have a social network around them – can tell us several things. It will give us an idea of how much support they have, but also the way that they talk about these things can give an indication of whether there is Heart *qi xu* or Liver *qi* stagnation. If they sound lonely and sad, this can indicate that there is Heart *qi xu*, because social contact, love and joy all help to nourish Heart *qi*. Being stuck in situations where there is frustration, irritation and dissatisfaction will create Liver *qi* stagnation. It requires respect and tact to ask about these issues, and, as described earlier, we must be conscious of our limitations as a therapist.

Medical history

This refers not to the current symptoms that the person has sought treatment for, but the diseases and disorders they have previously suffered from, the surgery they have had and the medication they have taken throughout their life. The diseases, surgeries and disorders that they have had will inform you about possible historical and current imbalance patterns. These patterns can also be instrumental in the development of their current patterns of imbalance. A severe febrile illness can have damaged their *yin* or created Phlegm. An operation will usually result in *xue* stagnation in the form of scar tissue. Medication, especially prolonged or repeated use of the medicine, is often a relevant aetiological factor. Antibiotics, for example, may have weakened their Spleen *yang* and created Dampness, whilst painkillers may have created Stomach Fire and damaged their *yin*. For more details about the energetic effects of Western medications, the reader is referred to Dr Stephen Gascoigne's *The Clinical Medicine Guide* (Gascoigne 2001).

It can also be relevant to ask about hereditary diseases. Some diseases and disorders are inherent in some families. Imbalances and diseases can be passed on in several ways. A person's constitution is dependent on the *jing* that they have inherited from their parents. This means that weaknesses can be passed on to the children in the same way that diseases are genetically inherited in Western medicine. A foetus is created and nourished for nine months by its mother's *qi, xue* and *jing*. It is physically and energetically a part of her body. This means that as the foster develops it may be significantly and fundamentally influenced by her patterns of imbalance. Another factor is that by growing up in the same climatic and psychological environment, as well as eating the same diet for years, a person will often develop some of the same imbalances as their parents and siblings. Finally, a small child resonates energetically with its mother and is not yet completely separated from her *qi*. This means that her patterns of imbalance can affect the child's *qi* and thereby produce the same patterns of imbalance.

Current medication

Enquiry should be made about a patient's current medication use, including which medicine they are taking, what they are taking it for, how long they have been taking it and in what dosages. This should include not only prescription medicine, but also over-the-counter medicines and herbal remedies. It is important to ask about everything a person takes. Amazingly, there are many patients who do not think of their sleeping pill as being medicine, even though it is prescribed by a doctor, nor the painkillers that they take because you can buy them from the supermarket. Nevertheless, these medicines will have a greater or lesser effect on their physiology. They can blur the relevant signs, such as insomnia for example, but they may well also be part of the aetiology of the patient's current imbalances. Herbal medicine and dietary supplements also have a physiological effect on the body, so it is important to ask about the patient's use of these. It is a good idea to familiarise yourself with the Chinese medicine dynamics of the most common medications, both those used in Western medicine and commonly used supplements. It is beyond the scope of this book's competence to go into detail about the energetic effects of the many and varied medications that people take. Reference is therefore made to relevant literature, such as Stephen Gascoigne's *The Prescribed Drug Guide* (Gascoigne 2003).

Disease history

We must ascertain how and when a disorder arose to get an idea about its aetiology, which will help us to reveal which patterns of imbalance can have initiated the disorder and which imbalances can have arisen as a consequence of it.

We must ask the patient how long they've had the symptoms and whether the symptoms appeared suddenly or slowly over a period of time.

A disease or symptom that develops slowly and gradually usually occurs due to a *xu* condition. An exception to this is *xue xu*. *Xue xu* can arise when there is heavy bleeding, such as there is in childbirth for example. A *shi* condition, on the other hand, will often result in symptoms that appear suddenly or over a shorter period of time. This therefore means that acute conditions are usually *shi* in nature.

Chronic disorders will almost always be pure *xu* conditions or, more commonly, combined *xu* and *shi* conditions. A condition that starts as a *xu* condition can easily develop a *shi* aspect. For example, Liver *yin xu* can also begin to manifest with ascending Liver *yang*, whilst Spleen *qi xu* will often result in Dampness, to name just two very common examples. Conversely, a *shi* condition can easily develop into a *xu* and *xu/shi* condition. Extreme Heat, such as in a febrile illness, can injure *yin*; *xue* stagnation can result in heavy menstrual bleeding, which then leads to *xue xu*, etc.

Enquiring about how the symptoms themselves have developed and how they have changed will also give you an idea of the nature of the disorder. Symptoms that rapidly change are usually more *yang shi* in nature, whereas *yin xu* symptoms tend to develop more slowly.

Enquiry should also be made into the circumstances surrounding the onset of symptoms. How was their life at that time, and were there any changes in their life in this period? Had they started taking a new medication? Did they have a febrile illness? Were there any significant climatic influences? Was there crisis in their relationship or a change of employment or had they made dietary or other changes in this period? The answers to these questions will give an idea of the aetiology of the disorder. If we know what the aetiology is, we will then have a good idea of the imbalances that may be present.

The patient's medical history is also relevant. What disorders have they suffered from over the years? Knowing this will give an indication of whether there is a particular pattern and whether the current situation could be a part of this pattern. A severe febrile illness could have weakened their *yin* or *qi* or it could have generated Phlegm. A gastrointestinal ailment that they picked up in India 10 years ago could help to explain the presence of Damp-Heat in the lower *jiao* and Spleen *qi xu*.

It is vital that the patient is asked about what makes their symptoms better or worse and when the symptoms occur. This requires the memorising of which aetiological factors can create which patterns of imbalance. The following examples are presented to give an idea of this way of thinking and are far from comprehensive. To learn more about which aetiological factors lead to the creation of the various patterns of imbalance, please see the sections on diagnosing patterns of imbalance in the second part of this book.

- A condition that is adversely affected by dietary factors is usually a Stomach/Spleen imbalance, but it could also indicate the presence of Phlegm, Damp-Heat, Heat, Cold, *yang xu* or *yin xu*.

- If the disorder is affected by climatic influences, then one or more of the six forms of exogenous *xie qi* will be involved. It can, though, also indicate a Lung disorder, *wei qi xu* or the presence of internally generated Damp-Phlegm.

- If the symptoms are provoked by activity, then it is probably often a *xu* condition, whilst a *shi* condition usually improves with activity. This, though, is just a rough rule of thumb. A *xu* condition can, for example, result in a stagnation, in which case the patient may well feel amelioration immediately after activity, but the symptoms or their general condition will usually feel worse later on in the day or the day after. The reason for this is that the physical activity will help to circulate *qi*, but will at the same time consume their *qi* and *xue*, so the condition will deteriorate in the long term. Conversely, *xue* stagnation can manifest with a strong, sharp pain when a joint is activated or extended beyond a limited range of movement, but will be less painful when the joint is at rest.

- Stress can create stagnation of Liver *qi*, generate Heat in the body and injure *yin*. This means that symptoms that are exacerbated by stress can be manifestations of these patterns.

- Emotional influences that provoke or exacerbate a disorder will indicate an imbalance in the organ that relates to these emotions.

- Certain symptoms arise at specific times during the day. Symptoms that come later in the day or in the evening can be a sign of a *xu* condition. If they come in the evening or at night, it will often be *yin xu*. Symptoms that are related to certain hours of the day can also be interpreted through the Chinese horary clock and whether an organ or channel is at its peak or ebb during this period. *Xue* stagnation symptoms are often worse or manifest at night, when *xue* is not being circulated by physical movement and activity. This is typically seen in joint pain and traumatic injuries.

- Symptoms that are worse in the premenstrual period are often related to Liver *qi* stagnation and symptoms that are worse immediately after the menstrual bleeding are more typically seen when there is *yin xu* or *xue xu*.

It is also important to determine whether there are other symptoms that arose concurrently with the symptoms or the disorder, as the more symptoms that relate to a certain organ, the more likely it is that this organ is directly or indirectly involved in the present imbalance.

Disease history

Symptoms	Significance
Symptoms that have arisen gradually	Usually a *xu* or a *xu*/*shi* condition
Symptoms that have arisen suddenly	Generally a *shi* condition, but can also be a *xu* condition
The symptoms that have changed rapidly	Usually a *yang* or *shi* condition
The symptoms have changed slowly and gradually	Usually a *yin xu* or a *xu*/*shi* condition

Temperature

This area of enquiry is used to determine how deep *xie qi* has penetrated into the body and whether the imbalance is Hot or Cold in nature, as well as to identify *yin* and *yang* imbalances. It is important to point out that in Chinese medicine the presence of Heat in the body is determined by the patient's subjective perception of their body temperature or by the practitioner's physical palpation of their skin and their observation of skin colour changes. This means that even if a thermometer reading says that they do not have an increased body temperature, if they themselves feel that they are warm or have a fever, or if the practitioner can feel that their skin is hot or see that the face it is red, then there is Heat, even though it cannot be measured physically by the thermometer. On the other hand, if they do have a measurable rise in body temperature, this is always a sign of Heat.

If a person feels cold or has an aversion to cold, it is important to ask them if they can get warm again by putting on more clothes or wrapping themselves in a blanket. If the increase in clothing or bedding makes them feel warmer, this is *yang xu* Cold. If they are *yang xu*, they will have difficulty maintaining the warmth of the body, but by packing the body into warm clothing they reduce the heat loss and no longer feel cold. If they have an invasion of exogenous *xie qi*, which blocks the circulation of *wei qi*, they will not be able to get warm again, even though they put more clothes on or lie beneath a duvet or blankets. This is because *wei qi*, as well as protecting the body and controlling the sweat pores, warms the muscles just below the skin. When *xie qi* invades the exterior, the warming *wei qi* is blocked and cannot circulate. This means that it does not help to increase the amount of clothing or bedding that is insulating the body. The *xie qi* must first be expelled so *wei qi* can circulate before the person will feel warm again.

When *xie qi* is in the exterior, as well as feeling cold and chilly, the person will often have a slight fever or feel feverish. This is because the exogenous *xie qi* will not only prevent the circulation of the warming *wei qi*, it will also give rise to a conflict with, and a stagnation of, *wei qi*, resulting in the generation of Heat. The difference between Wind-Cold and Wind-Heat is that in Wind-Cold there is a greater aversion to cold and little or no fever sensations, whereas in Wind-Heat the fever sensation is more predominant and the aversion to cold less noticeable.

When exogenous *xie qi* has penetrated the *yangming* aspect, it will generate a great amount of Heat. This is because there is a violent struggle between the body's *zheng qi* and the invading *xie qi*. One of the most important diagnostic differentiations between *xie qi* that is in the exterior and *xie qi* that has penetrated to the interior is the strength of the Heat and whether there is an aversion to cold. When *xie qi* is in the interior, it no longer blocks the circulation of *wei qi*. This means that the person no longer experiences chills and muscle soreness. The fever, on the other hand, will be much more virulent.

If the person experiences alternating fever and chills or an alternating sensation of heat and an aversion to cold, this will indicate that *xie qi* is located in the *shaoyang* aspect. *Xie qi* can become lodged in this hinge between the interior and the exterior. This results in symptoms that alternate between these two stages.

Internal Heat conditions can give rise to an aversion to heat, but it is not certain that the person is aware of it. Often, if you ask them how they feel they will say that they do not have an aversion to heat or feel hot, but you can often observe that they are more lightly clad than others.

A major difference between *xu* and *shi* Heat is that when there is *shi* Heat, there is a sensation of heat throughout the day. When there is *yin xu* Heat, the person will only feel warm in the evening and at night. Again, it is not certain that the person is aware of this. They do not think about whether their duvet is thinner than other people's or that they feel warm at night. Furthermore, a person with *yin xu* might not answer yes to feeling hot in the evening, because they are sensitive to cold during the day because they are also *yang xu*. In the evening and at night they just feel less cold and perhaps remove the jersey that they have worn all day.

Another difference between *xu* and *shi* Heat is that when there is *shi* Heat, the whole body feels warm. When there is *yin xu* heat, the person can experience what the Chinese call 'five palm Heat'. In 'five palm Heat', it is only the palms of the hand, the soles of the feet and the centre of the chest that feel hot. My own experience is that many European patients rarely report a sensation of heat in the chest in these situations. There are also many *yin xu* patients who only feel the heat in the palms of the hand. It is important when differentiating between *xu* and *shi*

Heat to ascertain whether it is the palm of the hand (*yin xu* Heat) or both sides of the hand (*shi* Heat) that feel hot.

A person who is *qi xu* can have difficulty controlling their temperature. Therefore, they may well experience an increase in temperature on exertion.

Cold hands and feet can be a sign of many different patterns of imbalance. One of the most common causes is Liver *qi* stagnation. When there is Liver *qi* stagnation there is sufficient heat in the body but the warmth cannot circulate out to the extremities. The difference between Liver *qi* stagnation and *yang xu* is that when there is Liver *qi* stagnation it is only the hands and feet (and sometimes only the hands) that are cold. When there is *yang xu*, it is the entire arm and leg that feel cold. The arm or leg will also feel increasingly cold, the further you get from the torso. *Xue xu* and *qi xu* can also manifest with cold hands and feet, because the warmth does not get transported from the torso.

When a person has cold hands and feet, they might say that they feel cold or have an aversion to cold. This can create confusion when there is, in reality, a diagnosis of Heat. One would expect that a person who has Heat would feel hot, have an aversion to heat or at least not say that they are cold or dislike cold. If they have Liver *qi* stagnation, which may well be the underlying cause of their Heat, their cold hands and feet mean that they have an aversion to cold and feel cold, whilst in reality the body itself is warm.

Temperature

Observation	Significance
Aversion to cold	*Shi* Cold or *yang xu*
	If there is an invasion of exogenous Cold, the person will freeze, no matter how much clothing and blankets they wrap themselves up in
	In *yang xu* Cold, the person can keep warm by wrapping themselves up in warm clothes or bedding
Aversion to heat	Heat
Simultaneous chills and fever	Invasion of Wind-Heat or Wind-Cold
	If there is Wind-Heat, the fever will be dominant; if there is Wind-Cold, the chills will be dominant
Prolonged or intense fever	Internal *shi* Heat
Fever that arises in the afternoon or evening	*Yin xu* Heat
A feeling of heat that arises on slight physical exertion	*Qi xu*
Alternating fever and chills	*Xie qi* located in the *shaoyang* aspect
'Five palm Heat' (hot sensation in the palms, soles of the feet and chest)	*Yin xu* Heat
Cold hands and feet	Liver *qi* stagnation, *yang xu*, *qi xu*, *xue xu*

Energy levels

It is important to remember that fatigue can be not only a *xu* condition, but also a *shi* condition. There are, however, fundamental differences in the underlying dynamics of the two types of fatigue. There are also significant differences in when and how the fatigue manifests.

In a *xu* state of fatigue, there is a genuine deficiency of energy in the body, which makes the person feel tired. The fatigue will last all day, become more apparent as the day goes on and will usually be worst in the late afternoon and evening. The fatigue will also be worse after physical and mental activity or exertion, because the physical and mental activity will consume the person's *qi* and make their deficiency greater. It is, however, important to be aware that the person might feel refreshed and more energetic immediately after physical activity. This is because the physical activity has created movement, thereby circulating and activating their *qi*. The fatigue will, though, resurface and be greater later on that day or the day after, as they have drawn on their reserves.

When there is fatigue, it is also important to determine whether the fatigue is due to an actual *xu* condition or whether the person has unrealistic expectations with regards to how much energy a person should have. It is not uncommon for a person to complain that they feel tired or exhausted, but when questioned you discover that they are constantly physically and mentally active from early morning to late evening, and they sleep too little. These patients are *qi xu*, but their *qi xu* is the consequence of unrealistic expectations of how much *qi* the body is capable of producing, rather than an imbalance in one or more of the *qi*-producing organs.

When there is a *shi* condition manifesting with tiredness, it is not because there is insufficient *qi*. The tiredness arises because there is something that is blocking the *qi*, so it cannot circulate around the body, resulting in the person experiencing fatigue. In these cases, the fatigue will be worst in the morning. This is because the person has been physically inactive all night and their *qi* has therefore not been circulated by the body's natural movement. This means that they feel tired and find it difficult to get going in the morning. Once they have been up and about for a while, the body's natural movements help to circulate *qi* and the tiredness is reduced. Fatigue due to *shi* conditions will also be relieved by physical activity such as running, biking, yoga, chopping wood and so on. They will, on the other hand, feel more lethargic and fatigued if there is a lack of physical movement.

There are differences not only in the overall underlying mechanisms of *xu* and *shi* tiredness, but also in the mechanisms within the two groups themselves. These differences mean that there are some characteristic signs that can be asked about when differentiating the various imbalances.

Qi xu fatigue

Qi xu fatigue arises when not enough *qi* is produced to carry out the various processes in the body.

The person may well feel tired already when they wake up in the morning, either because there is not enough *qi* or because their *qi xu* means that *qi* and *xue* have a tendency to stagnate due to a lack of propulsion. This condition is then exacerbated when the person has been inactive all night and the circulation of *qi* has not been assisted by the body's physical movement. The vital difference here between them and a person who has a pure stagnation condition, is that the fatigue worsens as the day goes on and is aggravated by activity and exertion.

A person with Spleen *qi xu* will often feel tired after meals, especially after eating a lot or eating rich food. This is because large or rich meals place a greater burden on the Spleen *qi* when the Spleen transforms the ingested food into *gu qi*. The weakening of Spleen *qi* will also often give rise to the emergence of Dampness, which blocks the pure *yang qi* from ascending upwards, whilst blocking the *shen* so the person becomes drowsy and lethargic.

Yang xu fatigue

One of the tasks that *yang* performs is to activate the body. When there is *yang xu*, a person will experience both physical and mental lethargy and fatigue. They will lack a fundamental sense of enthusiasm and motivation. The difference between *qi xu* fatigue and *yang xu* fatigue will be apparent in the other signs and symptoms. *Yang xu* conditions will simultaneously manifest with signs such as an aversion to cold, cold limbs and so on. *Yang xu* fatigue is sometimes more apparent in winter, the most *yin* period of the year. The person may also suffer from winter depressions.

A man with Kidney *yang xu* will feel more fatigued after he has had sex or ejaculated, because he loses both Kidney *jing* and Kidney *yang* on ejaculation. This is also the reason that many men fall asleep immediately after sex.

Xue xu fatigue

To be completely correct, neither *xue xu* nor *yin xu* directly result in tiredness. This is because they are more physical substances that nourish but do not activate the body. Nevertheless, most books state that tiredness is a symptom of both *xue xu* and *yin xu*. Fatigue arises in these conditions because *xue* and *yin* nourish the organs that produce *qi* and because *yin* is the fundamental substance that is transformed into *yang*. Furthermore, the brain is nourished by *xue*. This means that whilst too much mental activity depletes *xue*, a lack of *xue* will also result in a person feeling mentally tired and exhausted.

Both *xue xu* and *yin xu* fatigue can be exacerbated when the person has difficulty falling asleep or sleeps poorly at night, which is a typical consequence of *yin xu* and *xue xu*.

The difference between *xue xu* fatigue and *qi xu* fatigue will be seen in the accompanying symptoms and signs, such as dry skin, poor vision, scanty menstrual bleeding and so on when there is *xue xu*.

Yin xu fatigue

A person with *yin xu* fatigue will not always be conscious of their tiredness. This is because they are often restless. Their fatigue can be exacerbated when they do not go to bed at the proper time and when they sleep poorly. They will often feel tired during the day, but in the evening when *yin* should control *yang*, their *yang* starts to ascend because it is not anchored, resulting in their *shen* becoming more active. This means that they feel more awake and start to become more active. This is unfortunate, because by being active in the evening and at night, they will further consume their *yin*, worsening the condition. The inability to anchor their *shen* also means that they have difficulty in sleeping. This just exacerbates their fatigue the next day. People with *yin xu* can sometimes find that their fatigue feels worse or arises after they have started to receive acupuncture. This is because acupuncture controls the restless empty energy that they have and they then begin to become aware of their underlying fatigue. This is not dissimilar to small children who are overtired in the evening: the later it gets, the more restless and agitated they become. They do not feel tired but are, in fact, exhausted.

Qi stagnation fatigue

A person with *qi* stagnation fatigue will often feel tired in the morning and when they are physically inactive. They do not feel tired later in the day or when they have been physically active. This is the reason that many people with Liver *qi* stagnation play a lot of sport or exercise physically. Training excessively can, in fact, be a diagnostic sign of Liver *qi* stagnation. It can be a form of self-medication. A person with Liver *qi* stagnation will often experience fatigue when faced with the tasks or situations that they have an aversion to. They will also feel tired during stressful periods.

A person with Liver *qi* stagnation will not just be tired in the morning, but often will also be grumpy and bad tempered, because their Liver *qi* is stagnated. This is a significant difference from a person with a Damp-Phlegm stagnation, who will be mentally absent and hazy in the morning.

Heart *qi* stagnation can also cause tiredness but it will be more on the mental-emotional level. They will lack joy and vitality and they will often feel depressed.

Dampness or Phlegm stagnation fatigue

People with Phlegm or Dampness will often feel tired and lethargic in the morning. Dampness and Phlegm will accumulate around the body when it is not transformed and transported. When the person lies horizontally at night, *yin* substances such as Phlegm-Dampness will seep down to the head, blurring the brain. Furthermore, the lack of physical movement in the body will also add to the stagnation of Dampness and Phlegm at night. A person with Phlegm-Dampness will also have an increased desire to sleep. They will have trouble waking up in the morning and feel heavy and tired, both mentally and physically. They will have difficulty being mentally present at the start of the day, because their *shen* is blocked. A person with Phlegm must be careful not to sleep too much during the day. Sleeping will not usually ameliorate their fatigue and lethargy but will usually make it worse.

Humid weather and low pressure can cause a person with Phlegm-Dampness to feel more tired. This is because the external dampness will aggravate the inner condition of Dampness and thereby block the circulation of *qi* in the body.

Fatigue

Observation	Significance
Fatigue that is worse after activity or increases during the day	*Qi xu, yang xu, xue xu*
Fatigue that is the worst in the daytime but gets better in the evening	*Yin xu*
Fatigue that is worst in the morning and the person is irritable in the morning	Liver *qi* stagnation
Fatigue is worst in the morning and the person is mentally lethargic and not present in the morning	Dampness or Phlegm
Fatigue that is worse after exertion	*Xu* conditions
Fatigue that is better with activity	Stagnation conditions
Feeling tired and lethargic when not physically active	Liver *qi* stagnation
Fatigue that is worse or occurs after sex	Kidney *xu* conditions
Fatigue when there is low pressure or high atmospheric humidity	Dampness and Phlegm
Fatigue arising when frustrated or faced with challenges	Liver *qi* stagnation
Fatigue after meals, especially after eating rich food	Spleen *qi xu*

Sweating

Enquiring about perspiration is especially important in relation to a diagnosis according to the Six Stages and the Four Levels, but it also elicits important information for the differentiation of *xu* patterns. Sweating imbalances can be divided into three overall groups: Heart imbalances; *xu* conditions such as *qi xu, yin xu* and *yang xu*; and invasions of *xie qi*.

Sweat is the body fluid associated with the Heart and the Fire Phase, but many other organs' physiological relationships must also be taken into account when analysing abnormal patterns of sweating.

The pores in the skin are controlled by *wei qi*, which is the most *yang* aspect of *zhen qi*. *Wei qi* is controlled by Lung *qi* and created by Spleen *qi* and Kidney *qi*. This means that a *xu* condition in one or more of these organs, as well as an overall *yang xu* condition, can result in the pores not being controlled optimally. When there is physical activity in the body, heat is generated and this will drive the body fluids upwards and outwards. If *wei qi* or *yang qi* are weak, the pores will not be able to hold back the sweat and there will be spontaneous perspiration or sweating on light activity.

Sweat is created when heat evaporates *jin*. *Jin* is, amongst other things, a component of *xue* and *xue* is governed by the Heart. This means that imbalances in the Heart can lead to abnormal sweating. This can be seen in more chronic imbalances, such as Heart *yang xu* or Heart *xue xu*, Heart Fire and so on. It is also seen in more transient disturbances of *shen*, such as nervousness, which often results in spontaneous sweating. Spontaneous sweating due to Heart imbalances will often be observed in areas of the body that are controlled by the Heart channel, particularly the beginning and end of the channel i.e. the palms of the hands and the armpits.

Invasions of *xie qi* can interfere with sweating. Due to its *yang* nature, Wind can spread and disperse *wei qi*, opening the sweat pores and thereby allowing itself and other forms of *xie qi* such as Cold to enter through the skin. Cold will, due to its astringent *yin* nature, contract the pores, closing them shut so that the person cannot sweat (and thereby expel the *xie qi*). One of the main signs that there is an invasion of *xie qi* in the *taiyang* aspect is that there is soreness and stiffness in the skin and muscles. This is because *wei qi* has been blocked by exogenous Wind-Cold, the stagnation resulting in pain and discomfort, but also, importantly, a lack of sweating because the pores in the skin are contracted and closed shut. If the person is very *wei qi xu*, on the other hand, they will sweat but the sweating will not relieve the symptoms. This is because their *wei qi* is not strong enough to control the pores, so the person sweats spontaneously. Because the *wei qi* is so weak, it cannot expel the exogenous *xie qi* upwards and outwards.

If Wind-Heat has invaded the body, the *yang* nature of the Heat will force fluids and thereby sweat upwards and outwards. The pressure of the sweat will force the pores to open, resulting in sweating. Once again, because the exogenous *xie qi* has not been expelled, the sweating does not relieve the symptoms. The difference here, though, between an invasion of Cold when there is *wei qi xu* and an invasion of Wind-Heat is that there will be signs of Heat in the latter scenario. The pulse is often a good indicator when differentiating between the various types of invasion. An invasion of Wind-Cold will usually manifest with a Tight pulse, whereas the pulse will be Empty if there is *wei qi xu*. Invasions of Wind-Heat should be accompanied by a Rapid pulse. In all three situations, the pulse will be Superficial, because the imbalance is in the exterior aspect of the body.

If exogenous *xie qi* penetrates down to the *qi* or *yangming* aspect, the violent struggle between *zheng qi* and *xie qi* will generate a significant amount of Heat. The extreme Heat will force fluids up to the surface of the body, resulting in profuse sweating. Because *xie qi* has now penetrated deeper into the body, the profuse sweating does not relieve the symptoms. The difference between Wind-Heat and *qi* level or *yangming* Heat is that the pulse and the sweating will be much stronger when *xie qi* has penetrated to the interior.

If *xie qi* becomes locked in the *shaoyang* aspect, the person will alternate between periods where they spontaneously sweat and have a fever or feel hot and periods when they freeze and have chills. Importantly, there will be no sweating and fever sensations whilst they have chills, which is otherwise characteristic of invasions of exogenous *xie qi* in the *taiyang* aspect.

Yang xu and *qi xu* are not the only *xu* conditions that can cause sweating disturbances. A classic symptom of *yin xu* Heat is night sweats. This is because *yin* should be able to anchor *yang* and thereby control Heat. If *yin* is weak, it will not be able to control the Heat at night, which is the period in which *yin* should be dominant. The Heat will force fluids upwards and outwards during the night. The problem is compounded by the fact that *wei qi*, which controls the pores, does not circulate in the exterior at night but is in the interior. The pores are therefore not able to hold the sweat in the body. Night sweats due to *yin xu* can be a chronic condition or they can be acute when exogenous *xie qi* has penetrated down to the *ying* level in a diagnosis according to the Four Levels.

It is, however, important to note that night sweats are not always a manifestation of *yin xu* Heat; Damp-Heat can also result in night sweats. Damp-Heat sweat tends to be more yellowish. You can ask the patient whether the sweat stains their sheets or nightclothes a yellowish colour. Damp-Heat night sweats are also more predominant on the head than the torso and limbs, because Damp can block the pores of the skin in the body so the Heat funnels the sweat up to the head. Yellowish and sticky sweat is, in general, a sign of Damp-Heat, as is odorous sweat.

Sweat

Observation	Significance
Sweating during an invasion of exogenous *xie qi*, which does not relieve the symptoms	Wind-Cold with concurrent *wei qi xu* Wind-Heat
Lack of sweating during the invasion of exogenous *xie qi*	Wind-Cold
Spontaneous sweating	*Yang xu* or *qi xu*
Night sweats	*Yin xu*, *ying*-level Heat, Damp-Heat
Constant or profuse sweating	*Yangming* stage or *qi* level Heat *Shi* Heat
Alternating sweating and chills (not simultaneously)	*Shaoyang* stage
'Five palms sweating' (sweating from the palms of the hands, soles of the feet and the chest)	*Yin xu*
Yellowish or sticky sweat	Damp-Heat
Odorous sweat	Damp-Heat
Nervous sweating, especially in the palms of the hands and the armpits	Heart *qi xu*

Thirst, appetite and taste

Enquiring about a person's eating habits, thirst, taste preferences and appetite can tell us a lot about the condition of the internal organs and factors such as Heat, Cold, *yin* and *yang*. It will also help to identify possible aetiological factors among the substances that the person ingests. For example, a person whose diet consists primarily of salads, cheese and yoghurt will have a tendency to develop Spleen *yang xu* and Dampness, whilst a person who regularly drinks alcohol can have a tendency to develop Heat in the Liver and Stomach. The following sections will address a person's attraction to certain foods or drinks, their appetite, thirst and so on as a manifestation of possible patterns of imbalance, rather than possible aetiological factors.

Thirst

If there is Heat present in the body, it will both injure and expel body fluids. These fluids must then be replenished. This means that a person with Heat will experience thirst. One of the differences between *shi* and *xu* Heat is how powerful the thirst is. *Shi* Heat, being more substantial, results in a thirst that is stronger. A person with *shi* Heat will want to drink large amounts of cold fluids. They will also drink in large gulps, rather than sipping small mouthfuls, which is more typical of a person who is *yin xu*. When there is *yin xu*, the tissues in the body lack moisture. The person will often have a dry mouth and throat, especially at night. They will therefore not need to drink as often as a person with *shi* Heat. They do not have the same need either for cold drinks to cool the body down, and they do not need to drink as much at a time. A person with *shi* Heat will often have a large glass or a bottle of water nearby, which they quickly empty. A person who is *yin xu* is more likely to have a glass of water standing beside the bed, from which they only drink a couple of mouthfuls.

A person with Damp-Heat will be thirsty due to the presence of Heat, but the Dampness will mean that they still do not feel like drinking or that they forget to drink.

When there is *shi* Cold and *yang xu* Cold, the lack of transport and transformation of fluids in the body will mean that a person will have less need to consume fluids. They will, therefore, often have a lack of thirst. The presence of Cold or the lack of *yang* will result in a preference for hot beverages to help to warm the body up.

Thirst

Observation	Significance
Great thirst with desire for cold drinks, drinks in large gulps	Internal *shi* Heat patterns
Thirst or dryness of the mouth and throat, sips the water	*Yin xu* Heat
Lack of thirst or preference for hot drinks	Cold patterns, *yang xu*
Thirst with no desire to drink	Damp-Heat

Appetite, nausea and vomiting

The appetite should theoretically be a good indicator of the state of a person's Spleen *qi*, poor appetite being a key sign of Spleen *qi xu* in Chinese textbooks. Many of the clients we see in the clinic who are Spleen *qi xu* often say, however, that they have a healthy appetite. The reason for this is that people eat and drink for many reasons, most of which are not directly related to their nutritional needs. Eating food is closely connected to factors such as pleasure, comfort, bodily control, habits, boredom, upbringing, culture, procrastination and so on. This means that the answers given in relation to appetite and diet must also be seen in this context.

As stated, the Spleen and the Stomach have a determining influence on appetite. If there is Spleen and Stomach *qi xu*, the person will have difficulty transforming the food that is ingested and the *qi ji* (*qi* mechanism) in the middle *jiao* will start to stall. It will manifest with a reduced appetite or being easily sated. Despite this fact, it is more common that patients who are Spleen *qi xu* will say that they have a good appetite, as will patients with Dampness blocking the *qi ji* in the middle *jiao*. This is because people eat for many reasons other than hunger. If the patient consciously observes the sensation in their stomach, they will often discover that the sensation of hunger is located in the mouth or somewhere other than the physical stomach. You can ask the patient how their appetite is in the mornings. Many people with Spleen *qi xu*, especially those with Dampness or Phlegm, will have no appetite in the mornings. They will often skip breakfast and only eat later in the morning, maybe after they have arrived at their job. This is because the Stomach and Spleen's *qi ji* is inactive whilst they are sleeping. When they arise it will take a while for the Spleen and Stomach *qi* to start circulating if they are Spleen and Stomach *qi xu*, especially if Dampness blocks the movement of the *qi*.

Many people also express that they have a large appetite. This, again, is something that you have to be cautious about when drawing conclusions. A patient saying they have a large appetite is not always an indication of Stomach Fire. Many people, especially women, say their appetite is large, because they think that they eat too much but in reality their appetite is normal. The problem is that they think that they should be thinner than they are. Some people think that they have a large appetite because they are constantly nibbling at food and eating all day long. The question is whether they are constantly eating because they are actually physically hungry, as in Stomach Fire, or whether they eat because they are bored, mentally restless or to drown their feelings. These are more Heart imbalance patterns than they are Stomach Fire patterns. Stomach Fire will typically manifest with an insatiable appetite and the person will quickly feel hungry again soon after eating. This is typically seen in teenage boys, who immediately after having eaten a large meal will go into the kitchen to get a bowl of cornflakes or a sandwich. This is because their *mingmen* has flared up, creating Heat in the Stomach. Stomach Fire quickly burns up the food that has been consumed. The *yang* Heat also creates a need for something solid and *yin* to create a balance in the Stomach, especially something that is Cold in its dynamic.

Heart imbalances can also affect the appetite. Heart *qi xu* and Heart *qi* stagnation can lead to a person either comfort eating or losing their appetite entirely, such as when people are heartbroken or depressed.

Heat Patterns can manifest with an attraction to cold foods. This will be both food that is cold in temperature and food that is energetically cold. This is because the body needs to cool down when there is Heat. Consuming foods that are energetically hot will often have a negative effect on their symptoms. Conversely, people with Cold patterns will either prefer to eat warm meals or they will feel that it is unpleasant to eat food that is energetically cold or has a cold temperature.

Individuals with internal Heat and a stagnation of *qi* or *xue* will often be attracted to spicy food, which is often energetically hot. This is despite the fact that they should, theoretically, prefer cold food. This is because the hot and spicy food will help to alleviate and disperse the stagnation. Although the hot, spicy substances will ameliorate their symptoms in the short term, they will often have a negative effect in the long run, creating further Heat.

Food stagnation can manifest with an aversion to eating. This is because there is a physical accumulation in the digestive system that blocks the *qi ji*. Food stagnation can also generate Heat in the Stomach. This can mean that the person soon feels hungry again, even though the Stomach is still full.

Food stagnation can also cause the Stomach *qi* to become rebellious and manifest with acid reflux or burping, which can also be seen when there is Stomach Fire. This is because Heat has an ascendant energy, thereby sending Stomach *qi* upwards. Stomach Fire can also manifest with a stinging or burning sensation in the Stomach.

Nausea

Nausea can encompass anything from a lack of appetite to a feeling of wanting to vomit. Nausea is again a sign that the *qi ji* in the middle *jiao* is impaired. The reasons can be varied, and differentiation of the relevant patterns will often be based on when the nausea is worst. Nausea immediately after eating is mainly a manifestation of Spleen *qi xu* and food stagnation. The nausea arises due to the Spleen not being able to transform the food that has been consumed, which then accumulates in the Stomach and blocks the Stomach's *qi ji*.

If the nausea manifests in the premenstrual phase or arises when the person is stressed or emotionally affected, the nausea will be due to Liver *qi* stagnation, where the stagnated Liver *qi* invades the Stomach and Spleen, disturbing the movement of their *qi*.

Nausea is also seen in pregnancy and is caused by a disturbance of the *chong mai*. This is due to the physiological changes that the foetus initiates in the Uterus. *Chong mai* connects the Uterus and the Stomach. This means that disturbances of *qi* in the *chong mai* can disturb the Stomach's *qi ji*. This is only one of the causes of vomiting during pregnancy. Other causes of morning sickness can be Stomach and Spleen *qi xu*, Stomach *yin xu*, Liver *qi* stagnation, Liver Fire and Stomach Fire. If there is Stomach and Spleen *qi xu*, the nausea will be exacerbated when the woman is tired or if she has not eaten. Often, she can control the nausea by constantly nibbling at food. If she not only has nausea, but also has vomiting, the vomiting will not be explosive but more retching. If there is Liver Fire or Stomach Fire, the vomiting will be explosive and the vomit will be very sour in taste. Consuming ginger, which is often recommended to relieve nausea, will often worsen the condition if there is Fire. This is because it will add to the Heat in the Stomach. Ginger will, on the other hand, have a beneficial effect if there is Stomach and Spleen *qi xu.*

Most of these patterns can also be seen when there is vomiting that is not related to a pregnancy.

Acute vomiting will come from an invasion of exogenous *xie qi* or food stagnation. The exogenous *xie qi* can be Heat, Summer-Dampness, Summer-Heat or Cold. If there is an invasion of Cold in the Stomach, the vomit will be watery and contain undigested food. This is because the Cold has blocked or extinguished Spleen *yang*, which is the digestive fire. The person will often have a cold sensation in the Stomach and the skin in the epigastric region can feel cold on palpation.

Heat will cause the vomit to be sour or bitter in taste, and the vomit will be odorous. This will not be the case in a Cold condition. Summer-Heat and Summer-Dampness will result in the vomit being yellow and watery.

Observation of the tongue's coating and colour is important when differentiating between the above patterns. Heat patterns will manifest with the tongue having a yellow coating, whereas the Cold patterns will manifest with a white coating.

Damp-Phlegm in the Stomach will result in thin, slimy vomit.

Vomit that contains blood can be seen when there is Stomach Fire or *xue* stagnation in the Stomach. *Xue* stagnation can block the vessels so much that they eventually rupture. Fire can agitate *xue* so that it bursts the vessels' walls.

Appetite, nausea and vomiting

Observation	Significance
Preference for cold foods	Heat patterns
Preference for hot foods	Cold patterns
Poor appetite or easily satiated	Spleen *qi xu*
No appetite in the morning	Stomach and Spleen *qi xu*, Damp-Phlegm
Insatiable hunger or becoming hungry shortly after having eaten	Stomach Fire
Aversion to food	Food stagnation
Acid reflux	Stomach Fire
Nausea after eating	Spleen *qi xu*, food stagnation
Nausea caused by emotional pressure and stress	Liver *qi* stagnation
Nausea caused by hunger	Spleen *qi xu*
Nausea during the premenstrual period	Liver *qi* stagnation
Morning sickness	Rebellious *qi* in the *chong mai*, Stomach and Spleen *qi xu*, Liver and Stomach Fire, Liver *qi* stagnation, Stomach *yin xu*

Acute vomiting	Invasion of exogenous *xie qi*, food stagnation
Chronic vomiting	Food stagnation, Damp-Phlegm, Liver *qi* stagnation, Stomach Fire, Stomach and Spleen *qi xu*, Spleen *yang xu*
Explosive vomiting	*Shi* patterns
Thin, slimy vomit	Damp-Phlegm
Sour or bitter vomit	Heat in the Stomach, Liver or Gall Bladder
Clear and watery vomit that is odourless	Cold in the Stomach or Spleen *yang xu*
Blood in the vomit	*Xue* stagnation or Stomach Fire
Burping, with the taste of food that has been eaten earlier	Food stagnation

Taste

Imbalances in the various organs can result in a person being attracted to specific flavours. This is most typically seen when someone who is Spleen *qi xu* has a craving for sweets. The problem is that they often respond to this signal by eating sweets, cakes or other things that have a high sugar content and have a very concentrated sweet flavour. This will overload the Spleen and create Dampness, which further weakens the Spleen. This causes the weakened Spleen to crave more sweet food. The consequence will be that, because the Spleen is even weaker, the craving for something sweet will be greater and a vicious cycle begins. The craving for the other flavours are not as evident in imbalances of the other organs. It is, however, interesting how many people are attracted to the bitter flavour of coffee!

Certain flavours can be appealing to some people, not because of the organ that the flavour resonates with but due to the energetic dynamic of the flavour. For example, the spicy flavour is very dynamic and can help to disperse stagnant *qi*.

Imbalances in *zangfu* organs can also manifest with a person experiencing a certain taste in their mouth. Bitterness is the taste that relates to the Fire phase. If the person experiences a bitter taste in their mouth (often they will describe it as a bad taste or a metallic taste), it will not necessarily be a Heart imbalance. The Fire Phase resonates with Fire and Heat in general. This means that a bitter or metallic taste can be seen when there is Fire in the Stomach and Liver, as well as the Heart. Liver imbalances can manifest with a sour taste in the mouth. A sweet, sticky taste or sensation in the mouth will be a sign of Dampness or Phlegm. The person will sometimes brush their tongue to get rid of the sticky sensation that often accompanies a very greasy tongue coating (which in itself can be a sign of Dampness and Phlegm).

It is important to remember that some medicines can result in an unpleasant taste in the mouth. It is important to assess whether the taste is due to a change in the body's physiology, for example a bitter taste has arisen because medicine has created Heat in the body, or whether the taste itself is from the medicine and therefore has no diagnostic significance.

Lacking a sense of taste is mostly a manifestation of Spleen *qi xu* but can also result from Phlegm in the Lung that clogs the nose and sinuses or *xue* stagnation in the nose after a physical trauma. This is because aromatic flavours are discerned in the nose.

Taste

Observation	Significance
Craving for sweets	Spleen *qi xu*
No sense of taste	Spleen *qi xu*, Lung Phlegm or *xue* stagnation
Sweet, sticky taste in the mouth	Damp-Phlegm
Bitter or metallic taste in the mouth	Heart, Liver and Stomach Fire
Sour taste or taste of previously ingested food	Food stagnation

Stools and urination

Stools

Enquiry about the stool includes the stool's regularity, consistency and smell and whether there is pain associated with passing of the stool. Something that ought to be fairly straightforward and easy to get concrete answers about can sometimes be surprisingly difficult, because many people are not very conscious about their stools and can only provide vague answers.

It is also important to define for a patient what regular bowel movements are. Once a week is, technically, regular and so is six times a day, but both cases are signs of severe imbalances. Once to twice a day is considered normal, and less or more often than that is an expression of an imbalance.

The consistency of the stools can deviate from normal by being watery, sticky or dry.

Constipation

Constipation is when stool movements are less frequent than once daily. Knowing that a person is constipated is not enough; it is also important to ascertain the consistency of the stool and whether there is pain associated with passing the stool.

Acute constipation can be due to an invasion of exogenous *xie qi*. This will either be a direct invasion of Cold in the Intestines or *shi* Heat from an invasion of exogenous *xie qi* penetrating down to the *yangming* aspect. If the invading *xie qi* is Hot, the stools will dry out and the abdomen will feel tense. If the invading *xie qi* is Cold, the stools will not be dry, there will be cramping pain and the abdomen will feel cold on palpation.

Apart from *shi* Heat, *yin xu* and *xue xu* can cause the stools to be dry due to a lack of fluids. The difference between *xu* and *shi* conditions can be determined by whether there is pain or bloating, which will occur in a *shi* condition.

Liver *qi* stagnation can also result in the stool not moving freely and smoothly through the Intestines. Therefore, the stools will typically be pebble-like, similar to goat droppings. If *qi* stagnation has generated Heat, the stools will also be dry. *Qi* stagnation can cause the movement of the stool to be sluggish, taking a long time to pass through the Intestines. There may well also be pain, tension and bloating in the abdomen when there is *Qi* stagnation. This will be alleviated by the passing of the stool. It is important to remember that a stagnation of *qi* in the Intestines is not always due to Liver *qi* stagnation.

Liver *qi* stagnation can also manifest with alternating constipation and normal or loose stools.

Spleen *qi xu* can be indicated by stools that are long and thin like a pencil. The stools will have an otherwise normal consistency. *Yang xu* constipation will also manifest with a stool that has a normal consistency, the constipation arising from a lack of *yang* movement in the Intestines. The stool will take a long time to pass through the Intestines, and the person may feel exhausted and sweat after passing the stool. Lung *qi xu* can also manifest with exhaustion and sweating after bowel movements. Again, the person lacks the strength to transport the stool downwards through the Intestines. The effort of passing the stool will weaken the person's *qi* so much that they will feel exhausted and the Lung will temporarily lose control of the pores, resulting in spontaneous sweating.

Constipation

Observation	Significance
Constipation, dry stools, abdominal tension, pain	*Shi* Heat
Constipation, compact stools, abdominal tension, cramping pain	*Shi* Cold
Small lumpy stools, stools that resemble goat droppings	Liver *qi* stagnation
Long loose stools, not hard or dry	Spleen *qi xu*
Dried stool, the abdomen does not feel tense or tight	*Xue xu, yin xu*
Fatigue after defecation	Lung *qi xu*
Sluggish stools	*Qi* stagnation, *yang xu*
Constipation in a woman who has just given birth	*Xue xu*
Alternating constipation and loose or normal stools	Liver *qi* stagnation
Conditions that are better after defecation	*Shi* conditions
Conditions that are worse after a bowel movement	*Xu* conditions

Loose stools and diarrhoea

It is important to differentiate between an acute and a chronic condition. Acute diarrhoea will be due to an invasion of exogenous *xie qi* and will thus be a *shi* condition.

In acute conditions, it is important to differentiate between Heat and Cold. An invasion of Damp-Heat will cause the stool to be explosive, because there is an excess of *qi* present. The stools will also be strong smelling and sticky and there will be a burning sensation in the rectum due to the presence of Heat. If the Heat is very strong, it will cause *xue* to rupture the vessels in the intestinal walls, resulting in blood in the stools. Damp-Heat can be a chronic as well as an acute condition. The symptoms will be the same, but the aetiology will be different.

If the stool is very watery, does not smell and contains undigested food particles, it will be due to an invasion of Cold, which is an acute condition, or Spleen and/or Kidney *yang xu* if it is chronic. If it is an acute *shi* condition, the stools will also be explosive and the abdomen will feel cold and tense, and there will be a cramping pain. The tension and pain will be alleviated by passing stools.

Yang xu can manifest with the passing of watery stools early in the morning. The person will often feel exhausted after defecation.

When there is Spleen *qi xu*, the ingested food will not be transformed as it should, so the food will pass more quickly through the Intestines and the person will have a bowel movement soon after they have eaten. If there is Spleen *yang xu*, there will be undigested food in the stool because there has not been a transformation of the food. The stools will also be watery when there is Spleen *yang xu*. Neither Spleen *qi xu* nor Spleen *yang xu* will manifest with stools that smell strongly.

Enquiry should be made about which foods affect the stools negatively. Strong spices, alcohol, fried food, sugar and dairy products will have a negative effect on the Damp-Heat conditions. Spleen *qi xu*, Spleen *yang xu* and Dampness will all be aggravated by consuming raw vegetables, salad, too much fruit, cold foods, sugar, sweets, dairy products and the like.

If there is a lot of gas in the Intestines and the person has flatulence, this will be due to Liver *qi* stagnation, Spleen *qi xu* or Damp-Heat. Damp-Heat flatulence will be odorous.

Diarrhoea

Observation	Significance
Explosive diarrhoea	*Shi* pattern
Acute condition	*Shi* pattern
Chronic condition	*Xu* pattern
Passing of stools shortly after eating	Spleen *qi xu*
Passing of watery stools early in the morning	Kidney and Spleen *yang xu*
Burning sensation in the rectum and sticky, strong-smelling stools	Damp-Heat
Watery stools containing undigested food particles	*Yang xu*, *shi* Cold
Cramping pain that is alleviated by the passing of stools	Liver *qi* stagnation
Sticky stools	Damp-Heat
Bloody diarrhoea	Damp-Heat, Toxic-Fire
Pain or tension that is alleviated by defecation	Liver *qi* stagnation, Damp-Heat

Stools containing mucus	Damp-Phlegm
Flatulence without odour	Liver *qi* stagnation or Spleen *qi xu*
Flatulence which is odorous	Damp-Heat
Intestinal discomfort that is alleviated by the passing of stools	*Shi* conditions
The condition is aggravated by consumption of alcohol, fried food, dairy products, sugar and dried fruit	Damp-Heat
The condition is aggravated by consuming salad, raw vegetables, fruit, cold foods, dairy products, sugar, sweets and dried fruit	Spleen *qi xu*, Spleen *yang xu*, Dampness
Alternating diarrhoea and constipation/normal stools	Liver *qi* stagnation
Condition improves after the passing of stools	*Shi* conditions
The condition worsens after the passing of stools	*Xu* conditions

Urination

Urinary disturbances relate not only to Kidney and Urinary Bladder imbalances, but also to various forms of *xie qi*, such as Dampness and Hot and Cold conditions. It is important to ask about the frequency of urination, the amount, colour and odour of the urine and whether there is pain or discomfort upon urination.

If there is Kidney *yang xu*, the Kidneys will not perform their task of transforming and transporting fluids optimally. The untransformed fluids will therefore drain down to the Urinary Bladder due to their *yin* nature. Kidney *yang* should also control the lower orifices and hold the urine in the Urinary Bladder. These factors result in an increased amount of urine that is clear in colour, and the person will have difficulty retaining the urine in the body. This can manifest with symptoms such as frequent urination, urinary incontinence and nocturia.

Kidney *yang* is used to drive the urine out of the Urinary Bladder. This means that when there is Kidney *yang xu* there may be difficulty in voiding the urine or incomplete emptying of the Urinary Bladder. Incomplete and difficult urination can also be seen in stagnation conditions such as *shi* Cold, Damp-Heat, Phlegm and Liver *qi* stagnation.

If the urine is dark and/or strong-smelling, this is an indication of Heat. The Heat may be both *xu* or *shi* in nature The Heat will 'steam' the urine, so there will usually be a smaller volume of urine. The Heat may also agitate the urine and force it out of the Urinary Bladder, so even though there are only small amounts of urine, there is still frequent urination or an urge to urinate, despite the Urinary Bladder being almost empty.

The Heat can also cause the vessels in the Urinary Bladder to rupture so that there is blood in the urine. It is not only Heat that can result in there being blood in the urine; Spleen *qi* may be too weak to hold the *xue* inside the vessels and *xue* stagnation can block the vessels so that they finally rupture from the pressure of the *xue* that is being blocked from flowing. Heat can also manifest with a burning or stinging sensation when urinating.

If there is urinary pain that is ameliorated upon urination, it will be a stagnation condition. The urination itself is also likely to be difficult. Pain or discomfort after urination will be a sign of a *xu* condition.

Dampness tends to makes emissions, exudations and discharges become thicker, cloudy and less transparent. Therefore, oily or cloudy urine is a sign of Dampness or Damp-Heat in the lower *jiao*.

Urination

Observation	Significance
Dark, yellowish and/or odorous urine	Heat
Clear, voluminous urine	Cold or *yang xu* conditions
Frequent, scanty, yellow urine	Damp-Heat in the lower *jiao*
Frequent urination with clear urine	*Yang xu* or Cold in the lower *jiao*
Urinary difficulty or incomplete emptying of the Urinary Bladder	Damp-Heat in the Urinary Bladder, *yang xu*, Cold, Phlegm, *xue* stagnation and Liver *qi* stagnation
Blood in the urine	*Shi* Heat or Spleen *qi xu*
Nocturia (urination during the night)	Kidney *yang xu*
Pain or discomfort in urination	Stagnation conditions
Pain or discomfort during urination	Heat in the Urinary Bladder
Pain or discomfort after urination	*Xu* conditions
Cloudy urine	Dampness
Oily urine	Dampness

Heart, thorax and Lung

Heart

The main area of enquiry about the Heart is whether there are palpitations, cardiac pain or pain in the chest.

It is important to note that palpitations in Chinese medicine are not limited to a rapid heartbeat or a powerful heartbeat. Palpitations in Chinese medicine are all situations where the person can feel the beating of their heart, because normally you should not be conscious of your heart beating.

Palpitations where there is also a sense of emotional turmoil or anxiety will be due to Gall Bladder and Heart *qi xu*, Heart *yin xu*, Heart *xue xu* or *shi* Heat. Heart *yin* and Heart *xue*, as well as nourishing the physical aspects of the Heart, nourish and anchor the Heart's *shen* aspect, which means that it is not only the physical aspect of the Heart that becomes imbalanced when these are weak. Heat can agitate the *shen* and simultaneously over-activate the physical aspects of the Heart. This will also give rise to palpitations and emotional turmoil. Gall Bladder and Heart *qi xu* results in a person being very nervous and their *shen* lacks the ability to control their heartbeat when they are nervous.

If the palpations are of a more purely physical nature, it is more likely that there is Heart *qi* stagnation, Heart *qi xu*, Heart *yang xu* or Heart *xue* stagnation. If Heart *qi* or Heart *yang* are weak, they can no longer control the rhythmic beating of the Heart. *Xue* stagnation can block Heart *qi* and Heart *xue*, so they can no longer perform their functions.

Heart *xue* stagnation will also usually manifest with cardiac or chest pain.

Palpitations

Observation	Significance
Palpitations with a concurrent sense of emotional turmoil or anxiety	Heart *yin xu*, Heart *xue xu*, Heat, Gall Bladder and Heart *qi xu*
Palpitations with a tight sensation in the chest	Heart *qi* stagnation
Palpitations with stabbing pain in the chest	Heart *xue* stagnation

Thorax

Enquiry should be made about whether there is pain, tightness, heaviness and agitation in the thoracic region.

Pain in this thorax is often caused by Heart or Lung imbalances, but the Liver can also be involved.

Cramping, tight pain in the heart that feels as though the heart is being squeezed in a vice is due to Cold. If the pain is sharp, piercing or stabbing, there will be Heart *xue* stagnation. A burning pain is the result of Heat. The Heat can be both *xu* and *shi*.

If the chest feels tight – as if there is a metal rim or a piece of elastic around the chest, making it difficult to breathe in – this is a sign of *qi* stagnation. A similar sensation is that of having a large stone or weight on top of the chest. This will also inhibit the breathing and the chest will feel 'blocked'. This sensation results from the presence of Phlegm blocking the movement of *qi* in the upper *jiao*.

Heat in the upper *jiao* can give rise to a feeling of unease and turmoil in the chest because the Heat agitates the *qi*. The sensation may also be experienced when exogenous *xie* Heat penetrates deeper and affects the Pericardium.

Patients with acute cardiac and chest pain should immediately be referred to a Western doctor for further examination.

Thorax

Observation	Significance
Pain	Heart *xue* stagnation, Heat, Cold
Unrest and turmoil	Heat
Heaviness	Phlegm
Tightness	*Qi* stagnation
Pain radiating from the heart and down the left arm	Heart *xue* stagnation

Lung

Enquiry should be made about the respiration, coughing, whether there are exudations from the nose and whether there is mucus in the chest or in the throat. Breathing difficulties and coughing always indicate that there is a disturbance of Lung *qi*. The disturbance can be due to imbalances in the Lung itself or other factors affecting the Lung. This is because it is the Lung that controls the breathing by sending its *qi* downwards.

Heaviness and tightness in the chest have been described above.

Breathing

When a person becomes breathless, it is because the Lung is not able to send its *qi* downwards or because the Kidneys are not able to grasp the *qi*. Lung *qi xu*, possibly combined with the Spleen *qi xu*, can manifest with the Lung not being strong enough to descend and spread *qi* from the chest.

Lung *qi* can also be blocked in its movement by *xie qi*. This will typically be some form of Phlegm, but *qi* stagnation in the upper *jiao* may also be involved. Invasions by exogenous *xie qi* can also block the Lung *qi*.

Difficulty breathing can be due to Lung *qi xu* or Lung *yin xu*, resulting in the Lung being too weak to descend and disseminate *qi*. Kidney *qi xu* can mean that the Kidneys are not strong enough to grasp the *qi*. Phlegm, *xue* stagnation or *qi* stagnation can block the movement of Lung *qi*. Phlegm will often be the cause of wheezing or a rattling sound in the chest.

A person who frequently yawns or who has a need to sigh will often be manifesting Liver *qi* stagnation. The body yawns or sighs in an attempt to fill the Lung with air and thereby strengthen *zong qi* so it can forcibly disperse and circulate the stagnant *qi*.

Coughing

If the person has a cough, it is important to ask about how loud the cough is, how long they have had it, if there is sputum, the consistency and colour of the sputum and when the cough occurs.

A powerful, explosive or barking cough will be seen in a *shi* condition, usually Heat and/or Phlegm.

If the cough is acute and has recently arisen, it will probably be due to an invasion of exogenous *xie qi*.

Chronic coughs can be *xu* or *shi* or a combination of both. Lung *qi xu* and Lung *yin xu* coughs will be weak and will not be loud. Lung *yin xu* will manifest with a cough that is dry, ticklish and worse in the evening and at night. There may be dry, rubbery sputum that is difficult to expectorate. Both Lung *qi xu* and Lung *yin xu* coughs will be worse after the person has used their Lung *qi*, for example by talking, triggering a coughing fit. They will also cough more frequently when they are tired.

Exposure to a dry environment can result in a dry cough. The Lung fears dryness, because dryness will injure Lung *yin*. Dryness is not normally a climatic influence associated with Northern Europe, but it can be seen when there is poor indoor air quality, such as in buildings made of concrete.

Phlegm pattern coughs are usually worst in the morning. This is because the Phlegm will have accumulated in the Lung during the night whilst the person is lying down. There are several types of Phlegm and each will have its own characteristics. Phlegm-Heat results in a loud, sometimes barking cough with yellowish or greenish sputum. This mucus can be sticky and difficult to expectorate. This is a typical 'smoker's cough'. Damp-Phlegm and Phlegm-Cold will manifest with thin, watery sputum that is looser. Phlegm-Fluids manifest with sputum that is very watery; there will be a bubbling, rattling sound in the Lung and the person will have difficulty lying down because they start to suffocate.

Coughs with profuse sputum that are worse after consumption of certain foods, such as dairy products, are due to Damp-Phlegm in the Lung. The root of this Phlegm will often be Spleen *qi xu* with Dampness. It is said that 'Phlegm is stored in the Lung, but produced in the Spleen.'

If there is an element of *qi* stagnation, the cough or breathing difficulty will be worst in the morning or when the person is angry, frustrated, stressed or in the premenstrual phase.

The nose and sinuses

Sneezing is a sign of rebellious Lung *qi*. The nose is an aspect of the Lung and the Lung sends *qi* downwards. If the sneeze is acute, it will usually be due to an invasion of exogenous *xie qi*. The exudations from the nose will usually be clear and watery if there is Wind-Cold. If there is Wind-Heat, the nose will be more blocked and exudations will be yellowish and thicker. If there is Toxic-Fire the exudations will be thick and greenish and they will smell and taste foul.

There may be a chronic condition of runny nose with clear transparent and thin mucus. This is seen in Damp-Phlegm conditions. Phlegm-Heat can result in both an acute or a chronic blocked nose and sinuses. The mucus will be yellow or white and it will be thick and sticky. If there is Toxic-Heat, the mucus will be greenish and thick. Both Liver Fire and Stomach Fire may be involved in Phlegm-Heat conditions manifesting in the nose and sinuses. Fire conditions can also agitate *xue* so that it ruptures the walls of the vessels in the nose, resulting in blood in the mucus.

If there is Lung *qi xu*, the Lung can easily be invaded by exogenous *xie qi*. This can manifest as a chronic condition where the person sneezes after the slightest contact with the exogenous *xie qi*.

Coughing, dyspnoea, blocked or runny nose

Observation	Significance
Loud cough with white or clear sputum	Wind-Cold, Damp-Phlegm, Phlegm-Cold
Loud cough with yellow sputum	Wind-Heat, Phlegm-Heat
Loud and explosive cough	*Shi* condition

Observation	Significance
Barking cough	*Shi* Heat
Dry or ticklish cough	Lung *yin xu*, Dryness
Weak cough	*Xu* conditions
Weak cough with scanty Phlegm, dry, rubbery sputum or no sputum	Lung *yin xu*
Cough with sticky sputum that is difficult to expectorate	*Shi* Heat in the Lung
Loose, clear or watery sputum	Phlegm-Cold, Damp-Phlegm, Phlegm-Fluids
Cough that is worst in the evening and at night	Lung *yin xu*
Cough that is worst in the morning	Phlegm
Cough that is worst when a person speaks or is tired	Lung *xu* conditions
Cough that is worst after consuming dairy products	Phlegm
Shortness of breath, easily breathless	Lung *qi xu*, Lung *yin xu*, Kidney *xu*, Phlegm, *qi* stagnation
Difficulty breathing	Phlegm, Lung *qi xu*, stagnation of *qi*, *xue* stagnation in the Lung, invasions of exogenous *xie qi*
Wheezing or rattling sounds in the chest	Phlegm
Desire to yawn or sigh	*Qi* stagnation
Feeling that there is a heavy stone on top of the chest	Phlegm
Difficulty breathing in deeply because the chest feels tight	*Qi* stagnation
Sneezing	Invasion of exogenous *xie qi*, Lung *qi xu*
Runny nose with clear, watery mucus	Wind-Cold, Damp-Phlegm
The nose or sinuses are blocked with yellowish or greenish mucus	Wind-Heat, Phlegm-Heat, Toxic-Fire
Blood in the mucus	Fire

Dizziness

Dizziness encompasses everything from a slight dizziness when getting up, with dots in front of the eyes that quickly disappear again, to extreme vertigo, where the room spins around and there is difficulty maintaining balance.

The main differentiation of dizziness is between *xu* and *shi* conditions – whether there is enough *qi*, *xue* or *jing* to nourish the Brain or something is blocking their movement up to the Brain.

Enquiry should be made about what triggers the dizziness. If the dizziness comes when getting up, it is often due to *qi xu* and or *xue xu*, because *qi* and *xue* are not strong enough to ascend as quickly as the person getting up. In some situations, this can be due to Phlegm blocking the ascent of *qi* and *xue*.

Xue xu dizziness is often exacerbated during and after menstruation. This is because the woman is more *xue xu* due to bleeding. This type of dizziness is also common after childbirth. *Xu* types of dizziness are also worse when the person is tired after exertion and improve when the person has rested.

If the dizziness comes when the person is stressed, frustrated or irritated, it will be due to Liver imbalances, such as Liver Wind, Liver Fire or Liver *yang* rising. Liver Fire will also manifest with a hot sensation in the head during an attack of dizziness.

If the dizziness is worse after sexual activity, it will be an indication that Kidney *jing* is not nourishing the Brain.

A sensation that the room is spinning round indicates Wind-Phlegm. Sensations of nausea and heavy-headedness will also indicate Phlegm.

Dizziness and vertigo

Observation	Significance
Dizziness when getting up	*Qi xu*, *xue xu* or Phlegm
Acute dizziness, especially dizziness when lying down or sitting	Wind-Phlegm
Dizziness accompanied by nausea or a heavy sensation in the head	Phlegm
Dizziness and blurred vision, which is aggravated by exertion and when tired	*Qi xu* and *xue xu*
Dizziness that is worse after sexual activity	Kidney *jing xu*
Dizziness and ringing in the ears	Kidney *jing xu*
Dizziness with loud sound in the ears or headaches	Liver *yang* rising
Vertigo with heaviness in the body or head	Phlegm

Skin, hair and nails

Generally speaking, the skin is under the overall influence of the Lung, the hair of the head is under the influence of the Kidneys and the nails are an aspect of the Liver. In practice though, there are many other relevant aspects, in particular the condition of *xue*, that affect these types of tissue.

The skin

The skin is nourished and moistened by *xue* and *jin*. This means that imbalances manifesting in the skin are more often *xue* imbalances and patterns of Dampness, rather than being Lung imbalances. All channels traverse the skin. Changes in specific areas of the skin can therefore also relate to imbalances in specific channels.

If the skin is dry, it will be because the skin is not nourished and moistened. This will therefore be a sign of *xue xu* or *yin xu*. Oily or greasy skin can be seen when there is Dampness, Damp-Heat and Phlegm.

The skin can become dry and flaky when there is *xue* stagnation in the area below it. This is sometimes seen in the area of joints that have *xue* stagnation. *Xue* stagnation can block and thereby prevent fresh, nutritious *xue* from circulating in the skin in this area.

Damp-Heat and Phlegm can manifest with greasy or oily skin.

Itchy skin will indicate the presence of Wind in the area. It is important to identify the cause of the Wind. There will often be a combination of both exogenous and internally generated Wind simultaneously. Internal Wind may arise from factors such as *xue xu* or *shi* Heat. Exogenous Wind can be both Wind-Cold and Wind-Heat. Other factors that can be involved in itching are *xue* stagnation, Dryness and Dampness. It is important to observe and ask about other qualities of the skin, such as colour, moistness, texture and so on, to be able to differentiate the aetiology.

The hair

The hair on the head is created from Kidney *jing* but nourished and moistened by *xue*. This means that the quantity and quality of the head hair can be influenced by both *xue* and *jing*. If there is *jing xu*, there can be baldness, a receding hairline and thin hair. *Xue xu* can also result in hair loss, poor hair growth, dry hair or brittle hair. This is typically seen after childbirth and menstruation.

Phlegm, Damp-Heat and Dampness can make the hair greasy. The scalp can also be itchy when there is Damp-Heat. Dampness and Phlegm can also block *xue* from nourishing the hair so that it starts to fall out. A person can also suffer hair loss when Heat scorches the roots of the hair. The Heat may be generated internally or there may be invasions of Wind-Heat. If it is due to Wind-Heat, the hair loss will be sudden and defined patches will be missing.

The nails

The nails are an aspect of the Liver in the same way that the tendons are. Nails are nourished by Liver *xue*. Nails that are weak, break easily or are soft or ridged are a sign that Liver *xue* is not nourishing the nails. If the nails are very thick and yellowish, this can be a sign of Liver *xue* stagnation or Dampness. Typically, this is seen in the toenails, because Dampness seeps downwards.

Skin, hair and nails

Observation	Significance
Dry skin	*Xue xu*, *xue* stagnation
Greasy skin	Damp-Heat, Phlegm
Itchy skin	Wind, Dampness, Dryness, *xue* stagnation
Hair loss and baldness	*Jing xu*, *xue xu*, Fire, Wind-Heat, Dampness, Phlegm
Dry hair	*Xue xu*

Greasy hair	Damp-Heat, Phlegm
Oily, itchy scalp	Damp-Heat
Very thick nails	*Xue* stagnation
Weak, soft nails that break easily	Liver *xue xu*
Ridged fingernails	Liver *xue xu*

The ears and eyes

The ears are an aspect of the Kidneys and the eyes of the Liver, but again, there are several organs and vital substances that influence them.

The ears

The two organs that have the greatest impact on the ears are the Kidneys and the Liver. Kidney *jing* and Kidney *yin* nourish the ears, whilst the Liver has an influence on them because Liver *yang* imbalances can ascend to the ears via the Gall Bladder channel and disturb their functioning. The ears can also be directly and indirectly invaded by exogenous *xie qi*. In particular, Wind-Heat can directly invade the ear, as well as the *san jiao* channel. Invasions of exogenous *xie qi* will cause pain and the exudation of yellowish discharge from the ear. The invasion can also result in tinnitus with a loud sound or deafness. Because the condition is due to an acute invasion of exogenous *xie qi*, the symptoms will arise suddenly. It will typically be only one of the ears that is affected.

Kidney *jing xu* or Kidney *yin xu* can indicate that the ear lacks nourishment, meaning that the ear will not perform its functions optimally. Typical symptoms that may be due to Kidney *jing xu* or Kidney *yin xu* are deafness and tinnitus. Tinnitus due to a *xu* condition will typically manifest with a constant low tone and will be exacerbated by fatigue. If the tinnitus is alleviated by sticking fingers into the ears or pressing on the ears, this is a sign of a Kidney *xu* condition.

Tinnitus resulting from ascendant Liver *yang* or Liver Fire will be louder and will vary in strength. The tinnitus will also be adversely affected by stress and emotional influences. Liver *shi* tinnitus can also be exacerbated by sticking the fingers in the ears. It will often have arisen suddenly, whereas Kidney *xu* tinnitus will have developed gradually. These are general guidelines and it is actually most common that there are aspects of both. This is because Kidney and Liver *yin* have a common root, and Liver *yin xu* can result in ascending Liver *yang*.

Tinnitus that is worse at night is a sign of *yin xu* or *xue* stagnation. It is important to note that the tinnitus may not actually be louder at night, but because there is less noise in the room it is more noticeable.

Tinnitus that has arisen after exposure to loud noise will be classified as *xue* stagnation.

Deafness and hearing difficulties will often be due to Kidney *yin xu* or Kidney *jing xu* not nourishing the ear. However, a sudden loss or decrease in hearing will be due to an invasion of Wind-Heat or ascending Liver *yang*.

An increased production of earwax is usually due to Liver and Gall Bladder Damp-Heat. The exudation will be very sticky. Spleen and Kidney *yang xu* can also result in an increase in earwax, but it will be thinner and more watery. Phlegm and Dampness will, in general, result in increased and thicker exudations from the body's orifices. This also applies to the ears.

Liver and Gall Bladder Damp-Heat or Toxic-Fire can result in the formation of increased exudate in the middle ear. There will be pain and possibly yellowish discharge from the ear. Earache can also be seen in invasions of Wind-Heat, Liver Fire imbalances and when there is a local stagnation of *qi* and *xue*.

Ears that are itchy may be due to invasions of Wind-Heat, Gall Bladder Damp-Heat, Liver *xue xu* generating internal Wind or Kidney *yin xu* Heat.

The ears

Observation	Significance
Tinnitus with a loud noise or loud rushing sound	*Shi* conditions
Tinnitus with a low sound or faint rushing noise	*Xu* conditions
Tinnitus that has arisen gradually	Kidney *yin xu*, Kidney and Liver *yin xu*, Kidney *jing xu*
Tinnitus that has arisen suddenly	Liver Fire, ascending Liver *yang*, invasion of Wind-Heat, *xue* stagnation
Poor hearing	Kidney *xu* conditions
Hearing impairment (which occurs suddenly)	Wind-Heat, ascending Liver Wind
Earache	Wind-Heat, Liver and Gall Bladder Damp-Heat, *xue* and *qi* stagnation, ascending Liver *yang* or Liver Fire
Otitis or exudation of yellow discharge from the ears	Wind-Heat, Liver and Gall Bladder Damp-Heat, Toxic-Fire
Itchy ears	Wind-Heat, Gall Bladder Damp-Heat, Liver *xue xu*, which generates Wind or Kidney *yin xu* Heat
Increased production of earwax	Phlegm, Dampness, Liver and Gall Bladder Damp-Heat, Kidney and Spleen *yang xu*

The eyes

Although the eyes are nourished and moistened by Liver *xue* and Liver *yin*, there are many other factors that affect the eyes. Several channels emerge or terminate in the area of the eyes. The eyes can be disturbed by both exogenous and internally generated *xie qi*. Heat in particular can disturb the eyes. The eyes are physically located in one of the most *yang* areas of the body and Heat will always rise upwards due to its *yang* nature. This means that if there is internally generated Heat, such as Stomach or Liver Fire, the Heat can rise upwards resulting in red, stinging or itchy eyes. Invasions of Wind-Heat can also result in red and stinging eyes. This is typical of conjunctivitis and hay fever.

Ascending Liver *yang* and Liver Fire can also force an excess of *qi* up to the area. This will cause pain and pressure either behind or in the eyes. The increased amount of *qi* can also disturb the vision.

Phlegm can lead to there being a sensation of heaviness in and around the eyes. It can also block *xue* and *yin* from nourishing the eyes. This will result in visual isturbances.

Liver *xue xu* will also mean that the eyes lack nourishment. The eyes will feel dry and the vision will be poorer. The person may have difficulty focusing or there may be spots in front of the eyes. These symptoms will be exacerbated by fatigue. Liver *xue xu* can manifest with a sensitivity to bright light or poor nocturnal vision.

If a person is Liver *yin xu*, their eyes will also feel dry because they are not moistened by *yin*.

Tears are a body fluid that is directly influenced by the Liver, according to the theories of the Five Phases. This means that Liver imbalances can manifest with the eyes watering, especially when it is windy. Wind itself also has an adverse effect on the Liver. As with the other eye disorders, watering eyes can be a *xu* and a *shi* condition. Invasions of Wind-Heat and Wind-Cold can often cause the eyes to water. This is because the exogenous *xie qi* will disrupt the Lung and cause the Lung *qi* to become rebellious. The rebellious Lung *qi* will force the fluids that have accumulated in the Lung to ascend to the eyes.

Itchy eyes can arise when there is not enough *yin* or *xue* to nourish the eyes or when Heat rises upwards or invades from the exterior.

The eyes

Observation	Significance
Red eyes possibly with swelling and pain	Wind-Heat, Toxic-Fire, Liver Fire, Stomach Fire
Dry eyes	Kidney and Liver *yin xu*
Blurred vision, spots or floaters in front of the eyes	*Xue xu*
Visual disturbances	Liver *xue xu*, Liver *yin xu*, Liver Fire, ascending Liver *yang*, Phlegm
Pressure behind the eyes or feeling of pressure inside the eye	Ascending Liver *yang* or Liver Fire
Sensitivity to bright light	*Xue xu*
Poor night vision	*Xue xu*
Watering of the eyes, particular when it is windy	Liver imbalances, invasions of Wind-Cold or Wind-Heat
Itchy eyes	Liver *yin xu*, Liver *xue xu*, Liver Fire, Stomach Fire, Heart Fire, Wind-Heat

Sleep

Genuine insomnia is always caused by an imbalance involving a disruption of the *shen*.

A good night's sleep depends on the *shen* being anchored. This requires that *xue* and *yin* are strong enough to hold it down and that *shen* is not activated and agitated by Heat.

It is important to distinguish between genuine insomnia and insomnia that is caused by other factors such as the person being woken by, for example, pain, coughing, children, noisy neighbours, bedroom temperature, changing night shifts, coffee, tea or energy drinks.

Many of the questions that relate to the frequency and character of the insomnia are guidelines, not hard and fast rules. As always, multiple patterns are often present simultaneously.

An acute condition of insomnia that has arisen recently will usually be due to Liver *qi* stagnation, Liver Fire, food stagnation or *shi* Heat. Chronic insomnia will probably be related to *yin xu* or *xue xu*, but *shi* Heat can also be relevant.

Xue xu will usually manifest with a person having difficulty falling asleep. The person can also have difficulty remaining asleep. They may well feel that they do not sleep deeply and that they dream a lot. If they wake during the night, their mind will not be restless or full of thoughts, but they will often just lie awake. They may even be unsure in the morning if they were awake or not or for how long, because the mind was not active whilst they were awake.

People who wake after they have fallen asleep and have a restless mind or lucid thoughts will probably be *yin xu* and have Heat from Liver *qi* or food stagnation or some form of Fire.

Liver *qi* stagnation or Liver Fire patterns can be characterised by the person waking between 2 am and 4 am and having difficulty falling asleep again. Usually, a person who wakes early in the morning and cannot fall asleep again has some form of Heat or Heart and Gall Bladder *qi xu*.

Difficulty falling asleep or waking too early can also indicate an imbalance in the extraordinary channels *yin qiao mai* and *yang qiao mai*.

The more Heat that there is, the more restless and unstable the sleep will be. This is because Heat activates and agitates *shen*. The Heat can be *xu* or *shi* in nature. The Heat will also agitate the *hun* so there may be dream-disturbed sleep or many nightmares. Nightmares are also seen in Heart and Gall Bladder *qi xu*.

If sleep is affected by stress or the person's emotional condition, this is usually an indication that there is Liver *qi* stagnation or Liver Fire. Stress and too much mental activity can also worsen a condition of Heart *yin xu* or Heart *xue xu*, because the condition of stress will consume *yin* and *xue* whilst also generating Heat. It will be harder to sleep if they work or play on the computer late in the evening or if they go to bed too late.

Insomnia caused by food stagnation is closely linked to what they eat, how much they eat and at what time they eat.

Insomnia that is a manifestation of Heart and Kidney *yin xu* can often be accompanied by palpitations, mental agitation or anxiety. Palpitations can also be seen when there is Heart Fire.

Insomnia

Observation	Significance
Acute insomnia	Liver *qi* stagnation, Liver Fire, food stagnation, *shi* Heat
Difficulty falling asleep (but otherwise sleeps well)	Heart *xue xu*, Heart *yin xu*, Liver *qi* stagnation, disharmony of *yin qiao mai* and *yang qiao mai*
Wakes up frequently during the night	*Yin xu*, *xue xu*, food stagnation, Heat
Restless sleep with many dreams	Food stagnation, Heat
Wakes up early without being able to fall asleep again	Gall Bladder and Heart *qi xu*, Liver *qi* stagnation, Heat, disharmony of *yin qiao mai* and *yang qiao mai*
Nightmares and violent dreams	Liver or Heart Heat Fire
Waking up when stressed or under emotional pressure	Liver *qi* stagnation Heat
Insomnia with palpitations	Heart *yin xu*, Heart *xue xu*, Heart Fire
Difficulty sleeping after late meals or eating certain foods	Food stagnation

Pain

The category 'enquiring about about pain' has traditionally encompassed everything from headaches and menstrual pain to joint pains and hypochondriac tension. I have chosen to address some of these areas of pain individually. For example, I will discuss headaches, chest pain, menstrual pain and abdominal pain as unique areas of enquiry.

When enquiring about pain, it is important to locate where exactly the pain is experienced. This is to get an idea of which channels or which organs may be involved. For example, it is important when diagnosing joint pain to identify which channel is imbalanced. It is also important to investigate other aspects of the painful sensation, such as the quality of the pain, what improves or triggers the pain, how and when it arose, if the joint feels hot, whether there is swelling and so on. This is because the individual characteristics will help to differentiate one type of pain from another.

In general, all pain is due to a stagnation of *qi*: '*Bu tong ze tong, tong ze bu tong*' (where there is a stagnation, there is pain; where there is free movement, there is no pain). A stagnation of *qi* can arise when there is a *shi* condition and in *xu* conditions. In a *xu* condition, there will not be enough *qi* or *xue* to circulate *qi*, *xue* or *jinye*.

The pain seen in a *xu* condition will be milder. It will typically be described as being a dull or nagging pain or a tingling sensation. The pain will be relieved or ameliorated by palpating or putting your hand on the area. This is because the physical pressure will increase the amount of *qi* in an area that is *qi xu*. *Xu* types of pain should, in theory, feel worse after physical activity and improve with rest. Whilst this statement is true, it is also misleading. In some situations physical activity may well relieve the pain in a *xu* condition. This is because the physical activity will create a circulation of *qi*, temporarily relieving the stagnation and thereby the pain. *Xu* types of pain can be worse in the morning or if the person has been sitting still for a long time, which is otherwise characteristic of *shi* pain. Again, this is because there is too little *qi* to move the stagnant *qi* and *xue*, which stagnate when there is no physical activity. *Xu* types of pain are often worse after exertion or return later in the day when the person is tired. This is seen, for example, in lumbar pain, where the pain is worse if the person has been standing all day.

Xu pain will usually have arisen gradually. Acute pain, on the other hand, is almost always a manifestation of a *shi* condition.

Shi conditions will often be aggravated by inactivity, especially lying or sitting still for long periods of time, such as when sleeping. Contrary to what is written in standard TCM textbooks, activity does not necessarily relieve the pain. On the contrary, if there is a severe stagnation of *qi*, *xue* and *jinye*, such as when there is a sprain after a physical trauma or an operation, the movement of the joint will be severely limited and there will be extreme pain if the joint or muscle is moved beyond this range. *Shi* pain will typically be aggravated or feel greater if the area is palpated. This is because the increase in physical pressure will increase the amount of *qi* in an area that already has an excess. Something that can therefore seem counter-intuitive is when people with acute pain, such as a headache, press their fingers against certain spots, for example the temple, to relieve the tension. If you observe what they are doing you will often see that they are massaging the spot with very small movements of their fingers. They are therefore not increasing the amount of *qi* in the area, but spreading it with a draining finger technique and thereby relieving the pain. Because *shi* pain conditions are aggravated by pressure, the person will often have a dislike of wearing tight clothes in the relevant area. This is seen, for example, in some women with menstrual pain having an aversion to wearing tight jeans up to and during the start of the menstrual bleeding.

The descriptions of some of the individual types of pain can sound very similar. This is because the mechanisms involved in the generation of the pain can be fairly similar. *Xue* stagnation, for example, will manifest with a pain that is stabbing, piercing and sharp. The pain will be localised to a specific spot and will not move around. Cold can cause pain that is fairly similar to *xue* stagnation pain. Instead of being piercing and sharp, Cold stagnation pain is biting and cramping. The reason that the descriptions of these types of pain are so similar is that Cold contracts and thereby blocks the vessels, stagnating *xue*. When there is Cold stagnation, the area will feel either subjectively or objectively cold. Cold pain will be alleviated by heat. One should, however, be careful not to conclude that all pain that is alleviated by heat is Cold pain; it is not. Heat is *yang* and thereby creates movement and activity. This means that most types of stagnation, and therefore pain, will be relieved by warmth.

Pain from *xue* stagnation is often worse at night. This is because there is less movement of *qi* in the body whilst the person is sleeping, so *xue* is not circulated as effectively as during the day when the person is physically active. Furthermore, at night *xue* flows back to the Liver where it is stored. This means that there is less *xue* circulating in the channels and vessels, so there will be a greater tendency for *xue* to stagnate in places where there is already a stagnation.

Pain from *qi* stagnation will often move from place to place within a specific area. The person may not be able to localise the focus of the pain to a specific spot but will feel the pain in an area. Whereas a patient with Cold and *xue* stagnation will often point to a specific spot with their finger, a patient with *qi* stagnation pain is more likely to show you an area with their whole hand, possibly moving the hand at the same time. There will often be distension or even bloating in the area. The pain itself usually comes in waves or is variable in its intensity. It can also be described as tension or pressure.

Pain caused by Wind will also move from place to place, but in this instance the pain moves not only within a limited area of the body, but also from one area to another.

Heat will manifest with a pain that is burning or stinging. Pain caused by Heat can be relieved by putting something cold, such as ice, on the area. It can sometimes be relieved by the use of something hot like moxa, because the heat will help stagnated *qi*, *xue* and *jinye* to circulate.

Dampness will result in a pain that is heavy and dull.

Numbness and tingling sensations

Although numbness and tingling sensations are not actually pain, I have chosen to discuss them here for clarity. Numbness and tingling sensations occur when tissue is not nourished by *xue*. This means that a sensation of numbness or tingling can arise when there is either a genuine deficiency of *xue*, i.e. *xue xu*, or something that is blocking *xue* from reaching the area. Phlegm and *xue* stagnation can block the channel system so that *xue* cannot reach certain parts of the body. Tingling and numbness due to *xue xu* will usually be bilateral, whereas unilateral tingling or numbness is more typical of *xue* or Phlegm stagnation. *Xue xu* can manifest with numbness and tingling at night. This is because *xue* flows back to the Liver during the night when it is gathered and stored. This means that there is less *xue* in the channels and vessels to nourish the tissue. Liver *yin xu* and Liver *xue xu* can also result in cramping in the calf muscles in the evening and at night when *xue* flows back to the Liver, resulting in a deficiency of *xue* in the muscles in the extremities, meaning they lack nourishment so Wind can develop and manifest as cramps or restlessness.

Some organs have a special influence over certain areas or parts of the body. Pain in the lower back or knees can be caused by many factors such as trauma, invasion of exogenous *xie qi* and so on, but lumbar and knee pain can also be a reflection of a *xu* condition in the Kidneys. Kidney *xu* conditions typically manifest with either weakness, fatigue or stiffness in the lower back and knees. The pain or discomfort is worst when the person is tired, has stood a lot or has lifted heavy loads.

Hypochondriac tension is a classic symptom of Liver *qi* stagnation. Another sign of Liver *qi* stagnation is when *qi* stagnates in the throat. This will give a slightly suffocating sensation. If there is also Phlegm present, it will feel as if something that cannot be swallowed is stuck in the throat. Western clients will describe it as a lump in the throat. In China it is called 'plumstone *qi*', because it feels as if a plum stone is stuck in the throat.

Pain

Observation	Significance
Pain that is alleviated by pressure or by holding the area	*Xu* conditions
Pain that is aggravated by pressure	*Shi* conditions
Sharp or piercing pain (often localised to a specific area)	*Xue* stagnation
Cramping or biting pain	Cold
Burning pain	Heat, Damp-Heat
Dull, heavy pain	Dampness
Nagging or dull pain	*Xu* conditions
Tension and tightness	*Qi* stagnation
Pain that can 'come and go' or comes in waves	*Qi* stagnation
Pain that moves from one area to another	Wind
Pain that is localised and does not move	*Xue* stagnation
Pain that is alleviated by cold	Heat
Pain that is alleviated by heat	Cold (but because heat activates *qi*, most types of pain are relieved by heat)
Pain that is alleviated by rest	*Xu* conditions
Pain that is alleviated by movement	*Shi* conditions
Sudden pain	*Shi* conditions
Pain that has developed gradually	*Xu* conditions
Pain that is worse at night	*Xue* stagnation
Tingling or numbness	*Xue xu*, Phlegm stagnation, *xue* stagnation
Cramps in the calf muscles in the evening or at night	Liver *xue xu*, Liver *yin xu*
Soreness, fatigue or stiffness in the lower back and knees	Kidney *xu* conditions
Hypochondriac tension	Liver *qi* stagnation
Sensation of having a lump that cannot be swallowed in the throat	Liver *qi* stagnation and Phlegm

Headache

Headache has not traditionally been a separate enquiry area in terms of pain. Classically, it has been included in 'enquiry about the head and body'. Because it is such a common symptom and because there are so many different types of headaches, I have chosen to devote a separate category to this area of enquiry.

An acute headache in a person who does not normally suffer from headaches is usually caused by an invasion of exogenous *xie qi*. Wind-Cold can result in a tight or tense headache, Wind-Heat in a throbbing headache and Wind-Dampness in a heavy headache. This is because Cold is *yin* and has a contracting nature. Invasions of Cold will often create a stagnation in the *taiyang* channels in the head. Heat has a *yang* expansive nature and will cause *qi* to ascend and expand outwards. This will result in a throbbing sensation. Dampness is very *yin* and gives an oppressive sensation by blocking and slowing the movement of *qi*.

By asking about where in the head the pain is, you will be able to ascertain which channels are disrupted and possibly what the aetiology of the headache may be.

A unilateral headache will usually be due to an excess of *qi* or a stagnation of *qi* in the Gall Bladder channel. Typically, this is seen when there is ascending Liver *yang* or Liver Fire. It can also be seen in Liver Wind patterns. A stagnation of *qi* and *xue* due to physical trauma can also manifest with unilateral headaches. Liver *shi* imbalances will often manifest with pain in the temples and pressure behind or in the eyes. A nagging pain behind the eyes is typical when there is Liver *xue xu*.

A headache in the vertex of the head is usually a manifestation of a Liver imbalance. This is because there is a branch of the Liver channel that terminates in the acupuncture point Du 20. However, this type of headache can also be due to *qi* and *xue xu*.

Frontal headaches that are located in the forehead are often caused by Stomach imbalances, which can be both *xu* and *shi* in nature. Phlegm and Dampness are also typical causes.

A headache in the occiput region is often seen when there is an acute invasion of Wind-Cold. Chronic headaches in this region are sometimes seen when a Kidney imbalance manifests in the Urinary Bladder channel. Chronic headaches in this region will typically be due to stagnations of *qi* and *xue* resulting from physical trauma, for example whiplash injuries or due to stagnations of *qi* related to Liver *qi* stagnation.

Physical traumas can result in *xue* stagnating in the channels on the head. This will manifest with a headache that is localised in one or more fixed areas. The pain does not move and is sharp and stabbing. The trauma does not have to be recent – the *xue* stagnation can still manifest many years later.

Dull or nagging headaches are usually seen in *xu* conditions. There will be a nagging tiredness in the head. This type of headache is worse when the person is weary and is more likely to occur later in the day or in the evening. In women, it may manifest during or after the menstrual bleeding. This type of headache arises because there is not enough *qi* or *xue* to nourish the brain. *Xu* headaches can be triggered by activity or exertion but can be relieved with rest.

A throbbing headache occurs when too much *qi* rises to the head. This will usually be ascending Liver *yang* or Liver Fire.

Phlegm-Dampness can influence in a number of ways. It can block the *shen*, as well as preventing pure *yang qi* from rising up to the head. When *shen* is blocked by Phlegm-Dampness, the person will have difficulty thinking clearly. It will feel as if the head is full of cotton wool or that they are in a bell jar. Phlegm-Dampness is a *shi* condition, i.e. there is an excess of *qi* in the head. This means that there can be a throbbing or thumping sensation in the head. Phlegm-Dampness is *yin* in nature and the head can therefore feel very heavy. The person will also feel tired and exhausted, but the headache will often be aggravated by the person lying down. This is because Dampness seeps down to the head when the person is lying horizontally.

Headaches due to *shi* conditions can arise when there have been periods of physical inactivity, the lack of physical movement resulting in *qi* stagnation. A headache that comes from a person sleeping too much is due to *qi* or Phlegm stagnation.

Damp or humid weather is detrimental when there is Dampness and Phlegm and it can trigger a heavy or throbbing headache.

Headaches associated with the person's emotional condition are usually related to Liver *qi* imbalances.

Headaches arising after sex are seen in Kidney *xu* conditions or when there is ascending Liver *yang*.

A headache that is provoked by eating can be due to food stagnation, Phlegm-Dampness or Stomach-Heat. If the headache is relieved by eating, there will be *qi xu*.

Liver *qi* can have a tendency to stagnate in the premenstrual period. Headaches that have a pattern of occurring in this period are therefore probably due to ascending Liver *yang* or Liver *qi* stagnation.

Menstrual bleeding will exacerbate a condition of *xue xu*. If there is a tendency for the headache to occur immediately after or during the menstrual bleeding, it can indicate that there is Liver *xue xu*.

Headache

Observation	Significance
Acute	Invasion of exogenous *xie qi*
Unilateral	Ascending Liver *yang* or Liver Fire, it may also be due to Liver Wind
Temporal headache	Ascending Liver *yang* or Liver Fire, it may also be due to Liver Wind
Headache in the top of the head	Liver imbalances, *xue* or *qi xu*
Headache behind the eyes	Liver *xue xu* or ascending Liver *yang*
Frontal headache	Stomach imbalances, both *xu* and *shi*, Phlegm-Dampness
Headache in the occipital region	If the headache is acute, it will usually be Wind-Cold
	If the headache is chronic, it can be a Kidney imbalance manifesting in the Urinary Bladder channel
	It can also be due to muscular tension and tightness, resulting from either local stagnations of *qi* and *xue* or due to Liver *qi* stagnation

Whole head	It may be an invasion of Wind-Cold if the headache is acute, otherwise it is usually seen in *xu* patterns of imbalance
Localised in specific spots	*Xue* stagnation
Acute headache	*Shi* condition
Dull, nagging headache	*Xu* condition
Throbbing headache	Ascending Liver *yang* or Liver Fire, Wind-Heat, Phlegm
Heavy headache	Phlegm-Dampness
Stabbing or sharp pain	*Xue* stagnation
Arising from a lack of physical activity	Liver *qi* stagnation
Occurs when the person is tired or overworked	*Xu* conditions
Arising from weather changes and humid weather	Phlegm-Dampness
Triggered by stress and emotional influences	Liver imbalances
Triggered by sex	Kidney *xu* or ascending Liver *yang*
Premenstrual headache	Liver imbalances
Headache after menstruation	*Xue xu*

Enquiry that is specific to women

Menstruation

There are several areas of enquiry that can help to differentiate the diagnosis in women: the length, regularity, quality and quantity of her menstrual bleeding; pain associated with the cycle; physical and emotional changes during the cycle; irregular bleeding during the cycle. Enquiry must also be made into a woman's gynaecological history: the age she started to menstruate; whether there have been any births and pregnancies, and if so how these were; whether there were any complications and problems; whether there were any symptoms that arose concurrently or immediately afterwards. Enquiry must also be made into the use of contraception. Many forms of birth control can cause imbalances in themselves. Furthermore, the use of the contraceptive pill or the coil will directly affect her menstrual cycle and bleeding, and this must be taken into account when considering her replies.

If she is menopausal or post-menopausal, she should be questioned about when her menstruation ceased and whether there were any discomforts associated with it.

Finally, enquiry should be made about discharge from the vagina.

The information obtained about the menstrual cycle, as well as the gynae-cological history in general, will be relevant not only to the specific diagnosis of gynaecological imbalances, but also to the diagnosis in general. It is said that women are more difficult to treat because there are so many changes in their physiology and in the balance of *yin*, *yang*, *qi* and *xue* throughout the menstrual cycle. On the other hand, women are easier to diagnose, precisely because of these fluctuations during the menstrual cycle and the menstrual cycle and bleeding will act as a barometer for the whole body.

Asking about the menarche (the first menstruation) can give some indication of the woman's fundamental constitution. If she has never had a menstrual bleeding or if she had her first menstruation at a late age, it will be a sign of one or more imbalances. A girl should begin menstruating at the age of 13 (a woman's *jing* cycles are seven years long). The first *jing* cycle starts in utero, so a child is, in fact, one year old when born. The menstruation should start at the beginning of the third cycle, i.e. when she is 13). If menstruation does not start at around this age, it could indicate that she is *jing xu* or *xue xu*, i.e. there is a lack of substance to create bleeding. It can, though, also be a sign that there is a stagnation preventing the flow of the menstrual blood.

Enquiry into pregnancies and births will give an idea of the state of her *jing*. If there have been complications during pregnancies and births, this can indicate that there may be Kidney *xu*, Spleen *xu*, Heat, *qi* stagnation and so on.

Repeated and frequent abortions, miscarriages and births can weaken a woman's *jing* and *xue*. On the other hand, a woman who easily becomes pregnant will have strong *jing* and *xue*.

If she has had difficulty becoming pregnant, it can indicate *jing xu*, *xue xu*, Dampness and Phlegm stagnation, *qi* stagnation, Heat, Cold, Kidney *yin xu* or Kidney *yang xu*. Infertility is due to: a lack of potential – *jing xu*; a lack of activation of this potential – *yang xu*; a lack of nourishment to the fertilised egg or embryo – *qi xu* or *xue xu*; the nourishment being blocked by some form of stagnation – Dampness, Phlegm, *qi* stagnation or *xue* stagnation; Heat that agitates the egg so it does not unite with the sperm or the fertilised egg does not settle and attach to the wall of the uterus. If the woman has miscarried several times, it can be a sign that there is Kidney or Spleen *qi xu*, but Heat is also a possibility. A very rough rule of thumb is that if she miscarries in the first trimester, it can indicate Kidney *jing xu* (this will correspond to a genetic defect in Western pathology) and if she repeatedly aborts in the final two trimesters, it is either Kidney *qi xu* (the Kidneys failing to control the opening and closing the lower orifices) or Spleen *qi xu* (the Spleen failing to hold things up and in place).

Enquiry into the menstrual cycle can be difficult. Some women are very precise and know the regularity of the bleeding, the quality and quantity of the blood and so on. Other women take little interest in their cycle and sometimes even assume that you as the therapist know where she is in her cycle better than she does.

The length of the menstrual cycle is affected by many different imbalances. Spleen *qi xu*, Kidney *qi xu* and Heat can makes the cycle shorter. Heat will agitate *xue*, so the walls of the vessels rupture, whilst Spleen *qi xu* will not hold *xue* inside the vessels. The Kidney *qi xu* can result in the Kidney failing to hold the Uterus closed, so the bleeding comes earlier.

If there is too little *xue* to create menstrual bleeding or if anything blocks *xue* (such as Cold, *xue* stagnation or *qi* stagnation) the menstrual bleeding will be delayed.

Liver *qi* stagnation can cause the length of the cycle to be irregular.

A woman should menstruate approximately 45 ml of blood during the menstrual bleeding. Many women have difficulty judging whether they have normal bleeding, as they only have experience of their own bleeding and using tampon makes it difficult to gauge the amount of blood discharged. Asking about how often they have to change their tampon or pad and which type of pad or tampon they use can give an indication of the heaviness of the bleeding. Many women also have a reasonably good idea of the amount of blood there is, especially if they have heavy or scanty bleeding. Heavy menstrual bleeding can be seen when there is either Heat or Spleen *qi xu* due to the mechanisms explained above. *Xue* stagnation can block the vessels in the Uterus, causing them to rupture. This too will result in heavy bleeding. Scanty bleeding is due to *xue xu*, Cold or *xue* stagnation blocking the flow of *xue*.

Menstrual bleeding lasting longer than five days, spotting before the menstrual bleeding and bleeding in the middle of the cycle are all signs of Spleen *qi xu* resulting in *xue* not being held in the vessels. They can also be signs that Heat is agitating *xue* and rupturing the vessels or that there is *xue* stagnation creating a build up of pressure so that the walls of the vessels burst.

Enquiring about the quality of the menstrual blood is crucial. Again, some women can have difficulty answering this question, having seen only their own menstrual blood. Describing the differences between the various colours and qualities can be useful. Pale, watery or thin blood can be seen when there is *xue xu* and *qi xu*. Very dark, clotted blood is seen when there is *xue* stagnation. *Qi* stagnation will manifest with smaller clots, whilst Cold stagnation can result in very small, grainy clots that resemble coffee grounds. If there is a Kidney *xu* condition, the blood may contain thin 'threads' and if there is Damp-Phlegm, the blood will contain mucus.

Bright, red-coloured blood is seen when there is Heat. Heat can also result in the menstrual blood being sticky. Brown-coloured blood can be seen when there are *xue xu* conditions. *Xue* stagnation causes the blood to be very dark in colour. If there is a lot of *xue* stagnation, the blood will be almost black.

The presence of menstrual pain, its quality and when it occurs are important differential factors when determining which patterns of imbalance are present.

Pain that starts prior to the menstrual bleeding is seen when there is Liver *qi* stagnation. Liver *qi* stagnation pain is generally characterised by coming in waves and varying in its intensity. The word many women use for this is 'cramping'. The pain can be located in front and on both sides of the lower abdomen. It can also cause soreness or pain in the lower back and may radiate down the inside of the thigh. This is because Liver *qi* stagnation will stagnate *qi* and *xue* in *chong mai*.

The pain seen in *xue* stagnation is a stabbing pain that is sharper and more piercing than when there is *qi* stagnation. Furthermore, whilst *qi* stagnation pain is felt in a larger area, *xue* stagnation pain is localised to one spot, usually the same spot each time. The pain will be worst at the initiation of the menstrual bleeding and the pain can sometimes be relieved by the discharge of clots.

Menstrual pain caused by Cold will resemble *xue* stagnation pain in some ways. The pain will be biting and fixed. The similarity to *xue* stagnation pain is that Cold will stagnate the movement of *xue*.

Heat can cause stinging, searing or burning pain.

Dampness will cause a sensation of heaviness and dragging downwards, as if the uterus is falling out of the body.

Breast tension or pain in the premenstrual period is a sign of Liver *qi* stagnation. This is because the Liver channel has a branch that travels through the breasts. Liver *qi* stagnation will also often mean that a woman is more irritable during this period. If she tends to be tearful and weepy in the premenstrual period, it is usually a manifestation of Liver *xue xu*. Many women experience both of these types of mood swings. This just reflects that most women's Liver *qi* stagnation arises from a condition of Liver *xue xu*.

Some women's menstrual bleeding has a tendency to stop and start, for example starting with two days of bleeding, then a pause of a day or two, followed by two or three days of bleeding. This usually indicates that there is a stagnation of *qi* and/or *xue*.

Stagnant Liver *qi* can invade the Spleen and disrupt its functioning. This can manifest with symptoms such as alternating diarrhoea and constipation, nausea, cravings for sweets and oedema in the premenstrual phase.

The menstrual cycle and bleeding

Observation	Significance
Late menarche	*Jing xu*, *xue xu*, stagnation
Difficulty conceiving	*Jing xu*, *xue xu*, Dampness and Phlegm, *qi* stagnation, Heat, Cold, Kidney *yin xu* or Kidney *yang xu*
Repeated miscarriages	Kidney *xu* conditions, Spleen *qi xu*, Heat
Short cycle	Heat (both *xu* and *shi*), Spleen *qi xu*, Kidney *qi xu*
Long cycle	*Xue xu*, Cold stagnation, *xue* stagnation, *qi* stagnation
Irregular cycle	Liver *qi* stagnation, Spleen or Kidney *xu* conditions
Heavy menstrual bleeding	*Xu* or *shi* Heat, Spleen *qi xu*, *xue* stagnation
Scanty menstrual bleeding	*Xue xu*, *xue* stagnation, Dampness, Phlegm
Prolonged menstrual bleeding or spotting	Heat, *qi* stagnation, *xue* stagnation, Spleen *qi xu*
Menstrual bleeding that stops and starts	*Qi* stagnation, *xue* stagnation
Thick menstrual blood	*Shi* conditions
Thin menstrual blood	*Xu* conditions
Thin, watery blood	*Xue* or *qi xu*

Clots in the menstrual blood	Stagnation (fresh glistening clots suggest Heat and dark and dull clots suggest *xue* stagnation)
Murky menstrual blood (that looks as if it contains coffee grounds)	Stagnation due to Cold
Bright, red-coloured menstrual blood	Heat
Black-coloured or very dark menstrual blood	*Xue* stagnation
Brownish-coloured menstrual blood	*Xu* conditions
Sticky menstrual blood	*Yin xu* or Heat
Mucus in the menstrual blood	Phlegm
Strong, rotten or foul-smelling menstrual blood	Damp-Heat or Fire
Pain before menstruation	*Qi* or *xue* stagnation
Pain during menstruation	*Xue* Heat, *xue* stagnation
Pain or discomfort after menstruation	*Xue xu*
Strong, cramping pain just before or during menstruation	Stagnation conditions
Shooting, stabbing or piercing menstrual pain	*Xue* stagnation
Nipping or biting menstrual pain	Cold
Heavy or dragging menstrual pain	Dampness
Burning or searing menstrual pain	Heat
Bleeding occurs suddenly	*Xue* Heat
Delayed bleeding or prolonged bleeding but without the bleeding being heavy	*Xue* stagnation
Menstruation with a distended sensation, the menstrual bleeding takes a while getting started	Dampness, *qi* or *xue* stagnation
Premenstrual breast tension	Liver *qi* stagnation
Irritability and aggressiveness in the premenstrual phase	Liver *qi* stagnation
Tearful and sensitive in the premenstrual phase	Liver *xue xu*
Alternating diarrhoea and constipation, nausea, cravings for sweets or oedema in the premenstrual phase	Liver *qi* invading the Spleen

Vaginal discharge

A light vaginal discharge that is transparent and increases in volume, thickness and elasticity around ovulation is normal. It is also normal that the discharge increases in puberty and during pregnancy.

Vaginal discharge is differentiated according to its colour, consistency and smell.

Discharge that is heavier in volume than normal, not odorous and watery, transparent or white will be a manifestation of Kidney *yang xu* or Spleen *yang xu*. Kidney *yang* should control the lower orifices, as well as transforming and transporting the fluids in the body. If Kidney *yang* fails to do this, Dampness will arise and seep down to the lower *jiao*. Because the Kidneys are not able to control the lower orifices, the Dampness will leak out of the body. Spleen *yang xu* can also result in an increased volume of discharge from the vagina because Spleen *yang* is also involved in the transformation and transportation of fluids in the body. Spleen and Kidney *yang xu* are often seen together.

If there is *shi* Cold or Damp-Cold, the discharge will still be whitish, but it will be thicker in consistency and the discharge will smell slightly of fish.

If there is Heat present, the discharge will not only be thicker and stickier, but it will also be yellowish and odorous. The more Heat that there is, the thicker and more odorous the discharge. The colour of the discharge will also be darker. When there is Toxic-Fire, the colour of the discharge can become greenish.

Vaginal discharge

Observation	Significance
Yellowish and odorous discharge	Damp-Heat
Whitish or transparent discharge	Cold, Spleen *yang xu*, Kidney *yang xu*
White and red discharge	Damp-Heat
Greenish discharge	Damp-Heat in the Liver channel or Toxic-Fire
Discharge with a watery consistency	Damp-Cold or Kidney *xu* conditions
Discharge with a thick consistency	Damp-Heat
Odorous discharge	Heat

Sexuality

While not an outright gynaecological issue, and not an issue that was traditionally enquired about, a woman's sexual desire and functionality can reveal important information. It is not a question I always ask. Some clients, though, do give information that is relevant to the rest of the diagnosis. It is important to maintain the client's trust and respect and not overstep their boundaries. A woman who has come with tinnitus may not see the relevance of being asked about the moistness of her vagina and could feel violated.

Sexual desire

Our sex drive or libido is governed by the flaring up of the *mingmen* when it is activated by heat from the Heart. This is cooperation between the Imperial fire and the Ministerial fire. This is dependent on both the Heart and Kidneys being in balance.

When we are sexually aroused, there is an increase of heat in the body. This requires *yang*. The increase in heat is seen in the cheeks, lips, nails and so on becoming red, and the skin feels warmer when we are aroused. Heat and *yang* from the Heart and *mingmen* fills the genitals.

Clear and unimpeded communication between the Kidneys and Heart and a strong Kidney *yang* are essential. If Kidney *yang* is weak, there will be a lack of libido due to the lack of heat from the *mingmen*. If Kidney *yin* is weak, it will not be able to control the heat in the Heart, and there may be an excessive sex drive. Heat in the Heart can also arise from other sources.

If the Heart is *xu*, such as when there is sadness for example, the Heart will not activate the *mingmen*. This is typically seen in relationships where a woman believes she has lost her sex drive. If this relationship ends and she finds a new partner, often there are no longer problems with her libido.

Liver *qi* stagnation may also play a role in the lack of libido, because when Liver *qi* stagnates there can be a stagnation of *qi* on all levels.

Lack of self-confidence and low self-esteem may also be factors that affect the Heart *qi*.

Orgasm

Liver *qi* plays a major role in the orgasm and controls the muscles in the genitals. If there is Liver *qi* stagnation, a woman may have difficulty achieving orgasm. Her stagnant Liver *qi* causes her to have difficulty letting go. It often becomes a vicious circle. Orgasms are an excellent way to release stagnant *qi*. *Qi* accumulates more and more until the orgasm liberates it. If the woman does not achieve an orgasm, there is only the accumulation of *qi* without release. This in itself will stagnate Liver *qi*. At the same time, it can be emotionally frustrating not to achieve an orgasm. This will further stagnate Liver *qi*.

A lack of *yang* can also play a role. There needs to be sufficient *yang* heat to create sexual arousal and desire in the first place. To create an orgasm, this heat must be sent down from the Heart. If there is not enough *yang* or if the Heart is weak there can be difficulty in achieving orgasm.

A headache that arises immediately after the orgasm can be a sign of ascending Liver *yang*, rebellious *qi* in the *chong mai* or Heart Fire. This is because the sudden release of *qi* will rise up to the head.

Vagina

The Liver channel traverses the area around the genitals and its *luo* channel runs to and through the vagina. Stagnant Liver *qi* can cause the muscles in the vagina to become so tense that intercourse is painful or not possible, such as when there is vaginitis and vulvodynia.

If there is Kidney *yin xu*, the mucous membranes become dry. Many menopausal women suffer from dry mucous membranes in the vagina. This is because *yin* and *xue* have dried out in the *ren mai*, which passes through the vagina. This will result in the mucous membranes of the vagina not being lubricated. Dry mucous membranes can also be seen in younger women who are Kidney *yin xu* or *xue xu* or where Heat has damaged *jinye*.

Discharge from the vagina has been discussed in the section above.

Female sexual function

Observation	Significance
Lack of libido	Kidney *yang xu*, Heart *qi xu*, Heart *yang xu*, Liver *qi* stagnation
Excessive sex drive	Heat
Lack of orgasms	Liver *qi* stagnation, *yang xu*, Heart *qi xu*
Headache immediately after orgasm	Ascending Liver *yang*, rebellious *qi* in *chong mai*, Heart Fire
Tense vaginal muscles	Liver *qi* stagnation
Dry vaginal mucous membranes	*Yin xu*, *xue xu*, Heat

Enquiry that is specific to men

Potency, sexual desire and fertility

Potency and sexual desire is influenced not only by Kidney *jing* and Kidney *yang*, but also by other physiological and pathological factors.

In order to create and maintain an erection, *qi* and *xue* must flow out into the penis. This requires that there is sufficient *qi* and *xue*, and that these are not inhibited in their movement. The man's *shen* should be in harmony so that it can focus on his sexual desire. Heart fire travels down through *chong mai* to the penis, manifesting with a sensation of heat in the penis. Finally, Kidney *yang* sends Kidney *jing* through the penis, resulting in an ejaculation.

Kidney *yang* governs the functional activity involved in an erection. At the same time, sexual desire or arousal is dependent on Kidney *yang*. Heart *qi xu* and Liver *qi* stagnation can also manifest with a weak libido due to either a general lack of passion or a tendency to suppress emotions. A person with Heart *qi xu* will often be timid and nervous, which can affect their ability to achieve or maintain an erection.

Liver *yin*, and thereby to a certain degree Liver *xue*, shares a common root with Kidney *yin*. This means that Kidney *yin xu* can affect the Liver's ability to supply the penis with *xue* and thereby the ability to create an erection.

Kidney *jing* influences a person's reproductive ability. This manifests mainly in their sperm count and the quality of sperm, but it also influences the volume of the semen.

The Liver has several functions in relation to an erection. The penis itself is conceived of as being a tendon in Chinese medicine and thereby under the influence of the Liver organ, which nourishes and controls the tendons. The Liver channel traverses the genitals. Furthermore, the Liver ensures that there is enough *xue* to fill the penis so that it becomes rigid. Liver *qi* also ensures that *qi* and *xue* flow out into the penis. This is evident when periods of stress, frustration or anger affect some men's ability to achieve an erection.

The Heart governs *xue* in general, and during an erection the Heart sends *xue* down to the penis. An erection is also dependent on the Heart fire being sent down through *chong mai* to the penis. It is therefore important that a person's *shen* is harmonious. A typical example of an unsettled *shen* affecting the erection is seen when a man has performance anxiety.

Kidney *yin xu* and Heart *xu* conditions can also manifest in a man being able to achieve but not maintain an erection, with the penis quickly becoming limp.

The Stomach and Spleen ensure that there is a sufficient production of *qi* and *xue*. A *qi xu* condition in these organs could lead to there not being enough *qi* and *xue* to create an erection or to nourish the penis, which is a tendon, so it becomes weak and limp.

Damp-Heat can block the movement of *qi* and *xue* in the genitals

Uncontrolled ejaculation and low sperm count

Premature ejaculation or uncontrolled ejaculation can arise when there is either not enough *qi* and *yang* to hold the semen back or too much *yang* in the form of Heat, which drives the semen outwards. Too much *yang* can be a *shi* or *xu* condition.

Traditionally, sperm quality was not something that could be quantitatively measured. The only thing that could be observed was the consistency, colour and quantity of semen. By combining modern analytical techniques and traditional knowledge, it is now possible to differentiate the relevant imbalance patterns when diagnosing poor sperm quality. Kidney *jing xu*, and in some cases *xue* stagnation, can manifest with a low sperm count, sperm that are malformed or sperm that have a short lifespan. Kidney *yang xu* can manifest with poor sperm motility. Thin and watery seminal fluid can also be a sign of Kidney *yang xu*. Seminal fluid that is thick and sticky is more typical of Dampness, especially Damp-Heat. Damp-Heat can also make seminal fluid yellowish or too acidic.

The prostate

The prostate is not directly visible and was therefore not traditionally enquired about during diagnostic questioning. Nevertheless, many older male patients might report that they have an enlarged prostate, or it may even be the reason that they seek treatment. An enlarged prostate can become stiff and rigid. In Chinese medicine, this would indicate some form of stagnation, i.e. *qi* stagnation, *xue* stagnation, Dampness or Phlegm.

The muscles of the Urinary Bladder have to compensate for the prostate's narrowing of the urethra. From a Chinese medicine perspective, this means that it will require more Kidney *yang qi* to expel the urine from the Urinary Bladder. This, though, is a time in a man's life when his Kidney *yang qi* is in decline.

From the age of 40 onwards, many men experience various disorders resulting from the growth in size of the prostate. The prostate grows because there is an increasing stagnation of *xue* and Phlegm in the area. Typical symptoms of this increased growth are: nocturnal urination (nocturia); frequent and urgent, but at the same time scanty or incomplete, urination; dribbling after urination; cloudy urine, weak urinary flow and possibly blood in the urine. The fact that various symptoms associated with a Western medicine diagnosis of an enlarged prostate start to appear when a man is middle-aged or older harmonises with the Chinese medicine concept of a progressive weakening of the Kidney *yang* and a concurrent increase in the stagnation of Phlegm, Dampness, *xue* and *qi*, the older a man becomes.

Genitals

A man may report symptoms that relate directly to his genitalia.

Genital pain can result from Liver *qi* stagnation, Damp-Heat or *xue* stagnation. The Liver channel traverses the genitals, so a stagnation of Liver *qi* can result in soreness or pain in the genitals and inguinal area. *Xue* stagnation in the area will often arise from physical traumas or surgical operations in the area but can also be due to a stagnation of *qi*. *Xue* stagnation is more likely to manifest as a sharp, localised pain, rather than tenderness, tension or soreness in a larger area. Damp-Heat can seep down to the genitals and block the movement of *qi* and *xue* in the area. Damp-Heat is more likely to manifest with a burning pain or tenderness in the area.

Damp-Heat seeping down to the lower *jiao* can also manifest with sweaty or sticky genitals.

Cold genitalia can be seen when there is *shi* cold or *yang xu*.

Male imbalances

Observation	Significance
Lack of libido	Kidney *yang xu*, Heart *qi xu*, Heart *yang xu*, Liver *qi* stagnation
Excessive sex drive	Heat
Lack of orgasms	Liver *qi* stagnation, *yang xu*
Impotence	Kidney *xu* conditions, Heart *xu* conditions, Liver *qi* stagnation, *qi* and *xue xu*
Uncontrolled ejaculation	Kidney *xu* conditions, Heat conditions, Heart imbalances
Poor sperm quality	Kidney *xu* conditions, Damp-Heat, *xue* stagnation
Prostate problems	Kidney *xu* conditions, Phlegm, *xue* stagnation, Liver *qi* stagnation, Damp-Heat, Damp-Cold
Tenderness or pain in the genitalia or inguinal area	Liver *qi* stagnation, *xue* stagnation, Damp-Heat
Cold or moist genitals	*Shi* or *xu* Cold conditions
Sweaty and sticky genitals	Damp-Heat

Enquiry with regard to the emotions and mental state

Chinese medicine defines seven primary emotions that each have their own specific *qi* dynamics. These *qi* dynamics will resonate with, whilst affecting, the various *zangfu* organs. This means that the emotions are aetiological factors, as well as being manifestations of imbalances in specific organs. That Chinese medicine only defines seven emotions can sound slightly simplistic. These seven emotions should, though, be perceived of as being primary emotions in the same way that there are only three primary colours. The various combinations of the three primary colours can manifest as the infinite myriad of colours that we can see with our eyes. In the same way, all the emotions we experience contain varying elements and combinations of these seven primary emotions. The specific *qi* dynamics of the various emotions are described in *The Fundamentals of Acupuncture* (Ching 2016).

Enquiring about a person's emotional life can give an indication of the state of the various *zangfu* organs, as well as possibly revealing relevant aetiology. It is, though, important to be conscious of a person's boundaries and to exhibit tact when enquiring about a person's emotional universe. Furthermore, we must also be conscious of our therapeutic limitations. We are practitioners of Chinese medicine and not trained counsellors. That said, although we ask about the emotions from a diagnostic perspective, we will often affect the emotions therapeutically by our treatment of the organs involved. For example, by treating acupuncture points such as Liv 2 and Pe 6, we harmonise the Liver, drain the Heat from the Liver and Heart and help to get the *qi* flowing freely. This will affect the mood of a person with Liver and Heart *qi* stagnation, who is irritable, short tempered and impatient. It will often result in them acting and reacting differently in situations that previously resulted in conflict, which thereby increased their levels of Liver *qi* stagnation, thus breaking a vicious circle.

Shi conditions in an organ will often manifest with a certain emotion being dominant or difficult to control, such as anger when there is Liver Fire. A *xu* condition or a stagnation of an organ's *qi* can result in a person having difficulty manifesting certain emotions.

Generally, I tend not to ask directly about the seven emotions, but instead I enquire about various mental and emotional aspects of a person's life and in this way get a sense of how the seven emotions are manifesting.

The emotional aspects that I personally enquire most often about are:

- worry, speculation and obsessive thinking

- anger, irritability, quick temper and impatience

- mood swings

- depression

- anxiety

- the ability to say no and set boundaries and assertiveness.

Furthermore, I ask about their memory, ability to concentrate, mental restlessness and brain fog.

A person with Spleen *qi xu* or Dampness will often express that they have a tendency to worry a lot or that they speculate about things, pondering and thinking in circles. They will have difficulty letting go of thoughts again. Due to the weakness of their Spleen, they will have difficulty digesting information and transforming this information into knowledge. This will be reflected in the fact that they have to rerun the information through their head repeatedly in an attempt to extract what is relevant and useful.

Mood swings are often seen when there is Liver *qi* stagnation. There is no stability to the emotions because the Liver is not ensuring that the *qi* is flowing smoothly.

Heat in the Liver will manifest with irritability and the person can have a tendency to be temperamental and have a quick temper or be impatient. They will have a quick temper because anger is the emotion that resonates with Liver.

Severe stagnations of Liver *qi* can lead to a depressive condition. This is because Liver *qi* stagnation can prevent the movement of the *hun*. This will result in a person having difficulty seeing a future ahead of them. They cannot conceive of a future or a situation that is better than the emotional pain that they are feeling at the moment. When there is Liver *qi* stagnation, you can sometimes sense that there are pent-up emotions when the client describes their life.

Phlegm can also lead to depression. Here the *shen* becomes blocked and smothered. The person will have difficulty connecting to other people. The person can also seem torpid and difficult to engage.

Heart *qi* stagnation and *xue* stagnation can also result in a person's *shen* having difficultly emanating outwards and connecting to other people. At the same time, the stagnation of *qi* in the Heart can manifest with a lack of joy.

Heart *xu* conditions can also lead to depression or depressive conditions. When the Heart is harmonious, it manifests joy. If there is Heart *qi xu*, there will be a lack of joy and the person will be gloomy and sad. Conversely, if the client says that they have lacked joy or love in their childhood and in adult life, this can lead to Heart *qi xu*.

The Lung is affected by grief and melancholy. This can also be an aspect of a depressive condition. The person may mention a specific event that their condition can relate to, but it can also be something that is very far back in the past. Grief and loss do not, of course, have to manifest as depression. If a client talks of grief or loss, it may be something that has affected their Lung *qi*. The Metal Phase gives us the ability to experience but also let go of grief and loss so we can move on. If the Metal Phase is not in balance, its *qi* will not flow and the person will have difficulty letting go of grief.

I usually ask patients whether they are good at saying no and setting boundaries. Liver *xu* conditions and Liver *qi* stagnation can manifest, to some extent, in a person having difficultly saying no and setting boundaries. Conversely, by not being able to set their boundaries, they will often develop a stagnation of Liver *qi*.

Mental restlessness, and its extreme form – mania, is a sign of Heat agitating the *shen* so the person has difficulty concentrating and being tranquil.

Anxiety may be related to certain situations or objects. It may also be undefined. Anxiety will weaken Kidney and Heart *qi*, but in itself is often a manifestation of Heart and Kidney imbalances.

The memory depends on *jing*, *shen*, *xue*, *zhi* and *yi*. A poor memory can therefore be a reflection of imbalances in the Kidneys, Heart and/or Spleen. Usually it will be a *xu* condition, but Phlegm and *xue* stagnation can also block the *shen* and thereby the memory. Shock can also dissipate the *shen* and lead to amnesia.

Difficulty concentrating is seen when the Heart and the brain are undernourished, blocked or agitated. This means that Heart *qi xu*, Heart *xue xu* and Kidney *jing xu* can manifest in poor concentration. The person will often feel 'empty headed' and a bit dazed. Heat in the body will always ascend due to its *yang* nature. Heat will agitate *shen*, causing the person to have difficulty concentrating due to mental restlessness and many thoughts filling the head. Spleen *qi xu* can also cause a person to have difficulty concentrating, because the weakening of their *yi* will result in them having difficulty focusing their thoughts. Dampness and Phlegm can also mean that there is difficulty concentrating, because the person feels that their brain is wrapped in cotton wool. The blockage resulting from Phlegm-Dampness means that information and impressions have difficulty penetrating into the Heart. If I suspect that a client has Phlegm-Dampness, I ask them if they have a foggy or blurred sensation in the head as if there is a blanket smothering their mind or the sensation of being locked in a bell jar. This is the sensation most of us recognise from when we have had a heavy cold or have been hung-over.

Mental-emotional signs

Observation	Significance
Depression	Liver *qi* stagnation, Heart imbalances, Phlegm
Speculation, worry, thinking in circles	Spleen *qi xu*, Dampness
Anxiety	Heart and Kidney imbalances
Wrath, anger, quick temper, impatience	Heat in the Liver
Difficult saying no and setting boundaries	Liver *xu* patterns and Liver *qi* stagnation
Mental restlessness	Heat
Mood swings	Liver *qi* stagnation
Poor memory	Heart *xue xu*, Kidney *jing xu*, Spleen *qi xu*, Phlegm-Dampness
Difficulty concentrating	Heart *xue xu*, Kidney *jing xu*, Phlegm-Dampness, Spleen *qi xu*, Heart Fire, Phlegm Fire, Heat
Foggy and slurred sensation in the head	Phlegm-Dampness

Lifestyle and diet

Enquiry involves asking not only about physical and emotional signs and symptoms, but also the person's medical history. It is also relevant to ask about a person's lifestyle and diet, which includes: what they typically eat; how much and how often they eat; how much they exercise; how much stress they have; how much relaxation they get; their consumption of stimulants such as coffee, tobacco and alcohol. This information will inform us about possible aetiological causes. At the same time, it will give us an idea of what to recommend to the client with regard to supporting the treatment.

The diet is an incredibly important aetiological factor in many imbalances. It is therefore important to ask about what people eat in general. I usually get the client to tell me what they eat during a typical day and afterwards I ask more specifically about certain dietary factors such as dairy products, sugar, raw vegetables, hot spices, alcohol and so on that could have a relevance to their diagnosis. The dynamics of dietary factors is discussed in *The Fundamentals of Acupuncture* (Ching 2016).

Eating too much at a time, too often or too late in the day, as well as not chewing the food enough, can lead to food stagnation and weaken the Stomach and Spleen *qi*.

Exercise is extremely important, and a person who does not get enough physical movement will tend to develop stagnation conditions. If they have a certain working position, such as sitting still all day, it will put a strain on specific organs, in this case the Spleen.

Too much exercise, on the other hand, can weaken a person's *qi* and *xue*. Certain forms of exercise will have a negative effect on the specific imbalances. Lifting heavy weights will weaken Kidney *yang*. Swimming or playing sports in cold, damp environments will have a negative effect on Cold and Dampness conditions.[13] Exercise in which a person sweats profusely is not good for people who are *qi xu*, *yin xu* or *xue xu*, because *qi* and fluids are lost through the sweating. Extreme sports where the person gets an adrenaline rush consumes their *jing*. The 'mental rush' they experience is *jing* that has been transformed into *shen*.

Many people are conscious of the need to get sufficient exercise, but unfortunately fewer people are aware of the importance of getting enough rest – both physical and mental rest. We typically live very *yang* lifestyles and have little *yin* time in our daily lives. We need to balance all our *yang* activity with *yin* rest and contemplation. Unfortunately, many people think that they get relaxation and stress relief by watching television or sitting in front of a computer. Here, they only get physical rest but are still mentally stimulated. It is good to recommend that people begin to cultivate meditation, qi gong, tai ji or yoga. If you suspect that they will have difficulty accepting things that sound so foreign and mysterious, you can propose instead that they take time daily to really unwind by lying down or sitting completely still, emptying their head of thoughts and concentrating on their breathing. It is especially important in the evenings and at night to cultivate calm and tranquillity. One might be tempted to claim that the invention of electric lighting has in fact had a fundamentally negative impact on people's *yin*. In the past, people only had limited opportunities to be active after nightfall, often just staring into the flames of a fire. Now they can stay physically and, especially, mentally active throughout the *yin* period of the night.

Stimulants such as tobacco create Phlegm and Heat in the Lung and injure the *yin*. Alcohol creates Heat in the Liver and Stomach, as well as producing Dampness and Phlegm. Coffee activates Kidney *jing*, which is transformed into *yang qi*. Coffee therefore weakens both Kidney *yin* and Kidney *yang*. It overstimulates the Heart *yang* and thereby weakens the Heart *yin*. Illicit substances such as marijuana, cocaine, amphetamines and so on generally have a draining effect on the Kidney *jing*, spreading and thereby weakening Heart *qi*.

Part 2

THE DIAGNOSTIC MODELS

INTRODUCTION TO THE DIAGNOSTIC MODELS

Chinese medicine has developed various diagnostic models to classify and structure the information that has been gathered through the use of the four diagnostic pillars. Using the diagnostic models allows the practitioner to see connections and patterns in the diverse signs and symptoms that have been collected. In Chinese medicine it is the overall picture that is the most important, not the individual symptoms and signs. All signs and symptoms have relevance, but it is the context and the relationship between them that is the most important, not the individual components.

The diagnostic models can be used as a template that can be placed over the symptoms, enabling the practitioner to gain an impression of the correlation between the symptoms and signs.

Several diagnostic systems have arisen throughout the history of Chinese medicine. The various diagnostic models should not be seen as alternatives to each other, but as indispensable elements that supplement each other. The same situation, the same symptoms and the same signs can be analysed and described from several diagnostic perspectives at the same time. Using more than one diagnostic model at a time creates a more accurate and precise picture of the person and the imbalances that they are presenting. If, for example, a person coughs, we can use the model of *zangfu* diagnosis. In this diagnostic model, the person will be diagnosed as presenting with a Lung imbalance. This, in itself, is not a precise enough diagnosis upon which to base a treatment. It is necessary to know: whether it is a *xu* or *shi* condition (Eight Principles diagnosis); if there is Phlegm present (diagnosis according to *xie qi*); if there is Heat or Cold (Eight Principles diagnosis); whether there is *qi xu* or *qi* stagnation (diagnosis according to *qi*, *xue* and *jinye*); whether there is *yin xu* (Eight Principles diagnosis); whether the cough is due to an invasion of Wind-Cold or Wind-Heat (diagnosis according to *xie qi*, the Six Stages, or the Four Levels) and so on. Each time you add an aspect of another diagnostic model to the diagnosis, it does not complicate the picture; on the contrary, the image becomes clearer. By refining the picture as much as possible, it not only gives a more solid foundation for treating the disorder most effectively, it also helps to give an impression of how the condition may have arisen, i.e. what the cause of the disorder is. It is important to remember that the imbalance patterns we diagnose are not the cause of the disorder. The causes of the disorder are the factors that gave rise to these patterns of imbalance. These are the aetiological factors. There is often not just one aetiological factor but a mixture of several factors. This is especially the case in interior patterns of imbalance.

The diagnosis tells us how we should treat the patient. The diagnosis determines the treatment principle. If a person is diagnosed as being Lung *qi xu*, the treatment principle is to strengthen or tonify their Lung *qi*. When we have a treatment principle we can construct a treatment strategy. When we should strengthen Lung *qi*, as in the above example, we can use herbs or acupuncture points and techniques that tonify Lung *qi*. This could, for example, be achieved by needling the acupuncture points Lu 9 and UB 13 with a tonifying needle technique or prescribing the herbal prescription *Bu Fei Tang*. Furthermore, once we are also able to identify the aetiological factors that have led to creation of a pattern of imbalance, we can offer the client appropriate advice and this is often where the greatest possibility for healing is to be found.

The diagnostic models utilised in Chinese medicine are:

1. diagnosis according to the Eight Principles

2. diagnosis according to *xie qi*

3. diagnosis according to *qi*, *xue* and *jinye*

4. diagnosis according to the *zangfu* organs

5. diagnosis according to the Six Stages

6. diagnosis according to the Four Levels

7. diagnosis according to *san jiao*

8. diagnosis according to the channels

9. diagnosis according to the Five Phases.

It is important to remember that the symptoms and signs that are listed in each pattern of imbalance are the *possible* symptoms and signs. For example, the signs and symptoms listed in the diagnosis of Kidney *yin xu* are: dry mucous membranes, dry mouth and throat, night sweats, poor memory, nocturnal emissions, premature ejaculation, infertility, tinnitus, poor hearing, deafness, dry eyes, weak or sore knees, lumbar soreness or pain, thin body, scanty and dark urine, anxiety, depression, dizziness, a thin, dry tongue that lacks coating, possibly with cracks in the surface of the tongue, and an Empty or Fine pulse. It is highly unlikely that we will see someone with all these symptoms and signs. We will probably only see three or four of the signs and symptoms that are listed. Kidney *yin xu* can be diagnosed just by the person having lumbar soreness, sore knees, tinnitus and a dry, red tongue that has a cracked surface.

It is important to remember that a person will very rarely manifest only a single pattern of imbalance. It is normal that a person presents with several patterns of imbalance simultaneously. A client who seeks treatment will typically manifest between five and nine imbalances simultaneously.

If we continue with the example of a person who is Kidney *yin xu* and add two further patterns – ascending Liver *yang* and Phlegm – in addition to having some of the above symptoms, the person could have migraines, a quick temper, a slippery pulse, poor appetite, vertigo, lethargy and difficulty waking up in the morning.

Furthermore, several of these symptoms and signs will be worse after consuming dairy products. This, of course, makes diagnosing clients much harder and more complicated. The more chronic the disorder, the more complex the mixture of patterns of imbalance is likely to be.

It is important to remember that when we make a list of the various symptoms and signs, it is a snapshot, a static image. The body and the organs' relationships are dynamic processes where things are constantly influencing and being influenced by each other. Therefore we must not limit our understanding of an imbalance to only the possible aetiological factors, but should also understand how other organs and bodily substances could be involved, how the current situation may develop and what measures we should take in this case.

The acupuncture points that are discussed under each imbalance should be viewed as a treatment suggestion. You do not need to use all the points listed and other acupuncture points could be equally valid if their actions and indications are relevant. The same is true of the guiding herbal prescriptions.

DIAGNOSIS ACCORDING TO THE EIGHT PRINCIPLES

Diagnosis according to the Eight Principles is relatively new. It was first described as a single model in the early *Qing* dynasty, around the year CE 1680, by Cheng Zhong Ling. The differentiation of individual principles is, however, seen in books as old as the *Huang Di Nei Jing* and *Shang Han Lun*.

In the Eight Principle diagnosis, the patterns are differentiated in relation to four opposite pairs. These pairs are: *yin* and *yang*; Hot and Cold; interior and exterior; *xu* and *shi*. Each element has specific symptoms and signs that characterise it and these symptoms and signs are used to differentiate it from its counterpart. If there is Heat, for example, there may be symptoms and signs such as thirst, dark urine, a red face, a rapid pulse and a red tongue. If there is Cold, there will be no particular thirst, the urine will be clear, the face pale, the pulse slow and the tongue pale.

The Eight Principles are ultimately only two principles – *yin* and *yang* where the other six principles are subcategories or refinements of these two principles. Diagnoses would be incredibly simple but not very useful if we just differentiated between *yin* and *yang*, so it is necessary to further refine and differentiate the symptoms and signs. It also means that the six subcategories can be combined in many different ways. This makes situations more complex, because you can, for example, combine *yin* categories such as 'interior' with *yang* qualities such as 'Heat', and you can then combine this with *xu* or *shi*. The image becomes three dimensional and more intricate.

As described, the pairs can be combined in varying combinations. Furthermore, it is not necessary to utilise all four differentiations to create a diagnosis. It is enough, for example, in an invasion of Wind-Cold to state that it is 'exterior *shi* Cold' or, if there is *xue xu*, to state that there is an 'interior *xu*' condition. A diagnosis will frequently consist of multiple, simultaneous, individual diagnoses. There may also be contradictions within the same category. It's not an either/or differentiation, but can quite easily be a both/and diagnosis. For example, you can have both interior *xu* Heat and Exterior *shi* Cold at the same time (this could be a person who is Kidney *yin xu* who has been invaded by exogenous Wind-Cold).

Diagnosis according to the Eight Principles is the basis of all TCM diagnoses. The difference between this and other diagnostic models is that the Eight Principles can be and is used every time we make a diagnosis. All differentiation relies on the distinction between the Eight Principles. Other diagnostic models are relevant in specific situations and usually involve the Eight Principles in their diagnosis. If, for example, when making a diagnosis according to *qi*, *xue* and *jinye*, you have

.iagnosed *xue xu*, it is implicit in this diagnosis that it is an interior *xu* condition according to the Eight Principles.

The Eight Principles may appear to be very simplistic but because these principles are involved in all diagnostic scenarios and because the individual components of the situation are differentiated separately, there is no situation too complex to be analysed using the Eight Principles. On the contrary, when something appears to be complex and confusing, you can always take a step back and assess the entire situation from an Eight Principles perspective. There are often situations where there are many different symptoms and signs and it is difficult to gauge which organs are involved and whether it is *qi* or *xue* that has stagnated or whether there is Phlegm and so on. In these situations you can always ask yourself: What is the overall impression? Is it an interior or exterior condition? Is it *xu* or *shi*? Hot or Cold? and then proceed again.

The Eight Principles form the foundation of all treatment strategies and acupuncture point selections.

The Eight Principles are also a way of clarifying a diagnosis. For example, if a patient coughs, we know that it is a Lung imbalance. Because they cough, we also know that there is rebellious *qi*. To treat the cough though, it is important to know whether the imbalance is the result of interiorly generated or exogenous *xie qi*, whether it is a *xu* or a *shi* condition and whether there is Heat or Cold. All of these things will help to determine which acupuncture points or herbs are used and whether the acupuncture points should be tonified or drained.

Using the Eight Principles in practice requires flexibility. One must accept that there may be contradictions within the same diagnosis. One must learn to understand the dynamics and the relationship between the individual components. This means that it is then possible to accept contradictions such Heat and Cold, *xu* and *shi*, interior and exterior, not just in the same patient, but also in the same disorder. It is important to perceive and comprehend the imbalances as dynamic processes of change. Imbalances create new situations that in the final end can be the opposite of themselves. The following example considers Spleen *yang xu*: the Spleen is in the interior, so this is an interior imbalance; *yang xu* is a *xu* condition; because it is *yang* that is *xu*, there will be a lack of physiological heat. Spleen *yang xu* is therefore an interior *yang xu* Cold condition. Spleen *yang xu* will often lead to the formation of Damp. Dampness is a form of *xie qi* and is therefore something other and more than the body's *zheng qi*, so it is a *shi* condition. The Dampness is in the interior. This means that Dampness is therefore defined as being an interior *shi* condition. Dampness is *yin* in nature but, on the other hand, it is neutral in its temperature. Dampness is therefore an interior *yin shi* condition but is neither Hot nor Cold. Spleen *yang xu* resulting in Dampness is thereby a condition of interior *yang xu* Cold and interior *yin shi* at the same time.

Patterns of imbalance are not static but are dynamic and mutable. It is a fundamental principle of the Universe that *yin* and *yang* transform into each other. Therefore, one pattern can transform to another. Cold can transform to Heat; *shi* conditions can injure the body and thereby create a *xu* condition; exterior imbalances can become interior, and so on. In the above example, Spleen *yang xu* could easily have arisen after an Invasion of exterior *shi* Cold, and the resulting Dampness could lead to the creation of Damp-Heat.

Even though a diagnosis will usually comprise multiple components, for example interior *yin xu* Heat or exterior *shi* Cold, it is important to understand the dynamics of each separate aspect of the Eight Principles. For the sake of clarity, it is therefore necessary in the following sections to discuss each aspect separately. These individual aspects are, though, inextricably integrated with each other and the various combinations of these eight components will each have their own unique manifestations. There are, for example, significant differences, not only in the symptoms and signs of Cold and Heat, but also in the symptoms and signs that manifest when there is *xu* Heat and *shi* Heat or when there is interior Heat and exterior Heat, as differences between interior *shi* Heat and exterior *shi* Heat, interior *xu* Heat and interior *shi* Heat and so on. It is important to have this in mind when you read the following sections.

I have tried to be comprehensive in describing the aetiology, symptoms, signs and treatment of the various patterns, but, for the sake of space and clarity, I have chosen not to go into too much detail with regards to the various sub-patterns. Instead, I refer the reader to the relevant sections in the other diagnostic chapters.

Interior and exterior imbalances

The differentiation here is between where in the body the imbalance is located, not what it is that has created the imbalance. An invasion of Wind-Cold is an exterior imbalance, not because it is exogenous *xie qi* that has created the imbalance but because the imbalance is manifesting in the body's exterior aspect, more specifically in the *wei qi* aspect. This means that even if an imbalance is caused by the presence of an exterior pathogen, if this exogenous *xie qi* is located in the interior aspect of the body, it is by definition an interior pattern.

As well as identifying in which aspect of the body an imbalance is located, interior and exterior will often give an indication of how serious an imbalance is. Exterior imbalances are usually less serious than interior imbalances, because it is the *zangfu* organs and the vital substances that are affected when there is an interior imbalance.

Exterior imbalances

In exterior imbalances, the symptoms and signs are manifesting in the channels, between the skin and muscles (*wei qi* aspect) or in the skin, muscles and tendons. It is always necessary to incorporate other principles into the diagnosis of exterior imbalances, such as whether there is Exterior Heat or exterior Cold or whether it is an exterior *xu* or an exterior *shi* condition.

Exterior imbalances are often, but not always, acute. They are usually caused by invasions of exogenous *xie qi*. Typical examples of such patterns are invasions of Wind-Cold or Wind-Heat.

An example of a chronic exterior imbalance is when *xie qi* blocks the channels. This will result in '*bi* syndrome' or painful blockage syndrome. The Western diagnosis of arthritis would, for example, fall within this category.

Skin disorders are not necessarily exterior imbalances. Eczema, psoriasis, acne and so on are often caused by *xue* imbalances and interior Heat. This means that they are usually exterior manifestations of interior imbalances.

Exterior patterns will usually have little or no impact on the functioning of the *zangfu* organs.

Acute exterior imbalances

An exterior condition will typically be a *shi* condition. This is because acute exterior conditions are usually due to the presence of *xie qi*. There may well be a concurrent *xu* condition, for example *wei qi xu*, in which case it will be a *xu/shi* condition.[14] The symptoms and signs in an exterior *xu* condition will be milder than in an exterior *shi* condition. In addition to the symptoms and signs of an exterior condition being dependent on whether it is a *xu* or *shi* condition, they will also be different if the condition is a Hot or a Cold condition.

Exterior patterns will typically be acute and there will usually be tangible symptoms and signs that indicate that *wei qi* has been disrupted in its circulation and functioning. When *wei qi* is blocked by exogenous *xie qi*, it will not be able to warm the skin and muscles, resulting in the person having chills. The blockage of *wei qi* will also manifest with pain and tenderness of the skin and muscles. Cold in the exterior will often disrupt the *taiyang* channel. This is typically seen with there being stiffness and pain in the neck and head.

Invasions of Cold will block *wei qi* from controlling the pores in the skin. This will manifest with a person either not being able to sweat (*shi* condition) or sweating spontaneously without this relieving the symptoms (*xu* condition). Because *wei qi* is compromised, it cannot defend the body against exogenous *xie qi*. This will be seen in a person experiencing an aversion to cold, draughts and wind. This aversion is most pronounced in a *xu* condition. The conflict between *wei qi* and *xie qi* can generate Heat and therefore there may be a fever. This will be much more significant when there is exterior Wind-Heat.

An important differentiation in Chinese medicine is between the symptoms and signs seen in exterior Heat conditions and interior Heat conditions. A key symptom when differentiating these two patterns is whether there is a concurrent fever and aversion. In interior Heat, there is no aversion to cold, whilst there is fever. This will be the case when there is exterior Wind-Heat.

Headaches can be a symptom of an exterior imbalance, but there is a difference in the headaches seen in various exterior imbalances. Invasions of Heat in the exterior can manifest with a throbbing headache. This is due to the *yang* expanding nature of Heat. Exterior Cold can manifest with a tight and tense headache due to Cold's contracting dynamic. Invasions of Dampness in the exterior (exterior *yin shi*) can result in a heavy headache.

An invasion of Heat in the exterior can cause a person to feel thirsty, because the Heat will injure the body's fluids.

The pulse in exterior conditions will be Superficial, because there is increased activity in the superficial aspect of the body. The pulse that is felt when there is Wind-Heat will be Superficial and Rapid. Wind-Cold will manifest with a pulse that is Superficial and Tight, whilst a Wind-Dampness pulse will be Superficial and Slippery. The strength of the pulse will reflect whether it is a *xu* or *shi* condition. In *xu* conditions, the pulse will lack strength. Because these are acute imbalances, visible changes in the tongue will rarely be observed. If there are changes, these will manifest with changes in the coating on the front and at the edges of the tongue.

Differences between exterior Heat and exterior Cold

Exterior Cold	Exterior Heat
Immediate symptoms	Immediate/delayed/gradual symptoms
Strong aversion to cold	No or only a slight aversion to cold
Mild fever or no fever	Fever
Tight/tense headaches	Throbbing headache
No thirst	Thirst
Tight and Superficial pulse	Rapid and Superficial pulse

Differences between exterior *xu* and exterior *shi* conditions

Xu	*Shi*
Spontaneous perspiration or sweating that does not alleviate the symptoms	No sweating
Extreme aversion to Wind and draughts	Aversion to Cold
Milder symptoms	Strong symptoms
Empty pulse	Full and Superficial pulse

Aetiology
Invasion of exogenous *xie qi*.

Symptoms and signs
As written above, there will be considerable differences between the individual patterns depending on whether it is a Heat or Cold, and *xu* and *shi* condition.

Some of the common symptoms and signs are as follows:

- Symptoms in the *wei qi* aspect, skin, muscles, joints or tendons.

- When there is Wind-Heat, there can be a fever or a sensation of fever. If there is Wind-Cold, there may be only a slight fever or fever sensation.

- Headache.

- Aversion to Wind.

- Superficial pulse.

Key symptoms
Superficial pulse and aversion to wind and cold.

Treatment principle
Expel *xie qi* from the exterior, regulate *wei qi*.

If there is *wei qi xu*, you must simultaneously tonify *wei qi*.

Acupuncture points
Choose from: LI 4, Lu 7, GB 20, UB 10, SI 3, UB 62, SJ 5, Du 14, Du 16, UB 12 and UB 13.

- If there is Heat, add: LI 11.

- If there is *wei qi xu*, add: Lu 9, St 36, Sp 3.

Needle technique
Draining.

Explanation

- LI 4, Lu 7, SJ 5, Du 14, UB 12 and UB 13 activate *wei qi* and expel Wind.

- GB 20 and Du 16 expels Wind.

- SI 3 and UB 62 together activate *wei qi* and expel Wind from the *taiyang* aspect.

- LI 11 expels Wind-Heat.

- St 36, Lu 9 and Sp 3 tonify *wei qi*.

Herbal formula
The relevant herbal formula will depend on the exact exterior condition. The following are examples of such formulas, but there are many other formulas that could also be used, depending on the symptoms and signs.

- *Ma Huang Tang* (Expels Wind-Cold)

- *Gui Zhi Tang* (Expels Wind-Cold and regulates the *ying* and the *wei qi*)

- *Yin Qiao San* (Expels Wind-Heat)

- *Chuan Xiong Cha Tiao Tang* (Expels Wind-Cold and relieves headaches)

- *Xiao Qing Long Tang* (Expels Wind-Cold and transforms Phlegm-Fluids)

- *Huo Xiang Zheng Qi Tang* (Expels Wind-Cold and transforms turbid Dampness)

Relevant advice

When there is an acute invasion of exogenous *xie qi* in the exterior, it is advisable to consume beverages that are spicy and diaphoretic to open the exterior and expel *xie qi*. This could be ginger, garlic, whisky, brandy and chilli, for example, if there is an invasion of exogenous Wind-Cold, or mint, chrysanthemum, chamomile or elderflower if there is an invasion of exogenous Wind-Heat. Fasting is also advisable or only eating soup, such as onion soup. There are two reasons for this. First, when temporarily fasting *qi* will not be used to transform food and therefore can be used to combat the invading *xie qi*. Second, some sources say that the downward movement of food and *qi* in the Stomach can draw the exogenous *xie qi* inwards from the surface.

Similarly, the sour flavour should be avoided due to its astringent or centripetal dynamic. Vitamin C, lemon and other things that are very sour should not be consumed during an invasion of exogenous *xie* Cold, as they will draw the *xie* Cold inwards whilst closing the pores in the skin, thereby preventing the Cold from being expelled again. This also means that antibiotics are not recommended at this stage, as they are cold and drain downward.

Chronic exterior imbalances

Chronic exterior imbalances are typically *bi* syndromes. *Bi* syndromes arise from the simultaneous presence of three separate types of exogenous *xie qi* in the channels and collaterals. There may also be disruptions of the channels themselves due to trauma or repetitive movements that strain the joints, such as computer arm and tennis elbow. These disorders, with the exception of physical traumas, will often have arisen gradually, but there may also be episodes of acute flare-ups. These flare-ups will often be due to climatic influences or physical strain.

Aetiology

Invasion of exogenous Dampness, Heat, Cold and Wind. Repeated stress on the joint.

Symptoms and signs

- Pain in the joints and/or muscles.

Treatment principle

Expel exogenous *xie qi*, regulate *qi* and *xue* in the channel.
If there is *qi xu*, tonify *qi*.

Acupuncture points

Choose from: relevant channel points, local points, distal points, 'cross channel' points[15] and points to expel exogenous *xie qi*.

- If there is exogenous Wind, add: UB 12, Du 14, Du 16 and LI 4.

- If there is exogenous Cold, add: LI 4 and Du 14.

- If there is exogenous Dampness, add: Sp 6, Sp 9 and LI 4.

- If Exogenous Heat, add: Du 14, LI 4 or LI 11.

- If there is *xue* stagnation, add: Sp 10 and UB 17.

Needle technique
Draining.

Herbal formula
The relevant herbal formula will depend on the exact exterior condition. The following are examples of such formulas, but there are many other formulas that could also be used, dependent on the symptoms and signs.

- *Qiang Huo Sheng Shi Tang* (Expels Wind-Damp-Cold, activates channel *qi*)

- *Du Huo Ji Sheng Tang* (Expels Wind-Damp-Cold, activates channel *qi* and tonifies *qi* and *xue*)

- *Chuan Xiong Cha Tiao Tang* (Expels Wind-Cold and regulates *qi* in the head)

- *Huo Xiang Zheng Qi Tang* (Expels Wind-Damp-Cold and transforms turbid Dampness)

- *Bai Hu Jia Gui Zhi Tang* (Expels Wind-Damp-Heat)

Interior imbalances

Interior imbalances are de facto all imbalances that are not exterior.[16] Interior imbalances include all the imbalances where there is a change in the functioning of the *zangfu* organs and where the vital substances are affected. There may well be combined patterns in which there are imbalances in both the interior and the exterior. An example of this could be a person who is Kidney *yang xu* (interior *xu* Cold) who is also invaded by Wind-Heat (exterior *shi* Heat).

Imbalances in the interior can arise in one of three ways.

- Exogenous *xie qi* that has been located in the exterior penetrates downwards into the interior.

- Exogenous *xie qi* can directly invade certain *fu* organs.

- Interior imbalances can also arise due to other factors, such as diet, emotions and overexertion, affecting the *zangfu* organs and/or the vital substances.

Invasions of exogenous *xie qi* will usually be acute, whereas most other interior imbalances will be chronic in nature.

When an imbalance is in the interior, it will have affected one or more of the *zangfu* organs or the vital substances themselves. This means that the body's physiology will be affected and this will be apparent in the signs and symptoms that are manifesting. When there is an interior imbalance, certain organs and vital substances will not be carrying out their functions optimally. There will be observable changes in functions such as urination, defecation, appetite, sleep and so on. Because the imbalance will have lasted for longer than an exterior imbalance, and because the body's physiology is affected, there will not only be changes in the pulse, but the tongue will also show signs of change.

Differences between interior and exterior imbalances

Interior	Exterior
Mainly chronic	Mainly acute
May be due to the six forms of climatic *xie qi*, the seven emotions and the diverse causes	Usually caused by one or more of the six forms of climatic *xie qi*
Zangfu organs, *xue*, *qi*, *jinye* or *jing* will be disturbed	The channels, *wei qi*, skin, tendons or muscles will be affected
Disruption of the body's internal physiology	The body's internal physiology is not disrupted
Changes in pulse and tongue	Generally, only changes in the pulse
The pulse is generally not superficial	Superficial pulse
Usually there is no aversion to cold and wind	Usually there is an aversion to wind and cold

Aetiology

If exogenous *xie qi* is not expelled from the exterior, it can penetrate into the interior. This will occur because the *xie qi* is very virulent, *zheng qi* is weakened or the person has been treated improperly and *xie qi* has been dragged inwards and downwards. Initially, *xie qi* penetrating into the interior will be a *shi* and a Heat condition. The symptoms and signs will be powerful due to the struggle between *zheng qi* and *xie qi*. This corresponds to the *yangming* stage of the Six Stages or the *qi* level of the Four Levels. If the *xie qi* is not eradicated, if there are repeated invasions of exogenous *xie qi* or if the body's *zheng qi* is *xu*, the *xie qi* can penetrate even deeper into the body and will develop into a *xu* pattern. This will be similar to the *taiyin*, *shaoyin* and *jueyin* stages and the *ying* and *xue* levels. The patterns here can be Hot or Cold patterns. See 'Diagnosis According to the Six Stages' and 'Diagnosis According to the Four Levels' in Section 9 for a more detailed analysis of the symptoms and signs.

Exogenous *xie qi* can also directly invade into the interior. These invasions are almost exclusively into one of the *fu* organs. This will typically be when Cold or Dampness invades the Intestines, Stomach, Urinary Bladder or the Uterus, or when Damp-Heat invades the Intestines or the Urinary Bladder. Direct invasions of exogenous *xie qi* into the interior will manifest with acute symptoms, which will be *shi* conditions. The reader is referred to Section 8, 'Diagnosis According to *Zangfu* Organ Patterns', for more details about the relevant symptoms and treatment principles.

The internal organs and vital substances can be affected by the seven emotions and the so-called diverse or miscellaneous causes, such as diet, overwork, lifestyle and so on. These imbalances will be chronic, but there may still be acute symptoms. This is typically seen when there are combined *xu* and *shi* patterns. An example of this could be Liver *yin xu* with ascending Liver *yang*. Here, the person will often suffer from acute migraine attacks, even though the underlying patterns are chronic.

Symptoms and signs

There can often be a complex mixture of symptoms and signs resulting from several organs' functions being affected and there can also be a combination of *xu* and *shi* patterns. The symptoms and treatment of the individual patterns are described in 'Diagnosis According to *Qi*, *Xue* and *Jinye* Imbalances' (Section 7) and 'Diagnosis According to *Zangfu* Organ Patterns' (Section 8).

Knowing that the imbalance is in the interior is not precise enough. It is necessary, whenever possible, to locate the imbalance in the interior and find out what its nature is. There will be significant differences in the symptoms and signs between the various interior imbalances, depending on which organs and substances are affected and whether the condition is *xu* or *shi* and Hot or Cold. The reader is again referred to 'Diagnosis According to *Qi*, *Xue* and *Jinye* Imbalances' (Section 7) and 'Diagnosis According to *Zangfu* Organ Patterns' (Section 8) for more details about the relevant symptoms and treatment principles.

Hot and Cold imbalances

In the principal pair of Hot and Cold, the imbalance is differentiated according to the imbalance's energetic nature. Heat is *yang* in nature, it over-activates and accelerates the body's processes. Cold is *yin* and will do the opposite. It will slow down or weaken processes and, because it has a contracting nature, it will create blockages of *qi*, *xue* and *jinye*. The precise symptoms will again depend on whether it is a *xu* or *shi* condition and whether it is an interior or exterior condition.

There are often situations in which there is both Heat and Cold present simultaneously. There may be, for example, Heat and Cold in different organs at the same time. There may be Heat in the upper part of the body and Cold in the lower part. There can also be Heat and Cold in different aspects of the body, for example Wind-Cold in the exterior and Heat in the interior.

Differences between Heat and Cold conditions

Heat	Cold
Over-activates and accelerates the body's processes	Weakens the body and makes processes slower
Expands	Contracts and creates stagnations and blockage
Desiccates and concentrates the body's fluids	Disrupts the transformation and transportation of the body's fluids
Changes the colour of the skin to red and exudations to yellow or green	White or bluish skin colour

Causes exudations and discharges to become odorous, thicker and stickier	Exudations and discharges do not smell Clear, watery and more copious discharges from the body's orifices
Throbbing, stinging or burning pain	Biting or cramping pain
Red tongue	Pale tongue
Yellowish tongue coating (*shi* conditions) or no tongue coating (*xu* conditions)	Whitish tongue coating
Rapid pulse	Slow pulse
Rapid movements	Slow and languorous movements (*xu* conditions), stiff movements (*shi* conditions)
Restlessness, agitation	Lethargy
Sends *qi* upward (*shi* conditions) or does not root *qi* (*xu* conditions)	Blocks *qi* (*shi* conditions) or does not move *qi* (*xu* conditions)
Thirst	No thirst
Constipation with dry stool	Most frequently loose stools or diarrhoea, but there can be constipation The stools will not be dry
Insomnia	Possibly hypersomnia if there is *xu* Cold
Sleeps with limbs stretched outwards and with increased movement of the body whilst sleeping Sleeps with thin blankets and may have a tendency to kick the bedding off whilst sleeping	Sleeps with the body curled up and with thick bedding Does not move about in the bed whilst sleeping
The skin can feel warm on palpation	The skin can feel cold on palpation

Heat

It is necessary to further differentiate between *xu* and *shi* Heat, because the treatments are very different. Furthermore, it is very important to differentiate between interior and exterior Heat. This is because *xie qi* can be dragged deeper into the body by improper treatment. This is particularly important when treating with herbs.

Shi Heat

Shi Heat will often manifest with a sensation of heat in the body or an aversion to heat. The skin will feel warm and can become red in colour. Anywhere that the skin has changed colour and become red is a sign that there is Heat present. The Heat may be localised to this area, as is seen when there is a red, swollen joint due to a local stagnation of *qi*, *xue* and *jinye* when a joint is sprained. There may be Heat in an organ and its channel, as is seen when there are red and bleeding gums caused by Heat in the Stomach channel. The Heat can also be systemic, such as when there is a general condition of Heat in the body. When there is *shi* Heat, the face will often be red, as will the tongue. This is due to the *yang* nature of Heat, which means that it will ascend upwards in the body. When there is Heat in the body, the superficial vessels become more blood-filled, because the Heat drives *xue* up to the surface and therefore the skin appears more red in colour. It is not only the skin that changes colour when there is Heat – exudations and discharges from the body, such as mucus in the respiratory passages and nose, discharge from the vagina, urine, fluid from ulcers and so on will also change colour. When secretions are yellowish or greenish, it is a sign that there is Heat. Heat concentrates the exudations and this will result in a change in their consistency. Excretions become thicker and stickier. They will also begin to smell or taste different.

By driving fluids upwards and outwards, the *yang* nature of Heat can result in heavy sweating. Heat can also injure the body's fluids, in which case there may be a lack of sweating. By damaging fluids and dehydrating the body, Heat will result in a person having an excessive thirst, with a desire for cold liquids. Furthermore, by dehydrating the body, Heat can manifest with constipation.

Because the body feels warm, the person will often wear less clothing than other people. A patient who turns up wearing just a t-shirt and a jacket in the winter, when everyone else is walking around with sweaters and coats on, will often have *shi* Heat.

If there is a pain, the expansive energy of warmth will mean that the sensation is a throbbing pain. This is typically seen in certain types of headaches and joint pains. The sensation can also be stinging and burning, for example in the rectum or in the throat.

Some symptoms are more specific to interior or exterior *shi* Heat conditions. They are discussed separately below.

Interior shi Heat

Some people relate the bitter taste to the Heart. In reality, the bitter taste is an aspect of the Fire Phase, as is Heat. This means that a bitter taste in the mouth can be experienced in many Heat disorders, for example Liver Fire.

Heat activates and accelerates processes. In a person with Heat, this can be seen in the movements of their body, and their speech will be faster. Because interior *shi* Heat is an excess condition, the person's voice will be loud.

The nature of Heat is to rise upwards. This means that the Heart will become agitated when Heat rises upwards to the upper *jiao*. This can manifest on both the physical plane, with a faster pulse, and on the mental-emotional level, with the person being restless, agitated or downright manic. Heat opens and agitates the Heart so the person will often talk quicker and be more verbose than normal. When *shen* is agitated, there can be difficulty sleeping or just restless, dream-disturbed sleep. *Shen* and the Heart can also be affected when *xue*, which is governed by the Heart and is the residence for *shen*, is agitated by Heat.

Heat can also result in *xue* becoming so agitated and over-activated so that it bursts the walls of vessels and results in bleeding.

When there is Heat in the interior, the Heat will injure the body's fluids, resulting in thirst. The thirst seen in interior *shi* Heat will be different to the thirst seen when there is interior *xu* Heat. *Xu* Heat arises from a lack of *yin* and this manifests with a dryness of the mouth and throat as opposed to an actual thirst. This means that the person will have a desire to sip small amounts of liquid to moisten the mouth and throat. *Shi* Heat will injure fluids, resulting in a pronounced thirst and a desire to gulp copious amounts of cold fluids.

There will also be specific symptoms and signs that relate to the functions of specific organs when these organs are affected by Heat. For a detailed description of these symptoms and their treatment, the reader is referred to 'Diagnosis According to *Zangfu* Organ Patterns' (Section 7).

Exterior *shi* Heat

When there is exterior Heat, there will be signs relating to the disturbance of *wei qi* or to the muscles and joints, such as in *bi* syndrome. The only *zang* organ that can be affected immediately by an invasion of *shi* Heat in the exterior is the Lung. This is because exterior *xie* Heat will disrupt the functioning of *wei qi*, which is controlled by the Lung. When there is exterior *shi* Heat, there is no disturbance of other internal organs' physiology. The pulse will be Superficial and Rapid, because *xie qi* is in the exterior and because there is Heat. If there are any changes seen on the tongue, these will be visible on the tip and/or the sides, which will be red and there may be a thin yellowish coating in these areas. Exterior Heat symptoms and signs will be acute. Interior Heat's symptoms and signs will be more chronic in nature, but there may be acute episodes. There is often an aversion to wind and cold during an exogenous invasion of Heat, because *wei qi* is disturbed. This will not be the case when there is a condition of Heat in the interior; on the contrary, the person will often have an aversion to heat. The thirst will not be as strong if there is Heat in the exterior. This is because Heat is starting to injure the body's fluids but not to the same extent as when there is Heat in the interior.

Differences between interior and exterior Heat

Interior Heat	Exterior Heat
Most often chronic, but there may be acute episodes	Acute
May be due to one or more of the six climatic forms of *xie qi*, the seven emotions and diverse causes	Due to one or more of the six climatic forms of *xie qi*
Can be a *xu* or *shi* condition	*Shi* condition
Zangfu organs are affected	*Wei qi*, muscles or joints are affected
Disruption of the body's internal physiology	The body's internal physiology is not disrupted
The pulse can be Deep or Superficial	Superficial pulse

Interior Heat	Exterior Heat
The entire tongue can be red or the tongue can be red in an area that corresponds to a specific organ that is affected by Heat There can be both a yellow coating or a lack of coating, depending on whether it is a *shi* or *xu* condition	The tip and the sides may be red and there may be a thin yellowish coating in these areas
No aversion to wind and cold	Slight aversion to wind and cold
There may be a strong thirst	The thirst is not so pronounced
Rapid body movements	Normal body movements
Rapid and verbose speech	Normal speech
Shen may be affected	*Shen* not affected
There may be bleeding	No bleeding
Treatment principle: Either drain Heat or nourish *yin*	Treatment principle: Expel Wind-Heat

Aetiology
Shi Heat can arise in several ways.

- Excessive intake of foodstuffs, beverages and spices that have a Warm or Hot energy. Typical examples of these are chilli, garlic, pepper, alcohol, lamb, fried food such as chips, falafel, crisps and so on. This will be especially relevant when there is Heat in the Liver, Stomach and Intestines.

- Prolonged emotional imbalances: Stress, frustration and anger will create Heat in the Heart and Liver.

- Smoking tobacco creates Heat, especially in the Lung.

- Invasions of exogenous *xie qi*: Heat can directly invade the body. The invasion can be via the exterior or directly into the interior. Invasions of exogenous Cold can transform into Heat in the interior. Internally generated *xie qi*, such as Dampness, can transform and become Damp-Heat.

Symptoms and signs
- Thirst

- Aversion to heat

- The skin may feel warm when palpated

- The face can be red or ruddy

- Discharges and exudations that have changed colour and become yellowish or greenish

- Excretions that have become sticky or thicker

- Excretions that smell or taste strongly

274

- Pain that is throbbing, stinging or burning

- Excessive sweating or lack of sweating

- Constipation

- Red tongue

- Rapid pulse

Key symptoms
Thirst, aversion to heat, red face, red tongue and rapid pulse.

Treatment principle
Expel or drain Heat.

Acupuncture points

- If there is Heat in the exterior, choose from: Du 14, Du 16, LI 4, LI 11, SJ 5, Lu 11, GB 20 and *erjian* (Ex-HN 6).

- If there is Heat in the Lung, choose from: Lu 1, Lu 5, Lu 10, Du 14, LI 11, UB 13 and *erjian* (Ex-HN 6).

- If there is Heat in Heart, choose from: He 8, Pe 5, Pe 7, Pe 8, Du 14, UB 14, UB 15, Ren 15 and *erjian* (Ex-HN 6)

- If there is Heat in Liver, choose from: Liv 2, Liv 14, Du 14, UB 18 and *erjian* (Ex-HN 6).

- If there is Heat in the Stomach, choose from: St 43, St 44, St 45, LI 11, Du 14, UB 21, Ren 13 and *erjian* (Ex-HN 6).

- If there is Heat in Intestines, choose from: St 25, St 37, St 39, St 44 and *erjian* (Ex-HN 6).

- If there is Heat in Urinary Bladder, choose from: UB 28, Ren 3, Du 14 and *erjian* (Ex-HN 6).

- If there is *xue* Heat, choose from: Liv 1, Liv 2, Sp 10, Du 14, UB 17 and *erjian* (Ex-HN 6).

Needle technique
Draining. Bleeding can be applicable.

Herbal formula
The relevant herbal formula will depend on the exact Heat condition. The following are examples of such formulas, but there are many other formulas that could also be used, depending on the organ affected and the specific symptoms and signs.

- *Yin Qiao San* (Expels Heat and drains Toxic-Fire)

- *Huang Lian Jie Du Tang* (Drains Damp-Heat from all three *jiao* and drains Toxic-Fire)

- *Bai Tou Weng Tang* (Drains Damp-Heat from the Intestines and drains Toxic-Fire)

- *Long Dan Xie Gan Tang* (Drains Liver Fire and Liver and Gall Bladder Damp-Heat)

- *Ba Zheng Tang* (Drains Damp-Heat from the Urinary Bladder)

- *Dao Chi San* (Drains Fire from the Heart)

- *Xie Bai San* (Drains Heat from the Lung)

- *Qing Wei San* (Drains Fire from the Stomach)

Relevant advice

A person with *shi* Heat should avoid food and drinks that have a hot dynamic. Typical examples of these are chilli, garlic, pepper, alcohol, lamb, fried food such as chips, falafel, crisps and so on. They should try to avoid stress. If there is exterior Heat, you could recommend they drink mint tea or elderflower tea.

Xu Heat

There are significant differences between *xu* and *shi* Heat, both in their symptoms and signs and in how they arise. The treatment principle for these two types of Heat will also be different. If there is *shi* Heat, it must be drained or expelled. If there is *xu* Heat, *yin* must be nourished.

Yin has the task of cooling the body. If *yin* is *xu*, the body will not be able to control Heat, which is *yang*. Even though the nature of Heat is the same, because the Heat itself is not excessive and because it is not being controlled and balanced by *yin*, the symptoms and signs will not be the same as in *shi* Heat. It is not so much that there is a difference in the intensity of the symptoms and signs but more how and when the symptoms occur that is different. This is in contrast to the difference between *xu* and *shi* Cold, where there are significant differences in intensity of the symptoms themselves.

Difference between *shi* Heat and *xu* Heat

Shi Heat	*Xu* Heat
Powerful thirst with desire to drink cold drinks in large gulps	Dry mouth and throat, which results in a desire to sip rather than gulp
Red tongue with a yellow coating	Red tongue with little or no coating, possibly with cracks
Full and Rapid pulse	Fine, Rapid and possibly Superficial pulse
Loud voice	Weak and possibly nervous voice

Powerful and quick movements	Nervous and restless movements
Restless and dream-disturbed sleep	Wakes frequently, difficulty falling asleep
Restlessness, agitation, mania	Restlessness and anxiety
Profuse or lack of sweating Sweats throughout the day	Night sweats
Sensation of heat or fever throughout the day	Sensation of heat or feeling feverish in the evening and night, hot flushes
Heat in the whole body	Heat in the palms, soles of the feet and centre of the chest
Constipation with pain in the abdomen	Constipation or dry stools without pain in the abdomen
Bitter taste in the mouth	No bitter taste
Heat must be drained downwards or expelled through the skin	*Yin* must be nourished, so that Heat can be controlled

When there is *shi* Heat, its *yang* nature will drive the body fluids upwards and outwards as sweat. When there is *yin xu*, Heat will also make the person sweat, but it will usually only be in the evening and at night. This is because *yin* is the dominant energy at night. If *yin* is weak, it will not be able to control *yang* Heat in this period. Furthermore, *wei qi*, which controls the pores in the skins, circulates in the interior of the body at night. This means that the pores are not able to hold the sweat that has arisen from the uncontrolled Heat inside the body at night.

A person who is *yin xu* will experience sensations of heat or fever mainly in the evening and at night. The sensation of heat will not be as intense and sustained as it is when there is *shi* Heat. When there is *shi* Heat, the sensation of heat or fever is sustained throughout the day and the night. *Xu* Heat usually also comes in waves as hot flushes, rather than as a sustained sensation. When there is *xu* Heat, there is often only a sensation of heat in the palms of the hands, the soles of the feet and the centre of the chest,[17] whereas it is the whole body and particularly the head that feels hot when there is *shi* Heat. One of the ways to differentiate *xu* and *shi* Heat is to feel the patient's hands. If the whole hand feels warm, there is *shi* Heat. When only the palm feels hot, it is *xu* Heat.

The body will be dehydrated when there is *xu* Heat, but the mechanism is not quite the same as when there is *shi* Heat. *Xu* Heat is not as intense and does not injure the body fluids to the same extent that *shi* Heat does. When there is *yin xu*, the body fluids are not nourished and replenished by *yin*. *Xu* Heat will then further dry out the body fluids, but the Heat is not as intense as it is when there is *shi* Heat. This means that the thirst will not be as intense. Where there was a strong thirst with a desire to drink cold liquids in large gulps with *shi* Heat, there will instead be a dry mouth and throat that results in a person preferring to sip water, especially in the evening and at night. Often the person will have a glass of water standing beside the bed that they sip during the night and the glass will not always be emptied. This is in contrast with a person with *shi* Heat, who will empty more than one glass.

As with *shi* Heat, the dehydration of the body in *xu* Heat will result in dark and scanty urine. It can also result in constipation, but there is not the abdominal pain and discomfort that is seen in *shi* Heat conditions.

The face and the head will not be as red when there is *xu* Heat. In *shi* Heat, the whole head and face will be red. When there is *xu* Heat, there will be a malar flush, with the redness localised on the cheekbones, which is often more pronounced in the evening and when the person is tired. The is because when there is *xu* Heat, the Heat detaches itself because it is not anchored by *yin*, and then drifts up to the head. When there is *shi* Heat, there is an active flaring up of Fire. This means that the whole head turns red.

Tongue diagnosis is an essential tool in the differentiation of *xu* and *shi* Heat. In both cases the tongue is likely to be red and dry, but when there is *xu* Heat, there will be little or no coating on the tongue. The lack of nourishment and *yin* moisture can cause the tongue to crack. The pulse will also be weaker when there is *xu* Heat, but it can still be Rapid, because the Heat will have accelerated the beating of the Heart. Because *yang* is not rooted and anchored, the pulse can have a superficial quality when there is *xu* Heat.

Xu heat will also affect the Heart and *shen* but the impact will not be as great and the symptoms not as intense as when there is *shi* Heat. When there is *xu* Heat, the person is more nervous and unsettled than manic and agitated. They will often have a slight anxiety or a feeling that something is wrong without them being able to put their finger on what it is. If there are palpitations, they will not be as intense as when there is *shi* Heat. When there is *xu* Heat, the palpitations will often be accompanied by a feeling of nervousness or mild anxiety. *Xu* Heat often results in insomnia due to the *shen* not being anchored by *yin*. At the same time, the Heat will agitate and activate *shen*. Because *shen* is not anchored and because *shen* is agitated by Heat, the person's movements may well be nervous and fidgeting. Even though a person with *xu* Heat will be restless, they will not be as restless and agitated as a person with *shi* Heat. The nervousness and anxiety can sometimes be heard in their speech, both in the voice itself and what they talk about. The voice will not be as loud as it is when there is *shi* Heat, but because Heat agitates the Heart, the person can be very talkative and talk quickly.

Aetiology

Yin is weakened by old age, physical, mental and emotional overexertion (including stress), disease and illness, *shi* Heat conditions, too much sex, working at night, narcotics, energetically hot and spicy food, coffee, blood loss and profuse sweating.

Symptoms and signs

- Malar flush

- Fever or feeling hot in the evening and at night

- Night sweats

- Sweat or sensations of heat in the palms of the hands, the soles of the feet and the centre of the chest
- Dry mouth and throat
- Thirst with a desire to sip water
- Nervous, fidgeting movements
- Restlessness
- Slight feeling of anxiety
- Palpitations
- Nervous, rapid speech, talking a lot
- Dark, scanty urine
- Constipation or dry stools
- Red tongue with little or no coating, possibly a cracked tongue surface
- Rapid, Fine and possibly Superficial or Empty pulse

Key symptoms
Night sweats, malar flush, dry mouth, red tongue with little or no coating.

Treatment principle
Nourish *yin* and control Heat.

Acupuncture points
Choose from: Kid 2, Kid 3, Kid 6, Ren 4, UB 23, UB 52, Sp 6 and He 6.

Needle technique
Tonifying, except Kid 2, which can be treated with an even technique.

Explanation

- Kid 2, Kid 3, Kid 6, Ren 4, UB 23 and UB 52 nourish Kidney *yin*, which is the foundation of *yin* in the whole body.
- Sp 6 nourishes *yin*.
- He 6 nourishes Heart *yin*.

Herbal formula

- *Zhi Bai Di Huang Tang* (Nourishes Kidney *yin* and controls Heat)
- *Tian Wang Bu Xin Dan* (Nourishes Kidney and Heart *yin*, controls Heat and calms *shen*)
- *Da Bu Yin Wan* (Nourishes Kidney *yin* and controls Heat)

Relevant advice

A person with *xu* Heat should avoid food and drinks that have a Hot energy. They should also avoid stimulants such as caffeine drinks, for example coffee, Red Bull and green, black and white tea. Furthermore, they should avoid having too many spices in the diet. Stress and overwork will weaken *yin*. It is important that a person with *yin xu* makes sure that they go to bed early and sleep enough. They should avoid working on the computer too much, especially in the evening. Sweating is best avoided, as it results in the loss of fluid from the body. This means that they should preferably not sit in saunas and steam baths. Dynamic activities such as aerobics or action sports should also be avoided, as they will further consume the person's reserves. Meditation, qi gong, tai ji and yoga will, though, be beneficial.

Cold

The difference in when the symptoms and signs of *xu* Cold and *shi* Cold manifest, as well as the treatment itself, is not as pronounced as with Heat. The difference in symptoms between *xu* and *shi* Cold is seen more in the severity of symptoms and signs, the symptoms' and signs' intensity and whether the symptoms are acute or chronic. There is often an overlap between *xu* and *shi* Cold conditions, and one will frequently result in a person being more vulnerable to the other.

Both *shi* and *xu* Cold will result in the body's *yang qi* not being able to fulfil its functions. This will be because *yang* is either blocked, as it is in a *shi* Cold condition, or too weak, as it is in a *xu* Cold condition. This will compromise the body's ability to heat, transform, transport, protect and hold *yin* fluids inside the body.

Shi Cold

Shi Cold can arise when the body is invaded by exogenous Cold. The Cold can be located in the exterior, i.e. Wind-Cold, or there may be a direct invasion in the interior, when Cold invades a *fu* organ, such as the Stomach, the Intestines, the Urinary Bladder or the Uterus. There may also be a direct invasion of *xie* Cold in the Liver channel and in the *taiyin* and *shaoyin* stages of the Six Stages.

Exterior shi Cold

When there is *shi* Cold, it is necessary to differentiate between interior and exterior Cold. In exterior Cold, exogenous *xie* Cold will have invaded the body via the skin and blocked *wei qi*. This is reflected in the symptoms and signs. There will be shivering and an aversion to cold, because *wei qi* is blocked and cannot warm the skin and protect the body against the climatic cold. This is, in fact, a key symptom when differentiating between interior *xu* Cold and exterior *shi* Cold. In both cases, the person feels cold and has difficulty keeping warm. The difference, though, is that when the warming *wei qi* is blocked, the person cannot get warm, even though they wrap themselves up in blankets and put on extra clothing. There is actually enough heat in the body but it is prevented from circulating through the muscles and under the skin. When there is interior *xu* Cold, there is an actual deficit of heat in the body. This means that if the person puts on enough clothes or blankets, they can retain the heat they do have and will feel warm. The blockage of *wei qi* will result in a general soreness or aches in the skin, muscles and joints.

When Wind-Cold invades the exterior, it is the *taiyang* channels that are the first aspect to be invaded. There will be an acute headache and tension or stiffness in the shoulders and neck. This is because the circulation of *qi* in the Urinary Bladder and Small Intestine channels is blocked. There will also be tenderness and soreness in the muscles and joints in general, due to the blockage of *wei qi*.

The blockage of *wei qi* and the contracting nature of Cold will disrupt the pores in the skin so that the pores do not open. The person will therefore not be able to sweat.

An invasion of Wind-Cold will tend to disrupt and block the Lung in its spreading of *jinye*. This can manifest as acute oedema in the face and hands. The blocked fluids will ascend to the eyes and nose along with the rebellious Lung *qi* and cause watering eyes, puffy eyes or a runny nose. The fluids can also collect in the Lung and result in a cough with loose, watery sputum. The Lung *qi* will be rebellious, because the Cold has blocked the Lung's descending and spreading of *qi*. When Lung *qi* is rebellious, there may be coughing, sneezing or dyspnoea. When there is *shi* Cold in the exterior, the pulse will reflect this imbalance by being Superficial and Tight. The tongue will often not have had time to change. If the tongue has changed, it will have a thin, white and moist coating on the front.

Interior *shi* Cold

Interior *shi* Cold is a condition where the exogenous *xie qi* has invaded the interior of the body. *Fu* organs are in direct contact with the environment outside of the body via the body's orifices. This makes it possible for climatic *xie qi* to invade these organs directly. Furthermore, *xie* Cold can enter the body through the *yin* channels in the legs and thereby invade the organs of the lower *jiao*.

Cold has a crucial impact on an organ's physiology and it has an astringent nature. Cold's constricting dynamic results in stagnation, blockage and disruption of *qi*, *xue* and *jinye*. One of the dominant symptoms indicating the presence of Cold is pain. Where exterior Cold will manifest with pain such as headaches and muscle aches, interior Cold will manifest with cramping or biting pain. Examples of this could be menstrual pain, pain in the intestines or abdominal pain. Because the Cold is located in the interior, the aversion to cold will be different to when there is an exterior condition; there is not the same blockage of *wei qi*. The person will therefore not have the same aversion or fear of cold. The Cold will be more localised and internal. They will probably feel chilly and will seek heat, especially in the area of the body where Cold is located, but they will not freeze in the same way as when there is Wind-Cold. Their arms and legs can feel cold. Cold extremities are also seen when there is Liver *qi* stagnation but then only the hands and feet will be cold. When there is *shi* Cold, the whole arm and leg feel cold. The fingers and toes may become blue due to Cold blocking the movement of *xue*.

While there is a possibility of a slight fever or sensation of fever in the body when there is an invasion of Wind-Cold, this is not the case when there is interior *shi* Cold. Perspiration will be normal because *wei qi* is not blocked from controlling the pores in the skin. The pulse will be Deep because *xie qi* is in the interior and the Cold stagnation will make the pulse Tight or Confined. The tongue will be a key diagnostic factor. When there is interior *shi* Cold, there will be a thick, white tongue coating and the coating is often wet.

Interior *shi* Cold will disrupt and block fluid physiology. There will, therefore, be an increased volume of urine. The urine will be clear and there will be frequent urination. Cold can block the flow of *qi* in the Urinary Bladder and this can cause the person to have difficulty urinating. The disturbance of the fluid physiology can also result in the person having a lack of thirst.

Cold does not boil and condense excretions as Heat does; on the contrary, exudations and discharges from the body will be more copious. These excretions will be watery, clear and transparent, and they will not be odorous.

Cold can also prevent food from being transformed. If there is Cold in the Stomach, it can manifest with watery vomit, otherwise there will be watery diarrhoea with undigested food particles. The blockage by Cold will also manifest with pain in an organ. The pain and discomfort will be exacerbated by consuming cooling or cold drinks or food. In some cases, Cold can block the movement of the faeces through the Intestines. This can lead to constipation and cramping pains in the abdomen.

Palpation of the area of the body, or above the organ, that Cold has invaded will often reveal a cold sensation in the skin. The person will often also have a subjective sensation of cold in the area.

Where *yang xu* Cold will often result in a person having slow and lethargic movements, a person whose *qi* and *xue* is blocked by exogenous Cold will have movements that are stiff and limited due to *qi* and *xue* not being able to flow freely. This will usually be in a particular area of the body, such as the neck, the back or one or more of the joints in the limbs.

Shi conditions manifest with stronger colours than *xu* conditions. When there is *shi* Cold, the face will be white and shiny. It will not have the same dullness and lack of radiance that is characteristic of *xu* conditions. The face is white because Cold has the opposite dynamic of Heat. Where Heat's *yang* nature drives *xue* upwards and outwards, resulting in redness of the face, Cold has a *yin* dynamic and draws *xue* to the centre of the body. This is consistent with the Western physiological model, where when the body is cold, the blood is retained in the middle of the body to reduce cooling of the blood and keep the vital organs warm.

Cold's blockage of heat will also manifest with the person sleeping curled up to retain heat in the body.

Aetiology
Invasion of exogenous *xie qi*.

Symptoms and signs

- Aversion to cold

- Cold limbs

- White face

- Clear urine

- Diarrhoea or loose stools (constipation may be seen in some cases)

- Pain

- Stiffness

- No thirst

- Disinclination or discomfort when consuming cold beverages and foods

- Clear transparent excretions

- Oedema

- Slow, Tight or Confined pulse

- A white coating on the tongue

Key symptoms
Aversion to cold, clear urine, pain and stiffness, Tight pulse.

Differences between interior and exterior Cold

Interior Cold	Exterior Cold
No headache	Acute headaches
Pain in a *fu* organ	Skin, muscle and joint aches
Disruption of a *fu* organ's functions	No disturbance of the internal organs' functions
Attracted to warmth	Aversion to cold and wind
Normal perspiration	Lack of perspiration
Bluish fingers and toes	Normal coloured fingers and toes
No fever	Possibly a slight fever or fever sensation
Deep pulse	Superficial pulse
Pale or bluish tongue with thick, white, moist coating	The tongue is usually unchanged
Treatment principle: Warm the interior	Treatment principle: Expel Cold from the exterior

Treatment principle
If there is interior *shi* Cold: Expel Cold, warm the interior.
  If there is exterior *shi* Cold: Open to the exterior, expel Wind-Cold.

Acupuncture points
Point selection will depend on which organs or channels have been invaded by Cold.

- If there is Invasion of Wind-Cold (*taiyang* stage), choose from: SI 3, UB 62, UB 10, Du 14, Du 16, GB 20, LI 4, Lu 7, UB 12 and UB 13.

- If there is Cold *bi* syndrome, choose from: LI 4, Du 14 local and distal channel points, a-*shi* points.

- If there is Stomach Cold, choose from: Ren 12, Ren 8, St 21, St 34 and St 36.

- If there is Large Intestine Cold, choose from: St 25, St 37, St 28, Ren 6 and Ren 8.

- If there is Small Intestine Cold, choose from: St 25, St 39, St 28, Ren 6 and Ren 8.

- If there is Cold Uterus, choose from: Ren 4, Kid 12, Kid 13, St 30 and UB 32.

Needle technique
Draining. Moxa is recommended.

Herbal formula
The relevant herbal formula will depend on the exact Cold condition and where it is located. The following are examples of such formulas, but there are many other formulas that could also be used depending on the organ or the aspect of the body that is affected.

- *Ma Huang Tang* (Expels Wind-Cold from the exterior)

- *Chuan Xiong Cha Tiao Tang* (Expels Wind and Cold, circulates *qi*, relieves pain in the head)

- *Duo Huo Ji Sheng Tang* (Expels Wind, Cold and Dampness, circulates *qi* in the channels, stops pain)

- *Li Zhong Tang* (Dispels Cold from the middle *jiao*)

- *Huo Xiang Zheng Qi Tang* (Expels Wind-Cold and Dampness, regulates *qi* in the middle *jiao*)

- *Wen Jing Tang* (Expels Cold from the Uterus)

Relevant advice

A person who has been invaded by exogenous Cold will benefit from drinking hot ginger tea, a decoction of garlic or hot whisky with spices.

If they have interior Cold, they can use cinnamon in their diet, drink ginger tea and use warming spices, as well as avoiding food and beverages that are energetically and physically cold.

Differences between *xu* and *shi* Cold

Xu Cold	*Shi* Cold
The symptoms are usually chronic	The symptoms are often acute
The person freezes, but if they put on enough clothes or lie under a quilt, they can keep warm	The person freezes and cannot get warm, even if they put on enough clothes and blankets
Dull, pale facial colour	Shiny, white facial colour
Milder symptoms	Stronger symptoms
Dull pain that is alleviated by pressure	Biting or cramping pain that is aggravated by pressure
If there is diarrhoea or constipation, any discomfort or pain is not alleviated by the passing of stools	If there is diarrhoea or constipation, any discomfort or pain is alleviated by the passing of stools
Weak, Deep and Slow pulse	Full, Tight, Deep, Confined and Slow pulse
Thin, white tongue coating	Thick, white tongue coating
Treatment principle: Warm *yang*	Treatment principle: Expel Cold, warm the interior

Xu Cold

Xu Cold arises when there is insufficient *yang* to warm the body. The symptom picture will be characterised by physiological processes that are taking place more slowly or less effectively. There will be a poor transformation and transportation of the fluids and the food that has been ingested. This will manifest with symptoms such as oedema, loose stools or diarrhoea with undigested food particles, borborygmi, lack of thirst and frequent urination with copious amounts of clear urine.

Qi production will be diminished due to the poor transformation of the ingested food, air and *jing*. Fatigue and lethargy will therefore be key symptoms. This lassitude will be both physical and mental. The person will often have slow, ponderous movements, possibly dragging their feet and they will have a poor posture, due to the deficient *yang* failing to raise the body upwards and counteract gravity.

The person will feel cold and will freeze easily, because they lack the necessary *yang* to maintain the body's warmth. Unlike a person who has exterior *shi* Cold, a person who is *yang xu* Cold will be able to maintain a sensation of warmth in the body if they wear sufficient clothing. It is, therefore, a diagnostic sign of *yang xu* Cold when a person is noticeably more warmly dressed than others. They may, for example, be wearing a sweater when everyone else is in shirt sleeves. We must always be observant of whether a person's attire is appropriate for their surroundings, as this is a reliable way of diagnosing Heat and Cold.

The arms and legs of a person who is manifesting *yang xu* Cold often feel subjectively cold, as well as feeling cold when palpated. This is because there is not enough *yang* to circulate in the extremities. At the same time, there is a lack of heat in general and the priority of the body is to keep the internal organs warm and utilise *yang* here.

There will be frequent urination of copious amounts of clear urine, because fluids are not being transformed and transported and instead are seeping down to the lower *jiao*, and because there is not enough *yang* to hold the urine inside the Urinary Bladder. The deficiency of *yang* can also result in food and liquids that have been ingested not being optimally transformed, resulting in watery diarrhoea containing undigested food and borborygmi.

A person who is *xu* Cold will have a preference for hot food and drinks. This is one of the ways that the body tries to correct the imbalance.

Wei qi is an aspect of *yang*. When *yang* is weak, there may be spontaneous sweating or sweating on light activity. This is because *wei qi* will not be able to keep the pores in the skin closed. Likewise, there could be a tendency towards frequent invasions of exogenous *xie qi*, especially Wind-Cold.

Aetiology

Xu Cold arises when *yang* has been weakened. *Yang* is weakened by repeated invasions of Cold, excessive consumption of food and drinks that have a cold dynamic or are physically cold, medicine that has a cold dynamic such as antibiotics, too much sex, old age, chronic illnesses and physical exertion, such as too much sport.

Symptoms and signs

- Matt, white complexion

- Aversion to cold

- Cold limbs

- Slow, lethargic movements

- Poor posture

- Physical and mental fatigue

- Frequent urination with copious amounts of clear urine

- Loose stools or diarrhoea with undigested food in the stools

- No thirst

- Oedema

- Preference for hot food and drinks

- Freezes easily

- Wears warmer clothes than necessary

- Slow, Deep and Weak pulse

- Pale, swollen and wet tongue

Key symptoms
Aversion to cold, frequent urination, fatigue, Deep and Weak pulse.

Treatment principle
Warm and tonify *yang*.

Acupuncture points
Choose from: Du 4, Kid 3, Kid 7, UB 23, Ren 4, Ren 6 and Ren 8.

Needle technique
Tonifying. Moxa is recommended.

Explanation

- UB 23, Du 4, Ren 4, Kid 3 and Kid 7 tonify and warm Kidney *yang*.

- Ren 6 and Ren 8 tonify and warms *yang*.

Herbal formula

- *Jin Gui Shen Qi Tang* (Tonifies and warms Kidney *yang*)

- *You Gui Wan* (Tonifies and warms Kidney *yang*)

- *Li Zhong Tang* (Tonifies and warms Spleen *yang*)

Relevant advice
If there is *xu* Cold, the person should eat food and drinks that are both physically and energetically warm, such as ginger, cinnamon, garlic, lamb, venison, basil, chestnuts, shrimp, walnuts and so on. They should try to utilise cooking methods such as baking and grilling, which are more warming than steaming and boiling the food. Small changes in the diet can often make a big difference in the long run. They will, for example, benefit from eating lamb instead of pork and we can recommend that they use warming spices such as cinnamon, cloves, ginger and curry powder in their cooking. Furthermore, they should avoid foods and drinks that are physically and energetically cold, especially in the autumn and winter when *yang* is most challenged. In practice, this means avoiding eating fruit unless it is boiled or baked, avoiding salad and raw vegetables and drinking cold water. Although they are physically hot, mint tea, chamomile tea and elderflower tea are cooling in their energy, so the person should avoid these and drink beverages such as ginger tea. Green tea is cooling, whereas black tea is more warming, which means the latter will be preferable for a person who is *yang xu*. In the same way that a person who is *yin xu* should be careful not to challenge

their *yin* in the evening by using computers, smartphones and so on, a person who is *yang xu* should avoid straining their *yang* in the morning. Therefore, a good way to start the day would be to eat hot porridge sprinkled with cinnamon instead of yoghurt or cornflakes with milk. If they do not have Damp-Phlegm, a little cane sugar would also be good. A cup of black or ginger tea instead of cold orange juice will warm and support their Spleen *yang* in the morning instead of weakening it. Hot spices such as chilli and cayenne pepper are not necessarily good because they make a person sweat and thereby lose *qi*. Rebuilding a *xu* condition is something that takes time and cannot be forced, therefore making small, long-term changes is the best strategy.

Light exercise, especially in the morning just after waking up, is recommended because it will activate the lethargic *yang* and *qi*. The person must, however, be careful that they do not exercise to the extent that they become fatigued or feel tired afterwards. This means that they should not run long distances, swim 30 lengths of the swimming pool or spend hours in the gym. Again, yoga, tai ji and qi gong will be better for them. They can also cycle or go for walks. As stated, it is important that they do not exhaust themselves and that they get enough rest.

They will also benefit from a ginger or a mustard foot bath.

Combined Hot and Cold patterns

Combined Hot and Cold patterns have symptoms of Heat and Cold manifesting simultaneously. These patterns can occur when a person with a state of interior Cold is invaded by exogenous Heat or vice versa. There will be symptoms from both the exterior invasion and the interior imbalance.

There can also be a combination of Hot and Cold symptoms when an illness is changing character. This could, for example, be when Cold in the exterior is penetrating inwards and becoming *yangming* Heat.

Pure interior imbalances can also result in combined Hot and Cold patterns. There can be situations where there is Heat in the upper part of the body and Cold in the lower part. In this case there will be Heat symptoms in the top half of the body and Cold symptoms in the lower part. It could also be the other way round, but usually Heat will rise upwards and Cold will sink downwards due to their *yang* and *yin* dynamics. There can, though, be situations where there is Cold above and Heat below. This could be when there is an invasion of exogenous Cold in the Stomach, with such symptoms as watery vomit, abdominal cramps and no thirst, whilst there is Damp-Heat in the Urinary Bladder, with symptoms such as painful urination with dark, odorous urine.

Furthermore, there are also extreme situations where there is 'false Heat and true Cold' and 'false Cold and true Heat'. It is important to differentiate these two situations from the ones described above, in which there is just concurrent Heat and Cold. Furthermore, 'false Heat' or 'false Cold' is not the same as 'empty or *xu* Heat' or 'empty or *xu* Cold'. Empty Heat and empty Cold are when there is a deficiency of either *yin* or *yang*, resulting in a relative excess of Heat or Cold. When there is false Heat and false Cold, *yin* and *yang* are in the process of separating. This results in 'false' symptoms of Heat or Cold. When there is, for example, empty Heat (*yin xu* Heat), the deficient *yin* is not able to control Heat. This means that the person is hot at night and has red cheekbones, night sweats, a red tongue without coating and so on. In this situation, there is Heat present and it has arisen because *yin* cannot control *yang*. When there is false Heat and true Cold, there is almost no Heat, but the patient still manifests signs of Heat. This is because *yang* has become detached from *yin* and the little heat that there is rises upwards in an uncontrolled way. The tongue is the most reliable diagnostic tool in this context, because it will show the underlying imbalance. It is essential to treat the true state and not the false manifestation. Fortunately, these situations are rare and not something one encounters in a normal practice but are more likely to be seen in intensive care units in hospitals.

Xu and *Shi* imbalances

In *xu* and *shi* imbalances, we are differentiating between the relative strengths and weaknesses of *xie qi* and the body's *zheng qi*. When there is a *xu* condition, one or more of the vital substances or internal organs is in a weakened state. There is no *xie qi* present. A *shi* condition is characterised by there being either *xie qi* present or a blockage or stagnation of one or more of the vital substances, but the body's *zheng qi* is intact. In clinical practice, there will most often be a combination of *xu* and *shi*. Nevertheless, it is still crucial in these situations to gauge the relative ratio of how much *xu* and how much *shi* there is, and what it is that is *xu* and what it is that is *shi*.

Xu conditions

In a *xu* condition there is a deficiency of one or more of the vital substances. This will manifest with reduced activity of the body's physiological processes. How the symptoms manifest will depend on which substance has been weakened. The condition will typically be chronic.

Qi xu

A generalised *qi xu* condition can arise when there is a weakness in one or more of the *qi*-producing organs. There may also be a *qi xu* condition in a single organ, which is the consequence of an enfeeblement of the organ concerned. In addition to fatigue, the typical symptoms of a generalised *qi xu* condition will be a weak or low voice and disinclination to speak due to a lack of *zong qi*. Some people with *qi xu* may tend to have a poor posture and have difficulty keeping their back straight, because there is not enough *qi* to keep the body erect. The face will be pale, as will the tongue. The pulse will be Weak, reflecting the lack of *qi*. The fatigue will increase as the day goes on and will be worst in the afternoon and evening. It will be worse after physical and mental activity. If there is pain or discomfort, it will be relieved by pressure. Other symptoms will depend on which organ is weakened. Because the Lung, Spleen and Kidneys are often involved, there will usually be symptoms and signs such as loose stools, poor appetite, shortness of breath, spontaneous sweating and frequent urination.

As described above, other organs can be *qi xu*, not just the *qi*-producing organs. There will be signs of decreased activity in the organ's functioning. For example, Heart *qi xu* can manifest with symptoms and signs such as palpitations, spontaneous sweating and shyness. Again, these symptoms and signs of an imbalance in an organ will be most pronounced when the person is tired and after exertion or activity.

Aetiology
Qi xu arises either because one of the *qi*-producing organs are weakened or because the body is burdened by overexertion, lack of rest or disease.

Symptoms and signs

- Fatigue

- Pale face

- Loose stools

- Weak voice

- Reluctance to speak

- Spontaneous sweating

- Frequent urination

- Slumped posture

- Weak and slow movements

- Weak pulse

- Pale tongue

Key symptoms
Fatigue, pale face and a Weak pulse.

Treatment principle
Tonify *qi*.

Acupuncture points
Choose from: Ren 12, Ren 6, Lu 9, St 36, Sp 3, Sp 6, Kid 3, Kid 7, UB 13, UB 20, UB 21 and UB 23.

Needle technique
Tonifying. Moxa is recommended.

Explanation

- Ren 12, St 36, Sp 3, Sp 6, UB 20 and UB 21 tonify Spleen *qi*.

- Lu 9, and UB 13 tonify Lung *qi*.

- Kid 3, Kid 7 and UB 23 tonify Kidney *qi*.

- Ren 6 tonifies *yuan qi*.

Herbal formula

- *Liu Jun Zi Tang* (Tonifies Spleen *qi*)

- *Bu Zhong Yi Qi Tang* (Tonifies and raises Spleen *qi*)

- *Jin Gui Shen Qi Tang* (Tonifies Kidney *qi*)

- *Bu Fei Tang* (Tonifies Lung *qi*)

Relevant advice

If a person is *qi xu*, they will benefit from eating a diet that tonifies *qi*. They should eat as much prepared and hot food as possible. They should avoid raw vegetables, salads, cold drinks and ice cream. They should also avoid food that is unrefined, coarse and difficult to digest. This means that it is better for them to eat white rice instead of brown rice and to avoid too many wholemeal products. Even though these products are richer in minerals, fibre, vitamins and so on, they are more difficult to digest. They must also avoid foods that create Dampness, such as sweets, dairy products, bananas, dried fruit, honey, artificial sweeteners, stevia, etc., because they will further weaken the Spleen. It will be beneficial for the person to base their diet on soups, stews, steamed, boiled or sautéed vegetables and porridge in the morning, i.e. food that is easily digestible. They should also chew their food well so that it is easier to transform.

A person with Lung *qi xu* will benefit from being out in nature or anywhere else where there is fresh air. Yoga and qi gong often utilise breathing exercises. These will have a beneficial effect on Lung *qi*. It is important that a person with Lung *qi* is conscious of their posture, because sitting hunched forward or stooped will constrain Lung *qi*.

A person with *qi xu* must be careful that they do not overexert themselves and that they get adequate rest.

If a man is Kidney *qi xu*, he should avoid too much sex and ejaculating. A woman who is Kidney *qi xu* should try to avoid becoming pregnant. Both genders should avoid lifting heavy objects, as this strains the Kidney *qi*. The Kidneys contain our energetic reserves. It is therefore vital that a person who is Kidney *qi xu* does not overexert themselves, either through work or through sport. They should eat a diet that strengthens the Kidney (see section on Kidney imbalances on page 546 for more details).

Xue xu

When there is too little *xue* in the body, the tissues will lack nutrition and moisture. This will manifest with dry, pale skin. This will be most evident in the face, which will have a sallow complexion, but there will also be dry skin in general on the body. The hair will also be dry and can shed due to the roots lacking nourishment. Pallor and dryness will be seen on the tongue and lips, and the tongue will also be thin.

When the muscles in the limbs lack nourishment, numbness, tingling and muscle cramps can result. Women who are *xue xu* will often have sparse or even no menstrual bleeding. *Xue xu* can also be a cause of infertility.

Xue nourishes the brain. *Xue xu* will often manifest with dizziness, especially when the person gets up after sitting or lying down. The lack of nourishment to the brain can cause a person's memory to be poor.

A *xue xu* pulse is usually Choppy or Fine.

There are further symptoms and signs that are specific to Heart *xue xu* and Liver *xue xu* respectively. In practice, both of these organs are almost always affected in a *xue xu* condition. This means that there will nearly always be symptoms and signs of these imbalances when there is a general *xue xu*. Liver *xue* nourishes the eyes. Liver *xue xu* therefore typically manifests with spots in the visual field, blurred vision and poor night vision. Liver *xue* also nourishes tendons and nails. Brittle, weak nails that fray or nails that are dry and ridged are therefore always a sign of Liver *xue xu*. There will often be poor sleep, because the *hun* is not being anchored by Liver *xue*. When the *hun* is not anchored there can be dream-disturbed sleep. In extreme cases the person can have the feeling that they leave their body at night. The close relationship between the *hun* and Liver can also be observed in someone with Liver *xue xu* who has become depressed and has no vision in life because the *hun* is not being nourished.

Heart *xue xu* can be seen in symptoms such as palpitations. This is because the muscles of the Heart lack sufficient nourishment to be able to carry out their functioning optimally. At the same time, the *shen* lacks nourishment and is not strong enough to control the physical aspects of the Heart (the Emperor is losing control of the Kingdom). When the *shen* is not anchored and nourished by Heart *xue*, there will be symptoms such as insomnia and a slight feeling of unease or anxiety.

Aetiology

Xue xu can arise when not enough *xue* is being produced. This will be due to the person not consuming enough food that nourishes *xue* or the organs that produce *xue* being *qi xu*.

Xue xu can also arise when the body loses blood through haemorrhaging. This is typically seen after childbirth, surgery, physical trauma and heavy menstrual bleeding.

Furthermore, prolonged physical or mental-emotional stress consumes and thereby weakens *xue*.

Symptoms and signs

- Dizziness
- Palpitations
- Pale and sallow complexion
- Dry skin
- Dry and pale lips
- Insomnia
- Frayed, brittle or ridged fingernails
- Scanty or absent menstrual bleeding
- Infertility
- Numbness and tingling
- Muscle cramps
- Poor memory
- Spots in the visual field
- Blurred vision
- Depression
- Mild anxiety or unease
- Pale, thin and dry tongue
- Choppy or Fine pulse

Key symptoms
Pale and sallow complexion, dry skin, scanty menstruation, Choppy or Fine pulse.

Treatment principle
Nourish *xue*.

Acupuncture points
Choose from: UB 17, UB 20, UB 21, UB 23, Sp 3, Sp 6, St 36, Kid 3, Ren 4, Ren 6 and Ren 12.

- If there is Liver *xue xu*, add: Liv 3, Liv 8 and UB 18.
- If there is Heart *xue xu*, add: He 7 and UB 15.

Needle technique
Tonifying. Moxa is recommended, especially on St 36, Sp 6 and UB 17.

Explanation

- UB 17 nourishes *xue*.

- UB 20, UB 21, Sp 3, Sp 6, St 36 and Ren 12 tonify Spleen *qi*, which is needed to produce *gu qi*.

- UB 23, Ren 4, Ren 6 and Kid 3 nourish *jing* and tonify *yuan qi*.

- Liv 3, Liv 8 and UB 18 nourish Liver *xue*.

- He 7 and UB 15 nourish Heart *xue*.

Herbal formula

- *Si Wu Tang* (Nourishes *xue*)

- *Ba Zhen Tang* (Tonifies Spleen *qi* and nourishes *xue*)

- *Bu Gan Tang* (Nourishes Liver *xue*)

- *Gui Pi Tang* (Tonifies Spleen *qi*, nourishes *xue* and calms *shen*)

Relevant advice

It is important that a person who is *xue xu* eats a diet that is rich in food that nourishes *xue*. It will be good for them to eat foods that are rich in blood, such as red meat, bone marrow and blood sausages. Eating organic liver will be particularly good.[18] Green leafy vegetables will also be beneficial due to their high iron content. Other foods that nourish *xue* are beetroot, eggs, seaweed, watercress, avocado, dates and beans, particularly aduki beans, black beans and kidney beans. A person who is *xue xu* should avoid sugar, stimulants such as coffee and too much alcohol. Nettle tea will be good for them.

As well as being rich in *xue*-nourishing foods, their diet should strengthen their Spleen *qi*, as the Spleen must transform the ingested food into *gu qi*, the raw material of *xue*. This means they should consume warm, prepared food that is not cold in its energy and that does not create Dampness.

Yin xu

Yin, like *xue*, is nourishing and moistening and anchors *shen*. This means that there is a similarity in some of the manifestations of *yin xu* and *xue xu*. Dryness, for example, is a manifestation of both *yin xu* and *xue xu*. When there is *yin xu*, the dryness will be apparent in the mucous membranes of the orifices, especially the vagina, lips, mouth, nose and throat. The dryness often manifests as a slight thirst, but the thirst will not be as intense as it is when there is *shi* Heat. There will be a need to sip a glass of water, especially during the evening and at night, rather than drink a large glass in one go.

Yin controls *yang*. If there is *yin xu*, the uncontrolled, ascendant *yang* can cause night sweats and the person to feel hot at night. If *shen* is not anchored by *yin*, there can also be insomnia. When *yang* Heat is not controlled by *yin*, it will ascend to the head and visibly manifest as red cheekbones.

Dizziness can arise because there is not enough *yin* to nourish the brain and because if there is too little *yin* it can fail to anchor *yang*, which then ascends in an uncontrolled way up to the head causing dizziness.

The lack of moisture in the body that is characteristic of *yin xu* can also mean that the stools are very dry and that there is constipation.

Because *yin* is substantial, a person who is *yin xu* will typically have a thin, slender body. The tongue will also be thin. There can be a lack of coating on the tongue, as well as cracks in the surface of the tongue. If *yin xu* has resulted in *xu* Heat, the tongue will also be red, due to the Heat. The pulse will be Fine or Empty. If there is *xu* Heat, the pulse will be Rapid.

The person's movements can be restless and fidgety, especially if there is *xu* Heat. This is because the rootless Heat and *yang* will agitate *qi* in the muscles.

As was the case with *qi xu*, *yin xu* can be a generalised condition and it can be more specifically related to certain organs. The organs that typically are *yin xu* are the Kidneys, Liver, Lung, Heart and Stomach. Again, it will be possible to observe signs that indicate that there is a disturbance of their functioning. The reader is referred to Section 8 on *zangfu* imbalances for a more detailed analysis of the symptoms, signs and treatment of *yin xu* conditions in these specific organs.

Aetiology

Prolonged illness, stress, overexertion, working at night, coffee, narcotics, some forms of medicine such as steroids, a diet that is heating or stimulating, congenital weakness and old age can all weaken *yin*. Prolonged Fire imbalances and chronic *xue xu* will also injure *yin*.

Symptoms and signs

- Insomnia
- Dry mucous membranes
- Dry skin
- Dry mouth and throat
- Constipation or dry stools
- Night sweats
- Feeling warm in the evening and at night
- Malar flush
- Thin body
- Restless movements
- Dizziness

- The tongue can be thin, dry and lacking coating, possibly with cracks in the surface; if there is *xu* Heat, the tongue will be red
- Fine or Empty pulse; if there is *xu* Heat, the pulse can be rapid

Key symptoms
Dry mucous membranes, insomnia, malar flush, Fine or Empty pulse.

Treatment principle
Nourish *yin*.

Acupuncture points
Choose from: Kid 3, Kid 6, Ren 4, UB 23, UB 52, Sp 6 and Lu 7.

Needle technique
Tonifying. No moxa.

Explanation

- UB 23, UB 52, Ren 4, Kid 3 and Sp 6 nourish Kidney *yin*.
- Lu 7 and Kid 6 in combination open *ren mai* and *yin qiao mai* and thereby nourish Kidney *yin*.

Herbal formula

- *Liu Wei Di Huang Tang* (Nourishes Kidney *yin*)
- *Zou Gui Wan* (Nourishes Kidney *yin*)

Relevant advice
It is crucial that a person who is *yin xu* gets enough rest and relaxation. This means that they must get ample sleep and go to bed early at night. They must not work too hard or spend too much time in front of the computer, using a smartphone or watching television, as these stimulate the mind and thereby consume *yin*. A person who is *yin xu* should also avoid stimulants such as coffee, which will stress their system. Alcohol is not good for them because it is both spreading and heating in its dynamic. They should generally try to avoid food and beverages that are stimulating and heating, especially hot spices such as chilli and garlic. The way that food is prepared will affect its temperature. Raw food is the coldest, then steamed, boiled, sautéed, fried, baked, grilled, roasted and deep fried, which is the most warming. If there is *yin xu* Heat, the person should avoid the more heating cooking methods. Baked food can also be drying, which is not good for *yin xu*. Soups and stews will be the best preparation method, as these are not drying.

Concentrated proteins, green leaf vegetables, cereals and root vegetables will help to replenish *yin*. Foodstuffs that are rich in oil and minerals, for example nuts and seeds, will also nourish *yin*.

Sweating is to be avoided, because it will make the person lose body fluids. This means that they should not use saunas, Turkish baths or practise 'hot yoga'. Ordinary yoga, qi gong and tai ji are, on the other hand, beneficial forms of activity that nourish *yin,* whilst circulating *qi.* Dynamic activities such as aerobics or action sports will not be good and should be discouraged because they will further strain a person's *yin.* Shiatsu, massage and meditation are also good, because they bolster peace and tranquillity in the body and thereby replenish *yin.*

Men should avoid having too much sex, including masturbation, because there they lose *jing,* and thereby Kidney *yin,* when they ejaculate.

Yang xu

When there is *yang xu,* the body's fundamental warming, activating and energising aspect is weak. This will manifest as tiredness, feeling cold and lacking motivation. The person will be mentally and physically lethargic. Their body movements will be slow and limp and they will possibly drag their feet slightly when walking. The deficient *yang* will fail to lift the body upwards and counter gravity. This means that the person might be slightly slouched or that they will have a poor posture, the upper part of the body being slumped forward.

A person who is *yang xu* will need to wear warmer clothes than other people in order to keep warm. They will typically have cold limbs. The lack of heat in the body will manifest with a preference for hot food and beverages. Their face will typically have a pale colour, due to the lack of warmth and because *yang qi* is not strong enough to send *xue* up to the head.

Transformation and transportation of fluids in the body will be impaired when there is *yang xu* and *yang* is not capable of performing its functions. This will result in there being an increased volume of urine, which is clear in colour. There will be frequent urination because of the increased volume of urine and because Kidney *yang* is too weak to keep the urine inside the Urinary Bladder. *Yang qi* also helps to keep the sweat inside the body. *Yang xu* can therefore manifest with spontaneous sweating or sweating on light activity. The disruption of fluid physiology will also be seen in a lack of thirst and there can be a tendency to oedema.

Yang is utilised in the transformation of food that has been ingested. If *yang* is deficient, the person may have not only loose stools, which is typical of *qi xu,* but also watery stools, possibly containing undigested food particles. This is because the food and liquids consumed have not been transformed.

The tongue will be swollen and pale, and the pulse will be Deep and Weak.

The organs that are most likely to be *yang xu* are the Kidneys, Spleen and Heart. There will be tangible symptoms and signs that specifically relate to these organs' active functions if they are *yang xu.*

Aetiology

Yang xu can arise when *yang* has been overstrained through prolonged overexertion, old age, recurring cold invasions, improper diet, disease or congenital weakness.

Symptoms and signs

- Feeling cold or an aversion to cold
- Cold limbs
- Frequent urination
- Clear and copious amounts of urine
- Oedema
- Loose, watery stools, possibly containing undigested food
- Mental and physical fatigue
- Slow and lethargic body movements
- Slumped posture
- Spontaneous sweating
- Lack of thirst
- Preference for hot drinks and hot food
- Pale, white face
- Pale, swollen and possibly wet tongue
- Deep or Weak pulse

Key symptoms
Aversion to Cold, fatigue, pale and swollen tongue, Deep or Weak pulse.

Treatment principle
Tonify and warm *yang*.

Acupuncture points
Choose from: Du 4, UB 23, Ren 4, Ren 6, Kid 3 and Kid 7.

Needle technique
Tonifying. Moxa is recommended.

Explanation

- UB 23, Du 4, Ren 4, Ren 6, Kid 3 and Kid 7 tonify and warm Kidney *yang*.

Herbal formula

- *Jin Gui Shen Qi Tang* (Tonifies and warms Kidney *yang*)
- *You Gui Wan* (Tonifies and warms Kidney *yang*)

Relevant advice

A person who is *yang xu* should consume a diet that is warm, both in its physical temperature and energetic dynamic. They should try to avoid completely food that has a cooling quality, including food and beverages that are physically cold. This is especially relevant during the winter. This means that they should avoid fruit, unless it is stewed or baked and have no salads, raw vegetables or cold drinks. They should try to use more warming cooking methods, such as baked and grilled dishes. A good start to the day would be to eat hot porridge with a sprinkling of cinnamon. Hot spices such as chilli and cayenne pepper are not necessarily a good idea though, as they will cause the person to sweat and thereby lose heat and *yang qi*. Replenishing a *xu* condition is something that takes time and cannot be forced. Generally, spices in the diet will be beneficial, as they will awaken *yang*.

Exercise is important, but care must be taken. Light exercise is beneficial when there is *yang xu*, because it will activate *yang* and *qi*. However, the person must be careful that they do not train too hard, otherwise they will consume their *yang qi*. Starting the day with activities that can awaken and get *qi* moving, such as stretching and shaking the body, is a good idea.

Keeping warm is important, especially the lumbar area and the area just below the navel. Something that can be recommended is for the patient to wear a woollen 'belly-warmer'; alternatively they can tie a scarf or a shawl around their abdomen. No matter what, they should try to avoid these areas becoming exposed to the cold or draughts. A ginger or mustard foot bath is also something that can be recommended. It will also be beneficial for them to drink ginger tea during the day.

Patients who are Kidney *yang xu* should avoid activities that weaken the Kidneys and weaken *yang*. Apart from the general advice given above, men should avoid having too much sex, including masturbation, because *yang* is expended in the ejaculation and because the semen contains *jing*, which in the end is the root of Kidney *yang*. Lifting heavy objects weakens Kidney yang, so this should be avoided as much as possible.

Difference between *Shi* conditions and *Xu* conditions

Shi conditions	*Xu* conditions
Xie qi is present or there is a stagnation of *qi*, *xue* or *jinye*	Deficiency of *qi*, *xue*, *jinye*, *yin* or *yang*
Can be either acute or chronic	Usually chronic
Over-activity or a stagnation of an organ's *qi* or a vital substance	Lower level of functional activity in an organ or of a vital substance
If there is fatigue, it will be relieved by activity	Fatigue, exacerbated by activity
Symptoms often improve with physical activity	Symptoms often worsen with physical activity and when the person is tired
Severe symptoms	Milder symptoms
Strong pulse	Weak pulse

Shi conditions	*Xu* conditions
Thick tongue coating	Normal tongue coating or a lack of tongue coating
Pain or discomfort that is exacerbated by palpation	Pain and discomfort relieved by palpation
Loud voice	Weak voice

Shi conditions

Shi conditions are characterised by the presence of *xie qi* in the body. *Xie qi* will either be exogenous or internally generated. Furthermore, stagnation conditions are also defined as being *shi* conditions. The body's *zheng qi* is theoretically intact in a *shi* condition. In practice, though, a *shi* condition can be such a burden on a person's *zheng qi*, that it will often develop into combined *xu* and *shi* conditions. *Shi* conditions can also arise from *xu* conditions. These will therefore also be defined as being *xu/shi* conditions.

Shi conditions that are caused by invasions of exogenous *xie qi* will be acute, whereas internally generated *xie qi* is usually more chronic in its nature. Even though a condition is chronic, it can still flare up with acute symptoms.

The symptoms and signs seen in *shi* conditions tend to be more intense than those seen in *xu* conditions, which tend to be milder. For example, vomiting in a *shi* condition is often explosive, whereas regurgitation is more typical in *xu* conditions. If there is pain or discomfort, they will be more extreme. The pain will not be alleviated by palpation in the local area, but will usually be better with movement.

The voice of a person with a *shi* condition will be louder than if there is a *xu* condition. There is also less likelihood of fatigue. A person may feel fatigued when there are stagnation conditions, but this is a spurious form of fatigue. The fatigue that the person experiences is due to their *qi* not circulating around the body. When there is spurious fatigue, the person will usually feel fresher and more energetic after physical activity.

The pulse will be. powerful and the tongue will often have a thicker coating when there is a *shi* condition.

Shi conditions will often generate *xie* Heat in the body. This means that signs such as a red face, irritability, rough breathing and constipation are often seen.

In general, though, it can be difficult to generalise about how *shi* conditions will manifest. This is because there is so much variation in the types of *xie qi* that can be excessive. The reader is therefore referred to the relevant parts on *shi* Heat and *shi* Cold in this section (pages 271 and 280) and to the relevant parts of Section 6, 'Diagnosis According to *Xie Qi*'.

Shi conditions can be summarised as follows: invasions of exogenous *xie qi*, interior Cold, interior Heat, interior Wind, ascending *yang*, Dampness, Phlegm, *qi* stagnation, accumulation of fluids and *xue* stagnation.

Aetiology

Shi conditions arise when the body is invaded by exogenous *xie qi*, when there is internally generated *xie qi* or when there is a stagnation.

Symptoms and signs

- Symptoms that are acute (chronic symptoms can, though, sometimes also be *shi* in nature)

- Intense or severe symptoms

- Pain or discomfort that is not relieved by palpation

- Symptoms that are relieved by activity and movement

- Loud voice

- Heavy breathing

- Full pulse

- Thick coating on the tongue

Treatment principle
Expel, drain or transform *xie qi*, spread or dissolve stagnations.

Acupuncture points, herbal formula and relevant advice
See the relevant sections for the various types of *xie qi* and stagnation conditions.

Yin and yang imbalances

The categories of *yin* and *yang* can, in general, be seen as encompassing the other six categories. The differentiation of *yin* and *yang* can also be used as a specific diagnosis in certain situations. In general, the differentiations of exterior, Heat and *shi* can be defined as being *yang* qualities. Interior, Cold and *xu*, on the other hand, are *yin* qualities. In practice, though, it can often be difficult to say whether something is purely *yin* or *yang*. Wind-Cold, for example, is an exterior condition and a *shi* condition, both of which are defined as being *yang*, as is Wind, but Cold is *yin*. Liver Fire is an interior condition, i.e. *yin*, but it is also a Fire condition, which is *yang*.

Although it is often difficult to define a condition as being purely *yin* or *yang*, in situations where we are in doubt about our diagnosis we can simplify the diagnosis by taking a step backwards and asking ourselves whether the condition is essentially a *yin* or a *yang* condition and treat it as such.

We can also utilise *yin* and *yang* differentiation to be specific and focused when we want to define an imbalance precisely. For example, it is not enough to diagnose a person as being Kidney *xu*, but through the symptoms and signs that they are manifesting, we can explicitly define the imbalance as being either Kidney *yin xu* or Kidney *yang xu*.

The differentiation of *yin* and *yang* is especially relevant when diagnosing *yin xu* and *yang xu* conditions. *Yin shi* and *yang shi* conditions are generally the same as *shi* Cold and *shi* Heat but also encompass conditions' various other imbalances such as Dampness and internally generated Wind.

	Yang xu	*Yang shi*	*Yin xu*	*Yin shi*
Facial colour	Matt, white	Red	Red cheekbones	Bright white
Energy level	Tired and lethargic	Restless or manic	Tired or restless	
Movements	Sluggish and slow	Fast, powerful and hyperactive	Quick, restless and fidgety	Stiff and rigid
Mental state	Sluggish and lacks motivation Slow thinker	Manic, irritable, aggressive, restless, difficulty concentrating due to a cascade of thoughts	Mental restlessness, nervousness, unease	Can have difficulty thinking clearly and focusing when there is Damp-Phlegm
Stools	Loose stools or watery diarrhoea (it is possible that there is constipation when *yang qi* is too weak to move the stool through the Intestines)	Constipation	Constipation	Diarrhoea or loose stools
Urination	Frequent Copious amounts of clear urine	Dark, scanty urine Possibly painful urination	Dark, sparse urine	Either inhibited and painful urination or copious amounts of clear urine
The voice and speech	Weak and soft voice Talks slowly Reluctance to speak	Loud voice Garrulous and talks quickly	Nervous, quick Soft, weak and 'dry' voice	Can be nasal
Pulse	Slow, Deep and Weak	Large, Full and Rapid	Empty and Superficial or Fine Possibly Rapid	Tight
Tongue	Pale, swollen and wet	Red with yellow coating	Thin, red, cracked and/or peeled	Pale with a thick white coating
Body temperature	Aversion to cold, freezes easily, cold limbs	Fever or aversion to heat The skin feels hot	Hot in the evening and at night Palms of the hand and the soles of the feet can feel hot	Feels the cold The skin feels cold

Apart from *yin xu*, *yang xu*, *yin shi* and *yang shi*, there are also two conditions known as 'collapse of *yin*' and 'collapse of *yang*'. These are perilous and the life-threatening conditions in which *yin* and *yang* are separating from each other. These are therefore very serious conditions and often occur just before death.

Collapse of yin

Aetiology
Yin collapses when there is an extreme condition of *yin xu* Heat and *yin* is exhausted. This could be the end result of an initial invasion of *xie qi* that has penetrated down to the *xue* level of the Four Levels.

Symptoms and signs

- Profuse sweating
- The skin feels very hot
- Hot limbs
- Very dry mouth
- Dark, scanty urine that is difficult to void
- Constipation
- Mental restlessness and anxiety
- Thin, emaciated body
- Thin, short, dark red tongue without coating
- Fine, Superficial and Rapid pulse

Key symptoms
Hot skin, hot limbs, thin, dark red tongue without coating, Rapid and Fine pulse.

Treatment principle
Rescue *yin*.[19]

Acupuncture points
Acupuncture will not be enough in itself, but the following points can be tried.
    Choose from: St 36, Ren 4, Ren 6, Kid 3 and Kid 6.

Needle technique
Tonifying.

Explanation

- St 36, Kid 3, Kid 6 and Ren 4 nourish *yin*.
- St 36 and Ren 6 tonify *qi*.

Herbal formula

- *Da Bu Yin Wan* (Rescues collapsed *yin* and controls *yin xu* Heat)

Collapse of yang

Aetiology

Yang collapses when *yin* and *yang* are separating. This could happen when exogenous *xie qi* has penetrated to the deepest energetic aspects of the body and *yang* is exhausted.

Symptoms and signs

- Extreme sensitivity to cold

- The skin feels cold and clammy

- Cold limbs

- Shallow breathing

- Profuse sweating with beads of sweat like pearls

- Frequent urination or incontinence; the urine is clear

- Loose stools or faecal incontinence

- Mental confusion or loss of consciousness

- Pale, short and wet tongue

- Hidden, Slow pulse

Key symptoms

Cold and clammy skin, extreme sensitivity to cold, profuse sweating, Hidden pulse.

Treatment principle

Rescue *yang*.[20]

Acupuncture points

Choose from: St 36, Ren 4, Ren 6 and Ren 8.

Needle technique

Large amounts of moxa must be used.

Explanation

- Ren 4, Ren 6 and Ren 8 rescue *yang*.

- St 36 tonifies *qi*.

Herbal formula

- *Shen Fu Tang* (Rescues collapsed *yang*)

DIAGNOSIS ACCORDING TO *XIE QI*

In this diagnostic model, the symptoms and signs that are manifesting and the aetiological factors that are creating the symptoms and signs are one and the same. This means that when we diagnose say 'Dampness', there is an understanding both that the person will be manifesting specific symptoms and signs that are characteristic of the presence of Dampness and that the cause of the imbalance is that the person has been exposed to some form of *qi* that is intrinsically Damp in its nature or that some other aetiological factor or internal imbalance has resulted in the presence of internal Dampness. This stands in contrast to other aetiological factors and imbalances. Anger, for example, which is one of the seven internal or emotional causes of illness, is not a pattern of imbalance. Anger can be a cause of an imbalance, such as Liver Fire, but anger is not a pattern of imbalance with specific signs and symptoms. Liver Fire, on the other hand, is a pattern of imbalance with specific symptoms and signs that are characteristic of extreme Heat in the Liver, but Liver Fire is not an aetiological factor.

Like most medical systems, Chinese medicine has a shamanistic past. Initially it was believed that disease arose because the body was invaded by evil spirits. These spirits could, for example, be the person's ancestors who were dissatisfied with the person's behaviour or rootless spirits that were present in the local surroundings. Treatment at that time was based on either expelling the evil spirit from the body or trying to appease the disgruntled ancestor. These evil spirits that caused disease were termed *xie qi*. *Xie* can be translated as evil or perverse. These spirits were a perverse or evil form of *qi* because they were *qi* that only had a negative and disruptive effect on the body. This is in contrast to the body's own *qi*, which is exclusively benevolent, possessing only positive properties. *Xie qi* can also be translated as 'pathological *qi*', 'pathogenic *qi*' or simply 'pathogen', because it is a form of *qi* that can result in disease.

Many of the places where *xie qi* gathered and was predominant were places that were dark, damp or cold – places people instinctively feel are unpleasant. It was observed that people more often fell ill or developed disorders when they stayed in such places. Similar observations could also be made in other places where the climate was more extreme. Over time the perception started to change. Evil spirits were seen as the cause of illness less and instead the climate itself was viewed as being the culprit. The relationship between an individual and the world surrounding them became more apparent. The perception changed increasingly to being that people who dwelt in cold, dark, damp places became ill because of these conditions and not because they were where evil spirits resided. The dampness and the cold were the *xie qi*.

As analytical observers, Chinese scientists, scholars and doctors saw that there was a relationship between people becoming ill and being exposed to extreme or prolonged climatic influences. They also became aware that the condition of a person's own *qi* played an important role in their being susceptible to being affected by these climatic influences. It had already been observed that certain climatic conditions such as cold, dampness, heat and so on had specific, unique characteristics. These various forms of climatic *qi* were already known to affect the physical world in specific and thus predictable ways. For example, if there is an extreme or prolonged period of cold weather, water will freeze. Cold temperatures will also cause matter to contract due to the *yin* nature of cold. *Yang* heat, on the other hand, has a very drying quality and desiccates things that are moist. It was observed that when people were exposed to prolonged or extreme climatic influences, their body reacted in a similar way to the world outside the body. For example, it was observed that when the body was exposed to cold weather, *qi* stagnated in the same way that water does when it freezes.

The designation *xie* was not discarded though, because it was still an appropriate term. The idea is the same – the body is affected by a form of *qi* and this *qi* has negative characteristics and a pathological influence on body's own *qi*. Whereas before it was an evil spirit that had invaded the body, the new concept was that it was a form of negative *qi* that was disrupting the body's physiology. This is very typical for Chinese medicine and its way of thinking. An old theory is not rejected but is instead assimilated into the new understanding of how the body works.

Each *xie qi* has its own specific and unique *qi* dynamic. *Qi* dynamic is the directional movement that the *qi* has and the way in which it affects other forms of *qi*. This *qi* dynamic is a reflection of its relative *yin* or *yang* nature. For example, Heat is a *yang* form of *qi*. Heat's *yang* quality can be seen in the fact that it's a form of *qi* that ascends; it desiccates and it creates over-activity in the internal organs and the vital substances it is in contact with – it agitates. These *qi* dynamics are of great importance in relation to how the various *xie qi* affect *qi* in the body and what reactions they create. It is through observation of these changes that a diagnosis is made.

As stated, an invasion of exogenous *xie qi* is defined on the basis of its origin, i.e. how it has arisen. For example, you can be invaded by Damp-Cold if you get cold and wet after being drenched by the rain in winter. *Xie qi*, though, is also defined by how it manifests, i.e. how it affects the body's *qi*. If something affects the body in the same way as, for example, exogenous Cold does, it will be defined as being exogenous Cold even though the person has not been exposed to climatic cold. In general, there is no discrepancy between the way that symptoms and signs manifest and the climatic influences that a person has been exposed to. However, there are circumstances in which there has been no exposure to a climatic influence, yet the person still manifests symptoms and signs of an external invasion of *xie qi*. Allergic rhinitis is a typical example of this. This is because all pathogens, like climatic *qi*, have specific *qi* dynamics. This is of great importance when treating people who have been infected with bacteria, viruses and other 'invisible' forms of infection and when people react negatively to food additives, chemicals and allergens. If exposure to a particular virus makes the body temperature rise, the eyes become red, the thirst increase and the pulse beat faster, this virus is defined and thereby treated as Heat *xie qi*. This is because these physiological reactions are the reactions that occur when Heat is present in the body. Conversely, if a person feels very cold, has cramping intestinal and gastric pain and watery diarrhoea, this physiological reaction will instead be defined as being a Cold reaction. This will therefore indicate the presence of *xie* Cold in the body, even though the person has not necessarily been exposed to anything cold.

Something that is also important to remember is that when exogenous *xie qi* invades the body it can change character and transform into something else. It is, for example, very typical for invasions of Cold to transform into Heat patterns when the Cold has penetrated into the body.

As stated, each of the six exogenous forms of *xie qi* has its own unique symptoms and signs, which are manifestations of its specific *qi* dynamic. There are, however, some symptoms and signs that will be seen in all invasions of exogenous *xie qi*. This is because exogenous *xie qi* will have a disruptive effect on the body's *wei qi*. When *xie qi* invades the exterior aspect of the body, there will often be an aversion to cold and chills, even if the invasion of exogenous *xie* is Heat. This is because exogenous *xie qi* blocks *wei qi* so that it can no longer warm the skin. There can also be a slight fever or febrile sensation even though it is a Cold pathogen. This is because the conflict between *xie qi* and *wei qi* and the subsequent stagnation that arises will generate Heat. The febrile sensation may not be particularly pronounced and may well not be measurable with a thermometer. In Chinese medicine, fever is defined by the patient's own subjective sensation of warmth or the therapist observing signs of Heat, such as a red colour in the face or the skin feeling warm on palpation. An important diagnostic sign in invasions of exogenous *xie qi* is that chills and febrile sensations manifest simultaneously. In invasions of exogenous *xie qi*, the pulse will usually be Superficial.

An invasion of the body by exogenous *xie qi* will be due to one or more of the following factors:

- *Zheng qi* is weak or weakened: If *zheng qi*, including *wei qi*, is weak, the body will more easily be invaded. This is because the body will not be able to protect and defend itself. This means that *xie qi* does not need to be as strong or to have affected the body for a prolonged period of time. A weak or weakened *zheng qi* is typically seen in infants, older people, people who are physically run down and people who have been ill. To illustrate this, imagine that an old lady and a young man have to go out from their house to the corner shop, which is 400 metres away. It is freezing cold and both of them are only wearing a thin coat. It is much more likely that the old lady will catch a cold as a result of this trip than the young man. Her *wei qi* is not strong enough to withstand the onslaught of the wind and cold. It is typical that some people catch every bug that is going around whilst others rarely fall ill. This is usually a reflection of the relative strengths of their *wei qi*.

- *Xie qi* is very strong: If the body is subjected to a very strong influence of *xie qi*, it will have difficulty keeping it out, even though the *wei qi* is robust. Returning to the young man from the previous analogy – walking down to the shop in a thin jacket in winter will probably not result in him catching a cold or becoming ill. This is because his *wei qi* is robust. However, it is highly likely that he will catch a cold or fall ill if he falls through the ice on a lake into the freezing cold water below. Even though there is no difference in the length of time he is exposed to the cold, there is a difference in the intensity of the cold he is exposed to. This is also seen in some virulent diseases, where the majority of the population, including strong, healthy individuals, fall ill when exposed to the disease.

- Prolonged exposure to *xie qi*: A prolonged exposure to a certain form of *xie qi* will wear down the body's defences. Imagine the same young man – he will not become sick from walking to the shops in freezing weather in a thin jacket, but if he had to walk around town in freezing weather with only a thin jacket for two hours, it is more likely that he would become ill afterwards. This time it is not the strength of the cold that is crucial but the prolonged exposure to it. Imbalances that arise as a consequence of prolonged exposure to a certain type of *xie qi* are seen, for example, in people who live or work in an environment that is characterised by a particular climate, such as living or working in a place that is cold and damp.

- Sudden exposure to *xie qi*: Illnesses can arise when seasons change or when the weather is atypical for the season. It is as if *wei qi* does not have time to adjust to this atypical, climatic influence; as if it has prepared itself to protect the body against something that is, for example, *yin*, and all of a sudden there is something that is *yang*. We often see people catch a cold when there is a period of mild weather in winter or during a cold and wet period in summer. This is also the reason that many people get sore throats and colds from air-conditioning, especially in hot climates. The pores of the skin are wide open due to the heat and then they come into a building that is quite cold and the air-conditioning also creates a draught (Wind). In addition, many people fall ill in the transition from summer to autumn and from winter to spring – the classic spring cold.

- Presence of imbalances in the body: A person is more likely to be adversely affected by a specific form of *xie qi* if they already have a similar imbalance. A person with *yang xu* will be invaded by Cold more quickly than a person with *shi* Heat. A person with Spleen imbalances is more rapidly affected if there is Dampness than a person who is *yin xu*.

There are six exogenous forms of *xie qi*. Five of these forms of *xie qi* can also be internally generated. Summer-Heat is the only form of *xie qi* that is exclusively exogenous. Where exogenous *xie qi* can invade the body when it comes into contact with climatic influences, bacteria, viruses, allergens and so on, internally generated *xie qi* arises when there are internal imbalances in the body, especially *zangfu* organ imbalances. It is important to remember that *xie qi* is defined by its origin, but also how it manifests. This means that when an internal imbalance manifests with a person having a red face, being excessively thirsty, being mentally restless and having a Rapid pulse and a red tongue, this imbalance will be defined as Heat. The Heat here though has been internally generated, i.e. it is Heat that has arisen due to internal conditions and not because the person has been in contact with exogenous *xie qi*. As can be seen in this example, internally generated *xie qi* is in many ways similar to exogenous *xie qi*. The important difference being, as we saw previously, that internally generated *xie qi* is an aetiological factor in itself.

As well as there being a difference in their aetiology, the symptoms and signs of internally generated *xie qi* and exogenous *xie qi* are different in quality, intensity and duration. Exogenous *xie qi* tends to be acute and the symptoms more pronounced. The symptoms and signs of internally generated *xie qi* will usually be chronic and less intense. Exogenous *xie qi* will usually manifest with symptoms and signs relating to the exterior aspects of the body – *wei qi*, skin, muscles, joints and channels. There will probably be an aversion to cold and a slight febrile sensation. Internally generated *xie qi* can affect specific organs or vital substances or it can be systemic. There are, however, also situations where exogenous *xie qi* can manifest in the interior of the body. This will be because exogenous *xie qi* has penetrated deeper into the body or there has been a direct invasion of exogenous *xie qi* into the interior.

As stated, only five of the six forms of exogenous *xie qi* are generated in the interior. Furthermore, in addition to internal Heat, Cold, Wind, Dampness and Dryness, there are other forms of internally generated *xie qi* that do not exist as exogenous *xie qi*. These are Phlegm, *xue* stagnation and food stagnation, which are also classified as forms of *xie qi*. Like the other forms of internally generated forms of *xie qi*, Phlegm, *xue* stagnation and food stagnation are not defined as aetiological factors. This is because they themselves have resulted from one or more of the internal, external or miscellaneous aetiological factors.

Diagnosis according to *xie qi* in relation to diagnosis according to the Eight Principles

Xie qi imbalances are generally *shi* imbalances. This is because when there is *xie qi*, there is something extra present in the body. However, this does not exclude the possibility that there can be a combined *xu* and *shi* condition. This is seen, for example, when there is an invasion of Wind-Cold that has arisen because there is *wei qi xu* or when Phlegm-Dampness is generated because there is Spleen *qi xu*.

Xie qi imbalances can be both exterior and interior. When there is an invasion of exogenous *xie qi*, it will be an exterior imbalance, but if *xie qi* is internally generated, it will be defined as being an interior imbalance.

Wind

Wind is a very *yang* form of *xie qi*. Wind is the 'prevailing *qi* in spring', although invasions of Wind are not exclusive to this season. Both Wind and spring do have a powerful resonance with the Wood Phase and its dynamic – young *yang* energy. Wind's *yang* nature is seen in its mobility and speed. Wind has an expansive and thereby spreading dynamic. Imagine a pile of leaves lying in a heap on the ground: heat, dampness and cold will only result in the leaves drying out, becoming heavy and soggy or freezing into a solid mass, but a gust of wind will spread them in all directions and set them in motion. This ability of Wind to spread things apart enables it to penetrate through *wei qi*, whilst drawing other forms of *xie qi* into the body. This is the reason it is said that Wind is the spearhead that conveys other forms of *xie qi* into the body. This is very important for *yin* forms of *xie qi*, such as Cold. Cold has a contracting nature and therefore results in the pores in the skin contracting and closing, blocking its entry. Wind can spread open the pores and thereby lead Cold through the skin and into the body. This is similar to a draughty cabin in winter. If the temperature is sub-zero outside but it is completely windless, it is possible to warm the cabin with a small stove. If, on the other hand, the temperature is 10 degrees centigrade, it is still difficult to keep the cabin warm if the wind is blowing outside. This is because the wind will drive the cold into the cabin through the cracks in the walls.

Wind's *yang* nature means that it has a tendency to affect the head and the upper part of the body, as well as the outer aspects of the body, i.e. the *wei qi* aspect. Wind's dynamic *yang* nature also means that the symptoms and signs that are manifesting can have a tendency to migrate from place to place and to be variable in character. This is characteristic of the form of *bi* known as Wind *bi*, where the pain in the joints constantly changes character and location. Wind's *yang* nature also manifests in a sudden onset of its symptoms and signs. Wind creates movement because it is *yang*. Wind can often manifest as tremors, spasms and itching. Extreme stiffness and paralysis can also be a symptom of Wind, because when something vibrates very strongly and quickly, it becomes stiff and rigid.

Wind has a resonance with the *jueyin* aspect. This is shown by people's eyes watering when it is windy. Both the eyes and tears relate to the Liver through the Five Phases, as does Wind. Internally generated Wind can arise as a consequence of Liver imbalances. Many of the symptoms of internally generated Wind and exogenous Wind are similar, but the aetiology and the treatment principles will be very different.

The Liver is not the only *zang* organ to have a relationship with Wind. The Lung is easily affected by Wind, as it is the only *zang* organ that is in direct contact with the environment outside of the body. The Lung also controls *wei qi*. This means that the invasions of exogenous Wind will often affect the Lung and its sensory organ, the nose. Furthermore, if there is Lung *qi xu*, *wei qi* will also be *xu* and the person will be easily invaded by exogenous Wind.

Invasion of exogenous Wind

The patterns seen when there is an invasion of exogenous Wind are: Wind-Cold, Wind-Heat, Wind-Dampness, Wind-Water, Wind-Cold-Damp *bi*.

An invasion of exogenous Wind will nearly always be an acute pattern. The exception to this is Wind *bi*, which will often have developed into a chronic pattern.

Invasions of exogenous Wind will generally be relatively short-lived. The *xie qi* will either be expelled again or it will penetrate deeper into the body.

Aetiology

The invasion is due to there being a virulent *xie qi*, which has been strong enough to break through the defences of the body's *wei qi*. This could be when a person has been exposed to climatic wind, but it can also be that they have been exposed to an artificial indoor climate such as air-conditioning. Furthermore, some allergens and viruses can manifest as an exogenous Wind pattern.

There can also be an underlying *wei qi xu*, which means that *xie* Wind does not have to be that strong to be able to break through the defensive *qi*.

Symptoms and signs

The specific symptoms and signs will depend on the individual patterns.

Typical symptoms and signs that are seen when there is an invasion of exogenous Wind are:

- acute symptoms that arise suddenly

- stiffness, numbness, tremor and itching or tingling sensations in the skin

- pain in the joints

- pain that migrates from place to place and is variable in character

- headache

- aversion to cold and wind

- a disturbance of the functioning of the Lung, resulting in coughing and sneezing

- Superficial pulse.

Symptoms and signs of specific exogenous Wind pattern

Wind-Cold	Aversion to cold and wind; chills; headache; stiffness in the shoulders and neck; lack of sweating; coughing; sneezing; clear secretions from the nose; slight or no fever; itchy throat; no thirst; Superficial, Tight, Slow pulse.
Wind-Heat	Less aversion to cold than when there is Wind-Cold; chills; mild or high fever; thirst; red eyes; red and sore throat; yellowish secretions from the nose; cough, possibly with yellowish sputum; Superficial and Rapid pulse; the tongue may have a red tip or a yellowish coating.
Wind-Damp	Itchy skin disorders; skin diseases where there is swelling; aversion to wind and cold; heaviness in the arms and legs; heavy and painful muscles and joints; slight or no fever; Superficial and Slippery pulse; wet tongue.
Wind-Water	Acute oedema, especially in the face and around the eyes; cough with very watery sputum; wheezing; no thirst; Superficial and Slippery pulse; wet tongue.
Wind-Dryness	Dry throat; dry lips; dry mouth; dry eyes; dry skin; dry mucous membranes; dry tongue; Superficial pulse.
Wind *bi*	This is *bi* syndrome where Wind, Dampness and Cold have invaded the channel or the joint. Wind is the predominant of the three *xie qi*. There will be painful joints. The pain will be provoked by the wind or by drafts. The pain can migrate from joint to joint, be erratic and change character (sometimes sharp, sometimes throbbing, sometimes numb, sometimes heavy and so on). The pain can come and go very suddenly and will mainly affect the upper part of the body. There will often be aversion to wind, cold and drafts. There may be a slight fever and sweating. The pulse will be Superficial.
Invasion of Wind-Cold in the face	Wind-Cold can invade the channels in the face. It will often be the *yangming* channels that are affected. The invasion of Wind-Cold in the face will result in pain and especially paralysis of the facial muscles. The pulse will be Superficial and Tight.

Treatment principle
Expel Wind.

Acupuncture points
Choose from: UB 10, UB 12, LI 4, Lu 7, Du 14, Du 16, SJ 5 and GB 20.

- If there is Wind-Cold, add: SI 3 and UB 62.

- If there is Wind-Heat, add: LI 11.

- If there is Wind-Dampness, add: Sp 6 and Sp 9.

- If there is Wind-Water, add: Sp 9 and Ren 9.

- If there is Wind-Dryness, add: Kid 6 and Sp 6.

- If there is Wind *bi*, add: Local and distal points on the relevant channels.

- If the invasion of Wind is in the face, add: Local and distal points along the channels.

Needle technique

Draining technique. Moxa and cups are recommended.

Explanation

- UB 10, UB 12, LI 4, Lu 7, Du 14, Du 16, SJ 5 and GB 20 activate *wei qi* and expel Wind.

- UB 62 and SI 3 expel *xie qi* from the *taiyang* aspect.

- LI 11 expels Wind-Heat.

- Sp 6 transforms Dampness, drains water and can nourish *jinye* and *yin*.

- Sp 9 transforms and drains Dampness and water.

- Kid 6 nourishes *yin* and *jinye*.

Herbal formula

- *Ma Huang Tang* (Expels Wind-Heat)

- *Yin Qiao San* (Expels Wind-Heat)

- *Huo Xiang Zheng Qi Tang* (Expels Wind-Cold and Dampness).

- *Xiao Qing Long Tang* (Expels Wind-Cold and transforms Phlegm-Fluids)

- *Xing Su San* (Expels Wind-Cold and Dryness)

- *Sang Xing Tang* (Expels Wind-Heat and Dryness)

- *Juan Bi Tang* (Expels Wind-Cold and circulates *qi* in the channels)

Relevant advice

When there is an acute invasion of exogenous *xie qi* in the exterior, it is advisable to consume drinks that are spicy and diaphoretic to open the exterior and expel *xie qi*. This could be ginger, garlic, whisky, brandy and chilli if there is an invasion of exogenous Wind-Cold or mint, chamomile or elderflower if there is an invasion of exogenous Wind-Heat. It is also advised to abstain from eating or to only eat soups, for example such as onion soup. There are two reasons for this. First, when temporarily fasting *qi* will not be used to transform food and therefore can be used to combat the invading *xie qi*. Second, some sources say that the downward movement of food and *qi* in the Stomach can draw the exogenous *xie qi* inwards from the surface.

Similarly, the sour flavour should be avoided due to its astringent or centripetal dynamic. Vitamin C, lemon and other things that are very sour should not be consumed during an invasion of exogenous *xie* Cold, as they will draw the *xie* Cold inwards whilst closing the pores in the skin, thereby preventing the Cold from being expelled again. This also means that antibiotics are not recommended at this stage, as they are cold and drain downwards.

It is important that the person protects themselves from drafts and exposure to the elements.

Invasion of Wind can be caused by the following pattern of imbalance

- *Wei qi xu*

Invasion of Wind can result in the following pattern of imbalance

- This will depend on the individual pattern.

Internally generated Wind

The difference between internally generated and exogenous Wind is that internally generated Wind arises as a consequence of *zangfu* and *xue* imbalances. Invasions of Wind are seen when the body is invaded by exogenous *xie qi*. This difference is extremely important in relation to treatment strategies and treatment techniques. When there is exogenous Wind, you must 'open to the exterior' and expel *xie qi*. When there is Internally generated Wind, you must 'extinguish Wind' and treat the underlying *zangfu* or *xue* imbalance.

Wind in the body is similar to wind in nature in several ways and it can be just as destructive. There may be a slight breeze that just manifests with symptoms such as tics or a mild dizziness, or it can be like a hurricane and cause paralysis, spasms and stroke. This is particularly the case when the Wind has resulted from Heat; this can have very destructive and sometimes fatal consequences. One of the major problems with Wind is that it can whirl up Phlegm and send it up to the head, blocking the 'orifices'. This can result in the person losing their ability to talk and make the tongue stiff. The Phlegm can also block the channels and result in paralysis. Some of the disorders in Western medicine that are manifestations of internally generated Wind are meningitis, tetanus, febrile convulsions, epilepsy and stroke.

Wind can cause gentle movements, such as when a flag flaps gently back and forth on a summer's day, but it can also make the flag stand rigidly in the air, not moving to either side, such as in an autumn storm. In both scenarios it is characteristic that the flag's movements are involuntary, and this is the same in the body. All involuntary movements of the muscles and all forms of cramping and spasms will be due to Wind.

Aetiology
This will depend on the specific imbalances that have led to the generation of internal Wind (see the section on Liver imbalances on page 590 for the aetiology of these patterns).

Symptoms and signs
- Symptoms can be mild such as tremors, tics, numbness and dizziness.

- Symptoms can be more extreme, such as loss of consciousness, aphasia, extreme vertigo, coma, convulsions, paralysis.

- There will also be symptoms of the underlying imbalance.

Treatment principle
Extinguish Wind and harmonise the underlying imbalance.

Acupuncture points
Choose from: Du 20, Du 16, UB 10, GB 20 and Liv 3, as well as points to treat the underlying imbalance.

Needle technique
This depends on whether it is a *xu* or *shi* pattern of imbalance.

Explanation

- Du 20, Du 16, UB 10, GB 20 and Liv 3 all calm and extinguish Wind.

Herbal formula

- *Tian Ma Gou Teng Yin* (Extinguishes Liver Wind)

Relevant advice
This will depend on the underlying imbalance.

Internally generated Wind can be caused by the following patterns of imbalance

- Invasion of exogenous *xie qi*

- Liver Fire

- Ascending Liver *yang*

- Liver *yin xu*

- Liver *xue xu*

Internally generated Wind can result in the following pattern of imbalance

- Phlegm-Wind

Cold

Cold is referred to as 'the prevailing *qi* of winter'. This is because cold is the dominant climate at this time of year. This does not mean that Cold cannot or will not invade the body at other times of the year but that Cold is most prevalent in winter.

Cold is extremely *yin* in nature. This means that Cold can easily damage *yang*. Cold's *yin* nature can be seen in its *qi* dynamic, which is contracting. Its contracting nature means that Cold creates stagnations and blocks the movement of *yang*. This is seen in the world around us, where cold freezes water and stops it from moving; Cold does the same in the body. Cold will stagnate *qi, jinye* and *xue,* because it blocks their free movement. There is an aphorism in Chinese medicine: 'Where there is stagnation, there is pain, where there is free movement, there is no pain' ('*Bu tong ze tong, tong ze bu tong*'). This means that pain is a key symptom signifying the presence of Cold. The character of pain in Cold is typically cramping or biting in nature. Other typical symptoms are stiffness and a pronounced aversion to cold.

Exogenous *xie* Cold will often invade the body through the skin, where it will disrupt the circulation and the activities of the body's *wei qi*. This means that the symptoms and the signs of an invasion of Cold will be most apparent in the body's external aspects. Because Cold blocks the movement of *wei qi*, it will also block *wei qi* in its ability to open the pores and there will be a lack of sweating. Each of the six climatic *qi* has a resonance with specific organs and channels in the body. Cold has a resonance with the *taiyang* channel. *Taiyang* is the most exterior channel and it is in these channels that the initial reactions to an attack of Cold manifests according to 'Six Stage' theory.

Cold is often involved in the aetiology of *bi* syndromes. Here, Cold is combined with Dampness and Wind and will block the movement of *qi, xue* and *jinye* in the channels and in the joints.

There can be situations where exogenous *xie* Cold manifests with symptoms and signs in the interior of the body. This will typically be when there is an invasion of Cold in the Stomach and Intestines, Urinary Bladder or Uterus. An invasion of Cold in the interior is due to either climatic Cold penetrating through the skin to the channels or the consumption of food, liquids or medicaments that have a Cold nature.

Cold can block the movement and activity of *yang* and thereby prevent it from transforming and transporting fluids. This can result in clear, watery exudations from the nose, vagina or respiratory passages. Diarrhoea caused by Cold will also be watery.

The above are all *shi* Cold conditions. *Shi* Cold does not usually exist for very long. It will usually transform into Heat or it will weaken the *yang* and *xu* Cold will develop. *Xu* Cold may also arise from a condition of *yang xu*. The symptoms and signs of *xu* and *shi* Cold are very similar, but pain is more intense and the symptoms are more acute when there is *shi* Cold. The tongue will also have a thicker coating and the pulse will be Tight. *Xu* Cold pain is less intense and is more chronic. The tongue coating will be thinner. The principles of treatment are also different. When there is *xu* Cold, *yang* must be tonified and warmed. When there is *shi* Cold, the Cold must be expelled.

Aetiology
Exposure to Cold.

Symptoms and signs

- Pain that is biting or cramping in character
- Stiffness and soreness in the muscles and joints
- Aversion to or fear of Cold
- Chills
- No thirst
- White facial complexion
- Lack of sweating
- Stiff or impaired body movements
- No thirst
- Whitish, watery or clear secretions
- Tight pulse

Symptoms and signs of specific invasions of Cold patterns

Wind-Cold	Aversion to cold and wind; chills; headache; stiffness in the shoulders and neck; lack of sweating; coughing; sneezing; clear, watery secretions from the nose; slight or no fever; itchy throat; no thirst; Superficial, Tight and Slow pulse.
Cold *bi*	This is *bi* syndrome where *cold* is the predominant pathogen. The movement of the joints are inhibited and there will be severe pain due to the stagnation of *qi* and *xue*. The pain will be localised and will be intense. The pain is ameliorated by heat and motion and worse when exposed to cold and when there is inactivity. There will be a general aversion to cold, no sweating and therefore increased urination, chills and possibly muscle twitching. There will be a Superficial, Tight and Slow pulse.
Cold in the Stomach	Acute epigastric pain; explosive vomiting of clear fluids; acute sensitivity to cold. The symptoms will be provoked by the ingestion of cold foods and drinks, which often lead to vomiting. The symptoms are alleviated by heat. The Stomach area will feel cold on palpation. The tongue will have a thick, white coating and the pulse will be Deep, Tight, Confined and Slow, especially in the right *guan* positions.
Cold in the Intestines	Acute pain in the abdomen; painful, watery diarrhoea; acute sensitivity to cold; the skin of the abdomen may feel cold on palpation; there may be cold extremities; thick, white tongue coating; Deep, Tight, Confined and Slow pulse, especially in the *chi* positions.
Cold in the Uterus	Cramping and biting menstrual pain; long menstrual cycle; brown menstrual blood containing clots that look like coffee grounds; infertility; the area above the pubic bone will feel cold on palpation; thick, white tongue coating; Deep, Tight, Confined and Slow pulse, especially in the *chi* positions.

Treatment principle
Expel Cold.

Acupuncture points

- If there is Wind-Cold: Lu 7, LI 4, SI 3, UB 62, Du 14, GB 20, UB 10 and UB 12.

- If there is Cold *bi*: LI 4, Ren 6 and Du 14, as well as local and distal acupuncture points along on the appropriate channel.

- If there is Cold in the Stomach: St 21, St 34, Sp 4, Ren 6, Ren 13, UB 21 and Pe 6.

- If there is Cold in the Intestines: St 25, St 36, St 37, Ren 6, Ren 8, Sp 4, Sp 9 and UB 25.

- If there is Cold in the Uterus: Ren 4, Ren 6, Du 4, UB 23, Kid 3, Kid 7, Kid 13 and St 29.

Needle technique
Draining. Moxa is recommended.

Explanation

- Lu 7, LI 4, SI 3, UB 62, Du 14, GB 20, UB 10 and UB 12 all expel Wind and Cold, as well as activating *wei qi*.

- Kid 3, Kid 7, Du 4, Ren 4, Ren 6 and Ren 8 warm and activate *yang qi*.

- St 21, St 25, St 34, St 37, UB 21 and UB 25 expel Cold and regulate *qi* in the Stomach and Intestines.

- Sp 4 regulates *qi* in the Stomach and Intestines.

- Pe 6 regulates *qi* in the middle *jiao*.

- Sp 9 drains Damp-Cold.

- Kid 13 and St 29 expel Cold from the Uterus.

Herbal formula

- *Ma Huang Tang* (Expels Wind-Cold)

- *Juan Bi Tang* (Expels Wind-Cold-Damp and activates the channels)

- *Huo Xiang Zheng Qi Tang* (Expels Wind and Cold from the Stomach and Intestines)

- *Li Zhong Tang* (Warms the Stomach and Spleen, expels Cold)

- *San Wu Bei Ji Wan* (Warms the interior and drains Cold downwards)

- *Wen Jing Tang* (Warms and expels Cold from the Uterus)

Relevant advice

When there is Cold, it is best to avoid consuming food and beverages that are physically cold or have a cooling energy. It is beneficial to drink ginger tea or ingest other spices that have a warming and diaphoretic energy. It is important that the body is kept warm and dry.

Invasions of Cold can be caused by the following patterns of imbalance

- *Wei qi xu*

- *Yang xu*

Invasions of Cold can result in the following pattern of imbalance

- *Yang xu*

Dampness and Damp-Heat

A distinction is made in Chinese medicine between internally generated Dampness and exogenous Dampness, despite the fact that many of the symptoms are very similar. Exogenous Dampness is the result of climatic influences, such as living or working in a damp environment. Internally generated Dampness can arise when there is a *xu* condition in the Spleen or when there has been an excessive consumption of food and beverages that produce Dampness in the body.

If the Spleen does not transform the food and beverages consumed as it should, it will not separate the pure from the impure. The impure *qi* in the form of Dampness will be extracted from the food and liquid that has been consumed, whilst pure *qi* will be sent down to the Intestines and out of the body. Dampness will accumulate and initially disrupt the *qi* mechanism in the middle *jiao*, especially the functioning of the Spleen. Dampness, which is *yin*, will tend to seep downwards and accumulate in the lower *jiao*.

Exogenous Dampness often invades the body through the *yin* channels in the legs and can be drawn up into the body, again accumulating in the lower *jiao*.

The symptoms and signs of Dampness are varied and will depend on whereabouts in the body the Dampness is located and which organs are affected.

Dampness is extremely *yin*. It's heavy and sticky and creates stagnation. Dampness will block the movement of *qi* and burden *yang*. The Spleen loathes Dampness, which will rapidly block its *qi* mechanism. The accumulation of *qi* in the middle *jiao* will result in nausea and a loss of appetite. Fatigue arises because the production of *qi* in the middle *jiao* is disrupted and because *qi* is hindered in its movement by the Dampness. This will often result in a sensation of heaviness in the arms and legs.

Because the Spleen is disturbed in its transformation of the food, and because the body attempts to get rid of the accumulated Dampness, there is often loose stools or diarrhoea when there is Dampness.

Dampness will seep down to the lower *jiao* due to its *yin* nature. This can be seen in, amongst other things, increased vaginal discharge and cloudy urine. Dampness could also block the *qi* mechanism in the Urinary Bladder and this will result in difficult or blocked urination.

If Dampness is transformed into Damp-Heat, the secretions and exudations from the body become sticky, yellowish and odorous.

If Dampness is transported up to the head, it can block the *shen* and the Heart's orifices in the head. This will manifest with a fuzzy and heavy sensation in the head, as if the brain is wrapped in cotton wool.

Some skin disorders can have an aspect of Dampness. If there are vesicles, weeping skin or itching skin, this can be a sign that there is Dampness. Damp-Heat will make the vesicles and the exudation from the skin yellow, and the skin itself may be red.

If Dampness invades the channel system, the joints will be swollen and the pain will be dull or heavy. Dampness blocks the movement of *qi*. This can make joints feel numb. The pain will be localised to a single joint and it will not migrate from joint to joint.

As stated, distinction is made between exogenous Dampness and internally generated Dampness, but within each of these two categories there are several sub-categories depending on where the Dampness is located.

Exogenous Dampness

Exogenous Dampness can invade the exterior aspects of the body, i.e. *wei qi* and the channels and it can directly invade certain internal *fu* organs. Dampness can be Cold, neutral or Hot.

Aetiology

Exogenous Dampness can arise from an invasion of climatic Dampness or due to consuming a Damp-producing diet.

Contact with certain bacteria and viruses can result in Damp-Cold and Damp-Heat conditions. This could be anything from consuming spoiled food to cholera and salmonella. A pattern is defined by the symptoms and signs that are manifesting. If the symptoms and signs are those seen when there is Dampness, whatever has caused the imbalance will then be defined as Dampness and will be treated accordingly.

Symptoms and signs
Symptoms and signs of specific Exogenous Dampness patterns

Invasion of Damp-Heat in *wei qi* level	Fever that is worst in the afternoon; aversion to cold; heaviness in the arms and legs; no thirst; sticky taste in the mouth; skin feels warm on palpation; swollen glands in the neck; heavy and throbbing headache; head feels like a tight, wet towel has been wrapped around it; heaviness and obstructed sensation in the chest; sticky tongue coating; Slippery, Superficial or Soggy pulse.
Invasion of Wind-Damp	Itchy and swollen skin; aversion to wind and cold; heaviness in the arms and legs; heavy and painful muscles and joints; little or no fever; Superficial and Slippery pulse; wet tongue.
Invasion of Dampness in the Stomach	Bloating; nausea; vomiting; loss of appetite; heaviness in the body and head; fatigue; loose stools or diarrhoea that is watery and odourless; sticky taste in the mouth; no thirst; greasy white tongue coating; Slippery pulse. All symptoms and signs will be acute.
Invasion of Dampness in the Intestines	Diarrhoea or loose stools that are watery and odourless; borborygmi; heavy and blocked feeling in the abdominal cavity; bloating; nausea; vomiting; no thirst; thick, white greasy coating on the tongue; Slippery pulse. All symptoms and signs will be acute.
Invasion of Damp-Heat in Intestines	Diarrhoea that is explosive; sticky, odorous stools; burning or stinging sensation in the rectum; the stool may be bloody; thirst with no desire to drink; odorous flatulence; dark urine; oily or sticky sweat; Rapid and Slippery pulse; sticky, yellowish tongue coating. All symptoms and signs will be acute.
Invasion of Dampness in the Urinary Bladder	Cloudy or oily urine; difficult or obstructed urination; frequent but scanty urination; heaviness, tightness or obstructed sensation above the pubic bone; white, oily coating on the root of the tongue; Slippery or Tight pulse in the left *chi* position. All symptoms and signs will be acute.
Invasion of Damp-Heat in the Urinary Bladder	Dark, cloudy, odorous urine; there may be blood in the urine; frequent, scanty and burning urination; yellowish and oily coating at the root of the tongue; Rapid and Slippery pulse, especially in left *chi* position. All symptoms and signs will be acute.
Invasion of Damp-Heat in the Gall Bladder	Acute pain under the ribs; sensation of heaviness; nausea; sticky, bitter taste in the mouth; yellowish thick coating on one side of the tongue; Rapid, Slippery or Tight pulse, especially left *guan* postion.
Invasion of the Damp-Cold in the Uterus	Thin, watery, whitish vaginal discharge; vaginal discharge that is odourless or smells like fish; sticky white coating on the root of the tongue; Slippery pulse, especially in the *chi* positions. All symptoms and signs will be acute.
Invasion of Damp-Heat in the Uterus	Yellowish, sticky discharge from the vagina that is odorous and smells like leather; there may be vaginal itching and the mucous membranes may be red; sticky, yellowish coating on the root of the tongue; Rapid, Slippery pulse, especially in the *chi* positions. All symptoms and signs will be acute.

Invasion of Dampness in the channels or joints	This is *bi* syndrome where Dampness is the predominant pathogen. The pain will be heavy and dull and there will often be numbness. There will usually be swelling around the joint, possibly with puffiness or oedema. The pain is not sharp and will usually have arisen gradually. The symptoms will be affected by humid climates and locations. There will generally be fatigue and heaviness. The tongue can be wet with a thick, sticky coating. The pulse can be Slippery or Soggy. All symptoms and signs will be acute.
Invasion of Damp-Heat in the joints	Often, several joints at once will be affected. The joints will be sore, painful, swollen and red, and they will feel hot when palpated. The person will often have additional characteristic Heat signs, such as a red face, thirst, Rapid pulse and red tongue. All the symptoms and signs will be acute.

Treatment principle
Expel and transform Dampness, regulate *qi* and possibly drain Heat.

Acupuncture points
Choose from: Sp 6, Sp 9, Ren 9 and UB 22.

- If there is an invasion of Damp-Heat in the *wei* level, add: SJ 5, LI 4, LI 11, Du 14 and UB 12.

- If there is an invasion of Wind-Damp, add: Lu 7, LI 4, SJ 6, GB 31 and UB 12.

- If there is an invasion of Damp in the Stomach, add: St 21, St 34, St 36 and Ren 12.

- If there is an invasion of Damp-Heat in the Stomach, add: St 21, St 34, St 36, St 44, LI 11 and Ren 12.

- If there is an invasion of Damp in the Intestines, add: St 25, St 37 and St 39.

- If there is an invasion of Damp-Heat in Intestines, add: St 25, St 37, St 39, St 44 and LI 11.

- If there is an invasion of Dampness in the Urinary Bladder, add: Ren 3.

- If there is an invasion of Damp-Heat in the Urinary Bladder add: Ren 3, UB 39 and LI 11.

- If there is an invasion of Damp-Heat in the Gall Bladder, add: GB 24, GB 34 and GB 36.

- If there is an invasion of Damp in the Uterus, add: Pe 6, SJ 5, GB 26, GB 41 and Ren 2.

- If there is an invasion of Damp-Heat in the Uterus, add: LI 11, Pe 6, SJ 5, GB 26, GB 41 and Ren 2.

- If there is Damp *bi*, add: Local and distal points on the relevant channel. If there is Heat, also add LI 11 and Du 14.

Needle technique
Draining.

Explanation

- Sp 6, Sp 9, Ren 9 and UB 22 all drain and transform Dampness.

- Lu 7, SJ 5, LI 4, LI 11, Du 14 and UB 12 expel exogenous *xie qi* and activate *wei qi*.

- GB 31 and SJ 6 expel Wind from the skin and stop itching.

- St 21, St 34, St 36 and Ren 12 regulate Stomach *qi*.

- St 25, St 37 and St 39 regulate *qi* in the Intestines.

- LI 11 expels and drains Damp-Heat.

- St 44 drains Damp-Heat.

- Du 14 drains Heat.

- Ren 3 drains Dampness and Damp-Heat from the Urinary Bladder.

- UB 39 drains Damp-Heat from the Urinary Bladder.

- GB 24, GB 34 and GB 36 drain Damp-Heat from the Gall Bladder and regulate Gall Bladder *qi*.

- SJ 5 and GB 41 open *dai mai* and drain Dampness and Damp-Heat.

- GB 26 drains Dampness and Damp-Heat from *dai mai*.

- Ren 2 drains Dampness and Damp-Heat from the Uterus.

Herbal formula

- *Huo Xiang Zheng Qi Tang* (Expels Wind Dampness from the exterior, regulates Stomach and Intestine *qi*, transforms and drains Dampness)

- *Juan Bi Tang* (Expels Wind-Cold-Dampness and circulates *qi* in the channels)

- *San Ren Tang* (Expels and drains Damp-Heat)

- *Huang Qin Tang* (Drains Damp-Heat from the Intestines)

- *Bai Tou Weng Tang* (Drains Damp-Heat and Toxic-Heat from the Intestines)

- *Long Dan Xie Gan Tang* (Drains Damp-Heat from the Gall Bladder)

- *Bei Xie Shen Shi Tang* (Drains Dampness and Damp-Heat from the vagina)

- *Ba Zheng Wan* (Drains Damp-Heat from the Urinary Bladder)

Relevant advice

When there is an invasion of Dampness, it is important that the person does not consume food and beverages that can contribute to the condition of Dampness. This means that they should not consume dairy products, cold drinks, ice cream, sweets, dried fruit, cakes, wheat flour, sugar, lettuce, cucumber, tomato, melon, avocado and tropical fruit. Furthermore, if there is Damp-Heat, they should avoid alcohol, hot spices including chilli and fried food.

An invasion of Dampness can be caused by the following pattern of imbalance

- Spleen *qi xu*

An invasion of Dampness can result in the following patterns of imbalance

- Spleen *qi xu*

- Phlegm

Internally generated Dampness

Internally generated Dampness is primarily a consequence of Spleen *qi xu* or Spleen *yang xu*. It can also result from consuming foods, beverages and medicine that produce Dampness or Damp-Heat.

As with exogenous Dampness, it is important to differentiate between whether there is Damp-Cold or Damp-Heat, as well as where in the body the Dampness is.

Aetiology

Internally generated Dampness can arise when the Spleen or the Kidneys are too weak to carry out their functions of transforming and transporting fluids in the body. Dampness can also result from a prolonged or excessive consumption of foods, beverages and medicine that produce Dampness or Damp-Heat. Dampness can start as an acute invasion of exogenous Dampness that has penetrated into the interior and become a chronic interior condition.

Symptoms and signs

The general symptoms and signs of internally generated Dampness are:

- nausea

- loss of appetite

- heaviness in limbs

- fatigue

- abdominal bloating

- loose stools or diarrhoea

- increased vaginal discharge

- cloudy urine

- sticky taste in the mouth

- lack of thirst

- slippery pulse

- thick and sticky tongue coating.

Symptoms and signs of specific internally generated Dampness patterns

Stomach and Spleen Dampness	Poor appetite; no appetite in the morning; nausea; blocked or replete sensation in the epigastric region or abdomen; loose stools or diarrhoea; sticky taste in the mouth; lack of thirst; loss of sense of taste; heaviness in the arms and legs; white, sticky discharge from the vagina; oedema; fatigue; heaviness in the body and head; fuzzy thinking or feeling as if the head is full of cotton wool; dull, pale complexion; thick, white, sticky tongue coating on a pale tongue (in a chronic pattern the coating may not be so thick); Slippery, Slow pulse.
Dampness in the Intestines	Diarrhoea or loose stools that are watery and odourless; borborygmi; heavy, uncomfortable or replete sensation in the abdominal cavity; abdominal bloating; nausea; vomiting; lack of thirst; thick, white greasy coating on the tongue; Slippery pulse, especially in the *chi* positions.
Damp-Heat in the Intestines	Explosive diarrhoea; sticky, odorous stools; burning sensation in the rectum; the stool may be bloody; thirst without desire to drink; flatulence; odorous flatulence; dark urine; oily or sticky sweat; sticky, yellowish tongue coating; raised red papillae on the root of the tongue; Rapid and Slippery pulse, especially in the *chi* positions.
Dampness in the Urinary Bladder	Turbid or oily urine; difficult or obstructed urination; frequent but scanty urination; heaviness, tightness or obstructed sensation above the pubic bone; white, oily coating on the root of the tongue; Slippery and Tight pulse, especially in the left *chi* position.
Damp-Heat in the Urinary Bladder	Dark, cloudy, odorous urine; there may be blood in urine; frequent, scanty urination with burning sensation; yellowish and oily coating on the root of the tongue; there may be raised red papillae on the root of the tongue; Rapid and Slippery pulse, especially in the left *chi* position.
Dampness in the Uterus	Watery, whitish discharge from the vagina that is odourless or smells like fish; sticky white tongue coating on the root of the tongue; Slippery pulse, especially in the *chi* positions.
Invasion of Damp-Heat in the Uterus	Yellowish, sticky discharge from the vagina that is very odorous and smells of leather; there may be vaginal itch and the mucosa may be red; sticky yellowish coating on the root of the tongue; Rapid and Slippery pulse, especially in the *chi* positions. All symptoms and signs will be acute.
Dampness in the Liver	Sore, painful or swollen genitalia; weeping sores or itching in the genital region; hypochondriac tension; vaginal discharge; difficult urination; impotence; sticky coating on the root of the tongue; Slippery or Wiry pulse, especially in the left *guan* positions.

Dampness in the Gall Bladder	Costal pain; heaviness; nausea; sticky taste in the mouth; thick coating on one side of the tongue; Slippery or Wiry pulse, especially in the left *guan* positions.
Damp *bi*	This is *bi* syndrome in which Dampness is the predominant pathogen. The pain will be heavy and dull and there often will be numbness. There will usually be swelling around the joint, possibly also oedema. The pain is never sharp and will usually have arisen gradually. The symptoms will be affected by humid climates and environments. There will be a general sensation of fatigue and heaviness. The tongue can be wet with a thick, sticky coating. The pulse will be Slippery or Soggy.
Damp-Heat in the joints	There will often be several joints that are simultaneously affected. The joints will be sore, painful, swollen and red and will feel warm when palpated. The person will often have additional characteristic Heat signs such as a red face, thirst, rapid pulse and red tongue.
Dampness in the skin	Exuding skin disorders.

Treatment principle
Drain and transform Dampness, tonify the Spleen, regulate *qi* and possibly drain Heat.

Acupuncture points
Choose from: Sp 6, Sp 9, Ren 9, UB 20, UB 22, St 36 and Ren 12.

- If there is Stomach and Spleen Damp, add: UB 21 and Sp 3.

- If there is Dampness in the Intestines, add: St 25, St 37 and St 39.

- If there is Damp-Heat in Intestines, add: St 25, St 37, St 39, St 44 and LI 11.

- If there is Dampness in the Urinary Bladder, add: Ren 3.

- If there is Damp-Heat in the Urinary Bladder, add: Ren 3, UB 39 and LI 11.

- If there is Dampness in Gall Bladder, add: GB 24, GB 34 and GB 36.

- If there is Dampness in the Liver, add: Liv 8 and Liv 14.

- If there is Dampness in the Uterus, add: SJ 5, GB 26, GB 41 and Ren 2.

- If there is Damp-Heat in the Uterus, add: LI 11, Pe 6, SJ 5, GB 26, GB 41 and Ren 2.

- If there is Damp *bi*, add: Local and distal points on the relevant channel. If there is Heat, also add LI 11 and Du 14.

Needle technique
Drain Sp 9 and Ren 9, tonify the rest.

Explanation

- Sp 9 and Ren 9 drain and transform Dampness.

- Sp 3, Sp 6, St 36, Ren 12, UB 20, UB 21 and UB 22 tonify Stomach and Spleen *qi* and transform Dampness.

- St 25, St 37 and St 39 regulate *qi* in the Intestines.

- LI 11 expels and drains Damp-Heat.

- St 44 drains Damp-Heat.

- Du 14 drains Heat.

- Ren 3 drains Dampness and Damp-Heat from the Urinary Bladder.

- UB 39 drains Damp-Heat from the Urinary Bladder.

- GB 24, GB 34 and GB 36 drain Damp-Heat from the Gall Bladder and regulate Gall Bladder *qi*.

- SJ 5 and GB 41 open *dai mai* and drain Dampness and Damp-Heat.

- GB 26 drains Dampness and Damp-Heat from *dai mai*.

- Ren 2 drains Dampness and Damp-Heat from the Uterus.

- Liv 8 drains Dampness from the Liver channel.

- Liv 14 regulates the Liver channel.

Herbal formula

- *Ping Wei San* (Transforms Dampness in the middle *jiao*)

- *Er Chen Tang* (Dries Dampness and transforms Phlegm)

- *Huo Xiang Zheng Qi Tang* (Expels Wind Dampness from the exterior, regulates Stomach and Intestine *qi*, transforms and drains Dampness)

- *Wei Ling Tang* (Drains Dampness from the middle and lower *jiao*)

- *San Ren Tang* (Expels and drains Damp-Heat)

- *Huang Qin Tang* (Drains Damp-Heat from the Intestines)

- *Bai Tou Weng Tang* (Drains Damp-Heat and Toxic-Heat from the Intestines)

- *Long Dan Xie Gan Tang* (Drains Damp-Heat from the Gall Bladder)

- *Bei Xie Shen Shi Tang* (Drains Dampness and Damp-Heat from the vagina)

- *Ba Zheng Wan Yu Dai Wan* (Drains Dampness and Damp-Heat from the vagina)

- *Si Miao San* (Drains Damp-Heat)

- *Xiao Feng San* (Expels Wind, Dampness and Heat from the skin)

Relevant advice

When there is Dampness, a person should avoid foods and beverages that are both energetically cold and cold in their temperature. They should also avoid consuming foodstuffs and beverages that produce Dampness. Food and beverages that they should pay particular attention to avoiding are: dairy products, physically cold drinks, ice cream, sweets, dried fruits, honey, artificial sweeteners, cakes, wheat products, sugar, lettuce, cucumber, tomato, melon, avocado and tropical fruit. They will benefit from eating food that is prepared and warm in its energy. Ginger will be particularly good.

If there is Damp-Heat, they should also avoid alcohol, hot spices including chilli and garlic.

It is not good for a person with a pattern of Dampness to reside or work in places where the air is humid. This also includes buildings where there is a fungal infestation such as dry rot. These can often be an aggravating factor in their disorder or even an obstacle to therapy.

Dampness can be caused by the following pattern of imbalance

- Spleen *qi xu*

Dampness can result in the following patterns of imbalance

- Spleen *qi xu*

- Spleen *yang xu*

- Kidney *yang xu*

- Phlegm

Summer-Heat

This pathogen is *yang* in nature. It is 'the prevailing *qi* of summer', but the major difference between Summer-Heat and the other forms of climatic *qi* is that Summer-Heat is the only form of *xie qi* that is exclusively associated with a specific season. The other forms of exogenous *xie qi* can invade the body all year round, but Summer-Heat invasions are solely seen in the summer. Furthermore, all of the other five forms of climatic *qi* can manifest with related internal imbalances in the body. For example, signs of Cold manifest in a *yang xu* condition or signs of Heat manifest in a *yin xu* condition. This is not the case with Summer-Heat, which is exclusively an exogenous form of *xie qi*.

Summer-Heat can arise when a person has been over-exposed to the Sun, especially on their head. A contributing factor can be that the person has overexerted themselves in the Sun and has thereby weakened their *zheng qi*, which includes the *wei qi*. It is usually seen in people who physically overexert themselves playing sport, working, etc. on days when the Sun is very strong or in elderly people whose *wei qi* is weak.

There are three different kinds of Summer-Heat: Summer-Heat Warmth; Summer-Heat-Dampness and Summer-Heat Stroke. Summer-Heat is a very *yang* pathogen and has an upward and outward dynamic, which means that it tends to affect the head. Most of the signs of Summer-Heat are almost identical to Heat signs, because Summer-Heat is a Heat pathogen. Summer-Heat will therefore also injure *yin*. Typical symptoms and signs of an invasion of Summer-Heat are high fever, aversion to cold, profound thirst, excessive sweating, red face, headache, rapid, shallow breathing, mental restlessness and agitation. Summer-Heat will result in the heartbeat increasing and therefore a Rapid pulse. The pulse will also be Superficial. A sign of Summer-Heat that may require further explanation is that there is often an aversion to cold despite the fact that the person has extreme Heat signs and symptoms. This is because the Summer-Heat will have invaded the exterior and disrupted the circulation of the body's *wei qi*. This is the same pathomechanism that is seen in an invasion of Wind-Heat. Exogenous *xie qi* disrupts *wei qi* in its function of circulating and warming the area below the skin. The other symptoms all relate to Heat damaging *yin* and fluids in the body.

Although Summer-Heat is located in the *wei* aspect, it can quickly penetrate deeper into the body. It can penetrate down to the Pericardium blocking a person's *shen*. This can result in a loss of consciousness, incoherent speech or agitation. This is seen when there is Summer-Heat Stroke. The Heat is so intense here that it generates Wind in the body and the person may also have cramps and spasms.

If the weather or the environment is very humid while the sun is very intense, or if the person consumes large amount of cold fluids, the Dampness can combine with the Summer-Heat and create the pattern of Summer-Heat-Dampness. Here there will be symptoms and signs resulting from the exposure to Heat from the Sun, but at the same time there will also be perceptible signs that Dampness has disrupted the movement of *qi*, especially in the middle *jiao*.

Aetiology
Exposure to intense sunlight in the summer.

Symptoms and signs

- Fever
- Thirst
- Red face
- There may be aversion to cold
- Headache
- Dark urine
- Rapid and Superficial pulse

Symptoms and signs of specific types of Summer-Heat invasions

Summer-Heat Warmth	High fever; profuse thirst; profuse sweating (or no sweating if the body's fluids have been damaged by Heat); red face; headache; rapid, shallow breathing; restlessness and agitation; Rapid and Full pulse.
Summer-Heat Dampness	Persistent low fever; no strength; heaviness in the arms and legs; bloated abdomen; nausea; loose stools; sparse and yellowish urine; thick, greasy, yellow tongue coating; Rapid, Full and Slippery pulse.
Summer-Heat Stroke	Dizziness; headache; tightness in the chest; dry mouth; thirst; fatigue; nausea; in extreme cases there may be a loss of consciousness, spasms or convulsions; Rapid and Wiry pulse.

Treatment principle
Expel Summer-Heat.

Acupuncture points
Choose from: UB 40, LI 4, LI 11, SJ 5, Du 14 and Du 20.

- If the person has lost consciousness, bleed: Pe 9 and He 9.

Needle technique
Draining. Bleeding on Du 14, Pe 9 and He 9.

Explanation

- LI 4, LI 11 and SJ 5 expel Summer-Heat from the exterior.

- UB 40 and Du 14 clear and expel Summer-Heat.

- Du 20 sinks *xie* Heat from the head.

- Pe 9 and He 9 drain Heat from the Heart and revive consciousness.

Herbal formula

- *Bai Hu Tang* (Drains Summer-Heat Warmth)

- *Qing Luo Yin* (Expels Summer-Heat)

- *San Shi Tang* (Clears Heat and drains Dampness)

- *An Gong Niu Huang Wan* (Clears the Heat from the Pericardium, opens the orifices and revives consciousness)

Relevant advice
With these patterns, prevention is important. This means that it is important to avoid prolonged exposure to strong sunlight, especially on the head. It is therefore advisable to wear a hat or scarf on the head in the summer. It is also important to consume ample fluids when it is hot in the summer. This is because if you become dehydrated, or *jinye xu* in Chinese medicine, Heat will more easily create an imbalance and further injure *yin*. Chrysanthemum tea is particularly recommended.

Summer-Heat can be caused by the following pattern of imbalance

- *Wei qi xu*

Summer-Heat can result in the following pattern of imbalance

- Internally generated Wind

Heat and Fire

Before discussing Heat and Fire imbalances, it is important to differentiate between pathological Heat and physiological heat. All of the body's *qi* functions are dependent on physiological heat. There would not be any kind of transformation or transportation in the body without this heat. Physiological heat is an aspect of the body's *yang qi*. Pathological Heat does not have any beneficial physiological qualities; on the contrary, pathological Heat only has a negative effect on the body. Pathological Heat, which includes Fire, will over-activate the functioning of various organs. It will agitate *shen* and *xue*, as well as desiccating and injuring *yin* substances in the body. Furthermore, Fire can generate Wind and create Phlegm.

The difference between Heat and Fire is mainly a question of intensity. Fire is a stronger and more aggressive form of Heat. Fire is described as being more 'solid' than Heat. It is more drying, damages body tissues and can agitate *xue* to such an extent that the walls of the vessels rupture, resulting in bleeding. Fire will also agitate *shen* to a greater extent than Heat does.

There are various forms of pathological Heat and Fire in the body. I will briefly outline the various forms and how they arise, before going into detail and describing their specific signs and symptoms.

Heat can arise from an exogenous invasion, such as when the body is invaded by Wind-Heat, Damp-Heat and Summer-Heat. Furthermore, exogenous *xie qi* such as Cold and Dampness can transform and become internal Heat or Fire when they penetrate deeper into the body. This is because of the clash between *zheng qi* and *xie qi*. The body itself is warm in nature. This means that *xie qi* will eventually be affected by, and take on the character of, its host and its surroundings.

Heat and Fire can also arise from internal imbalances. Consuming food or drink that is hot in its dynamic, such as alcohol and hot spices, will generate *shi* Heat or Fire. Smoking can also result in internal Heat. Heat and Fire can also arise from emotional imbalances, particularly when *qi* stagnates over a period of time. Any stagnation in the body, whether it is *qi*, Dampness, Phlegm or *xue* stagnation, will in the end begin to generate Heat. The difference will be in how intense and systemic heat is.

Fire and Heat are desiccating and will injure fluids and *yin* in general. Therefore there will be symptoms and signs such as thirst, a dry mouth, dark urine, dry stools and constipation. Other classic Heat signs are a red face, sweating (because body fluids are driven upwards and outwards), a Rapid pulse and a red tongue.

Another form of pathological Heat is *yin xu* Heat. It is extremely important to differentiate between *xu* and *shi* Heat. This is because the treatment strategies for each are very different. *Yin xu* Heat does not arise due to the presence of *shi* Heat, but the presence of *shi* Heat will certainly accelerate the process. *Yin xu* Heat arises when the body or specific organs are *yin xu*. *Yin* when it is weak is unable to control Heat, which then up flares up. There are some fundamental differences in how the two types of Heat manifest in the body and this can be seen in the table below. When there is *shi* Heat, the treatment must be aimed at draining the pathogenic Heat. This means that the acupuncture points used need to have a Heat-draining action and draining needle techniques should be used. In herbal medicine, herbs and prescriptions that either drain or expel Heat should be used.

When there is *yin xu* Heat, the treatment aim is primarily to nourish *yin*. This means that acupuncture points that nourish *yin* are used. These points should be stimulated with a tonifying needle technique. In herbal medicine prescriptions, herbs that are *yin* nourishing are used together with herbs that clear the *xu* Heat.

Apart from differentiating between *xu* and *shi* Heat, it is also important to identify where in the body the Heat is and which organs are affected. This applies to both *xu* and *shi* Heat.

Differences between *shi* and *xu* Heat

Shi Heat	*Xu* Heat
Constant sensation of heat in the body	Sensation of heat primarily in the evening and at night
The entire face is red	Only the cheekbones are red
The person either sweats all the time or not at all	The person sweats at night
The person sweats all over the body and especially on the head	The person sweats mainly on the palms of the hands and the soles of the feet
The entire hand feels warm when palpated	Only the palm feels warm when palpated
Strong thirst with a desire for cold drinks, which are drunk in large gulps	The person experiences a dry mouth and throat, which is most apparent at night They will generally sip water
Bitter taste in the mouth	No bitter taste in the mouth
Mental restlessness, agitation, manic behaviour	Mild restlessness or unrest in the evening
The pulse is Full and Rapid	The pulse is Fine and Rapid
The tongue is red and has a yellowish coating	The tongue is red and lacks coating

Another form of pathological Heat that must be mentioned here, is Toxic-Fire. Toxic-Fire is a very intense form of Fire. The Fire is so intense that it damages not only the fluids in the body, but also tissue. All conditions in which there is inflammation with pus, greenish secretions or erosion of the skin or mucous membranes are defined as being Toxic-Fire. There will often be some degree of swelling in the area.

The area itself will be extremely red in colour and the skin above the area will be hot to the touch. Due to the concentration of extreme *yang* Heat in the area, the pain will often have a different characteristic and will be very intense. Toxic-Fire can arise from chronic internal conditions and acute invasions in the exterior, such as by staphylococcal infection, mumps, herpes and so on.

Shi Heat and Fire

Aetiology

Shi Heat can arise in several ways. It will mainly result from dietary and emotional influences.

Hot food and beverages such as hot spices, lamb, alcohol, fried food and so on will create Heat. These will generate Heat in the Liver, Stomach and Intestines in particular.

Prolonged emotional imbalances such as stress, frustration and anger will typically generate Heat in the Heart and Liver.

Tobacco smoking creates Heat in the Lung.

Exogenous *xie* Heat can directly invade the body. The invasion can be located in the exterior, but there can also be direct invasions of exogenous Heat into the interior.

Yin pathogens can transform and turn into Heat. Invasions of Cold can transform into interior Heat, whilst Dampness can transform and turn into Damp-Heat.

Symptoms and signs

- Thirst

- Aversion to heat, unless the pathogenic Heat is in the *wei* aspect, in which case there will be an aversion to cold

- The skin may feel warm on palpation

- The face can be red

- Secretions and exudations can change colour and become yellowish or greenish

- Secretions and exudations become thicker and more sticky

- Secretions and exudations can become odorous or taste strongly

- Pain that is throbbing, stinging or burning

- Excessive sweating or no sweating

- Constipation

- Red tongue

- Rapid pulse

Symptoms and signs of specific Fire and Heat patterns

Heat in the exterior	Mild or high fever; thirst; red eyes; red and sore throat; yellowish secretions from the nose; cough, possibly with yellowish sputum; aversion to cold; shivering; Superficial and Rapid pulse; possibly a red tip to the tongue or yellowish coating on the tongue.
Stomach Fire	Thirst; excessive appetite; stinging or burning sensations in the Stomach; indigestion; bad breath; bleeding gums; mouth ulcers; constipation; red tongue with dry, yellow coating; Rapid and Full pulse, especially in the right *guan* position.
Liver Fire	Thirst; irritability; anger; headache; bitter taste; red eyes; dizziness; red sides of the tongue; dry, yellow coating; Fast and Wiry pulse, especially in the left *guan* position.
Heart Fire	Mental agitation; restlessness; mania; insomnia; palpitations; ulcers on the tongue; thirst; red tongue tip; Rapid pulse, especially in the left *cun* position.
Lung Fire	Cough; thick, sticky and yellowish sputum that possibly contains blood; thirst; redness in the front third of the tongue; Rapid, Full and Slippery pulse, especially in the right *cun* position.
Heat in the Intestines	Constipation; pain or discomfort in the abdomen; the abdomen is distended and tense; dry, yellow coating on the tongue; Rapid and Full pulse, especially in the *chi* positions.
Heat in the Urinary Bladder	Dark, yellowish urine that is odorous; the urine may contain blood; frequent scanty and burning urination; yellowish coating on the root of the tongue with raised, red papillae; Rapid and Full pulse, especially in the left *chi* position.
Toxic-Fire	Inflammation with pus or greenish secretions; erosion of the skin or mucous membrane; swelling in the area that will be extremely red in colour and feel warm on palpation; the area will be painful; red tongue with a dry and yellowish coating; Rapid and Wiry pulse.

Treatment principle
Expel or drain Heat.

Acupuncture points
Choose from: *Erjian* (Ex-HN 6), Du 14 and LI 11.

- If there is Heat in the exterior, add: Du 16, LI 4, SJ 5, Lu 7, Lu 11 and GB 20.

- If there is Heat in the Lung, add: Lu 1, Lu 5, Lu 10 and UB 13.

- If there is Heat in the Heart, add: He 8, Pe, 5, Pe 7, Pe 8, UB 14, UB 15 and Ren 15.

- If there is Heat in the Liver, add: Liv 2, Liv 14 and UB 18.

- If there is Heat in the Stomach, add: St 43, St 44, St 45, Ren 12, UB 21 and Ren 13.

- If there is Heat in the Intestines, add: St 25, St 37, St 39 and St 44.

- If there is Heat in the Urinary Bladder, add: UB 28, UB 32 and Ren 3.

Needle technique

Draining. If there is extreme Heat, Du 14 and *Erjian* (Ex-HN 6) can be bled.

Explanation

- *Erjian* (EX-HN 6), LI 11 and Du 14 drain and expel Heat.
- Du 16, Lu 7, LI 4, SJ 5 and GB 20 expel Heat from the exterior.
- Lu 1, Lu 5, Lu 10, Lu 11 and UB 13 drain Heat from the Lung.
- He 8, Pe 5, Pe 7, Pe 8, UB 14, UB 15 and Ren 15 drain Heat from the Heart.
- Liv 2, Liv 14 and UB 18 drain the Heat from the Liver.
- St 43, St 44, St 45, UB 21 and Ren 12 drain Heat from the Stomach.
- St 25, St 37, St 39 and St 44 drain Heat from the Intestines.
- UB 28, UB 32 and Ren 3 drain Heat from the Urinary Bladder.

Herbal formula

- *Yin Qiao San* (Expels Wind-Heat and drains Toxic-Heat)
- *Huang Qin Tang* (Drains Heat from the Intestines)
- *Long Dan Xie Gan Tang* (Drains Heat from the Liver and Gall Bladder)
- *Ba Zheng Tang* (Drains Heat from the Urinary Bladder)
- *Huang Lian Tang* (Drains Heat from the Intestines and drains Toxic-Fire)
- *Dao Chi San* (Drains Heat from the Heart)
- *Xie Bai San* (Drains Heat from the Lung)
- *Qing Wei San* (Drains Heat from the Stomach)

Relevant advice

A person with *shi* Heat must avoid food and drinks that have a Hot energy. They must also avoid stress. When there is Heat in the exterior, it is recommended to drink mint, chrysanthemum, elderflower or chamomile tea.

Heat and Fire can be caused by the following patterns of imbalance

- Invasions of *xie qi*
- *Qi* stagnation

Heat and Fire can result in the following patterns of imbalance

- *Yin xu*
- Phlegm

- Wind
- *Xue* Heat

Xu Heat

Aetiology
Yin is weakened by old age, physical, mental and emotional overexertion (including stress), disease, *shi* Heat conditions, too much sex, dietary imbalances, blood loss and excessive sweating.

Symptoms and signs

- Malar flush
- Fever or warm sensation in the body in the evening and at night
- Night sweats
- Sweating or hot sensation in the palms of the hands, soles of the feet and the centre of the chest
- Dry mouth and throat
- Thirst with desire to sip water
- Nervous, fidgety movements
- Restlessness and unease
- Slight sensation of anxiety
- Palpitations
- Nervous, rapid speech, talks a lot
- Dark, scanty urine
- Constipation or dry stools
- Red tongue with little or no coating, possibly with cracks in the surface
- Rapid, Fine and possibly Superficial pulse

Key symptoms
Malar flush, evening fevers or night sweats, dry mouth and throat, red tongue with little or no coating.

Treatment principle
Nourish *yin* and control Heat.

Acupuncture points
Choose from: Kid 2, Kid 3, Kid 6, Ren 4, UB 23, UB 52, Sp 6 and He 6.

Needle technique
Tonifying apart from Kid 2, which should be drained.

Explanation

- Kid 2, Kid 3, Kid 6, Ren 4, UB 23 and UB 52 nourish Kidney *yin*, which is the foundation of all *yin* in the body.

- Sp 6 nourishes *yin*.

- He 6 nourishes Heart *yin*.

Herbal formula

- *Zhi Bai Di Huang Tang* (Nourishes Kidney *yin* and clears *xu* Heat)

Relevant advice
When there is *xu* Heat, the person should avoid food and drinks that have a Warming energy such as alcohol, garlic and chilli. They should also avoid stimulants such as drinks that contain caffeine. Furthermore, they should avoid too many spices in the diet. Stress and overwork will weaken *yin*. It is important that a person who is *yin xu* goes to bed early and gets enough sleep.

Xu Heat can be caused by the following patterns of imbalance

- *Shi* Heat

- *Xue xu*

Xu Heat can result in the following pattern of imbalance

- Internally generated Wind

Dryness

Dryness is 'the prevailing *qi* in autumn'. Whilst it is quite logical that Cold is defined as being the prevailing *qi* in winter, it seems less logical in North-Western Europe that Dryness should be the prevailing *qi* in the autumn. Autumnal weather in Britain is often very damp. The reason that Dryness has been ascribed this definition is that in autumn many parts of China are extremely dry, because the prevailing wind is from the West. The Gobi Desert is located in West China, which means that the air is extremely dry. Furthermore, autumn is the season of the Metal Phase and west is the compass direction of this phase. Dryness is extremely deleterious for the

Lung, which is the Metal Phase organ. In addition, dryness has a resonance with the *yangming* aspect, which the Metal organs and channels are a part of. Constipation and dry stools are a classic symptom of Dryness in the body.

The British Isles have a damp climate because of their geographical location. This means that external Dryness has not traditionally been a problem here. Invasions of Dryness can, however, be observed in people who live and work in buildings that have a very dry indoor climate such as buildings made of concrete.

Dryness is defined as being *yang*. This is because the dominant negative effect that Dryness has is that it desiccates and injures fluids, i.e. Dryness injures *yin*. The most typical manifestations of an invasion of Dryness are dry mucous membranes, dry throat, dry eyes, dry mouth, dry nose, dry stool and sparse urinations.

A distinction is made between the exogenous and internally generated Dryness.

Interior Dryness is a precursor of *yin xu*.

Exogenous Dryness
Aetiology
Exposure to an excessively dry climate.

Symptoms and signs
- Dry throat
- Dry lips
- Dry mouth
- Dry eyes
- Dry skin and mucous membranes
- Dry tongue
- Superficial pulse

Key symptoms
Dry mucous membranes, Superficial pulse.

Treatment principle
Expel Dryness.

Acupuncture points
Choose from: LI 4, LI 20, Lu 7, Kid 6 and GB 20.

Needle technique
Draining, apart from Kid 6, which is tonified.

Explanation

- LI 4, Lu 7 and GB 20 expel exogenous *xie qi* and activate *wei qi*.

- LI 20 circulates *qi* and *jinye* in the nose and expels *xie qi*.

- Kid 6 nourishes *yin* and *jinye*.

Herbal formula

- *Xing Su San* (Expels Wind-Cold and Dryness)

- *Sang Xing Tang* (Expels Wind-Heat and Dryness)

Relevant advice

The person should avoid places where the air is very dry.

Exogenous Dryness can be caused by the following patterns of imbalance

- Wind-Heat

- *Yin xu*

Exogenous Dryness can result in the following pattern of imbalance

- *Yin xu*

Internal Dryness

The aetiology here will be different from Exogenous Dryness, but the way the symptoms and signs manifest will be almost the same.

Aetiology

Exposure to an excessively dry climate, smoking, eating foods that are drying such as baked food, talking a lot and excessive sex.

Symptoms and signs

- Dry throat

- Dry lips

- Dry mouth

- Dry eyes

- Dry skin and mucous membranes

- Dry stool

- Scanty urination

- Dry tongue

- Superficial pulse

Key symptom
Dry mucous membranes.

Treatment principle
Nourish *yin* and *jinye*.

Acupuncture points
Choose from: Lu 7, Kid 6, Sp 6 and Ren 4.

Needle technique
Tonifying.

Explanation

- Lu 7 and Kid 6 open *ren mai*.

- Ren 4 and Sp 6 nourish *yin* and *jinye*.

Herbal formula

- *Mai Men Dong Tang* (Nourishes *yin* and moistens Dryness)

Relevant advice
When there is internally generated Dryness, the person should avoid places where the air is very dry. They should limit their consumption of baked food or spices, as these can be drying.

Internal Dryness can be caused by the following patterns of imbalance

- Heat and Fire

- *Yin xu*

Internal Dryness can be the result of the following pattern of imbalance

- *Yin xu*

Phlegm
Phlegm is a very comprehensive concept in Chinese medicine. Phlegm is both an aetiological factor and a pathological condition.

Phlegm can be difficult to diagnose for novices. This is because Phlegm symptoms and signs are often not as tangible as they are in other patterns. Phlegm signs can be as varied as they are subtle. Phlegm is often involved in, or is directly responsible for, many complex and chronic conditions. In Chinese medicine there are a couple of relevant aphorisms: 'Phlegm is the root of the 100 disorders' and 'All the strange symptoms and diseases are caused by Phlegm'.

The signs and symptoms of Phlegm can be difficult to recognise in the beginning because they are so subtle and varied. Textbooks that are published in China, and those that are inspired by these textbooks, tend to describe only a few, gross Phlegm symptoms and signs, but Phlegm is not usually as obvious as this. Phlegm is something you have to train yourself to see. It is often difficult to define precisely why there is a diagnosis of Phlegm; it is usually the sum of many small, subtle signs.

Phlegm is fluids that have congealed, coagulated or thickened. Because these body fluids have changed their form or structure, they have none of the nourishing or moistening qualities that *jinye* has. They have thus gone from being an aspect of *zheng qi* to becoming a form of *xie qi*.

Phlegm can be substantial, i.e. it can be seen, or insubstantial, i.e. it is not visible to the naked eye. Substantial Phlegm can be observed as sputum and mucus in the respiratory passages, stool or menstrual blood. Non-substantial Phlegm can be observed or palpated below the surface of the skin as nodules, ganglion cysts, deformations of bones and cartilage, uterine fibroids, lumps and other physical accumulations in the tissues such as gallstones and kidney stones. Non-substantial Phlegm can also manifest as a sensation of heaviness in the body and the head, numbness, fatigue, mental confusion, depression, dizziness, nausea and chest oppression. The pulse can be Slippery or Wiry. The tongue can be swollen and have a greasy coating.

Phlegm is a heavy and sticky *yin* pathogen. It shares characteristics with Dampness, but Phlegm is stickier and even more disruptive of the body's *qi ji* (*qi* mechanisms), because both Phlegm and Dampness block the *cou li* (the space between the body tissue and between the cells, i.e. the space in which *qi* moves). This has important consequences. First, it will result in the blockage of *qi*, *xue* and *jinye*. This means that there may be signs of stagnation – of these substances in general and of the various *qi ji* around the body. This could be symptoms and signs such as nausea, loss of appetite and a heaviness in the chest, as if there is a large stone on top of the chest. Phlegm's blockage of *qi* in the upper *jiao* can also result in palpitations and a shortness of breath. The stagnation of *qi* can cause the person to feel fatigued and lack energy. The feeling of fatigue will be worst in the morning, because the lack of movement of *qi* during the night will increase the stagnation of Phlegm. They will often feel very tired in the morning and can have difficulty waking up. The fatigue and heaviness can also result in an increased need for sleep. The problem is that the person will often find that the more they sleep, the more tired and heavy they feel. This is because Phlegm will stagnate even more whilst they are lying down. As well as fatigue, they may feel that they are a bit fuzzy and heavy-headed and are not fully present mentally. This will be especially apparent in the mornings, when they will often be slightly absent and go around in a bubble. They may also lack appetite in the morning, and if they have a cough it will also be worst in the mornings. Once they get going and are physically active, the signs and symptoms will improve.

Phlegm can also manifest with areas of skin that are numb, because Phlegm will block *xue*, and thereby *shen*, so that it does not circulate in an area. This is also why Phlegm can result in numbness elsewhere in the body.

As well as stagnation, the body can be characterised by heaviness. This will also be seen on the mental and emotional level, because Phlegm will block the Heart's 'orifices'. This means that *shen* is restricted in its movement, which is why Phlegm can often be a contributing factor when a person suffers from depression. When Phlegm is very pronounced it can be seen in the person's eyes. There can be a tendency to have blobs of sleep in the eyes and the eyes can seem glazed. The *shen* in their eyes is not bright and lucid. It can be difficult to make clear eye contact. They may look into space whilst they are talking to you, which is not because they are shy and have difficulty looking you directly in the eye, as is the case when there is Heart and Gall Bladder *qi xu*, or because their gaze is restless and shifting, as it is when there is Heart Fire or Phlegm-Fire, rather, it is because their *shen* is smothered and blocked and they are in a bubble of their own. Their vision 'does not come out of their head'. These eyes and gaze can be observed when someone has drunk excessive alcohol or taken narcotics.

They may also have the feeling that they are in a bell jar. It's a feeling most people will have experienced when they have a heavy cold. Because *shen* is blocked, the person may seem confused and unclear in their thinking. They may have difficulty finding words. If the blockage is severe, they will have incoherent speech or will think one thing but say something else. In extreme cases, for example in some mental illnesses, a person can sit and talk to themselves or to a person who is not there.

A person with a lot of Phlegm will have difficulty concentrating. There is a difference in how a difficulty in concentrating manifests itself in various imbalance patterns. When there is Heat, the person will find it hard to concentrate because they are mentally and physically very restless. New thoughts and ideas will constantly arise, which makes it hard for them to remain focused. When there is Heart *xue xu* and Spleen *qi xu*, *shen* will lack nourishment, resulting in the mind feeling empty. When they read something, they cannot remember what they have just read. When there is Phlegm, it is hard to concentrate because the head feels as if it is full of cotton wool and the thoughts are very blurred. It is difficult to think clearly. Again, this can be recognised from when you have had a heavy cold or a bad hangover.

Due to its obstructive nature, Phlegm can also be a cause of dizziness. The difference between dizziness in a *xu* condition and Phlegm is that when there is Phlegm there will also be a heavy sensation in the head and possibly even nausea. Moreover, the dizziness can arise completely at random and it often feels as if the room is spinning round. The dizziness will often feel worse when the person is lying down, or lying down will not ameliorate the condition.

Physically, Phlegm can be seen in a person's skin and the flesh below, which appears dough-like and lacks tone. This can sometimes be seen in the face. The skin will be 'pasty'. There may be a lack of lustre to the skin. The skin and the hair can also be greasy or oily.

There can be a tendency to be slightly overweight or even obese. The person may be stocky and portly without being muscular. There can also be excessive growth of body hair. This will be especially noticeable in women.

The fingers of a person with chronic Phlegm may be a little too thick and appear to be slightly chubby.

Phlegm, because it blocks the movement of *xue*, can manifest with a dark, sooty colour around the eyes.

A person with Phlegm can sometimes have a special odour. The odour is difficult to describe precisely, but it is easily recognisable when it has been smelt a couple of times. The smell is heavy and lingers in the air a long time after the person has left the room. It can sometimes smell a bit like a wet leather jacket.

The saliva in the mouth will be thicker and stickier. The person can have a sticky taste or sensation in their mouth.

Phlegm can also manifest with a gravelly voice or the person can can be slightly nasal. There can be a need to clear the throat a lot.

The tongue can be swollen or slightly limp and can have an oily or sticky coating.

The pulse is usually Wiry or Slippery.

Symptoms and signs that are triggered or provoked by perfume, petrol or solvents will be due to Phlegm-Dampness. This is because Phlegm has a heavy and greasy nature. The above substances dissolve and dilute things that are oily and they will dissolve and dilute Phlegm in the body. This will result in Phlegm that was previously stagnant and embedded in the body's tissues being set in motion and circulating around the body. Although this dilutes the Phlegm, it still has a disrupting and obstructive affect. Phlegm-Dampness can also be provoked by scents and odours that are heavy, such as certain perfumes and flowers like hyacinths and lilies. Phlegm-Dampness symptoms are also often provoked by weather fronts, especially when there is low pressure, thundery weather and very humid weather. Symptoms that are triggered or exacerbated by consuming Phlegm- or Damp-producing food and drinks will, of course, indicate that there is Phlegm.

Looking through the symptoms and signs can give the impression that we and most of our clients have Phlegm. This is not far from the truth. Both the climate and diet in northern Europe mean that there can be a tendency to develop Phlegm-Dampness, but Phlegm is also something that accumulates throughout life and is often a consequence of most chronic patterns of imbalance. Therefore, the older you get, the more Phlegm you will probably have in your body.

Aetiology

Phlegm often arises when Heat thickens and condenses body fluids, when Spleen *qi* *xu* creates Dampness, when there is stagnation of *qi* or *xue* resulting in a stagnation of the body's fluids or when there is lack of *yang* to transport and transform fluids. Phlegm can also be a consequence of the diet that a person consumes.

This could be foods that weaken the Spleen, create Dampness or Heat or have a Phlegm-producing dynamic.

Symptoms and signs

- Fatigue that is worse in the morning
- Difficulty getting going, and being mentally absent in the morning
- Increased need for sleep
- Lack of appetite, especially in the morning
- Nausea or vomiting
- Heaviness in the chest
- Cough in the morning, the sputum can be loose or sticky depending on whether or not there is Heat present
- Shortness of breath
- Dizziness
- Heaviness in the head
- Glazed vision and dull eyes
- Sleep in the eyes
- Dark, sooty colour around the eyes
- Depression, melancholy
- Mental confusion and difficulty thinking, especially in the morning
- Incoherent speech or talking to themselves
- Difficulty concentrating
- Skin and flesh tissue can lack tone and be 'doughy'
- The skin lacks lustre
- The fingers can be thick and chubby
- Increased growth of body hair
- Tendency to obesity and plumpness
- Symptoms and signs that are triggered or provoked by weather changes, perfume, petrol or solvents
- Symptoms that are provoked by consuming Phlegm-producing foods and beverages

- Numbness

- Greasy or oily skin and hair

- Sticky taste or sensation in the mouth

- Thick saliva or saliva in the mouth

- Mucus in the menstrual blood

- Fibroids and nodules

- Fat nodules under the skin

- Deformed joints

- Heavy, sticky odour

- Repeated need to clear the throat

- Gravelly or nasal voice

- Swollen tongue, a tongue that lacks tone, sticky or greasy tongue coating

- Slippery or Wiry pulse

Key symptoms
Fatigue and mental absence in the mornings, lack of appetite in the morning, sticky sensation in the mouth, symptoms and signs that are triggered or provoked by weather changes, perfume, petrol or solvents.

Treatment principle
Transform and drain Phlegm.

Acupuncture points
Choose from: St 40, St 36, Ren 12, Sp 3, Sp 6, Sp 9, UB 20 and UB 21.

Needle technique
Drain St 40 and Sp 9. Tonifying on the rest of the points.

Explanation

- St 40 drains Phlegm.

- Sp 9 drains Dampness.

- Sp 3, Sp 6, St 36, Ren 12, UB 20 and UB 21 tonify Spleen *qi* and transform Phlegm.

Herbal formula

- *Er Chen Tang* (Drains and transforms Phlegm)

- *Wen Dan Tang* (Drains and transforms Phlegm-Heat)

- *Qin Qi Hua Tan Tang* (Drains Phlegm-Heat from the Lung)

- *Di Tan Tang* (Transforms and clears Phlegm misting the orifices)

Relevant advice

The relevant advice will depend on which individual patterns have been involved in the creation of Phlegm. Nevertheless, there are some general guidelines that are relevant for all individuals who present with Phlegm imbalances. Diet is very important, and the patient should avoid foodstuffs and beverages that produce Dampness and Phlegm. This will include avoiding dairy products, bananas, sugar, things that taste sweet such as dried fruits, honey, stevia and so on, wheat, fried food and alcohol. Nuts are interesting in this context, because eating too many nuts creates Phlegm, but eating small amounts of almonds or walnuts can transform Phlegm in the Lung. In general, a person with Phlegm will benefit from eating foods that have a slightly spicy flavour such as watercress, radishes, turnips, daikon, garlic, pepper, herb and so on. It is also important that they do not eat too much at a time and do not eat too late in the evening.

Physical activity and movement are important to counteract Phlegm's tendency to stagnate.

Phlegm can be caused by the following patterns of imbalance

- Spleen *qi xu*

- Lung *qi xu*

- Dampness

- *Yang xu*

- *Yin xu*

- Heat

- Cold

- *Qi* stagnation

- *Xue* stagnation

- Food stagnation

Phlegm can result in the following patterns of imbalance

- Heat

- *Qi* stagnation

- *Xue* stagnation

- Spleen *qi xu*

- Lung *qi xu*

Xue stagnation

Xue should flow freely and unhindered throughout the body. *Xue* can stagnate for a variety of reasons. *Xue* and *qi* have an extremely close relationship, with *xue* being dependent on *qi* for its movement. This means that *qi* stagnation can result directly in *xue* stagnation. *Qi xu* can also be a cause of *xue* stagnation when *qi* lacks the strength to circulate and spread *xue*. In this way, *xue xu* can also be the cause of *xue* stagnation. The movement of *xue* can also be blocked by Phlegm and by physical traumas, including surgery, because when there is physical trauma or surgery *xue* will leave the vessels, will no longer be circulated by *qi* and will therefore stagnate. Heat can 'condense' *xue* so that it becomes sticky and clots. Cold can freeze and congeal *xue*.

Just as Phlegm and Dampness have none of the moistening or lubricating qualities that *jinye* has, *xue* stagnation has none of the moistening and nourishing qualities that physiological *xue* has. In fact, stagnant *xue* blocks the passage of *qi* and *xue* in the *cou li* (the microscopic spaces in the tissue) and thereby prevents fresh, nutritious *xue* from circulating to or through an area. This means that some of the symptoms and signs of *xue* stagnation and *xue xu* can be very similar. There is, though, a significant difference between them, which is that the signs of *xue xu* will be limited to a very localised area and will not be systemic, as is the case when there is *xue* stagnation.

In China, many doctors focus on treating *xue* stagnation in elderly patients. This is because *xue* stagnation is part of the ageing process and *xue* stagnation is often a consequence of most chronic imbalances. The consequences of *xue* stagnation can often be observed in elderly patients. Their movements can be stiff and painful, and they often have visible signs of *xue* stagnation in the form of spider naevi and visible purple capillaries in the skin.

Like Phlegm, *xue* stagnation is something that is very common, but many people overlook it when they diagnose. This is because, like Phlegm, the symptoms and signs that are described in Chinese textbooks are slightly over-simplified and gross. In reality, a diagnosis of *xue* stagnation will be based on many small signs and symptoms that are less tangible and thus more difficult to spot unless you consciously search for them

One of the main symptoms that Chinese textbooks define as being characteristic of *xue* stagnation is pain that is stabbing, sharp or piercing in character. The pain will be fixed, localised to a specific place and will not move about. The pain has this character because *xue* stagnation creates a physical blockage that prevents the movement of *qi*, *xue* and *jinye*. This results in *qi* accumulating in a small and limited area where it cannot circulate. Where there is stagnation, there is pain. The pain in *xue* stagnation is unlike *qi* stagnation pain. *Qi* stagnation pain is more fluctuating and less fixed. When there is *qi* stagnation, there will be stagnation in a much larger area, but *qi* will be able to move about within this area. It means that the pain is more undulating and spasmodic. The pain will also be able to move slightly from place to place. *Qi* stagnation will also manifest with a more tense or distended sensation.

Xue stagnation can manifest as physical accumulations, lumps or hard knots in the muscle or tissue. This is because there is a stagnation of physical substance. Fibroids and myoma are examples of *xue* stagnation, but it is important to remember that Phlegm can also create lumps in the tissue. This is because Phlegm is also a physical substance. The difference between lumps and accumulations that are manifestations of *xue* stagnation and Phlegm is that *xue* stagnation accumulations will be harder and have more clearly defined but rougher edges. Phlegm accumulations are less clearly defined and smoother. Furthermore, *xue* accumulations will be more painful.

The menstrual cycle is totally dependent on *xue* flowing freely and unhindered. *Xue* stagnation will therefore often manifest with a disruption of the menstrual cycle. The cycle may be longer because *xue* does not flow freely and thereby stagnates in *chong mai*. There will be dysmenorrhoea and the menstrual blood will be dark and clotted. There can also be heavy or extended bleeding, with the bleeding continuing for longer than the normal four to six days. *Xue* stagnation can be a factor in bleeding anywhere in the body, because stagnated *xue* will create a blockage in a vessel. This will lead to an increase of pressure in the vessel, because *xue* and *qi* cannot get past the blockage. Eventually, the pressure becomes so great that the wall of the vessel ruptures. When there is bleeding – whatever the cause – it will itself become a further source of a *xue* stagnation, because when *xue* exits the vessels and channels it is no longer circulated and governed by Heart *qi*. It will then stagnate and further disrupt the movement of *qi*, *xue* and *jinye*.

The Heart has the function of governing *xue*. The Heart can easily be affected by *xue* stagnation, which will manifest as a sharp pain in the chest and a disturbance of the cardiac rhythm.

Stagnated *xue* does not have any of the nourishing qualities of *xue*; on the contrary, *xue* stagnation blocks fresh, nutritious *xue* from circulating through an area. This can result in the skin above an area where there is stagnated *xue* being dry, flaking or thickened. There may also be changes in skin pigmentation. By blocking the circulation of *xue* in area, *xue* stagnation will prevent *shen* – which is anchored by and thereby circulates together with *xue* – from flowing through the area. This can result in a sensation of numbness. This is typically seen when there is scar tissue. The stagnated *xue* from the trauma or the operation will have accumulated in the tissue around the operation site or the injured area. The tissue is often hard and thickened, and there is either numbness or sensory disturbance in the area, all of which are characteristic of *xue* stagnation.

Stagnated *xue* moves more slowly, if at all and is therefore less oxygenated. This can be seen in generalised signs such as a dark facial complexion, dark lips, dark or purple nails, purple tongue and swollen veins on the underside of the tongue. Wherever there is tissue, skin or blood vessels that are purple in colour, this is a sign of *xue* stagnation. Typical examples of this are bruising, varicose veins and spider naevi, but it could also be the tissue around a joint.

The pulse can be Choppy, Wiry or Confined when there is *xue* stagnation. It can also be Knotted if there is Heart *xue* stagnation.

On the mental-emotional level, *xue* stagnation can impede the movement of *shen*. This may mean that the person is psychotic, depressed or has difficulty staying awake.

One way of testing whether someone has *xue* stagnation is to fold their ear and squeeze it tightly together with your fingers. The more stagnation of *xue* there is, the more painful it will be. You can also press your fingers into the skin in the area where you suspect that there may be *xue* stagnation and then release them again. The more stagnation there is, the longer it will take before the white imprint of the fingers in the colour of the skin fades away.

Aetiology

Xue stagnation can arise as a consequence of virtually all chronic patterns of imbalance. *Qi* stagnation, Heat, Cold, Phlegm, *qi xu* and *xue xu* are often precursors to *xue* stagnation. Physical traumas and operations will always create a stagnation of *xue*.

Symptoms and signs

- Sharp pain that is localised in one place, pain that is sharp, piercing or stabbing
- Pain that is worse at night or after the person has been physically inactive
- Limited or stiff movements
- Bleeding
- Long menstrual cycle
- Painful menstrual bleeding
- Dark and clotted menstrual blood
- Sharp chest pains
- Irregular cardiac rhythm
- Dark facial complexion
- Altered pigmentation
- Dark lips
- Dark nails
- Rough, flaky, thickened or dry skin

- Physical lumps and knots in the body's tissue

- Numbness or sensory disturbances

- Purple skin, purple blood vessels, spider naevi or varicose veins

- Psychosis

- Depression

- The ear is tender or painful when it is bent double and squeezed

- Purple or dusky tongue

- Swollen, purple sub-lingual veins

- Choppy, Wiry, Confined or Knotted pulse

Key symptoms
Sharp, piercing or stabbing pain, limited or stiff movements, dark lips, swollen, purple sub-lingual veins.

Treatment principle
Circulate *xue*, disperse *xue* stagnation.

Acupuncture points
Choose from: UB 17, Sp 6, Sp 10, *jing*-well points and local points.

Needle technique
Draining. Bleed *jing*-well points and small purple vessels in the skin. The use of cupping, moxa, *gua sha* and seven-star needles is also relevant.

Explanation

- UB 17, Sp 6 and Sp 10 move *xue* in general.

- *Jing*-well points activate *xue* in their own channel when they are bled.

- Bleeding spider naevi and stagnated blood vessels disperse *xue* stagnation in the local area.

Herbal formula
There are a great many relevant formulas. The choice of formula will be dependent on, amongst other things, where the *xue* stagnation is and what the root cause is. The following are examples of some of these formulas.

- *Tao Hong Si Wu Tang* (Spreads *xue*)

- *Tao He Cheng Qi Tang* (Invigorates and disperses *xue* stagnation in the lower *jiao*)

- *Xue Fu Zhu Yu Tang* (Invigorates and disperses *xue* in the upper *jiao*)

- *Shao Fu Zhu Yu Tang* (Invigorates and disperses *xue* and dispels Cold in the lower *jiao*)

- *Gui Zhi Fu Ling Tang* (Invigorates and disperses *xue* and Phlegm accumulations in the lower Uterus)

- *Shen Tong Zhu Yu Tang* (Invigorates *qi* and *xue* in the channels and collaterals)

Relevant advice

As with Phlegm, it is vital that the underlying pattern that has been involved in the creation of *xue* stagnation is addressed.

Xue stagnation can prevent the circulation of *wei qi* in an area where there has been a physical trauma. It is therefore important that this area is protected from the environment so Wind, Cold and Dampness cannot invade the area. It is typical that joints that have been injured or operated on are often sensitive to changes in the weather.

Physical activity is beneficial because it will circulate *qi* and *xue*, but it is also important not to overburden the area or force a joint to move more than it will. A joint or a limb should not be forced to move beyond the spot where there is a sharp pain, because doing so may cause further *xue* stagnation.

Xue stagnation can be caused by the following patterns of imbalance

- *Qi* stagnation

- Phlegm

- *Xue xu*

- *Qi xu*

- Cold

- Heat

Xue stagnation can result in the following patterns of imbalance

- *Qi* stagnation

- Heat

- Phlegm

- *Xue xu*

Food stagnation

Food stagnation is similar to *xue* stagnation and Phlegm in that it is often overlooked. Food stagnation tends to be a contributory factor to other imbalances rather than being a consequence of them. However, several imbalances can lead directly to food stagnation.

As with *xue* stagnation and Phlegm, the symptoms and signs of food stagnation can be easily overlooked. This is because you have to ask about specific signs and symptoms that the client often does not even realise that they have or they do not see as relevant, because it is something they have always had and regard as being normal. Food stagnation can be seen on the tongue and in the pulse, but these signs are often overlooked because they get interpreted as Dampness, Phlegm or *qi* stagnation.

Food stagnation arises when food physically and energetically accumulates in the middle *jiao*. Food stagnation generally has two consequences that can lead to further imbalances and complications. Food stagnation can block the *qi ji* (*qi* dynamic) of the middle *jiao* and it can create Heat. By physically and energetically blocking *qi* in the middle *jiao*, food stagnation will disrupt and burden the Stomach and Spleen's *qi ji*. This can lead to Stomach and Spleen *qi xu*, rebellious Stomach *qi*, Dampness, Damp-Heat and Phlegm. In addition, a blockage of *qi* in the middle *jiao* can disrupt the communication of *qi* between the lower and upper *jiao* and between the Kidneys and the Heart. Food stagnation can also disrupt Liver *qi* in its spreading function. Heat will quickly arise as a consequence of Food stagnation. This can initially lead to Stomach Fire and Stomach *yin xu* and contribute to the creation of Damp-Heat and Phlegm-Heat.

When food stagnates in the Stomach, it will manifest with a turgid and distended sensation in the epigastric region. Food stagnation creates Heat. At the same time, it blocks the Stomach *qi* from descending. Both of these factors can cause the Stomach *qi* to rebel. This can manifest as burping, heartburn and acid regurgitation a while after eating. The belching will usually taste of the food that has been consumed and sometimes will also be accompanied by a small amount of semi-digested food. The disruption of the Stomach and the Spleen *qi ji* can result in nausea or poor appetite. When the food is stagnant, it will not be transformed properly and will instead have a tendency to rot and ferment. The combination of untransformed food and Heat can also result in the stool being loose and sticky. The stool can also smell rotten like sewage. Food stagnation can cause constipation by stagnating *qi* in the Stomach and the Intestines.

Food stagnation can manifest on the tongue with a thick, greasy coating in the middle of the tongue. The pulse will often be Wiry and Slippery in the middle or *guan* positions.

Aetiology

Food stagnation can arise as an acute imbalance when too much food is consumed at one time, when food is eaten too frequently or too late in the evening or when inappropriate food is eaten, i.e. food that is difficult to transform. Food stagnation can also be a chronic condition due to the Spleen and Stomach being too weak to be able to perform their respective functions. Dampness, Phlegm and Liver *qi* stagnation can also be involved. In this case, even smaller amounts of food and even more types of food will result in Food stagnation. The foundation for food stagnation can have been laid very early when the person was a baby due to the diet they were fed and the way they were fed. Many babies and toddlers are fed food that is too coarse and unrefined, is too sweet, creates Dampness and Phlegm and is too cold. Moreover, many babies are often fed too frequently. This is problematic because their Spleen is not capable of transporting and transforming optimally. This can lead to food stagnation, a subsequent weakening of the Spleen and the formation of Dampness, Heat and Phlegm.

Symptoms and signs

- Stuffed or turgid sensation in the Stomach after consuming food
- Abdominal distension after eating
- Discomfort after eating
- Loss of appetite
- Nausea
- Acid reflux
- Belching
- Belching or burping with the taste of previously ingested food
- Hiccup
- Bad breath
- Loose stools, stools with undigested food particles, constipation
- Stools smell rotten
- Thick, greasy coating in the middle of the tongue
- The pulse is Slippery or Wiry in one or both *guan* positions

Key symptoms
Full sensation or discomfort in the epigastric region, belching that tastes of previously ingested food, thick, greasy tongue coating.

Treatment principle
Disperse and dissolve Food stagnation, tonify and regulate *qi* in the middle *jiao*.

Acupuncture points
Choose from: Ren 11, Ren 12, Ren 13, Ren 22, St 21, St 34, St 36, Sp 4 and Pe 6.

- If there is Heat, add: LI 11 and St 44.

Needle technique
Draining or even.

Explanation

- Ren 11, Ren 12, Ren 13, Ren 22, St 21, St 34, St 36, Sp 4 and Pe 6 regulate Stomach *qi* and *qi* in the middle *jiao*.

- LI 11 and St 44 drain heat from the Stomach and Intestines.

Herbal formula

- *Bao He Wan* (Dissolves Food stagnation)

- *Jian Pi Wan* (Dissolves Food stagnation and tonifies Spleen *qi*)

Relevant advice
A person with food stagnation should avoid eating too quickly, too much at a time, late in the evening and foods that are difficult to transform. They must chew their food thoroughly. They will benefit from massaging their abdomen with light downward strokes from Ren 16 down to Ren 8 immediately after they have eaten. They can also massage the abdomen in a clockwise direction a few times throughout the day. As well as avoiding the consumption of foods that are difficult to transform, they will benefit from using aromatic herbs in their diet and possibly consuming a little bit of cardamom, aniseed and other aromatic seeds immediately after they have eaten. This will help the Stomach and Spleen to move *qi* in the middle *jiao*.

Food stagnation can be caused by the following patterns of imbalance

- Stomach and Spleen *qi xu*

- Dampness

- *Qi* stagnation

Food stagnation can result in the following patterns of imbalance

- *Qi* stagnation

- Heat

- Damp-Heat

- Dampness

- Phlegm

- Spleen *qi xu*

- Stomach *yin xu*

- Stomach Fire

Section 7

DIAGNOSIS ACCORDING TO *QI, XUE* AND *JINYE* IMBALANCES

In this diagnostic model, patterns are differentiated in relation to changes in the qualities, amounts and functioning of *qi*, *xue* or *jinye*.

From an Eight Principles point of view, these imbalances will, by definition, be interior imbalances and they can be either *xu* or *shi*.

Differentiating in relation to the vital substances alone is usually not precise enough to be able to treat a patient effectively. When there is, for example, *qi xu*, it is important to determine which organs are *qi xu* and what type of *qi* is deficient. This, however, works both ways. It is not enough to know that there is a Heart imbalance. For the treatment to be effective, we have to determine whether there is a Heart *qi*, Heart *xue*, Heart *yin*, Heart *yang*, Cold or Phlegm imbalance. This though is still not precise enough. If we determine there is a Heart *qi* imbalance, we need to know whether there is Heart *qi xu* or Heart *qi stagnation*. Similarly, if there is a Heart *xue* imbalance, we need to determine whether there is Heart *xue xu* or Heart *xue* stagnation or whether *xue* Heat is agitating the Heart. These differentiations are important, because the treatments required in each situation will be different, as will the advice that is given to the client.

Diagnosis in relation to the vital substances is a key aspect of other diagnostic models, especially the diagnosis according to *zangfu* organs.

The treatment strategy is implicit in a diagnosis according to *qi*, *xue* and *jinye*. When something is *xu*, it must be tonified or nourished. When there is a stagnation, that which is stagnant must be dispersed and circulated. If *qi* is rebellious, it must be regulated, etc.

The following patterns are differentiated in the model 'diagnosis according to *qi*, *xue* and *jinye*'.

There are four kinds of *qi* imbalances:

- *qi xu*

- *qi* sinking

- stagnant *qi*

- rebellious *qi*.

There are four kinds of *xue* imbalances:

- *xue xu*

- *xue* loss

- *xue* stagnation

- *xue* Heat.

There are four kinds of *jinye* imbalances:

- *jinye xu*

- accumulation of fluids

- Damp

- Phlegm.

Qi imbalances

When there are *qi* imbalances, there will be signs that there is a disturbance of one or more of *qi*'s functions in the body. These signs will arise either because there is too little *qi* available for *qi* to be able to perform its tasks – *qi xu* – or because there is *qi* stagnation. *Qi* stagnation can prevent the free movement of *qi*, *xue* and *jinye*. This will often result in pain, discomfort, bloating and so on.

Qi can also move in the wrong direction, i.e. the opposite direction that it should be moving in. For example, when there is harmony, the Stomach sends its *qi* downwards. If Stomach *qi* is rebellious, Stomach *qi* will ascend upwards. This will manifest with symptoms such as nausea, vomiting, hiccups, belching and acid regurgitation.

If there is '*qi* sinking', *qi* is no longer able to lift and hold things in place. *Qi* lifts and holds structures in the body in place, so if there is *qi xu*, there can be prolapse of organs or a sinking, downward-dragging sensation in the body.

Qi xu

Any *zang* organ can be *qi xu*, but when there is a diagnosis of *qi xu*, there will usually be a *xu* condition in one or more of the *qi*-producing organs – the Lung, the Spleen and the Kidneys. This does not mean that other organs cannot be *qi xu* – Heart *qi xu* is, for example, a very common pattern of imbalance, but in this case the condition of *qi xu* is related to a specific organ's functioning and it will not necessarily affect the state of *qi* and the functioning of the body in general. When there is a diagnosis of *qi xu*, there is a systemic deficiency or lack of *qi*, and this is seen in the accompanying symptoms and signs in the whole body. When a specific organ is *qi xu*, there will be symptoms and signs that this organ is unable to perform its functions properly due to a lack of *qi*. This condition will, though, be differentiated as a *zangfu* imbalance.

A generalised condition of *qi xu* will arise when more *qi* is consumed than the body is able to produce. This may be due to overusing and straining *qi*, such as when there is illness, overwork, excessive sport and fitness training, excessive physical and mental activity, too much sex and lack of sleep. *Qi xu* will also arise when not enough food has been consumed or if the food that has been consumed and air that has been inhaled are of poor quality, so that sufficient *qi* to replenish the *qi* that has been consumed is not produced. There can also be a deficiency or weakness of *jing*, the inherited essence that is the foundation of *qi*. Finally, *qi xu* can be due to a weakness of one of the three *qi*-producing organs, i.e. Kidney *qi xu*, Spleen *qi xu* or Lung *qi xu*, or a combination of these. For a more detailed analysis of the aetiology of *xu* conditions in these organs, please see the relevant parts of Section 8 on *zangfu* imbalances.

The key symptom of *qi xu* is fatigue, but even though *qi xu* will always result in fatigue, not all fatigue is the result of *qi xu* or a *xu* condition at all. The fatigue will manifest both physically and mentally.

Apart from fatigue, the person may have a pale face. This is because there will be too little *qi* to send *xue* up to the head. That is why the tongue will also be pale. Fluids will not be transported and transformed as they should be; this will manifest with the tongue being swollen or having teeth marks on the sides.

Qi is needed to maintain control of the pores in the skin. Therefore, if there is a lack of *qi,* there can be spontaneous sweating or perspiration on light activity.

A person who is *qi xu* will often be short of breath and quickly become breathless. This is because the Lung is too weak to disseminate *qi*. *Zong qi* can also be weakened and this will be apparent when a person has a weak voice and a disinclination to talk. They can also have a sunken chest and poor posture, because *zong qi* is not strong enough to expand and open the thorax.

The Spleen is supposed to transform the food and beverages that are ingested. If there is Spleen *qi xu*, the Spleen will fail to perform these functions adequately. This can be seen when a person has a poor appetite and loose stools.

Dizziness can also be seen when there is *qi xu*. This is because *qi* and *xue* are not able to ascend up to the head and nourish the brain.

The pulse will be Weak, because there is not enough *qi* to drive *xue* through the vessels.

Aetiology

Qi xu can arise when the body uses more *qi* than it is able to produce. This will be because the person places too great a demand on their *qi* or they are not able to produce sufficient *qi*.

Qi can be burdened by working too much and too hard or by being too physically active, for example by playing too much sport or doing too much fitness training, as well as through excessive sex.

Illnesses, both chronic and acute, will strain and weaken *qi*, because *qi* is used to combat the *xie qi*, but also because *xie qi* can disrupt the production of *qi*.

The Lung, Spleen and Kidneys are all involved in the production of *qi*. If one or more of these organs are out of balance, it will affect *qi* production and thereby the *qi* levels in the whole body. For a more detailed explanation of the aetiology of imbalances in these organs, please see the relevant parts of Section 8 on *zangfu* imbalances.

Poor production of *qi* can also be due to the quality and quantity of the food and beverages consumed and poor-quality air being breathed in.

The person may be born *jing xu*, which will negatively affect the quality and quantity of their *qi*. *Jing xu* can also arise or be exacerbated if a man has too many ejaculations. Chronic *qi xu* and *xue xu* conditions will also deplete *jing*.

Symptoms and signs

- Mental and physical fatigue

- Pale face

- Spontaneous sweating

- Sweating on light activity

- Poor appetite

- Loose stools

- Weak voice

- Reluctance to speak

- Dizziness

- Pale and swollen tongue

- Weak pulse

Key symptoms
Fatigue, pale tongue and Weak pulse.

Treatment principle
Tonify *qi*.

Acupuncture points
Choose from: St 36, Sp 3, Sp 6, UB 13, UB 20, UB 21, UB 23, Lu 9, Kid 3, Ren 4, Ren 6, Ren 12 and Ren 17.

Needle technique
Tonifying. Moxa is recommended.

Explanation

- St 36, Sp 3, Sp 6, UB 20, UB 21 and Ren 12 tonify the Spleen and thereby the production of post-heaven *qi*.

- Lu 9, Ren 17 and UB 13 tonify the Lung and thereby the production of post-heaven *qi*.

- Kid 3, UB 23 and Ren 4 tonify the Kidneys and thereby pre-heavenly *qi*.

- Ren 6 tonifies *yuan qi*.

Herbal formula

- *Liu Jun Zi Tang* (Tonifies Spleen and Lung *qi*)

- *Bu Fei Tang* (Tonifies Lung *qi*)

Relevant advice

When there are *qi xu* conditions, it is important that the person ensures that the air that they breathe and the food that they eat are *qi* tonifying. They must ensure that they do not consume more *qi* than they produce. In practice, this means that they need to eat a diet and eat in a way that tonifies Spleen *qi*, i.e. foods that are fresh, easily digestible, prepared and warm. They should eat small, frequent meals. They should avoid foods that are cold and hard-to-digest and have not been prepared. Soups, puréed vegetables and stews are particularly recommended. They must also eat slowly and chew their food well. Lung *qi* is tonified by fresh air and breathing exercises. Qi gong, tai ji and yoga will be beneficial, as they tonify and circulate *qi* at the same time. Caution should otherwise be observed with regards to physical activity, fitness training and sport. It is important that the person does not engage in activities that make them feel tired. On the whole, they must ration their energy and avoid working too much and for too long. Men who are Kidney *qi xu* should avoid having ejaculations.

Qi xu can be caused by the following patterns of imbalance

- Lung *qi xu*
- Spleen *qi xu*
- Kidney *qi xu*
- Invasions of *xie qi*
- *Xue xu*
- Phlegm-Dampness
- *Yang xu*
- *Jing xu*

Qi xu can result in the following patterns of imbalance

- *Xue xu*
- Phlegm-Dampness
- *Qi* stagnation

- *Xue* stagnation

- *Yang xu*

- *Yin xu*

Qi sinking

When there is 'qi sinking', there is not enough *yang qi* to rise and ascend. Rather than being a specific pattern of imbalance, it should perhaps be seen as an aspect of *qi xu*, where *qi* is not able to perform one of its functions – lifting. In this pattern, there may be prolapse of organs and a heavy, sinking or dragging-down sensation in the body. It will mainly be Spleen *qi* that is deficient in this pattern.

Aetiology
The aetiology for this pattern is the same as for *qi xu*.

Symptoms and signs

- Dizziness

- Prolapse of organs (stomach, uterus, intestines, anus, vagina or urinary bladder)

- A feeling of heaviness or sinking in the body

- Mental and physical fatigue

- Bleeding

- Frequent urination

- Bruising

- Stooping posture

- Pale, swollen tongue

- Weak pulse

Key symptoms
Organ prolapse, sensation of heaviness, Weak pulse.

Treatment principle
Raise and tonify qi.

Acupuncture points
Choose from: Du 20, Ren 6, Ren 12, St 36, Sp 3, UB 20 and UB 21.

Needle technique
Tonifying. Moxa can be used on Du 20 and Ren 6.

Explanation
- Du 20 and Ren 6 raise *qi* in the whole the body when treated with moxa.
- St 36, Sp 3, Ren 12, UB 20 and UB 21 tonify Spleen *qi*.

Herbal formula
- *Bu Zhong Yi Qi Tang* (Tonifies and lifts Spleen *qi*)

Relevant advice
In addition to the advice given above for *qi xu*, the person must avoid lifting and carrying heavy objects, and they should avoid standing up too much.

Qi sinking can be caused by the following patterns of imbalance
- *Qi xu*
- Spleen *qi xu*
- Spleen *yang xu*

Qi sinking can result in the following pattern of imbalance
- *Yang xu*

Qi stagnation
When there is *qi* stagnation, *qi* is not flowing as it should. There can be a local stagnation of *qi* in a specific place in the body or the stagnation of *qi* can be general and systemic.

A local stagnation of *qi* can manifest as tension and spasmodic or fluctuating pain that is not completely fixed in its location. There can be a feeling of distension or bloating in the area. When there is *qi* stagnation, the feeling of distension or bloating is more dominant than the pain itself. However, this does not mean that the pain experienced when there is *qi* stagnation cannot be very intense. There can be a physical swelling in the area, but it can also simply be a subjective sensation of bloating and distension.

A generalised *qi* stagnation will often cause symptoms such as abdominal bloating, irritability, mental depression and mood swings.

There can often be a need to yawn or to sigh. This is the body attempting to disperse the stagnant *qi*. By yawning or sighing the body draws in extra air or *da qi* and thereby can create more *zong qi*, which can move and disperse the stagnant *qi*.

Belching or breaking wind can relieve *qi* stagnation in the digestive system.

An important symptom seen in *qi* stagnation is fatigue. Even though there is in reality enough *qi* in the body, fatigue is experienced because the *qi* is stagnated. It will be experienced as fatigue and lack of energy, and also as a lack of motivation and laziness. When there is *qi* stagnation, the fatigue will usually be the worst in the morning and after the person has been sitting still for a long while, because the lack of physical movement will also cause *qi* to stagnate. This type of tiredness should not be confused with *qi xu* fatigue. *Qi xu* fatigue gets worse during the day as *qi* is consumed. *Qi* stagnation fatigue is often worse during periods when the person is under emotional strain or faced with situations that they are dissatisfied with.

Not only can a person with *qi* stagnation have difficulty getting going in the mornings due to feeling tired, they can also be more irritable in the morning until the *qi* starts flowing more harmoniously.

Qi xu may be a contributing factor in *qi* stagnation. In the same way that water in a stream can stop flowing if the water level becomes too low, *qi* can stagnate in the channel system when there is too little *qi*.

The symptoms and signs seen in *qi* stagnation are characterised by whether there is a localised stagnation of *qi* in the channel system, for example elbow pain, or when the *qi* stagnation is on the *zangfu* level. When the *qi* stagnation is on the *zangfu* level, the symptoms are characterised by signs that organs are not carrying out their functions optimally. When there is a general state of *qi* stagnation, the Liver will usually be involved. This is because one of the primary functions of the Liver is to ensure the free and unhindered movement of *qi* in the whole body. Stagnant Liver *qi* can also invade other organs, especially the Stomach, Spleen, Lung and Intestines. This invasion of Liver *qi* will disrupt the functioning of these organs. One must, however, be careful not to diagnose all *qi* stagnations as Liver *qi* stagnation. The *qi* of other organs can also be stagnated without the Liver being involved.

Aetiology

Qi stagnation can arise when there is emotional turmoil, frustrations, unresolved emotions, repressed anger and irritation or stress. It can also arise from a lack of physical activity. Many other patterns of imbalance can directly lead to *qi* stagnation, such as food stagnation, Cold, Dampness, Phlegm and so on.

Localised *qi* stagnation will usually be due to a physical trauma or when *xie qi* blocks the movement of *qi* in the channel system.

Symptoms and signs

- Bloating and distension
- Distending, spasmodic or throbbing pain, which can come and go
- Pain that is not localised to a particular spot
- Physical or subjective sensation of swelling in an area
- Irritability

- Mood swings

- Depression

- A need to yawn or sigh

- Symptoms that are relieved by belching, passing wind or yawning

- Fatigue, especially in the morning and when physically inactive

- The sides of the tongue may be swollen

- Wiry pulse

Key symptoms
Distension, swelling, Wiry pulse.

Treatment principle
Spread *qi*.

Acupuncture points
Choose from: LI 4, Liv 3, Liv 14, GB 34, SJ 6, UB 18, Ren 6, Ren 17 and local points.

Needle technique
Draining.

Explanation

- The combination of LI 4 and Liv 3 spreads stagnant *qi* and *xue* in the whole body.

- Liv 14, GB 34 and UB 18 spread Liver *qi*.

- SJ 6 circulates *qi* in all three *jiao*.

- Ren 6 circulates *qi* in the middle and lower *jiao*.

- Ren 17 circulates *qi* in the upper *jiao*.

Herbal formula

- *Chai Hu Shu Gan Tang* (Spreads stagnant Liver *qi*)

Relevant advice
When there is stagnant *qi*, it is important that the person gets enough physical activity. Exercise and dynamic exercise will help the body to move the stagnant *qi* physically. Massage and stretching will also be beneficial.

If there are emotional issues beneath the imbalance, whenever possible the person must try to resolve these. If it is not possible to resolve these issues, reaching a position of acceptance is important.

Qi stagnation can be caused by the following patterns of imbalance

- Liver *qi* stagnation

- *Qi xu*

- *Xue* stagnation

- Damp

- Phlegm

- Accumulation of fluid

Qi stagnation can result in the following patterns of imbalance

- *Xue* stagnation

- Heat

- Phlegm

Rebellious qi

In this pattern there are symptoms and signs indicating that an organ's *qi* is moving in the wrong direction. It is always necessary to differentiate which organ is involved.

Qi can become rebellious when:

- it is forced to move in the wrong direction (usually upwards by Heat)

- it is prevented from moving in the right direction (usually because it is blocked by *xie qi*)

- an organ is too weak to send its *qi* in the right direction (a *qi xu* condition).

Aetiology

This will mainly depend on which organ is involved. It will often be due to invasions of exogenous *xie qi*, consuming too much or the wrong foods or emotional imbalances. Heat, *qi* stagnations and *qi xu* conditions are often involved.

Symptoms and signs

When there is rebellious Lung *qi*:

- coughing

- sneezing

- tightness of the chest
- shortness of breath.

When there is rebellious Stomach *qi*:

- belching
- reflux and acid regurgitation
- nausea
- vomiting
- hiccups.

When there is rebellious Spleen *qi*:

- diarrhoea
- organ prolapse
- dragging or sinking sensation.

When there is rebellious Liver *qi*:

- headache
- dizziness
- nausea
- abdominal bloating
- alternating diarrhoea and constipation.

Treatment principle
Regulate *qi*.

Acupuncture points

- If there is rebellious Lung *qi*: UB 13, Ren 22, Ren 17, Lu 1 and Lu 7.
- If there is rebellious Stomach *qi*: Ren 13, St 21, St 34, St 36 and Pe 6.
- If there is rebellious Spleen *qi*: Sp 3, St 36, Ren 6 and Du 20.
- If there is rebellious Liver *qi*: LI 4, Liv 2, Liv 3, Liv 14, GB 20, GB 34 and GB 43.

Needle technique
Draining, with the exception of the points for rebellious Spleen *qi*, which should be tonified and heated with moxa.

Explanation

- UB 13, Ren 22, Ren 17, Lu 1 and Lu 7 regulate Lung *qi*.

- Ren 13, St 21, St 34, St 36 and Pe 6 regulate Stomach *qi*.

- Sp 3, St 36 and Ren 6 tonify and lift Spleen *qi*.

- Du 20 lifts *qi*.

- LI 4, Liv 3, Liv 14 and GB 34 regulate Liver *qi*.

- Liv 2, GB 20 and GB 43 drain Liver *yang*.

Herbal formula

- *Ding Chuan Tang* (Regulates Lung *qi*, clears Heat and resolves Phlegm)

- *Su Zi Jiang Qi Tang* (Regulates Lung *qi* and tonifies Kidney *yang*)

- *Ban Xia Hou Po Tang* (Regulates Stomach *qi*)

- *Ju Pi Zhu Ru Tang* (Regulates Stomach *qi* and tonifies Stomach *qi*)

- *Bu Zhong Yi Qi Tang* (Raises and tonifies Spleen *qi*)

- *Chai Hu Shu Gan Tang* (Regulates Liver *qi*)

Relevant advice

This will depend on which organs are affected and the relevant aetiology. Please see the relevant parts of Section 8 on *zangfu* imbalances.

Rebellious *qi* can be caused by the following patterns of imbalance

- Invasions of *xie qi*

- *Qi* stagnation

- *Qi xu*

- *Xue* stagnation

- Phlegm

- Food stagnation

- Heat

- Cold

- *Yang xu*

- *Yin xu*

Xue imbalances

When there are *xue* imbalances, there will be observable disturbances in one or more of the functions performed by *xue* in the body. It will either be because there is too little *xue* to perform the function, i.e. *xue xu*, or because *xue* has stagnated and therefore cannot fulfil its functions. Stagnations of *xue* will also prevent the free passage of *qi*, *xue* and *jinye*, and this will often result in pain.

Xue can also become too hot – *xue* Heat – and there can be a physical loss of *xue* through bleeding – loss of *xue*.

Xue xu

As we saw with *qi xu*, there can be a general condition of *xue xu* with accompanying signs and symptoms, as well as a *xue xu* condition in specific organs – Liver *xue xu* and Heart *xue xu*. In this section I will discuss a general condition of *xue xu*. For a detailed discussion of Liver *xue xu* and Heart *xue xu*, please see the parts of Section 8 on *zangfu* imbalances.

The main function of *xue* is to nourish and moisten the tissues of the body and to nourish and anchor *shen*. This means that when there is a condition of *xue xu*, any of the following signs and symptoms could be experienced.

The skin, especially the skin in the face, can be pale, sallow and dry. This is due to a lack of moisture and nourishment. *Shen* is anchored and thereby circulates together with *xue*. *Xue xu* can therefore also result in the complexion lacking lustre and radiance.

The lack of nourishment and moisture can also manifest with: dry hair; ridged, brittle or soft fingernails; pale and dry lips. The hair can also be very fine and there can be a tendency to lose hair due to the hair roots lacking nourishment.

Dizziness is often seen when there is *xue xu*, especially when the person gets up from a sitting or lying position. The dizziness arises because the brain lacks nourishment. The brain's lack of nourishment can also manifest as a poor memory. This is, for example, a common complaint of women whilst they breastfeed their baby. The breast milk is produced from *xue*, so they are often *xue xu* as a consequence.

When there is *xue xu*, there can be insufficient *xue* to nourish the extremities. *Shen* (consciousness) is anchored by *xue* and thereby circulates together with *xue*. The lack of *xue* in the extremities can therefore result in numbness, sensory disturbance and tingling sensations in the extremities. There can also be muscle cramps in the legs in the evenings when *xue* returns to the Liver.

The eyes are nourished by Liver *xue*. A person who is *xue xu* can have poor vision (especially at night), difficulty focusing their eyes when they are tired, spots in front of the eyes, and a sensitivity to bright light.

Women who are *xue xu* will often have scanty menstrual bleeding or even amenorrhoea.

If there is Heart *xue xu*, there can be palpitations, as well as insomnia, anxiety or a sense of unease and nervousness. This is because *shen is* not being anchored and nourished by *xue*.

The tongue will be pale, thin and dry because it is not saturated by *xue*. The pulse will be Fine or Choppy.

Aetiology

There are three main causes of *xue xu*: there may be an inadequate intake of food that creates *xue*; there may be a *xu* condition in one or more of the *xue*-producing organs, i.e. the Spleen or Kidneys; there may be loss of *xue* through bleeding or because it is consumed by mental or physical over-activity.

Symptoms and signs

- Pale or sallow complexion
- Dry skin
- Dry and pale lips
- Dry hair
- Hair loss
- Fine, thin hair
- Numbness, tingling sensations or sensory disturbance in the arms and legs
- Dizziness
- Poor memory
- Visual disturbances, spots in the visual field
- Night blindness
- Difficulty focusing the vision
- Sensitivity to bright light
- Ridged, soft or brittle fingernails
- Palpitations
- Insomnia
- Nervousness or anxiety
- Scanty or absent menstrual bleeding
- Thin, pale and dry tongue
- Fine or Choppy pulse

Key symptoms
Pale, sallow complexion, dry skin, scanty menstrual bleeding, dizziness, Fine or Choppy pulse.

Treatment principle
Nourish *xue*.

Acupuncture points
Choose from: St 36, Sp 3, Sp 6, Ren 4, Ren 12, UB 17, UB 20 and UB 21.

Needle technique
Tonifying. Moxa is recommended and should be used on UB 17.

Explanation

- UB 17 nourishes *xue*.

- St 36, Sp 3, Sp 6, Ren 12, UB 20 and UB 21 tonify the Spleen and thereby the production of *xue*.

- Ren 4 nourishes *jing* and thereby *xue*.

Herbal formula

- *Ba Zhen Tang* (Nourishes *xue* and tonifies Spleen *qi*)

Relevant advice
It is important that a person who is *xue xu* eats a diet that is rich in foods that nourish *xue*, such as red meat, chicken, liver, green leafy vegetables, beetroot, seaweed, dates, nettles, aduki beans, kidney beans and black beans. Furthermore, they should eat a diet that tonifies Spleen *qi*.

Xue xu can be caused by the following patterns of imbalance

- *Xue* loss

- Spleen *qi xu*

Xue xu can result in the following patterns of imbalance

- Spleen *qi xu*

- *Xue* stagnation

- *Yin xu*

Xue stagnation

Xue should flow freely and unhindered throughout the body. *Xue* can stagnate for a variety of reasons. *Xue* and *qi* have an extremely close relationship, with *xue* being dependent on *qi* for its movement. This means that *qi* stagnation can directly result in *xue* stagnation. *Qi xu* can also be a cause of *xue* stagnation when *qi* lacks the strength to circulate and spread *xue*. *Xue xu* can, in this way, also be the cause of *xue* stagnation. The movement of *xue* can also be blocked by Phlegm and by physical traumas, including surgery, because when there is a physical trauma or surgery, *xue* will leave the vessels and no longer be circulated by *qi* and will therefore stagnate. Heat can 'coagulate' *xue* so that it becomes sticky and clots. Cold can freeze and congeal *xue*.

Just as Phlegm and Dampness have none of the moistening or lubricating qualities that *jinye* has, *xue* stagnation has none of the moistening and nourishing qualities that physiological *xue* has. In fact, stagnant *xue* blocks the passage of *qi* and *xue* in the *cou li* (the microscopic spaces in the tissue) and thereby prevents fresh, nutritious *xue* from circulating to or through an area. Therefore, some of the symptoms and signs of *xue* stagnation and *xue xu* can be very similar. There is, though, a significant difference between them, which is that the signs of *xue xu* will be limited to a very localised area and will not be systemic, unlike in *xue* stagnation.

The treatment of *xue* stagnation is often relevant in elderly patients. This is because *xue* stagnation is part of the ageing process and *xue* stagnation is often a consequence of most chronic imbalances. The consequences of *xue* stagnation can often easily be observed in elderly patients. Their movements can be stiff and painful and they often have visible signs of *xue* stagnation in the form of spider naevi and visible purple capillaries in the skin.

As we saw with Phlegm, *xue* stagnation is very common but is often overlooked in diagnosis. This is because, like Phlegm, the symptoms and signs that are described in Chinese textbooks are crude and slightly over-simplified. In reality, a diagnosis of *xue* stagnation will be based on many small signs and symptoms that are less tangible and thus more difficult to spot unless you consciously search for them.

One of the main symptoms that Chinese textbooks defines as being characteristic of *xue* stagnation is pain that is stabbing, sharp or piercing in character. The pain will be fixed and localised in a specific place and will not move about. The pain has this character because *xue* stagnation creates a physical blockage preventing the movement of *qi*, *xue* and *jinye*. This results in *qi* accumulating in a small and limited area, because it cannot circulate here. Where there is stagnation, there is pain. The pain in *xue* stagnation is unlike *qi* stagnation pain. *Qi* stagnation pain is more fluctuating and less fixed. When there is *qi* stagnation, there will be stagnation in a much larger area, but *qi* will move about within this area. It will mean that the pain is more undulating and spasmodic. The pain will also be able to move slightly from place to place. *Qi* stagnation will manifest with a tense or distended sensation.

Xue stagnation can manifest as physical accumulations, lumps or hard knots in the muscle or tissue. This is because there is a stagnation of a physical substance. Fibroids and myoma are examples of *xue* stagnation, but it is important to remember that

Phlegm can also create lumps in the tissue. This is because Phlegm is also a physical substance. The difference between lumps and accumulations that are manifestations of *xue* stagnation and Phlegm is that *xue* stagnation accumulations will be harder and have more clearly defined but rougher edges. Phlegm accumulations are less clearly defined and are smoother. Furthermore, *xue* accumulations will be more painful.

The menstrual cycle is dependent on *xue* flowing freely and unhindered. *Xue* stagnation will therefore often manifest with a disruption of the menstrual cycle. The cycle may be longer because *xue* does not flow freely and thereby stagnates in *chong mai*. There can be dysmenorrhoea and the menstrual blood can be dark and clotted. There can also be heavy or extended bleeding, with the bleeding continuing for longer than the normal four to six days. *Xue* stagnation can be a factor in bleeding anywhere in the body. This is because stagnated *xue* will create a blockage in a vessel. This will lead to an increase of pressure in the vessel, because *xue* and *qi* cannot get past the blockage. Eventually, the pressure becomes so great that the wall of the vessel ruptures. When there is bleeding, whatever the cause, the bleeding will itself become a further source of a *xue* stagnation, because when *xue* exits the vessels and channels, it will no longer be circulated and governed by Heart *qi*. It will then stagnate and further disrupt the movement of *qi*, *xue* and *jinye*.

The Heart has the function of governing *xue*, and can easily be affected by *xue* stagnation. This will manifest as a sharp pain in the chest and a disturbance of the cardiac rhythm.

Stagnated *xue* does not have any of the nourishing qualities of *xue*. On the contrary, *xue* stagnation blocks fresh, nutritious *xue* from circulating through an area. This can result in the skin above an area, where there is stagnated *xue*, being dry, flaking or thickened. There may also be changes in skin pigmentation. By blocking the circulation of *xue* in area, *xue* stagnation will prevent *shen*, which is anchored by and thereby circulates together with *xue*, from flowing through the area. This can result in a sensation of numbness. This is typically seen when there is scar tissue. The stagnated *xue* from the trauma or the operation will have accumulated in tissue around the operation site or the injured area. The tissue is often hard and thickened and there is either numbness or sensory disturbance in the area, all of which are characteristic of *xue* stagnation.

Stagnated *xue* moves more slowly, if at all, and is therefore less oxygenated. This can be seen in generalised signs, such as a dark facial complexion, dark lips, dark or purple nails, purple tongue and swollen veins on the underside of the tongue. Wherever there is tissue, skin or blood vessels that are purple in colour, this will be a sign of *xue* stagnation. Typical examples of this are bruising, varicose veins and spider naevi.

The pulse can be Choppy, Wiry or Confined when there is *xue* stagnation. It can also be Knotted if there is Heart *xue* stagnation.

On the mental-emotional level, *xue* stagnation can impede the movement of *shen*. This may mean that the person is psychotic or depressed or that they may have difficulty staying awake.

A way of testing whether someone has *xue* stagnation is to fold their ear and squeeze it tightly together with your fingers. The more stagnation of *xue* there is, the more painful it will be. You can also press your fingers into the skin in area where you suspect that there may be *xue* stagnation and then release them again. The more stagnation there is, the longer it will take before the white imprint of the fingers in the colour of the skin fades away.

Aetiology

Xue stagnation can arise as a consequence of virtually all chronic patterns of imbalance. *Qi* stagnation, Heat, Cold, Phlegm, *qi xu* and *xue xu* are often precursors of *xue* stagnation. Physical traumas and operations will always create a stagnation of *xue*.

Symptoms and signs

- Sharp pain that is localised to one place, pain that is sharp, piercing or stabbing
- Pain that is worse at night or after the person has been physically inactive
- Limited or stiff movements
- Bleeding
- Long menstrual cycle
- Painful menstrual bleeding
- Dark and clotted menstrual blood
- Sharp chest pains
- Irregular cardiac rhythm
- Dark facial complexion
- Altered pigmentation
- Dark lips
- Dark nails
- Rough, flaky, thickened or dry skin
- Physical lumps and knots in the body's tissue
- Numbness or sensory disturbances
- Purple skin, purple blood vessels, spider naevi or varicose veins
- Psychosis
- Depression

- The ear is tender or painful when it is bent double and squeezed
- Purple or dusky tongue
- Swollen, purple sub-lingual veins
- Choppy, Wiry, Confined or Knotted pulse

Key symptoms
Sharp, piercing or stabbing pain, limited or stiff movements, dark lips, swollen, purple sub-lingual veins.

Treatment principle
Circulate *xue*, disperse *xue* stagnation.

Acupuncture points
Choose from: UB 17, Sp 6, Sp 10, *jing*-well points and local points.

Needle technique
Draining. Bleed *jing*-well points and small purple vessels in the skin. The use of cupping, moxa, *gua sha* and seven-star needles is also relevant.

Explanation
- UB 17, Sp 6 and Sp 10 move *xue* in general.
- *Jing*-well points activate *xue* in their own channel when they are bled.
- Bleeding spider naevi and stagnated blood vessels disperse *xue* stagnation in the local area.

Herbal formula
- *Tao Hong Si Wu Tang* (Spreads *xue*)
- *Tao He Cheng Qi Tang* (Invigorates and disperses *xue* stagnation in the lower *jiao*)
- *Xue Fu Zhu Yu Tang* (Invigorates and disperses *xue* in the upper *jiao*)
- *Shao Fu Zhu Yu Tang* (Invigorates and disperses *xue* and dispels Cold in the lower *jiao*)
- *Gui Zhi Fu Ling Tang* (Invigorates and disperses *xue* and Phlegm accumulations in the lower Uterus)
- *Shen Tong Zhu Yu Tang* (Invigorates *qi* and *xue* in the channels and collaterals)

Relevant advice
As with Phlegm, it is vital that the underlying pattern that has been involved in the creation of *xue* stagnation is addressed.

Xue stagnation can prevent the circulation of *wei qi* in an area where there has been a physical trauma. It is therefore important that this area is protected from the environment, so Wind, Cold and Dampness cannot invade the area. It is typical that joints where there has been an injury or an operation are often sensitive to changes in the weather.

Physical activity is beneficial because it will circulate *qi* and *xue*, but it is also important not to overburden the area or force a joint to move more than it will. A joint or a limb should not be forced to move beyond a spot where a sharp pain is experienced. Doing so may cause further *xue* stagnation.

Xue stagnation can be caused by the following patterns of imbalance

- *Qi* stagnation
- Phlegm
- *Xue xu*
- *Qi xu*
- Cold
- Heat

Xue stagnation can result in the following patterns of imbalance

- *Qi* stagnation
- Heat
- Phlegm
- *Xue xu*

Xue Heat

Xue Heat can arise when exogenous *xie qi* invades the body and penetrates into the interior or it can be internally generated. Like *xue* stagnation, *xue* Heat will manifest with symptoms and signs that indicate that *xue* has lost its physiological properties and now has a pathological influence on the body.

One of the main negative effects that Heat in general has is that it agitates *xue*. This can cause *xue* to become frenetic and rupture the walls of the vessels, resulting in bleeding. Bleeding anywhere in the body can be due to *xue* Heat, but it is especially prominent in heavy and prolonged menstrual bleeding or bleeding mid-cycle. The menstrual blood will be bright red in colour, sticky and usually with fresh, shiny clots, because it is Heat that is causing *xue* to stagnate.

Xue normally anchors and nourishes *shen*. If there is *xue* Heat, *shen* becomes agitated. This will manifest as mental restlessness, irascibility and insomnia. If *xue* Heat is more extreme, there can be manic behaviour, delirium or even coma.

Many skin disorders are a direct result of *xue* Heat, or *xue* Heat is a major contributing factor. This is because *xue* should nourish and moisten the skin. If there is *xue* Heat, *xue* will no longer be able to perform these functions and it will instead negatively affect the skin. This can be seen in skin disorders, where the skin is dry, red and swollen and feels hot to the touch. The Heat can generate Wind. This will cause the skin to be itchy.

Xue Heat, in common with other forms of *shi* Heat, can manifest with a sensation of heat in the body, fever or an aversion to heat. When there are invasions of *xie qi* that have penetrated into the interior, the sensation of heat or fever will be worst at night, because the *yin* aspect of the body is injured.

Xue Heat will also cause a person to be thirsty, because the Heat injures and desiccates the fluids in the body.

The tongue will be red and the pulse will be Rapid.

Aetiology

Xue Heat can arise when an invasion of exogenous Heat penetrates from the exterior aspect of the body down to the *ying* or *xue* level in the Four Levels. There can also be a residue from previous invasions of *xie qi* that have not been expelled from the body or from vaccinations. These residues or residual *xie qi* can generate Heat in the *xue*. The Liver is a reservoir for *xue*. If the Liver is Hot, it will cause *xue* to become Hot. This means that factors such as consumption of food and beverages that are energetically hot, particularly alcohol, and emotional imbalances can be contributing factors.

Symptoms and signs

- Skin disorders where the skin is red, hot, dry, swollen or itchy
- Bleeding
- Short menstrual cycle
- Prolonged menstrual bleeding or mid-cycle bleeding
- Heavy menstrual bleeding
- Menstrual blood that is bright red, sticky and possibly clotted
- Mental restlessness
- Mania or delirium
- Coma

- Insomnia

- Fever, which may be worse at night

- Aversion to heat

- Thirst

- Red facial colour

- Red tongue

- Rapid pulse

Key symptoms
Red complexion, bleeding, bright red menstrual blood, mental restlessness, Rapid pulse.

Treatment principle
Drain *xue* Heat.

Acupuncture points
Choose from: UB 17, UB 18, UB 40, Du 14, Sp 10, LI 11, Liv 2 and Pe 3.

Needle technique
Draining. Bleed UB 40, Pe 3 and Du 14.

Explanation

- UB 17, UB 18, UB 40, Du 14, Sp 10, LI 11, Liv 2 and Pe 3 all drain *xue* Heat.

Herbal formula

- *Xi Jiao Di Huang Tang* (Drains Heat from the *xue* level)

- *Qing Ying Tang* (Clears Heat from the *ying* level and cools *xue*)

- *Si Sheng Wan* (Drains *xue* Heat and stops bleeding)

- *Long Dan Xie Gan Wan* (Drains Heat from the Liver and thereby cools *xue*)

- *Xiao Feng San* (Drains *xue* Heat, drains Dampness and expels Wind in skin disorders)

Xue Heat can be caused by the following patterns of imbalance

- Invasions of exogenous *xie qi*

- Liver Fire

- Stomach Fire

- Heart Fire

Xue Heat can result in the following patterns of imbalance

- Liver Fire

- Stomach Fire

- Heart Fire

- _Yin xu_

- _Xue_ stagnation

- _Xue_ loss

Xue loss

This differentiation includes all forms of abnormal bleeding, whether it is from the nose, the gastrointestinal system, the urinary system, the respiratory system or menorrhagia.

There are three main causes of bleeding:

- The walls of vessels are not strong enough to keep _xue_ within the vessels – Spleen _qi xu._

- _Xue_ is agitated and frenetic in its movement, so it ruptures the walls of the vessels – _shi_ or _xu_ Heat.

- There is a blockage in the vessel, which results in a build-up of pressure in the vessel, which finally bursts – _xue_ stagnation.

Often, there will actually be a combination of two or more of these factors at the same time. There will be a difference in the quality, colour and amount of the blood that is lost depending on the cause.

Bleeding usually leads to _xue xu_, and if the bleeding is internal, it will create _xue_ stagnation in the local area.

When there is blood loss, it is important to not only treat the underlying pattern of imbalance that has led to the bleeding, but also to invigorate _xue_. This is because the bleeding will have created a local condition of _xue_ stagnation. Furthermore, it is important to subsequently nourish _xue_ in order to replenish the _xue_ that has been lost.

Aetiology

For a detailed aetiology, see the parts on Spleen _qi xu_, _yin xu_ Heat, _shi_ Heat and _xue_ stagnation in Sections 6 and 8.

Symptoms and signs

- Bleeding and blood loss.

When there is *qi xu* bleeding:

- bleeding and blood loss

- the blood will be paler and more watery

- pale tongue

- Weak pulse.

When there is *shi* Heat bleeding:

- bleeding and blood loss

- the blood will be fresh red or bright red and possibly sticky

- heavy blood loss

- red tongue

- Rapid and Full pulse.

When there is *xu* Heat bleeding:

- bleeding and blood loss

- the blood will be a fresh red colour

- low volume blood loss

- red tongue without coating

- Rapid and Fine pulse.

When there is *xue* stagnation bleeding:

- bleeding and blood loss

- the blood will be dark and probably clotted

- low volume blood loss

- dark purple and swollen sub-lingual veins

- Choppy or Confined pulse.

Key symptom
Blood loss.

Treatment principle
Stop the bleeding.

Acupuncture points

Choose from: Sp 1, Sp 8, Sp 10, UB 17, Liv 1 and Kid 8, as well as points relevant to the underlying pattern of imbalance.

Needle technique

Even technique. Moxa should be used on Sp 1 and Liv 1.

Explanation

- Sp 1 and Liv 1 are points that, empirically, can stop bleeding.

- Sp 10 and UB 17 stop bleeding and invigorate *xue*.

- Sp 8 and Kid 8 stop bleeding from the Uterus.

Herbal formula

- *Shi Hui San* (Drains Fire and Heat and stops bleeding)

- *Si Sheng Wan* (Drains *xue* Heat and stops bleeding)

- *Huang Tu Tang* (Tonifies Spleen *qi* and stops bleeding)

Relevant advice

This will depend on the underlying pattern of imbalance – please see the relevant sections for specific advice. It is important that a person who has suffered from bleeding makes sure that they eat a diet that nourishes *xue*, i.e. red meat, chicken, liver, green leafy vegetables, beetroot, seaweed, dates, nettles, aduki beans, kidney beans and black beans. They should also eat a diet that tonifies Spleen *qi*.

Xue loss can be caused by the following patterns of imbalance

- Spleen *qi xu*

- *Yin xu* Heat

- *Shi* Heat

- *Xue* stagnation

Xue loss can result in the following patterns of imbalance

- *Xue xu*

- *Xue* stagnation

- *Yin xu*

- *Jinye xu*

- *Qi xu*

Jinye imbalances

Jinye imbalances include patterns where *jinye* is weakened or stagnated, but also patterns where *jinye* has transformed into Dampness or Phlegm.

Jinye xu

More than being a pattern in itself, *jinye xu* is involved in and is a consequence of other imbalances. *Jinye* is an aspect of *yin*. *Yin xu* and *jinye xu* are like the chicken and the egg. They often lead to one another. The lack of body fluids means that the body dries up and this injures *yin*. There will be symptoms and signs such as a dry mouth, dry lips, dry throat, dry skin, dry cough, constipation and scanty urination due to the lack of moisture.

The tongue will be thin and dry. The pulse will be Fine.

Aetiology

Jinye xu can arise when there has been profuse sweating, acute Heat in the body (as in a high fever), chronic Heat imbalances, bleeding, *xue xu*, frequent and heavy urination, vomiting and diarrhoea, as well as excessive consumption of spicy food or medicine that has a spicy dynamic.

Symptoms and signs

- Dry mouth
- Dry lips
- Dry skin
- Dry eyes
- Dry throat
- Dry cough
- Dry nose
- Dry mucous membranes
- Scanty urination
- Constipation
- Thin and dry tongue
- Fine pulse

Key symptoms

Dry mouth, dry eyes, dry throat, dry mucous membranes, dry tongue.

Treatment principle
Nourish *jinye*.

Acupuncture points
Choose from: Lu 7, Kid 6, Sp 6, Ren 4 and Ren 12.

Needle technique
Tonifying.

Explanation

- Lu 7 and Kid 6 open *ren mai* and *yin qiao mai*.

- Sp 6, Ren 4 and Ren 12 nourish Stomach and Kidney *yin*.

Herbal formula

- *Mai Men Dong Tang* (Moistens Dryness)

Relevant advice
As well as following the appropriate advice that is relevant for the underlying patterns of imbalance, a person who is *jinye xu* must also make sure that they consume adequate fluids, avoid drinks that are diuretic and avoid sweating.

Jinye xu can be caused by the following patterns of imbalance

- *Yin xu*

- *Shi* Heat

- *Xu* Heat

- *Xue xu*

- Stomach Fire

- Stomach *yin xu*

Jinye xu can result in the following patterns of imbalance

- *Yin xu*

- *Xue xu*

Accumulation of fluids

If there is a disturbance of the Lung, Spleen or Kidney's functions with respect to the transformation and, especially, the transportation of fluids, these will stagnate and accumulate in the body. This will correspond to a condition of oedema in Western medicine.

Accumulation of fluids can also occur when there is *qi* stagnation. This will be because *qi* does not move the fluids, which will cause them to stagnate, creating Dampness and Phlegm, which in themselves can block the movement of fluids.

If the condition is due to a disorder of the Lung, there will most often be oedema in the face and the upper part of the body. This condition is often acute and will usually be due to an invasion of exogenous *xie qi*.

Spleen *yang xu* can result in oedema accumulating in the middle of the body and in the limbs.

Kidney *yang xu* can manifest with oedema that is predominantly in the ankles and legs. Both Kidney *yang xu* and Spleen *yang xu* oedema will be chronic conditions.

One way to distinguish whether the oedema is due to a *xu* condition of the Lung, Spleen or Kidneys and oedema that is due to *qi* stagnation or Damp is by pressing a finger down into the area where there is oedema. If the oedema has arisen because of a Kidney, Spleen or Lung *xu* imbalance, an imprint of the finger will remain after the pressure is released.

Aetiology
This condition arises when there is a disturbance in the transportation and transformation of fluids in the body. Acute oedema is usually seen when the Lung's function of spreading fluids is disrupted by exogenous *xie qi*. More chronic conditions of oedema usually arise from Spleen and/or Kidney *yang xu*, *qi* stagnation or Phlegm-Dampness conditions. For a description of the aetiology of these patterns, please see the relevant parts of Sections 6 and 8 where these patterns are discussed.

Symptoms and signs

* Oedema

* The tongue will be swollen and wet

* The pulse will be Slippery

Key symptom
Oedema.

Treatment principle
Drain fluids.

Acupuncture points
Choose from: Ren 9, Sp 6, Sp 9 and UB 22.

* If there is invasion of exogenous *xie qi* in the Lung, add: GB 20, Lu 7, LI 4 or LI 6.

* If there is Spleen *yang xu*, add: Sp 3 and St 36.

* If there is Kidney *yang xu*, add: Kid 7 and Du 4.

- If there is *qi* stagnation add: Liv 3 and LI 4.

- If there is Phlegm and Damp stagnation add: St 40.

Needle technique
Drain Ren 9, Sp 6, Sp 9, Lu 7, LI 4, GB 20 and UB 22. Tonify the remaining points. Moxa is recommended on Sp 3, St 36, Kid 7 and Du 4.

Explanation

- Ren 9, Sp 6, Sp 9 and UB 22 drain fluids and Dampness.

- GB 20, Lu 7, LI 4 and LI 6 expel exogenous *xie qi* and regulate the water passages.

- Sp 3 and St 36 tonify Spleen *yang*.

- Kid 7 and Du 4 tonify Kidney *yang*.

- Liv 3 and LI 4 disperse stagnant *qi*.

- St 40 transforms Phlegm.

Herbal formula

- *Wu Ling San* (Drains Dampness and expels Wind-Cold)

- *Wu Pi San* (Drains Dampness and regulates *qi*)

- *Ji Sheng Shen Qi Wan* (Tonifies Kidney *yang* and drains Dampness)

- *Fang Ji Huang Qi Tang* (Tonifies Spleen *qi*, expels Wind and drains Dampness)

- *Xiao Qing Long Tang* (Expels Wind-Cold and transforms Phlegm-Fluids)

Relevant advice
This will depend on the underlying pattern of imbalance. Please see the appropriate sections for advice.

Accumulation of fluid can be caused by the following patterns of imbalance

- Invasion of *xie qi*

- Lung *qi xu*

- Spleen *yang xu*

- Kidney *yang xu*

- *Qi* stagnation

- Dampness

Accumulation of fluid can result in the following patterns of imbalance

- Spleen *yang xu*

- Kidney *yang xu*

- Dampness

- Phlegm

Internally generated Dampness

Internally generated Dampness will often but not always be the result of Spleen *qi xu* or Spleen *yang xu*. It can also result from the excessive consumption of Damp-generating substances.

There may be a general condition of Dampness or there may be Dampness in specific organs. In this section I will only discuss Dampness as a general condition. For discussions on Damp-Heat, Damp-Cold and Dampness in specific organs, please see the relevant parts for these in Section 6, 'Diagnosis According to *Xie Qi*'.

Aetiology

Internally generated Dampness may be due to the Spleen or Kidneys being too weak to carry out their functions of transforming and transporting fluids. It can also be the result of excessive consumption of food, beverages or medicine that have a Damp dynamic. Furthermore, Dampness can initially have started as an acute exogenous invasion that has penetrated into the interior and become a chronic interior imbalance.

Symptoms and signs

- Nausea

- Loss of appetite

- Heaviness in limbs

- Fatigue

- Abdominal bloating

- Loose stools or diarrhoea

- Increased vaginal discharge

- Cloudy urine

- Sticky taste in the mouth

- No thirst

- Slippery pulse

- The tongue will have a thick and sticky coating

Key symptoms
Poor appetite, fatigue, heaviness in limbs, sticky tongue coating, Slippery pulse.

Treatment principle
Drain and transform Dampness, tonify the Spleen.

Acupuncture points
Choose from: Sp 3, Sp 6, Sp 9, Ren 9, UB 20, UB 21, UB 22, St 36 and Ren 12.

Needle technique
Drain Sp 9 and Ren 9, tonify the other points.

Explanation

- Sp 9 and Ren 9 drain and transform Dampness.

- Sp 3, Sp 6, St 36, Ren 12, UB 20, UB 21 and UB 22 tonify Stomach and Spleen *qi* and transform Dampness.

Herbal formula

- *Ping Wei San* (Tonifies Spleen *qi* and transforms Dampness)

Relevant advice
When there is Dampness, a person should avoid food and drinks that are cold, both energetically and in their temperature. They should also avoid consuming anything that generates Dampness. Food and drinks they must pay particular attention to avoiding are: dairy products, cold drinks, ice cream, sweets, dried fruit, stevia, artificial sweeteners, cakes, wheat products, sugar, lettuce, cucumber, tomato, melon, avocado and tropical fruit. They will benefit from eating foods that are prepared and warming in their energy. Ginger will be particularly beneficial.

Furthermore, when there is Damp-Heat, they should avoid alcohol, fried food and hot spices including chilli.

When there is Dampness it is best to avoid living and working in humid environments. This will also include buildings with fungal damage, such as dry rot. These can often be an aggravating factor or can even be an obstacle to the therapy.

Internally generated Dampness can be caused by the following patterns of imbalance

- Spleen *qi xu*

- Spleen *yang xu*

Internally generated Dampness can result in the following patterns of imbalance

- Spleen *qi xu*

- Spleen *yang xu*

- Kidney *yang xu*

- Phlegm

Phlegm

Phlegm is a very comprehensive concept in Chinese medicine. Phlegm is both an aetiological factor and a pathological condition.

Phlegm can be difficult for novices to diagnose. This is because the symptoms and signs are often not as tangible as they are in other patterns. Phlegm signs can be as varied as they are subtle. Phlegm is often involved in, or is directly responsible for, many complex and chronic conditions. In Chinese medicine there are two relevant aphorisms: 'Phlegm is the root of the 100 disorders' and 'All the strange symptoms and diseases are caused by Phlegm'.

The signs and symptoms of Phlegm can be difficult to recognise in the beginning because they are so subtle and varied. Textbooks that are published in China, and those that are inspired by these textbooks, tend to describe only a few, gross Phlegm symptoms and signs, but Phlegm is not usually as obvious as this. Phlegm is something you have to train yourself to see. It is often difficult to define precisely why there is a diagnosis of Phlegm; it is usually the sum of many small, subtle signs.

Phlegm is fluids that have congealed, coagulated or thickened. Because these body fluids have changed their form or structure, they have none of the nourishing or moisturising qualities that *jinye* has. They have thus gone from being an aspect of *zheng qi* to becoming a form of *xie qi*.

Phlegm can be substantial, i.e. it can be seen, or insubstantial, i.e. it is not visible to the naked eye. Substantial Phlegm can be observed as sputum and mucus in the respiratory passages, stool or menstrual blood. Non-substantial Phlegm can be observed or palpated below the surface of the skin as nodules, ganglion cysts, deformations of bones and cartilage, uterine fibroids, lumps and other physical accumulations in the tissues such as gallstones and kidney stones. Non-substantial Phlegm also manifests as a sensation of heaviness in the body and the head, numbness, fatigue, mental confusion, depression, dizziness, nausea and chest oppression. The pulse can be Slippery or Wiry. The tongue can be swollen and have a greasy coating.

Phlegm is a heavy and sticky *yin* pathogen. It shares characteristics with Dampness, but Phlegm is stickier and even more disruptive of the body's *qi ji* (*qi* mechanisms), because both Phlegm and Dampness block the *cou li* (the space between the body tissue and between the cells, i.e. the space in which *qi* moves). This has important consequences. First, it will result in the blockage of *qi*, *xue* and *jinye*. This means that there may be signs of stagnation – of these substances in general and of the various *qi ji* around the body. This could be symptoms and signs such as nausea, loss of appetite and a heaviness in the chest as if there is a large stone on top of the chest. Phlegm's blockage of *qi* in the upper *jiao* can also result in palpitations and a shortness of breath. The stagnation of *qi* can cause the person to feel fatigued and lack energy. The feeling of fatigue will be worse in the morning, because the lack of movement of *qi* during the night will increase the stagnation of Phlegm. They will often feel very tired in the mornings and can have difficulty waking up. The fatigue and heaviness can also result in an increased need for sleep. The problem is that the person will often find that the more they sleep, the more tired and heavy they feel. This is because Phlegm will stagnate even more whilst they are lying down. As well as fatigue, they may feel that they are a bit fuzzy and heavy-headed and are not fully present mentally. This will be especially apparent in the mornings, when they will often not be fully present and will go around in a bubble. They may also lack appetite in the morning, and if they have a cough it will be worse in the mornings. Once they get going and are physically active, the signs and symptoms will improve.

Phlegm can also manifest with areas of skin that are numb, because Phlegm will block *xue* and thereby *shen*, so that it does not circulate in the area. This is also why Phlegm can result in numbness elsewhere in the body.

As well as stagnation, the body can be characterised by heaviness. This will also be seen on the mental and emotional level, because Phlegm will block the Heart's 'orifices'. This means that *shen* is restricted in its movement, which is why Phlegm can often be a contributing factor when a person suffers from depression. When Phlegm is very pronounced it can be seen in the person's eyes. There can be a tendency to have blobs of sleep in the eyes and the eyes can seem glazed. The *shen* in their eyes is not bright and lucid. It can be difficult to make clear eye contact. They may look into space whilst they are talking to you, not because they are shy and have difficulty looking you directly in the eye, as is the case when there is Heart and Gall Bladder *qi xu*, or because their gaze is restless and shifting, as it is when there is Heart Fire or Phlegm-Fire, rather, it is because their *shen* is smothered and blocked and they are in a bubble of their own. Their gaze 'does not come out of their head'. These eyes and their vision can be observed when someone has drunk excessive alcohol or taken narcotics.

They may also have the feeling that they are in a bell jar. It's a feeling most people will have experienced when they have had a heavy cold. Because *shen* is blocked, the person may seem confused and unclear in their thinking. They may have difficulty finding words. If the blockage is severe, they will have incoherent speech or think one thing but say something else. In extreme cases, for example in some mental illnesses, a person can sit and talk to themselves or to a person who is not there.

A person with a lot of Phlegm will have difficulty concentrating. There is a difference in how a difficulty in concentrating manifests itself in various imbalance patterns. When there is Heat, the person will find it hard to concentrate because they are mentally and physically very restless. New thoughts and ideas will constantly arise, which makes it hard for them to remain focused. When there is Heart *xue xu* and Spleen *qi xu*, *shen* will lack nourishment, resulting in the mind feeling empty. When they read something, they cannot remember what they have just read. When there is Phlegm, it is hard to concentrate because the head feels as if it is full of cotton wool and the thoughts are very blurred. It is difficult to think clearly. Again, this can be recognised from when you have had a heavy cold or a bad hangover.

Due to its obstructive nature, Phlegm can also be a cause of dizziness. The difference between dizziness in a *xu* condition and Phlegm is that when there is Phlegm there will also be a heavy sensation in the head and possibly even nausea. Moreover, the dizziness can arise completely at random and it often feels as if the room is spinning round. The dizziness will often feel worse when the person is lying down, or lying down will not ameliorate the condition.

Physically, Phlegm can be seen in a person's skin and the flesh below, which appears dough-like and lacks tone. This can sometimes be seen in the face. The complexion will be 'pasty' and the skin slightly loose. There may be a lack of lustre to the skin. The skin and the hair can also be greasy or oily.

There can be a tendency to be slightly overweight or even obese. The person may be stocky and portly without being muscular.

The fingers of a person with chronic Phlegm may be a little too thick and appear to be slightly chubby.

There can be increased growth of body hair.

Phlegm, because it blocks the movement of *xue*, can manifest with a dark, sooty colour around the eyes.

A person with Phlegm can sometimes have a special odour. The odour is difficult to describe precisely, but it is easily recognisable when it has been smelt a couple of times. The smell is heavy and lingers in the air a long time after the person has left the room. It can sometimes smell a bit like a wet leather jacket.

The saliva in the mouth will be thicker and stickier. The person can have a sticky taste or sensation in their mouth.

Phlegm can also manifest with a gravelly voice, a slightly nasal quality to the voice or the need to clear the throat a lot.

The tongue can be swollen or lacking in tone and can have an oily or sticky coating.

The pulse is usually Wiry or Slippery.

Symptoms and signs that are triggered or provoked by perfume, petrol or solvents will be due to Phlegm-Dampness. This is because Phlegm has a heavy and greasy nature. The above substances dissolve and dilute things that are oily and they will dissolve and dilute Phlegm in the body. This will result in the Phlegm that was previously stagnant and embedded in the body's tissues being set in motion and circulating around the body. Although this dilutes the Phlegm, it still has a disrupting and obstructive effect. Phlegm-Dampness can also be provoked by scents and odours that are heavy, such as certain perfumes and flowers such as hyacinths and lilies. Phlegm-Dampness symptoms are also often provoked by weather fronts, especially when there is low pressure, thundery weather and very humid weather. Symptoms that are exacerbated by consuming Phlegm- or Damp-producing food and drinks will, of course, also indicate that there is Phlegm.

Looking through the symptoms and signs can give the impression that we and most of our clients have Phlegm. This is not far from the truth. Both the climate and diet in northern Europe mean that there can be a tendency to develop Phlegm-Dampness, but Phlegm is also something that accumulates throughout life and is often a consequence of most chronic patterns of imbalance. Therefore, the older you get, the more Phlegm will probably have in your body.

Aetiology

Phlegm often arises when Heat condenses body fluids, when Spleen *qi xu* creates Dampness, when there is stagnation of *qi* or *xue* that stagnates the body's fluids or when there is lack of *yang* to transport and transform fluids. Phlegm can also be created by the diet that a person consumes. This could be foods that weaken the Spleen, create Dampness or Heat or have a Phlegm-producing dynamic.

Symptoms and signs

- Fatigue that is worse in the morning
- Difficulty getting going and being mentally absent in the morning
- Increased need for sleep
- Lack of appetite, especially in the morning
- Nausea or vomiting
- Heaviness in the chest
- Cough in the morning, the sputum can be loose or sticky, depending on whether there is Heat present
- Shortness of breath
- Dizziness
- Heaviness in the head
- Blurred vision and dull eyes
- Sleep in the eyes
- Dark, sooty colour around the eyes
- Depression, melancholy
- Mental confusion and difficulty thinking, especially in the morning
- Incoherent speech or talking to themselves

- Difficulty concentrating

- Skin and flesh tissue can lack tone and be 'doughy'

- The skin lacks lustre

- The fingers can be thick and chubby

- Increased growth of body hair

- Tendency to obesity and plumpness

- Symptoms and signs that are triggered or provoked by weather changes and perfume, petrol or solvents

- Symptoms that are provoked by consuming Phlegm-producing foods and drinks

- Numbness

- Greasy or oily skin and hair

- Sticky taste or sensation in the mouth

- Thick saliva or saliva in the mouth

- Mucus in the menstrual blood

- Fibroids and nodules

- Fat nodules under the skin

- Deformed joints

- Heavy, sticky odour

- Repeated need to clear the throat

- Gravelly voice

- Nasal voice

- Swollen tongue, tongue that is limp or has a flabby tone, sticky or greasy tongue coating

- Slippery or Wiry pulse

Key symptoms
Fatigue and mental absence in the mornings, lack of appetite in the morning, sticky sensation in the mouth, symptoms and signs that are triggered or provoked by weather changes, perfume, petrol or solvents.

Treatment principle
Transform and drain Phlegm.

Acupuncture points
Choose from: St 40, St 36, Ren 12, Sp 3, Sp 6, Sp 9, UB 20 and UB 21.

Needle technique
Drain St 40 and Sp 9. Tonify the rest of the points.

Explanation

- St 40 drains Phlegm.

- Sp 9 drains Dampness.

- Sp 3, Sp 6, St 36, Ren 12, UB 20 and UB 21 tonify Spleen *qi* and transform Phlegm.

Herbal formula

- *Er Chen Tang* (Drains and transforms Phlegm)

- *Wen Dan Tang* (Drains and transforms Phlegm-Heat)

- *Qin Qi Hua Tan Tang* (Drains Phlegm-Heat from the Lung)

- *Di Tan Tang* (Transforms and clears Phlegm misting the orifices)

Relevant advice
The relevant advice will depend on which individual patterns have been involved in the creation of Phlegm. Nevertheless, there are some general guidelines that are relevant for all individuals who present with Phlegm imbalances. Diet is very important, and they should avoid foods and beverages that produce Dampness and Phlegm, including dairy products, bananas, sugar, things that taste sweet such as dried fruits, honey, stevia and so on, wheat products, fried food and alcohol. Nuts are interesting in this context, because eating too many nuts creates Phlegm, but eating a small, limited amount of almonds or walnuts can transform Phlegm in the Lung. In general, a person with Phlegm will benefit from eating foods that have a slightly spicy flavour, such as watercress, radishes, turnips, daikon, garlic, pepper, herbs, etc.

It is also important that they do not eat too much at a time and do not eat too late in the evening.

Phlegm can be caused by the following patterns of imbalance

- Spleen *qi xu*

- Lung *qi xu*

- Dampness

- *Yang xu*

- *Yin xu*
- Heat
- Cold
- *Qi* stagnation
- *Xue* stagnation
- Food stagnation

Phlegm can result in the following patterns of imbalance

- Heat
- *Qi* stagnation
- *Xue* stagnation
- Spleen *qi xu*
- Lung *qi xu*

Section 8

DIAGNOSIS ACCORDING TO *ZANGFU* ORGAN PATTERNS

In this diagnostic model, patterns are differentiated in relation to changes in the functioning of the *zangfu* organs. What has elicited these changes can both be external influences, such as climate, diet, emotions and lifestyle, as well as internally generated imbalances, such as Heat, Dampness, *yang xu*, etc., that are affecting the functioning of the organ. When a *zangfu* organ is negatively affected it will manifest symptoms and signs that relate to a disturbance of its physiology, as well as signs and symptoms that relate to the tissues, sense organs, emotions, vital substances, etc. that are influenced by this organ. The diagnosis will be based both on changes in the organ's physiological processes and changes that are manifesting on the exterior of the body, such as changes in the skin colour, sound of the voice, pulse, tongue, etc. *Zangfu* diagnoses are often central to most TCM diagnoses.

Lung imbalances

The Lung has several functions, the most important being that it controls *qi* and respiration. Along with the Kidneys and Spleen, the Lung is responsible for the production of *qi* in the body. *Zong qi*, which is created by the Lung, is the foundation for *zhen qi*. This means that all the organs are dependent on the Lung as well as the Kidneys and the Spleen. If the Lung *qi* is weak, it will affect all other organs of the body.

The Lung is the only *zang* organ that is in direct contact with the world outside of the body. The Lung is in contact with the environment through the upper respiratory tract and through its related tissue, namely the skin. *Wei qi*, which is spread by the Lung, circulates under the skin and is the first aspect of *qi* that is affected when there are invasions of exogenous *xie qi*. This makes the Lung vulnerable to exogenous influences. It is for this reason that the Lung is called the 'sensitive' or the 'delicate' organ.

The aetiology of Lung imbalances

As described above, the Lung is in direct contact with the environment through the respiratory tract, the skin and *wei qi*. This means that exogenous *xie qi* can be a very important aetiological factor in Lung imbalances. Wind is the spearhead that can pierce through *wei qi* and lead other forms of exogenous *xie qi* into the body. *Xie qi* will initially be combated by, but will also block, *wei qi*. Because it is the Lung that spreads *wei qi*, the blockage of *wei qi* will have a stagnating effect on the Lung *qi*. If *xie qi* is not expelled, it can penetrate deeper and affect the Lung more directly.

Wind, Cold, Damp and Heat are the forms of exogenous *xie qi* that we most often meet in the clinic in North-Western Europe. It is important to remember that the Lung is also very vulnerable to Dryness, because it is a *zang* organ that is in direct contact with the air. If the air is dry, it can desiccate the Lung and injure Lung *yin*. Although this has not traditionally been a problem in a maritime climate, it is something that has become more relevant over the years due to the interior environment of modern buildings, especially buildings made of concrete. Furthermore, it may be a problem in very cold regions where the air can be very dry in the winter.

Damp and Phlegm in the Lung can arise when exogenous *xie qi* condenses and congeals *jinye* in the Lung so that it transforms into Phlegm. Chronic Phlegm in the Lung, though, is often the result of an imbalance in the Spleen. There is a Chinese medicine saying: 'Phlegm accumulates in the Lung, but is created in the Spleen.' This is because the Spleen sends *gu qi* up to the upper *jiao*, where the Lung creates *zong qi*. If there is Spleen *qi xu* or if Cold or Damp- and Phlegm-creating foods are excessively consumed, the Damp and Phlegm that are generated will ascend together with the pure *qi* up to the Lung from the middle *jiao*. This has great importance in relation to the treatment strategy when treating Lung Phlegm imbalances.

Food and drinks that create Heat in an organ can also affect the Lung, due to its physical position in the body. The Lung is a 'canopy' that arches across the other organs in the top of the body. If these organs are affected by Heat or if there is Heat generated by one of these organs, the Heat can rise up to the Lung, due to the *yang* nature of Heat.

The spicy flavour is very dynamic and moves from the centre to the periphery. The spicy flavour is therefore used, amongst other things, to 'open to the exterior', i.e. the spicy flavour can induce a sweat. This is fine when *wei qi* is blocked by exogenous *xie qi*, but if the spicy flavour is excessively consumed it will weaken Lung *qi* and Lung *yin*.

Lack of nourishment, such as eating too little or eating food that is of poor quality, can lead to a generalised *qi xu* condition and thereby also Lung *qi xu*.

The Lung inhales air from the environment. This air is known as '*da qi*' or 'great *qi*' in English. This means that the quality of the air that is inhaled is of great importance for the Lung, as Lung *qi* is dependent on whether the air is fresh and pure. This is the reason that people get tired and sleepy in rooms where the air is heavy. Air pollution can also create imbalances in the Lung. This can be seen in allergic reactions, as well as in chronic ailments. Although air pollution does not fall within the traditional Chinese categories of exogenous *xie qi*, it can still be defined in relation to these imbalance categories by analysing how it affects the body. If an allergen or a pollutant creates symptoms and signs, such as those seen in Wind-Heat for example, this allergen or pollutant will be defined as having a Warm nature and will be treated accordingly. In this context, it is appropriate to mention tobacco smoke. This is a form of pollution that many patients will have been exposed to, both voluntarily and involuntarily. Tobacco smoke is warming and drying in its energy. This means that it is likely to injure Lung *yin*, create Heat in the Lung and boil fluids in the Lung so that they congeal into Phlegm. Furthermore, the combination of Heat and Phlegm can lead to the creation of *xue* stagnation and Toxic-Fire in the Lung. *Xue* stagnation, Toxic-Fire and Phlegm in the Lung, are three of the most important precursors to Lung cancer.

The Lung descends and spreads *qi* and *jinye* throughout the body. When there is an inhalation, the chest opens and *qi* is sent downwards and outwards. Poor posture can impede this function. If a person sits or stands in a stooped way with a sunken chest, this will burden the Lung, because it has to use more force to spread *qi* out from the chest.

The Lung is emotionally affected by sorrow, melancholy and worry. These emotions encompass many other and more nuanced emotions, but common to many of these is that they debilitate and bind Lung *qi*. Therefore, emotions such as a powerful, prolonged or unprocessed grief, worry or speculation can weaken Lung *qi* and stagnate *qi* in the chest.

The Lung cooperates closely with several of the other *zang* organs, as well as its partner organ, the Large Intestine. There are, therefore, often combined patterns when there is a chronic Lung imbalance. The Lung and Liver are both involved in spreading *qi* and thereby also *xue* through the body. Disturbances of these organs' *qi* can therefore affect one and the other. Furthermore, Liver Fire can invade the Lung. The Heart and the Lung have a very close relationship, in terms of their physical location, and especially in relation to *zong qi* and moving *xue* through the channels and vessels. The Kidneys, Urinary Bladder and Lung cooperate in relation to fluid physiology, and Lung *yin* is nourished and moistened by Kidney *yin*. Furthermore, Lung *qi* is grasped by Kidney *yang*. The Spleen, Stomach and Lung are closely involved in the transformation and transportation of *qi* and *jinye*. Finally, the Lung and the Large Intestine's relationship is seen not only in that Lung *qi xu* can lead to constipation, but also in that constipation can disrupt the Lung's sinking function, leading to difficulty in breathing.

Lung imbalance pattern's pathology

If exogenous *xie qi* invades the body, *wei qi* is the first aspect or level to be attacked. *Wei qi* is controlled and spread by the Lung. This means that when *wei qi* is disturbed in its activity and movement, Lung *qi* is also disturbed. This can lead to the Lung not descending and spreading *qi* as it should. Lung *qi* will then accumulate and eventually become rebellious and ascend upwards. This rebellious Lung *qi* can manifest as coughing and sneezing. The Lung also spreads *jinye* throughout the body. When Lung *qi* is impaired it can no longer spread these fluids, which will then accumulate in the Lung and form thin Phlegm. When Lung *qi* becomes rebellious, this will force the thin Phlegm up to the nose, resulting in an exudation of thin, clear, watery mucus as a consequence. The stagnated fluids and thin Phlegm will also be driven up to the face by the rebellious Lung *qi* and can give a slight puffiness to the face. This puffiness is often apparent in the area around the eyes. The disturbance of the Lung's ability to transform and spread fluids can be so extreme that as well as there being oedema and thin, watery sputum in the Lung, there can be problems with urination because the Lung is not sending fluids down to the Urinary Bladder.

If Heat is present in the Lung because Wind-Heat has invaded the Lung, exogenous *xie qi* has penetrated down to the *qi* level or Heat has been transmitted to the Lung from another organ, the fluids in the Lung can be condensed by the Heat. This will result in the fluids becoming thicker and sticky. If the Heat is mild, the Phlegm will be viscous and white. If the Heat is more intense, the Phlegm will be yellowish or greenish. The Heat can be so intense that it causes vessels in the Lung to rupture. If this is the case, there will be blood in the sputum. *Shi* Heat will also cause the upward movement of the rebellious *qi* to be more powerful. This will mean that the cough will be louder and barking. Heat can ascend to the nose, throat and eyes and cause these to become red and irritated.

When there are invasions of exogenous *xie qi*, *wei qi* will be blocked, as described above. When *qi* stagnates, pain arises. In this situation there will be aches and stiffness in the muscles and joints. Because *wei qi* circulates in the *taiyang* aspect and because Wind tends to invade the upper parts of the body, the soreness and stiffness will be most pronounced in the neck and shoulders where the *taiyang* channels traverse. The blockage of *qi* in the *taiyang* channels can also result in there being a headache. As well as protecting the body against invasions of exogenous *xie qi*, *wei qi* warms the skin. If *wei qi* is blocked, especially by exogenous Cold, *wei qi* will not be able to warm the skin, even though there is sufficient heat in the body itself. This will manifest with the characteristic symptom of a person freezing and not being able to get warm, even though they pack themselves into clothes and under blankets. This is in contrast to *yang qi xu* where the person cannot generate enough warmth in the body and is very sensitive to the cold, but if they put on sufficient warm clothing they will not feel cold. The inability to warm the skin when there are invasions of exogenous *xie qi* will manifest with a pronounced aversion to Cold. This is most marked when there is Wind-Cold and less so when there are invasions of Wind-Heat. When *wei qi* is weak, as is typically the case when a person is Lung *qi xu*, the person will be vulnerable to invasions of exogenous *xie qi* and Wind. This will mean that they have an aversion to drafts in particular and to cold in general. They will also suffer from frequent colds and other respiratory disorders.

The Lung controls the pores in the skin via its relationship to *wei qi*. When *wei qi* is blocked by exogenous Cold, it will not be able to open the pores. It is actually through the pores that *wei qi* should expel the exogenous *xie qi*. This means that one of the key symptoms of an invasion of Wind-Cold is that the person does not sweat. Conversely, if there is Lung *qi xu* and *wei qi* is thereby weak, the pores in the skin will not be controlled and the person will sweat spontaneously or on light exertion.

Invasions of exogenous *xie qi* take place in the exterior aspect of the body. This is reflected in the pulse, which will be Superficial. As an invasion of exogenous *xie qi* is an acute condition, there will not normally be major changes in the tongue presentation.

The Lung is very sensitive to Dryness. This can be exogenous Dryness or Dryness that arises when there is *yin xu*. Dryness arises when there is *yin xu* because *jinye* is an aspect of *yin*. If the Lung become desiccated, its *qi* mechanism will become disrupted and Lung *qi* will become rebellious. This will manifest with a dry, ticklish cough, with no sputum or only small amounts of thick, rubbery sputum that is difficult to expectorate. When there are *yin xu* conditions, the cough will also be weak, due to the lack of *qi*. In these situations, the cough will be worse in the evening and at night or when the person speaks. Dryness will also be seen in the fact that the skin can be dry. The voice will often be hoarse and the throat will feel dry.

Shi Heat coughs are explosive and loud. This is because there is an accumulation of *xie qi* in the Lung and because Heat has an ascending nature. This means that there is a more powerful and more dynamic, ascending movement of rebellious *qi* in the Lung. At the same time, Heat condenses *jinye* in the Lung so it turns into Phlegm. This will manifest as sputum that is usually sticky, yellow or green, but it can also be white, thick and viscous. The cough will usually be worse in the morning because Phlegm will have accumulated and stagnated in the Lung during the night. The Phlegm will often be difficult to expectorate because the sputum is so thick and sticky, even though it is copious. A smoker's cough is a typical example of this type of cough.

Both *xu* and *shi* Heat can agitate *xue* so much that the vessels in the Lung rupture, which produces bloody sputum.

Damp-Phlegm or Phlegm-Cold will also disrupt the *qi* mechanism in the Lung and result in a cough. The sputum here will be thinner and more fluid. This type of sputum will be easy to expectorate.

If the Lung is blocked by Phlegm-Fluids, which is a very watery form of Phlegm, there will be very thin, watery sputum that is easily expectorated. There will also be wheezing. The sputum will be so thin that the person will find it difficult to lie flat on their back, as they will quickly feel suffocated. They will also vomit thin, frothy mucus when they cough.

If the Lung is too weak to send *qi* downwards, *qi* will eventually become rebellious and rise upwards. This will manifest with a weak cough, because the deficiency of *qi* will mean that there is not much force behind it.

The Lung descends and spreads *qi*. If this *qi* mechanism is disrupted, the person will be breathless or they will have superficial, shallow respiration. They can also have a stuffy, distended or oppressed sensation in the chest. There will, however, be differences in how and when these symptoms are experienced, depending upon whether it is a *xu* or *shi* condition. When there are *xu* conditions, the Lung will lack the strength to be able to descend and spread *qi*. This will mean that the person quickly becomes breathless, even on light exertion. When there is Lung *qi* or Phlegm stagnation, they will also be breathless, but it will feel as if there is something that is blocking their breathing. When *qi* stagnates in the chest, it can be hard to inhale fully and it will feel as if there is a strap or an elastic band around the chest, making it difficult for them to inhale deeply. When there is Phlegm stagnation, it will feel as

397

if there is a heavy weight, like a rock, that is lying on top of their chest. They will, therefore, find it difficult to inhale deeply and get enough air into the chest.

The voice is created by *zong qi* and is thereby affected by the state of the Lung. If there is Lung *qi xu*, the person's voice will be weak. They will often be disinclined to talk. This is not the same as when there is Heart *qi xu*. When there is Heart *qi xu*, their taciturnity is due to shyness, rather than talking requiring an effort. Lung *yin xu* can cause the voice to be low or weak. The voice will also sound dry or hoarse when there is Lung *yin xu*. When there is Phlegm-Heat, the voice can be loud but also gravelly or hoarse.

Because the Lung is fundamentally involved in the production of *qi*, a key symptom of Lung *qi xu* is fatigue. There can also be a pale face because the weakness of *qi* will result in less *xue* circulating in the skin of the face. When there are Cold conditions, the face will be a brighter white that is almost shiny rather than just lacking colour as it does when there is Lung *qi xu*. When there are Heat conditions, the face can be red either only on the cheekbones, as is seen when there is Lung *yin xu*, or the entire face can be red or ruddy when there are *shi* Heat conditions. Heat will also make the person thirsty because it consumes and injures fluids.

There is a close relationship between the Lung and its partner organ, the Large Intestine. This is seen in the process of defecation. The Large Intestine is dependent on the Lung sending *qi* downwards to expel the stool out of the body. If there is Lung *qi xu*, the person will have difficulty defecating. They will feel exhausted and they will often sweat afterwards. They will often feel that the defecation was incomplete.

The Lung resonates with the emotions of sorrow and melancholy. These emotions will affect the Lung *qi*. At the same time, if the Lung is *qi xu*, the person can also experience an underlying or pervasive sense of sorrow and melancholy.

General symptoms and signs of a Lung imbalance

- Cough

- Runny or blocked nose

- Shortness of breath

- Sweating disturbances

- Fatigue

- Chest oppression

Shi patterns

Invasion of Wind-Cold in the Lung

An invasion of Wind-Cold is an acute pattern that does not usually last for extended periods of time, the Wind-Cold either being quickly expelled from the body or transforming into Heat and penetrating deeper into the body. It is nevertheless important to diagnose and treat this condition correctly.

Furthermore, it is important to remember that it is th.
a pattern of imbalance. If a person manifests with sympton.
there is Wind-Cold. This is relevant, for example, in the diagn.
other allergic reactions.

Aetiology
There will be a powerful *xie qi* that has been potent enough to pierce .
qi. The invasion can arise if the person has been exposed to climatic W.   .d,
but it can also arise after exposure to artificial air-conditioning. Furtherm. .c, some
allergens and pollutants can also provoke a Wind-Cold pattern of imbalance.

There may be an underlying *wei qi xu*, which means that *xie qi* does not require
the same strength to be able to penetrate the body's defences.

Symptoms and signs

- Acute headache

- Stiffness in the neck and upper back

- Joint pain

- Skin and muscle aches

- Aversion to cold and wind

- Lack of sweating in a *shi* condition and perspiration that does not relieve the
  symptoms when there is *wei qi xu*

- Possibly a slight fever

- Coughing

- Sneezing

- Slight breathlessness

- Itchy throat

- The person will pack themselves into warm clothing

- Stooped posture

- Thin, white, moist coating on the tongue

- Superficial and Tight pulse

Key symptoms
Sore, aching muscles and joints, aversion to cold, Superficial and Tight pulse.

Treatment principle
Open to the exterior, expel Wind and Cold, activate *wei qi*.

cture points
oose from: Lu 7, LI 4, GB 20, UB 10, UB 12, UB 62 and SI 3.

Needle technique
Draining. Vacuum cups on UB 12 or *gua sha* on the upper back is recommended.

Explanation

- Lu 7 and LI 4 regulate the Lung's function of descending and spreading, activate *wei qi* and expel Wind and Cold.

- GB 20, UB 10 and UB 12 expel Wind and activate *wei qi*.

- SI 3 and UB 62 expel exogenous *xie qi* from the *taiyang* aspect.

Herbal formula

- *Ma Huang Tang* (Expels Wind-Cold)

- *Chuan Xiong Cha Tiao Tang* (Expels Wind-Cold and relieves headache)

- *Gui Zhi Tang* (Expels Wind-Cold and harmonises *wei* and *ying qi*)

Relevant advice
When there are invasions of Wind-Cold, it is advisable to consume beverages that are hot and spicy to open the exterior and expel *xie qi*. This could be, for example, ginger, garlic, whisky, brandy or chilli. Fasting is also advisable or only eating soup, such as onion soup. There are two reasons for this. First, when temporarily fasting *qi* will not be used to transform food and therefore can be used to combat the invading *xie qi*. Second, some sources say that the downward movement of food and *qi* in the Stomach can draw the exogenous *xie qi* inwards from the surface.

Similarly, the sour flavour should be avoided due to its astringent or centripetal dynamic. Vitamin C, lemon and other things that are very sour should not be consumed during an invasion of exogenous *xie* Cold, as they will draw the *xie* Cold inwards whilst closing the pores in the skin, thereby preventing the Cold from being expelled again. This also means that antibiotics are not recommended at this stage, as they are cold and drain downward.

Invasion of Wind-Cold can be caused by the following pattern of imbalance

- Lung *qi xu*

Invasion of Wind-Cold can result in the following patterns of imbalance

- Wind-Heat

- Phlegm-Heat in the Lung

- Phlegm-Fluid in the Lung

- Lung Heat

- *Yangming* Heat

- *Shaoyang* disorders

Invasion of Wind-Heat

Like an invasion of Wind-Cold, an invasion of Wind-Heat is usually an acute pattern. Whilst an invasion of Wind-Cold will often, but certainly not always, arise from climatic influences such as Cold or drafts, an invasion of Wind-Heat can be caused by exposure to climatic influences and also by infectious pathogens, such as bacteria and viruses. Where Wind-Cold invades the body via *wei qi* in the skin, Wind-Heat can also invade the body via the mucous membranes in the nose and mouth. Again, allergens and other influences from the outside of the body can give rise to a Wind-Heat reaction and, as described earlier, it is the symptoms and signs that define the pattern.

Aetiology

Exposure to climatic factors or to bacteria, viruses, allergens and so on that have a Wind-Heat dynamic. There may be an underlying Lung *qi xu*, which makes it easier for exogenous *xie qi* to invade the body.

Symptoms and signs

- Cough

- Sore throat, the throat is red and there are possibly swollen tonsils

- Blocked nose or sinuses

- Sticky, yellowish mucus

- Headache

- Sweats easily

- Fever[21]

- Thirst

- Aversion to cold (not as pronounced as it is when there is Wind-Cold)

- The nose or the area around the nose may be red

- The forehead may feel warm when palpated

- The eyes may be red or irritated

- The tongue can be slightly red on the front third and have a thin yellow coating

- Rapid, Superficial pulse especially in the right *cun* position

Key symptoms
Fever, aversion to cold, Rapid and Superficial pulse.

Treatment principle
Expel Wind-Heat, activate *wei qi*, regulate Lung *qi*.

Acupuncture points
Choose from: Lu 7, LI 4, SJ 5, LI 11, UB 12, Du 14 and GB 20.

Needle technique
Draining. Vacuum cups can be used on UB 12 or *gua sha* on the upper back.

Explanation

- Lu 7 and LI 4 regulate the Lung's function of descending and spreading. They enable *wei qi* and expel Wind and Heat.

- GB 20, SJ 5 and UB 12 expel Wind and activate *wei qi*.

- LI 11 and Du 14 expel Heat.

Herbal formula

- *Yin Qiao San* (Expels Wind-Heat)

Relevant advice
When there is an acute invasion of exogenous *xie qi* in the exterior, it is advisable to consume beverages that are cooling and spicy, such as mint, chamomile, chrysanthemum or elderflower, to open the exterior and expel Wind-Heat. Fasting is also advisable. Fasting temporarily means that *qi* will not be used to transform food and can therefore be used to combat the invading *xie qi*. Furthermore, some sources are also of the opinion that the downward movement of food and *qi* in the Stomach created by eating food can draw the exogenous *xie qi* inwards from the surface.

Similarly, the sour flavour should be avoided due to its astringent or centripetal dynamic. Vitamin C, lemon and other things that are very sour should not be consumed during an invasion of exogenous *xie* Cold, as they will draw the *xie* Cold inwards whilst closing the pores in the skin, thereby preventing the Cold from being expelled again. This also means that antibiotics are not recommended at this stage, as they are cold and drain downward.

Invasion of Wind-Heat can be caused by the following pattern of imbalance

- Lung *qi xu*

Invasion of Wind-Heat can result in the following patterns of imbalance

- Wind-Heat

- Phlegm-Heat in the Lung

- Lung Heat

- *Yangming* Heat

- *Shaoyang* disorders

Invasion of Wind-Water

This is also an acute pattern. The difference between this pattern and an Invasion of Wind-Cold is that exogenous *xie qi* has blocked *wei qi* and the Lung's ability to spread and transform fluids. This will be apparent in the oedema and the disruption of urination. The urination will be scanty, because the Lung is not sending impure fluids down to the Urinary Bladder.

Aetiology
Exposure to climatic influences such as Wind, Cold and Damp.

Symptoms and signs

- Facial oedema

- Puffy eyes

- Scanty urination

- Aversion to wind, cold and dampness

- Breathlessness

- Cough

- Puffy and shiny face

- Greasy, white tongue coating

- Superficial and Slippery pulse

Key symptoms
Facial oedema, aversion to cold, Superficial and Slippery pulse.

Treatment principle
Expel Wind, Damp and Cold, activate *wei qi*, open the water passages, regulate Lung *qi*.

Acupuncture points
Choose from: Lu 7, LI 4, LI 6, GB 20, UB 12, UB 62, SI 3, Ren 9 and Sp 9.

Needle technique
Draining.

Explanation

- Lu 7 and LI 4 regulate the descent and spreading function of the Lung. They activate *wei qi* and expel Wind, Damp and Cold.

- SI 3 and UB 62 expel exogenous *xie qi* from the *taiyang* aspect.

- GB 20 and UB 12 expel Wind and activate *wei qi*.

- LI 6 and Ren 9 regulate the water passages.

- Sp 9 drains Damp.

Herbal formula

- *Xiao Qing Long Tang* (Expels Wind-Cold and transforms Phlegm-Fluids)

Relevant advice
When there are invasions of Wind-Water it is advisable to fast and consume spicy, hot (both energetically and in their temperature) beverages to induce a sweat. This could, for example, be a hot whisky toddy with ginger or a ginger and garlic infusion. It will be particularly beneficial to use the skin of the ginger in these infusions when there is acute oedema and urinary blockage due to an invasion of Wind-Cold.

Invasions of Wind-Water can be caused by the following pattern of imbalance

- Lung *qi xu*

Invasion of Wind-Water can result in the following patterns of imbalance

- Phlegm-Fluids in the Lung

- Damp and Phlegm

Damp-Phlegm in the Lung

This pattern can occur when the *qi* mechanism of the Lung is disrupted by repeated invasions of exogenous *xie qi* or when the Spleen is not able to separate the pure from the impure, resulting in Damp and Phlegm arising in the middle *jiao*, which are then sent upwards along with the pure *gu qi* to the Lung. According to Chinese medicine, 'Phlegm is created by the Spleen and stored in the Lung.' This means that in chronic conditions when there is Damp-Phlegm in the Lung, the Spleen must also be tonified at the same time.

The presence of Damp-Phlegm will block the Spleen and Lung's *qi* mechanism and this blockage can then lead to the further formation of Phlegm-Dampness.

Aetiology

Damp-Phlegm in the Lung can arise from invasions of exogenous *xie qi* that disrupt Lung *qi* and block the transformation and spreading of fluids.

As described above, Spleen *qi xu* and Dampness are often at the root of an accumulation of Damp-Phlegm in the Lung. The Spleen is particularly burdened when the diet contains a lot of food that has a Cold or Damp energy or when the food and liquids consumed are physically cold. The pattern can also arise through the use of medicines that are energetically Cold.

Posture can be a contributing factor. If the person has a tendency to sit stooped or slumped, it will block both the Spleen and Lung *qi* mechanisms. This will lead to the formation of Damp-Phlegm in the middle *jiao* and the accumulation of Damp-Phlegm in the upper *jiao*.

Emotional factors such as sorrow or worry can affect the Lung and Spleen and this may be a contributing factor to this pattern.

Symptoms and signs

- Chronic cough with loose sputum

- Copious amounts of white sputum that is easy to expectorate

- Chest oppression

- There may be a sensation as if there is a heavy weight or a rock lying on the chest

- Slight breathlessness

- The symptoms are worse in the supine position

- Mucus or sputum in the throat

- The voice may be slightly gravelly or nasal

- Wheezing

- Dull, pale complexion

- The flesh in the face may be slightly doughy

- The flesh in general may be doughy

- Difficulty thinking clearly

- Tiredness and heaviness of the body

- Nausea or poor appetite

- Swollen tongue with white greasy coating

- Floating and Slippery pulse

Key symptoms
Cough with loose sputum, sputum is clear or white in colour, greasy white tongue coating.

Treatment principle
Transform and drain Dampness and Phlegm, regulate Lung *qi*.

Acupuncture points
Choose from: Lu 1, Lu 5, Lu 7, Lu 9, Ren 12, Ren 17, Ren 22, Sp 3, Sp 9, St 36, St 40, UB 13 and UB 20.

Needle technique
Tonifying on Lu 7, Lu 9, Sp 3, St 36, UB 20 and Ren 12. Draining or even technique on the other points. Moxa is applicable to Sp 3, St 36 and UB 20.

Explanation

- Lu 1, Lu 5, Lu 9, UB 13 and Ren 22 drain Phlegm and regulate Lung *qi*.

- Lu 7 and Ren 17 regulate Lung *qi*.

- Ren 12, UB 20, Sp 3 and St 36 tonify Spleen *qi* and transform Damp and Phlegm.

- Sp 9 drains Damp.

- St 40 drains Phlegm and opens the chest.

Herbal formula

- *San Zi Yang Qin Tang* (Descends Lung *qi* and resolves Phlegm)

- *Er Chen Tang* (Drains and transforms Damp-Phlegm)

- *Ling Gan Wu Wei Jiang Xin Tang* (Resolves Phlegm and fluids and tonifies Spleen *yang*)

Relevant advice
It is essential that a person with Damp-Phlegm in the Lung avoids consuming Damp- and Phlegm-creating foods and beverages, especially dairy products, sweets, wheat, sugar, bananas, avocados, dried fruit and so on. They should also avoid consuming cold, refrigerated foods, foods that have not been cooked and eating irregularly, as these will strain the Spleen and can lead to the formation of Dampness and Phlegm.

Correct body posture and exercise are important in order to avoid stagnation and blockage of the *qi* mechanism in the upper and middle *jiao*.

Repeated invasions of exogenous *xie qi* can be a contributing factor in the formation of Dampness and Phlegm in the Lung. This means that the patient must make sure that they are suitably dressed and do not expose themselves to invasions of exogenous *xie qi*.

Beating the chest and the upper back with a loose fist or a wooden spoon will help to activate *qi* in the chest and thereby help to resolve stagnations of Phlegm and Dampness.

Damp-Phlegm in the Lung can be caused by the following patterns of imbalance

- Lung *qi xu*

- Spleen *qi xu*

- Spleen *yang xu*

- Kidney *yang xu*

- Invasions of exogenous *xie qi* in the Lung

Damp-Phlegm in the Lung can result in the following patterns of imbalance

- Phlegm-Heat in the Lung

- Lung *qi xu*

- Spleen *qi xu*

Phlegm-Fluids blocking the Lung

The difference between this pattern and the previous one is that the Phlegm here is very watery, not thick as in the previous pattern. This pattern often has its root in a condition of *yang xu*.

Aetiology

Old age and long-term physical overexertion. The ingestion of Cold and Phlegm-creating foods can lead to the formation of this pattern. Repeated invasions of Wind, Cold and Damp can also be contributing factors.

Symptoms and signs

- Cough with thin, watery and frothy sputum

- Wheezing

- Shortness of breath

- Superficial breathing

- Vomiting of white foamy mucus

- Aversion to cold

- Fuzzy sensation in the head

- Chest oppression

- Dizziness

- Lack of thirst

- Scanty but pale urine

- The patient feels suffocated if they lie on their back and must sit upright in bed

- Bright white complexion

- Wet and white tongue coating

- Slippery, Wiry or Soggy pulse

Key symptoms
Cough with watery sputum, cannot lie flat on their back, chest oppression.

Treatment principle
Drain Phlegm-Fluids from the Lung, regulate Lung *qi*, tonify *yang*.

Acupuncture points
Choose from: Lu 5, Lu 9, Ren 9, Ren 12, Ren 17, UB 13, UB 23, UB 43, Kid 7, St 36, St 40, Sp 3 and Sp 9.

Needle technique
Tonifying, moxa is recommended, except on Lu 5, St 40, Sp 9 and Ren 9, which should be drained.

Explanation

- Lu 9, UB 13 and UB 43 tonify Lung *qi* and transform Phlegm.

- Lu 5 drains Phlegm from the Lung and regulates Lung *qi*.

- Ren 9, Sp 9 and St 40 drain Phlegm and fluids.

- Ren 17 regulates Lung *qi*.

- Ren 12, St 36 and Sp 3 tonify Spleen *yang* and transform Phlegm and fluids.

- Kid 7 and UB 23 tonify Kidney *yang* and transform fluids.

Herbal formula

- *Xiao Qing Long Tang* (Transforms Phlegm-Fluids in the Lung)

- *Su Zi Jiang Qi Tang* (Regulates Lung *qi*, transforms Phlegm and tonifies Kidney *yang*)

Relevant advice

The advice that was given for Damp-Phlegm in the Lung is relevant here. The person should also try to strengthen their *yang qi*. They can do this by consuming foods that are warm and avoiding cooling foods and cooling of the body in general.

Phlegm-Fluids blocking the Lung can be caused by the following patterns of imbalance

- Lung *yang xu*

- Spleen *yang xu*

- Kidney *yang xu*

- Invasions of Wind, Cold and Damp

Phlegm-Fluids blocking the Lung can result in the following patterns of imbalance

- Lung *yang xu*

- Spleen *yang xu*

- Kidney *yang xu*

- Kidney *yang xu*, Water overflowing to the Heart

Phlegm-Heat in the Lung

Phlegm-Heat in the Lung will often have developed from other Lung imbalances. Damp-Phlegm in the Lung can easily transform into Phlegm-Heat in the Lung, because either there is already Heat in the Lung or the stagnation that is created by the Phlegm will generate Heat in the Lung. The difference between this pattern and Damp-Phlegm in the Lung is that there are Heat symptoms and signs.

The pattern of Lung Heat can also be a precursor of this, because Heat in the Lung can condense fluids and thereby lead to the formation of Phlegm-Heat.

It is important to note that Phlegm-Heat does not necessarily manifest with yellow or green sputum. The sputum can be white, thick and sticky. This is due to the Heat condensing fluids so that they become thick and sticky. When the Phlegm is yellow or greenish, the Heat will be more intense.

Aetiology

Phlegm-Heat in the Lung can arise if there is an excessive consumption of foods that create Phlegm or Heat. Examples of these foods are dairy products, sweets, sugar, alcohol, wheat, fried food, too much red meat, spicy food and chocolate. Very cold food and beverages or raw vegetables can be involved indirectly, because they can weaken Spleen *yang* and *qi* thereby leading to the creation of Dampness and Phlegm.

Invasions of exogenous *xie qi* can create both Phlegm and Heat in the Lung.

Air pollution, especially tobacco smoke, can be an important aetiological factor. This is seen in many people who smoke tobacco developing a 'smoker's cough', having difficulty breathing and easily becoming breathless.

Stress can create Heat in the body, and emotions such as anger, irritation and frustration can generate Heat in the Liver that then rises to the Lung and creates Heat here.

Symptoms and signs

- Loud and noisy cough with sticky sputum, the cough is worst in the mornings
- Yellow or greenish sputum, the sputum can also sometimes be white, but it will not be watery or loose, the sputum is thick and sticky
- There may be blood in the sputum
- Chest oppression
- Sensation of a heavy weight or a stone lying on the chest
- Shallow breathing or wheezing
- Shortness of breath or slight breathlessness
- Gravelly or hoarse voice
- Phlegm in the throat
- Thirst
- Foggy or heavy sensation in the head, especially in the morning
- Aversion to heat
- Red face
- Red lips
- Red tongue with thick, sticky, yellowish coating
- Fast, Slippery and Full pulse, especially in the right *guan* position

Key symptoms

Loud, productive cough, shortness of breathing, yellow sticky tongue coating.

Treatment principle
Drain Phlegm and Heat from the Lung, regulate Lung *qi*.

Acupuncture points
Choose from: Lu 1, Lu 5, Lu 7, Lu 10, LI 11, UB 13, Du 12, Du 14, St 40 and Ren 17.

Needle technique
Draining.

Explanation

- Lu 1, Lu 5 and UB 13 regulate Lung *qi* and drain Phlegm and Heat from the Lung.

- Lu 10 and Du 12 drain Heat from the Lung and regulate Lung *qi*.

- Lu 7 and Ren 17 regulate Lung *qi*.

- LI 11 and Du 14 drain Heat.

- St 40 transforms Phlegm and opens the chest.

Herbal formula

- *Qing Qi Hua Tan Tang* (Drains Phlegm-Heat from the Lung and regulates Lung *qi*)

Relevant advice
A person with Phlegm-Heat in the Lung should avoid consuming food that creates Heat, Dampness and Phlegm. This includes dairy products, sweets, dried fruits, sugar, alcohol, fried food, chilli, pepper, garlic, chocolate and lamb.

Smoking should be discouraged and the person should avoid other forms of air pollution.

Phlegm-Heat in the Lung can be caused by the following patterns of imbalance

- Damp-Phlegm in the Lung

- Lung Heat

- Spleen *qi xu*

- Invasions of exogenous *xie qi*

Phlegm-Heat in the Lung can result in the following patterns of imbalance

- Spleen *qi xu*

- *Xue* stagnation

- Lung *yin xu*

Lung Heat

This can be both an acute and a chronic pattern. Acute patterns will be caused by invasions of exogenous *xie qi* that have penetrated into the '*qi* level'.

Aetiology

Invasions of exogenous *xie qi* can directly generate Heat in the Lung. Smoking or exposure to tobacco smoke can also create Lung Heat.

Ingestion of food and beverages that are Hot can indirectly create Heat in the Lung.

Symptoms and signs

- Barking cough

- Dry throat

- Painful lungs

- Flaring nostrils

- Rapid and shallow breathing

- Shortness of breath

- Bitter or metallic taste in the mouth

- Intense thirst

- Aversion to heat

- Red face

- Red lips

- Dark and scanty urine

- Constipation

- Restlessness

- Red tongue with yellow coating

- Rapid and Full or Rapid and Superficial pulse, especially in the right *cun* position

Key symptoms

Barking cough, thirst, aversion to heat, red tongue and Rapid pulse.

Treatment principle
Drain Heat from the Lung, regulate Lung *qi*.

Acupuncture points
Choose from: Lu 1, Lu 5, Lu 7, Lu 10, LI 11, UB 13, Du 12, Du 14 and Ren 17.

Needle technique
Draining. Bleed Du 14.

Explanation

- Lu 1, Lu 5, Lu 10, Du 12 and UB 13 regulate Lung *qi* and drain Heat from the Lung.

- Lu 7 and Ren 17 regulate Lung *qi*.

- LI 11 and Du 14 drain Heat.

Herbal formula

- *Xie Bai San* (Drains Heat from the Lung)

Relevant advice
A person with Heat in the Lung should avoid eating or drinking anything that has a hot dynamic.
Tobacco smoke is hot and drying so the person should avoid exposure to this.

Lung Heat can be caused by the following patterns of imbalance

- Invasions of exogenous *xie qi*

- Liver Fire

Lung Heat can result in the following patterns of imbalance

- Phlegm-Heat in the Lung

- Lung *yin xu*

Xu patterns

Lung *qi xu*

Lung *qi xu* can arise independently, but will most often be seen together with Spleen *qi xu* or Heart *qi xu*. When there is Lung and Spleen *qi xu*, there will be a general condition of *qi xu* characterised by a poor production of *qi*, whereas Lung and Heart *qi xu* will be a more emotional imbalance with sorrow, grief and a lack of joy as the dominant symptoms.

Aetiology

Lung *qi xu* can be caused by a respiratory illness in childhood.

Poor posture, where the person sits slumped forwards, can inhibit the *qi* mechanism of the Lung and thereby weaken Lung *qi* over time. Furthermore, a lack of exercise will mean that the *qi* mechanism in the upper *jiao* is not supported by physical movement.

Lung *qi* can be weakened by repeated invasions of exogenous *xie qi* or if there has been an invasion of exogenous *xie qi* that has not been properly resolved, for example through the use of antibiotics.

The Lung is emotionally affected by grief, sorrow and melancholy. If the person has experienced repeated or excessive grief and sorrow, especially if the grief remains unresolved, it will bind and weaken Lung *qi*.

Lung *qi* is weakened by excessive talking or singing. This is because *zong qi* is used to create the volume of the voice. This means that teachers, lecturers, actors and singers can have a tendency to develop Lung *qi xu*.

Excessive consumption of spicy food can spread and expel Lung *qi* through the pores in the skin.

Finally, as described above, Lung *qi* can be an aspect of other *qi xu* patterns and therefore their aetiology can also be involved in the generation of Lung *qi xu*.

Symptoms and signs

- Fatigue

- Shortness of breath

- Shallow breathing

- Slight cough, possibly with watery sputum

- Weak voice

- Reluctance to speak

- Sweating spontaneously or sweating on slight exertion

- Aversion to cold and drafts

- Frequent colds and respiratory infections

- Bright white complexion

- The person may have a slouching posture, the chest can appear sunken and the shoulders slumped forwards

- Pale or normal-coloured tongue, the front third of the tongue can be depressed and hollow

- Deep and Weak pulse, especially in the right *cun* position

Key symptoms
Fatigue, slight breathlessness, spontaneous sweating, weak voice and a Weak pulse.

Treatment principle
Tonify Lung *qi*.

Acupuncture points
Choose from: Lu 1, Lu 7, Lu 9, UB 13, St 36, Sp 3, Ren 6 and Ren 17.

Needle technique
Tonifying. Moxa can be used.

Explanation

- Lu 1, Lu 7, Lu 9 and UB 13 tonify Lung *qi* and regulate Lung *qi*.

- St 36, Sp 3 and Ren 6 tonify *qi* in general.

- Ren 17 tonifies *zong qi* and regulates *qi* in the upper *jiao*.

Herbal formula

- *Bu Fei Tang* (Tonifies Lung *qi*)

- *Bu Zhong Yi Qi Tang* (Tonifies Lung and Spleen *qi*)

Relevant advice
Because this is a *qi xu* condition, the advice given for Spleen *qi xu* and Kidney *qi xu* will also apply here, i.e. the person should eat a diet that is nutritious but does not weaken the Spleen. Food that is white in colour will often have an affinity with the Lung and can be used to focus *qi* tonics on the Lung. The person should avoid consuming food that is very spicy because it will spread and thereby weaken Lung *qi*. Foods that particularly strengthen Lung *qi* are: turnips, daikon, radishes, parsnips, parsley, onion, garlic, tofu, herring, walnuts, almonds, cauliflower, dates, figs, duck, tuna, grapes, thyme and ginseng. Ginger tea will also be beneficial.

It is important that a person who is Lung *qi xu* does not strain their voice, because it will weaken the Lung *qi*.

A person with Lung *qi xu* must ensure that they get enough rest and do not overexert themselves. However, light exercise and movement will be beneficial because they will open the chest and support the Lung's *qi* mechanism. Going for walks in fresh air will be salutary because the person will get some light exercise and the fresh air will nourish the Lung. Yoga and qi gong often utilise breathing exercises that have a beneficial effect on Lung *qi*. It is important that a person who is Lung *qi xu* is conscious of their posture, because a slouched, slumped posture and sunken chest will strain Lung *qi*.

If there is an emotional aspect to the Lung *qi xu*, the person should try to resolve these issues.

Lung *qi xu* can be caused by the following patterns of imbalance

- Spleen *qi xu*
- Heart *qi xu*
- Kidney *qi xu*
- Invasions of exogenous *xie qi*
- Stagnation of *qi* in the upper *jiao*

Lung *qi xu* can result in the following patterns of imbalance

- Spleen *qi xu*
- Heart *qi xu*
- Kidney *qi xu*
- *Wei qi xu*
- Lung *yin xu*
- Stagnation of *qi* in the upper *jiao*
- Phlegm in the Lung

Lung *yang xu*

Lung *yang xu* is seen when the Lung lacks the necessary activating heat to perform its activities and functions. It is a pattern that is not commonly described or listed in many textbooks, its symptoms and signs being attributed to the combined pattern of Lung *qi xu* and Kidney *yang xu*. Treating these two patterns simultaneously will also provide excellent results.

Aetiology

Lung *yang xu* will arise from the same aetiological factors that cause Lung *qi xu*. Factors such as repeated invasions of exogenous Cold, overexertion and consuming cooling foods will often be involved.

Symptoms and signs

- Fatigue
- Breathlessness
- Shallow breathing
- Slight cough, possibly with watery sputum
- Oedema in the face, arms and hands

- Frequent urination with copious amounts of pale urine

- Cold limbs

- The person is sensitive to Cold and has an aversion to draughts

- The person wears warmer clothes than is normal for the season or room temperature

- Weak voice

- Sunken chest or slumped posture

- Reluctance to speak

- Pale lips

- Spontaneous sweating

- Frequent colds and respiratory infections

- Bright white complexion

- Pale or normal coloured tongue with a wet coating, the front third of the tongue may be hollow

- Deep and Weak pulse, especially in the right *cun* position

Key symptoms
Aversion to cold, fatigue, breathlessness, spontaneous sweating and a pale and wet tongue.

Treatment principle
Tonify and warm Lung *yang*.

Acupuncture points
Choose from: Lu 1, Lu 9, UB 13, Du 4, Du 12, Ren 6, Ren 17, Kid 3 and Kid 7.

Needle technique
Tonifying. Moxa is recommended on Lu 9, Du 4, Du 12 and Kid 3.

Explanation

- Lu 1, Lu 9, Du 12 and UB 13 tonify Lung *qi* and Lung *yang*.

- Kid 3, Du 4 and Ren 6 tonify *yang* in general.

- Ren 17 tonifies *zong qi*.

- Kid 7 tonifies Kidney *yang*, thereby helping to transform and transport fluids in the body.

Herbal formula

- *Gan Jiang Ling Zhu Tang* (Warms and tonifies Spleen and Lung *yang*)

- *Li Zhong Tang* (Warms *yang* in the middle *jiao*, but three of the four herbs also directly tonify the Lung)

- *Su Zi Jiang Qi Tang* (Regulates Lung *qi* and tonifies Kidney *yang*)

Relevant advice

In addition to the advice that is relevant for Lung *qi xu*, it is important that the person keeps warm, avoids consuming cold foods and drinks (both physically and energetically cold) and does not overexert themselves physically. They will benefit from getting enough rest and drinking ginger tea.

Lung *yang xu* can be caused by the following patterns of imbalance

- Kidney *yang xu*

- Lung *qi xu*

Lung *yang xu* can result in the following patterns of imbalance

- Kidney *yang xu*

- Phlegm-Cold in the Lung

- Damp-Phlegm in the Lung

- Phlegm-Fluids in the Lung

Lung *yin xu*

Unlike most *yin xu* patterns of imbalance, Lung *yin xu* can be both a chronic and a more acute and temporary condition. This is because the Lung is a 'delicate' *zang* organ and its *yin* aspect can be easily injured by Dryness and Heat, for example when there is a *shi* Heat condition in the Lung, such as an invasion of exogenous *xie* Heat.

Aetiology

Lung *yin* can be injured by exogenous *xie qi*, for example Dryness and Heat. Exogenous Dryness can invade the Lung when a person lives or works in a building with a dry interior climate, such as buildings made of concrete. Lung *yin* will also be injured by a condition of *shi* Heat in the Lung. Tobacco smoke is both Hot and Dry. This means that smoking can be an aetiological factor in chronic Lung *yin xu* patterns.

Prolonged use of the voice can strain Lung *yin*, which can be a problem for teachers and singers.

Lung *yin* will eventually be adversely affected by the same emotions that are involved in the generation of Lung *qi xu*, i.e. sorrow and melancholy.

Old age will weaken Kidney *yin* and can therefore be a factor.

Symptoms and signs

- Dry, ticklish cough that is worse at night or on exertion
- Sticky or rubbery sputum in the Lung that is difficult to expectorate, there can even be blood in the sputum
- Insomnia
- Dry mouth, nose and throat
- Weak or hoarse voice
- Dry skin
- Fatigue
- Thin body, with a thin or sunken chest
- Thin, dry tongue with a lack of coating on the front third
- Superficial and Fine pulse, especially in the right *cun* position

If there is Lung *yin xu* Heat, there may also be:

- malar flush
- hot sensation in the palms of the hands, soles of the feet and chest
- night sweats
- slight fever or sensation of heat in the evening and at night
- red, thin and dry tongue
- Rapid, Fine and possibly Superficial pulse.

Key symptoms
Dry, ticklish cough, hoarse voice, dry throat.

Treatment principle
Nourish Lung *yin*, possibly control *xu* Heat.

Acupuncture points
Choose from: Lu 7, Lu 9, UB 13, UB 43, Sp 6, Kid 6 and Ren 4.

- If there is *xu* Heat, add: Lu 10.

Needle technique
Tonifying, except Lu 10, which should be drained.

Explanation

- Lu 9, UB 13 and UB 43 nourish Lung *yin*.

- Sp 6 and Ren 4 nourish *yin* in general.

- Kid 6 combined with Lu 7 opens *ren mai* and *yin qiao mai* and thereby nourishes *yin*, regulates Lung *yin* and opens communication between the Kidneys and the Lung.

- Lu 10 drains *xu* Heat from the Lung.

Herbal formula

- *Sha Shen Mai Men Dong Tang* (Nourishes Kidney and Lung *yin*)

- *Bai He Gu Jin Tang* (Nourishes Lung *yin* and drains Phlegm-Heat from the Lung)

Relevant advice

A person who is Lung *yin xu* should not smoke and they should avoid others' smoke. Living and working in concrete buildings or other buildings or places where there is a dry climate will injure their Lung *yin*. Like a person who is Lung *qi xu*, a person who is Lung *yin xu* must be careful not to overuse their voice. In general, they should avoid straining their body and make sure that they get enough rest and sleep.

Strong and spicy foods promote sweating and expel *qi*. The excessive consumption of spicy food should therefore be avoided. This is especially important if there is *xu* Heat, as many spices are also Hot. Milk nourishes Lung *yin*, but caution should be exercised as it also can create Phlegm in the Lung.

Lung *yin xu* can be caused by the following patterns of imbalance

- Lung Dryness

- Lung *qi xu*

- Kidney *yin xu*

- Stomach *yin xu*

- Lung Heat

- Phlegm-Heat in the Lung

Lung *yin xu* can result in the following pattern of imbalance

- Kidney *yin xu*

Lung Dryness

The Lung is the only *zang* organ that is in direct contact with the environment outside of the body. This means that the Lung is very vulnerable to Dryness, because it will injure the fluids and the *yin* aspect of the Lung. In many parts of China the climate in the autumn is very dry. This resonates with autumn being the season where Lung imbalances can be more common.[22]

Lung Dryness is a precursor of Lung *yin xu*, the difference being that in Lung Dryness there are signs of Dryness without there being decidedly *yin xu* symptoms.

Aetiology

In North-Western Europe, Lung Dryness is not specifically related to a particular season; it can be experienced in northern Scandinavia and mountainous areas in the winter when the air is extremely dry and when it is very cold. Dryness can be experienced throughout the year in buildings with very dry indoor climates, especially in concrete buildings with central heating.

Symptoms and signs

- Dry cough, possibly with dry and sticky sputum
- There may be pain in the chest if the cough is bad
- Dry mouth
- Dry throat
- Dry skin
- Thirst
- Hoarseness
- Dry tongue
- The pulse can be Rapid or it may be Fine in the right *cun* position

Key symptoms

Dry, ticklish cough, hoarseness, dry mouth, dry nose and dry throat.

Treatment principle

Moisten the Lung and nourish Lung *yin*.

Acupuncture points

Choose from: Lu 7, Lu 9, Ren 4, Ren 12, Kid 6 and St 36.

Needle technique

Tonifying.

Explanation

- Lu 9 nourishes Lung *yin* and *jinye*.

- Ren 4 and Kid 6 nourish *yin* and *jinye*.

- Ren 12 and St 36 nourish Stomach *yin*, which is the root of *jinye*.

- Lu 7 and Kid 6 open *ren mai* and *yin qiao mai*, nourish *yin* and thereby lead *yin* fluids up to the Lung, mouth, throat and respiratory passages.

Herbal formula

- *Bai He Gu Jin Tang* (Nourishes Lung *yin*, cools the Lung and resolves dry Phlegm in the Lung)

Relevant advice
The advice given for patterns of Lung *yin xu* will also be relevant when there is Lung Dryness, especially the advice not to stay in places where the air is very dry.

Lung Dryness can be caused by the following patterns of imbalance

- Stomach *yin xu*

- Lung *yin xu*

Lung Dryness can result in the following pattern of imbalance

- Lung *yin xu*

Combined patterns

Lung and Spleen *qi xu*
The Lung and the Spleen create *zong qi* and *zhen qi* together. It is very common to see a combined pattern of Lung and Spleen *qi xu* where a deficiency in one of the organs will be instrumental in the creation of a deficiency in the other due to the resultant decrease in the production of *qi*.

Aetiology
As described above, this pattern will usually start with a deficiency of either Lung or Spleen *qi*, while the decreased production of *qi* and the resultant *qi* deficiency will lead to a weakening of the other organ. Otherwise, the aetiology is the same as that seen in Lung *qi xu* and Spleen *qi xu*.

Lung *qi* is weakened by poor posture, repeated or unresolved invasions of exogenous *xie qi* and excessive use of the voice.

Spleen *qi xu* arises from consuming foods and beverages that are cold in nature and temperature, raw foods and foods and beverages that create Dampness. Eating too much at a time or too quickly will also strain the Spleen. Excessive consumption of spicy food can weaken Lung *qi*.

The Lung and Spleen are affected by emotions such as sorrow, melancholy, worry and pondering.

Prolonged illness and overexertion of the body can weaken both Lung and Spleen *qi*, because they then have to work harder to replenish the *qi*.

Symptoms and signs

- Fatigue

- Loose stools

- Pale face

- Disinclination to speak and the voice lacks strength

- Breathlessness

- Bloating after meals

- Feeling drowsy after meals

- Poor appetite or no appetite in the morning

- Slight cough, possibly with watery sputum

- Spontaneous sweating or sweating on light activity

- Weakness or fatigue in the limbs

- Craving for sweets

- Aversion to cold and draughts

- The person looks tired and worn out

- Possibly slumped posture

- Excessively worries and speculates about things, difficulty letting go of thoughts

- Pale, swollen tongue, possibly with teeth marks on the sides or near the front, the tongue can also be sunken in the front third

- Weak pulse, especially in the right *guan* and *cun* positions

Key symptoms

Fatigue, loose stools, breathlessness, pale complexion, pale tongue with teeth marks and a weak pulse.

Treatment principle

Tonify Lung and Spleen *qi*.

Acupuncture points
Choose from: Lu 9, St 36, Sp 3, Sp 6, Ren 12, UB 13, UB 20 and UB 21.

Needle technique
Tonifying. Moxa can be used.

Explanation

- Lu 9 and UB 13 tonify Lung *qi*.

- St 36, Sp 3, Sp 6, Ren 12, UB 20 and UB 21 tonify Spleen *qi*.

Herbal formula

- *Bu Zhong Yi Qi Tang* (Tonifies Lung and Spleen *qi*)

Relevant advice
The advice given for both Lung *qi xu* and Spleen *qi xu* is relevant here.

The diet should ideally consist of foods that are slightly warming (both in temperature and energetically) and prepared (boiled, steamed, stir-fried, baked and so on), and the diet should not be Damp and Phlegm creating.

Fresh air and breathing exercises will strengthen the Lung.

Both the Lung and Spleen will benefit from good posture and gentle exercise, because they will support their *qi* mechanisms.

Lung and Spleen *qi xu* can be caused by the following patterns of imbalance

- Lung *qi xu*

- Spleen *qi xu*

- Invasions of exogenous *xie qi*

Lung and Spleen *qi xu* can result in the following patterns of imbalance

- *Wei qi xu*

- Spleen *yang xu*

- Spleen *qi* sinking

- Spleen *qi* not holding *xue* inside the vessels

- Stagnation of *qi* in the upper *jiao*

- Heart *qi xu*

- Phlegm-Damp in the Lung

- Food stagnation

- Damp

- Phlegm

- *Xue xu*

- Lung *qi xu*

- Heart *qi xu*

Lung and Heart *qi xu*

There is a very close relationship and cooperation between the Lung and the Heart. They support each other in their functions. Lung *qi* is used to circulate *xue* around the body and in the Heart. Heart *xue* nourishes the Lung. Furthermore, both the Lung and Heart are dependent on *zong qi*. Therefore, a *qi xu* condition of either *zong qi*, Lung *qi* or Heart *qi* can result in this pattern.

Aetiology

There are two main aetiological factors in this pattern. One of the main elements will often be emotional imbalances that affect the Lung and Heart. Grief, sorrow and melancholy will have a negative impact on both organs. Grief, sorrow and melancholy bind and stagnate Lung *qi* and thereby *zong qi*. The stagnation of *zong qi* will have a negative effect on both the Lung and the Heart. The Heart will also be weakened by the lack of joy that is characteristic for these emotional conditions.

Overexertion generally exhausts *qi*. When *qi xu* arises, all organs in the body can become *qi xu*. Excessive talking and overusing the voice directly burden *zong qi*. People whose work requires them to use their voice a lot, such as singers, actors and teachers, can have a tendency to develop this pattern.

Symptoms and signs

- Palpitations

- Shortness of breath

- Weak cough

- Insomnia

- Being easily startled

- Tendency to have sorrow and melancholy

- Lack of joy

- Depression

- Poor posture

- Hollow chest

- Fatigue

- Low or weak voice

- Reluctance to speak

- Fatigue in their voice

- Pale face

- Spontaneous sweating

- Pale tongue

- Weak pulse in both *cun* positions

Key symptoms
Weak voice, disinclination to talk, sunken chest, palpitations, Weak *cun* pulse on both sides.

Treatment principle
Tonify Lung and Heart *qi*.

Acupuncture points
Choose from: Ren 17, Lu 7, Lu 9, He 5, He 7, Pe 6, UB 13 and UB 15.

Needle technique
Tonifying. Moxa can be used.

Explanation

- Ren 17 tonifies *zong qi*.

- Lu 7, Lu 9 and UB 13 tonify Lung *qi*.

- He 5, He 7, Pe 6 and UB 15 tonify Heart *qi* and calm *shen*.

Herbal formula

- *Sheng Mai San* (Tonifies Lung *qi* and Heart *qi*)

- *Bu Zhong Yi Qi Tang* (Tonifies Lung *qi* and *zong qi*)

Relevant advice
Lung and Heart *qi xu* should be tonified on both the emotional and physical plane.

On the emotional level, it is important that the person tries to address the emotional issues that may be present. It is also important that the person cultivates joy in their lives. They can try to spend some time each day doing something that gives them pleasure or sit and meditate on something that they associate with joy.

Lung *qi* can be tonified through the use of breathing exercises, and fresh air in general will be salutary. Tonifying *qi* will also benefit the patient, which could be done through the diet, fresh air and by getting enough rest and avoiding overexertion.

Light exercise, yoga, tai ji and qi gong will be beneficial, as they will help to circulate *qi* in the upper *jiao*. This is important, as the deficiency of Heart and Lung *qi* can also lead to a stagnation of *qi* in the upper *jiao*.

Lung and Heart *qi xu* can be caused by the following patterns of imbalance

- Lung *qi xu*
- Heart *qi xu*
- Spleen *qi xu*
- Kidney *qi xu*
- Gall bladder *qi xu*
- Heart *qi* stagnation
- *Xue xu*
- Damp-Phlegm

Lung and Heart *qi xu* can result in the following patterns of imbalance

- Heart *yang xu*
- Heart *qi* stagnation
- Lung *qi xu*
- Spleen *qi xu*
- Damp-Phlegm
- Heart *yin xu*
- Heart *xue xu*

Liver Fire invades the Lung
See Liver imbalance patterns (page 590).

Large Intestine imbalance
The Large Intestine's functions are to receive the dross that remains after the food and beverages that have been ingested have been transformed by the other organs, extract the last usable fluids out of the remaining contents and send the untransformed residues out of the body as faeces. These functions are influenced by the Spleen, the Stomach and the Kidneys. This means that the Large Intestine is the stage in which these activities take place, but a disruption of these functions will usually be addressed by treating an imbalance in the Spleen, Stomach or Kidneys whilst using points that directly influence the Large Intestine.

The Large Intestine can also be affected negatively without other organs being involved. This is seen when there has been an invasion of exogenous *xie qi*. Invasions of exogenous Cold or Damp will disrupt the movement of *qi* in the Large Intestine. The blockage of *qi* will manifest with pain. An invasion of exogenous Cold can result in constipation, because Cold can block the movement of the stool through the Large Intestine, but also the blockage of *qi* can mean that exogenous Cold and Damp prevent the Large Intestine from extracting fluids from the stool and in these situations the invasion of Cold will manifest with watery diarrhoea.

Damp-Heat can also invade the Large Intestine. This will also cause diarrhoea, but the diarrhoea in this situation will be sticky and odorous. The Heat will scorch the mucous membranes, resulting in a stinging, burning sensation in the rectum. The Heat can be so intense that *xue* is agitated to the extent that the walls of the Large Intestine rupture. This can result in blood in the stools.

When *qi* stagnates in the Large Intestine, it will result in abdominal bloating, distension or pain. In a purely *shi* condition, the pain will be alleviated by the passing of stools, because the stagnation will thereby be alleviated. *Qi* in the Large Intestine can stagnate when there are invasions of exogenous *xie qi* or when stagnated Liver *qi* invades the Large Intestine, interfering with the downward movement of *qi* in the Large Intestine. *Xue* stagnation in the Large Intestine can also block the free downward movement of *qi* and stools.

There is close cooperation between the Large Intestine and its partner organ, the Lung. The Large Intestine is dependent on Lung *qi* being sent down so that it can force the faeces out of the rectum. Lung *qi xu* can manifest with there not being enough force to expel the stool from the body. In these situations, the person will typically feel very exhausted after they have passed the stool and will possibly sweat spontaneously afterwards.

A condition of *yang xu* can lead to Cold more easily invading the Large Intestine and to there not being enough *yang qi* to move the stool through the Large Intestine. This will result in constipation.

General symptoms and signs of a Large Intestine imbalance

- Constipation or diarrhoea

- Abdominal pain

- Abdominal bloating

Shi patterns
Damp-Heat in the Large Intestine

This pattern will frequently be combined with other patterns – usually Spleen and Stomach imbalances. What makes this pattern difficult to treat is that there is *yin* and *yang xie qi*, which are bound together. Exactly how the symptom picture manifests will depend on which of these two elements is dominant.

Damp-Heat in the Large Intestine will be defined in an Eight Principle diagnosis as an 'interior *shi* Heat' condition. The pattern can arise when there has been an invasion of exogenous Damp-Heat, for example after the ingestion of spoiled food. In this case, it will be a purely *shi* condition. Usually, however, the pattern arises in the background of Spleen *qi xu* or Spleen *yang xu* conditions. This makes the situation more complicated because there will be a condition of interior *shi* Heat that has arisen from a concurrent 'interior *xu*' condition (which will in fact be an interior *xu* Cold condition if there is Spleen *yang xu*). This requires a treatment strategy that will require both tonification and draining at different stages, as well as the clearing of Heat and the warming of *yang*.

Aetiology
Diet plays a significant role in this pattern. The diet itself can directly create Damp-Heat when foods that create Dampness and Heat are excessively consumed. The diet can, though, also create imbalances in the middle *jiao* that subsequently result in the generation of Dampness. The Damp stagnation will then begin to 'ferment' or combine with an existing Heat condition. This is typical when Liver *qi* stagnation Heat is also present.

The pattern can also occur after consumption of foods that are spoiled or infected, for example with salmonella.

Summer-Heat can directly invade the Large Intestine and create Damp-Heat.

Worry and speculation can bind and weaken Spleen *qi*, leading to the generation of Dampness, which can then transform into Damp-Heat. Anger and frustration can create Heat or stagnate Liver *qi*, which then invades the Spleen.

Symptoms and signs
- Diarrhoea
- Frequent defecations
- The stools are sticky, malodorous and possibly contain blood or mucus
- The defecation may be explosive
- Stinging or burning sensation in the rectum
- Abdominal pain that is not alleviated by the passing of stools
- Abdominal bloating
- The abdomen feels tight or distended when palpated
- Dark and scanty urine
- Thirst with no desire to drink
- Fever, feeling feverish or an aversion to heat
- Heaviness in the body

- Red tongue with a yellow sticky coating on the root, possibly with elevated, red papillae on the root

- Rapid and Slippery pulse, possibly Full in both *chi* positions

Key symptoms
Diarrhoea with strong-smelling, sticky stools, yellowish sticky tongue coating.

Treatment principle
Drain Damp-Heat from the Large Intestine.

Acupuncture points
Choose from: LI 11, St 25, St 27, St 37, St 44, Sp 6, Sp 9, UB 22 and UB 25.

- If there is blood in the stool, add: Sp 1 and Sp 10.

Needle technique
Draining. Moxa on Sp 1.

Explanation

- LI 11, St 25, St 27, St 37, St 44 and UB 25 drain Damp-Heat from the Large Intestine.

- Sp 6, Sp 9 and UB 22 drain Dampness.

- Sp 1 and Sp 10 stop bleeding.

Herbal formula

- *Huang Lian Jie Du Tang* (Drains Damp-Heat from the Intestines)

- *Bai Tou Weng Wan* (Drains Damp-Heat from the Intestines)

- *Shao Yao Tang* (Drains Damp-Heat from the Intestines)

Relevant advice
If there is Damp-Heat in the Large Intestine, the patient should avoid consuming food and beverages that create Dampness, Heat or Damp-Heat. Deep-fried foods, alcohol, hot spices, dairy products and sugar should be avoided completely.

Damp-Heat in the Large Intestine can be caused by the following patterns of imbalance

- Spleen *qi xu*

- Spleen *yang xu*

- Food stagnation

- Invasions of *xie qi*

Damp-Heat in the Large Intestine can result in the following patterns of imbalance

- Spleen *qi xu*

- *Qi* stagnation in the Intestines

- *Xue* stagnation

Heat in the Large Intestine

Unlike the previous pattern, this will always be a pure *shi* pattern of imbalance. All the symptoms and signs will be due to the presence of Heat, which desiccates and scorches.

Aetiology

Heat can arise in the Large Intestine due to prolonged intake of substances that have a Hot energy, such as lamb, alcohol, chilli and fried food.

Exogenous *xie qi* can penetrate into the *yangming* aspect and generate Heat in the Large Intestine.

Symptoms and signs

- Constipation with dry stool

- Burning sensation in the rectum

- Bloated abdomen that resists pressure when palpated

- Thirst

- If the condition is due exogenous *xie qi* that has sunk to the *qi* level, there will be profuse sweating

- Fever or aversion to heat

- Scanty, dark urine

- Dry mouth

- Red tongue with dry yellow, brown or black coating

- Rapid and Full pulse

Key symptoms

Constipation with dry stools, yellow, brown or black tongue coating.

Treatment principle

Drain Heat from the Large Intestine.

Acupuncture points

Choose from: LI 11, St 25, St 27, St 37, St 44, SJ 6 and UB 25.

Needle technique
Draining.

Explanation

- LI 11, St 25, St 27, St 37, St 44 and UB 25 drain Heat from the Large Intestine.

Herbal formula

- *Ma Zi Ren Wan* (Drains Heat and moistens the Large Intestine)

Relevant advice
If there is Heat in the Large Intestine, the patient should avoid consuming food and beverages that are hot in their energy. Spinach, bean sprouts, bananas, cucumber, fig, rhubarb and bamboo shoots all drain Heat from the Large Intestine and are therefore beneficial. Spinach is especially salutary because it moistens and lubricates the Large Intestine. This will enable the stool to move more easily through the Large Intestine.

Heat in the Large Intestine can be caused by the following patterns of imbalance

- Stomach Heat

- Invasions of exogenous *xie qi*

Heat in the Large Intestine can result in the following patterns of imbalance

- *Yin xu*

- *Ying* level Heat

- *Xue* stagnation

Damp-Cold in the Large Intestine

This is, again, a purely *shi* pattern of imbalance, but there may well be an underlying *yang xu* condition which means that the body has difficultly protecting itself from exogenous Cold or transforming Cold foods that have been ingested.

Aetiology
The Large Intestine can be directly invaded by exogenous *xie qi* through the skin if the person, for example, has had cold, wet clothes on the abdomen after they have been swimming or has sat on the cold, wet earth.

Damp-Cold can also result from consuming cold or cooling food and beverages (both thermally or energetically cold).

Symptoms and signs

- Diarrhoea

- Stools are watery and explosive

- Borborygmi

- Cramping pain in the abdomen

- The skin of the abdomen feels cold when palpated

- The abdomen can feel tense or distended when palpated

- Aversion to cold

- Thick, white and wet tongue coating

- Slow and possibly Tight pulse

Key symptoms
Watery diarrhoea, cramping pain in the intestines.

Treatment principle
Drain Damp and Cold from the Large Intestine.

Acupuncture points
Choose from: St 25, St 36, St 37, Ren 8, Sp 4, Sp 9 and UB 25.

Needle technique
Draining, except for Ren 8, which should be treated with moxa. Moxa or a moxa box on the abdomen is recommended.

Explanation

- St 25, St 36, St 37, Sp 4, Sp 9 and UB 25 drain the Damp-Cold from the Large Intestine.

- Ren 8 with moxa expels Dampness and Cold from the Large Intestine.

Herbal formula

- *Huo Xiang Zheng Qi Tang* (Expels Wind, Damp and Cold and regulates *qi* in the Intestines)

- *San Wu Bei Ji Wan* (Vigorously purges Cold downwards)

Relevant advice
When there is Damp-Cold in the Large Intestine, the person should avoid consuming food and beverages that are cold or have a cooling energy. They will benefit from

drinking ginger tea or other spices that are warming and spreading in their dynamic. It is important to keep the abdomen warm and dry.

Damp-Cold in the Large Intestine can be caused by the following pattern of imbalance

- Spleen *yang xu*

Damp-Cold in the Large Intestine can result in the following pattern of imbalance

- *Yang xu*

Xu patterns

Large Intestine Dryness

This imbalance pattern is a precursor of *yin xu*. There will be perceptible symptoms and signs of Dryness but not decidedly *yin xu* symptoms and signs.

Aetiology
This pattern may be due to exogenous Dryness, which can arise when a person is living in a very hot and dry climate. The most common cause, though, is irregular diet. Eating late, eating whilst working, irregular eating or eating whilst stressed will all injure the Stomach *yin*, which is the root of *jinye*.

Symptoms and signs

- Dry, pellet-like stools
- Difficulty defecating
- Dry mouth and throat
- Dry skin
- Thin body
- Thin and dry tongue
- Fine pulse

Key symptoms
Dry, pellet-like stools.

Treatment principle
Moisten and activate the Large Intestine.

Acupuncture points
Choose from: St 25, St 36, St 37, Sp 6, Sp 15, Ren 4, Ren 12, Kid 6 and UB 25.

Needle technique
Tonifying.

Explanation

- St 25, St 37, Sp 15 and UB 25 moisten and activate the Large Intestine.

- St 36 and Ren 12 nourish Stomach *yin*.

- Sp 6, Kid 6 and Ren 4 nourish *yin*.

Herbal formula

- *Run Chang Wan* (Moistens and lubricates the Large Intestine)

Relevant advice
When there is Large Intestine Dryness, the patient should eat foods that are moistening and lubricating. This includes foods that are rich in oils and fats, such as nuts and seeds, as well as vegetable oil. Prunes, bananas, avocados, spinach and plants from the cabbage family moisten and lubricate the Intestines.

Large Intestine Dryness can be caused by the following pattern of imbalance

- Stomach *yin xu*

Large Intestine Dryness can result in the following pattern of imbalance

- *Yin xu*

Large Intestine *xu* Cold

The difference between this pattern and Damp-Cold in the Large Intestine is that this is a *xu* pattern of imbalance, whereas Damp-Cold in the Large Intestine is a *shi* pattern. The stools here will not be explosive and there will not be cramping pain in the abdomen. Instead, the pain will be a dull, nagging pain that is not alleviated by the passing of a stool.

Aetiology
This pattern can arise due to excessive consumption of food and beverages that are cold or cooling (both energetically and thermally) or from prolonged exposure to climatic cold and repeated invasions of exogenous Damp-Cold. Physical and sexual overexertion can also be involved in the generation of the underlying *yang xu* patterns.

Symptoms and signs

- Unformed stools

- Dull, nagging or gnawing pain in the abdomen that is not alleviated by the passing of stools

- Borborygmi

- Frequent urination with a large quantity of pale urine

- The skin of the abdomen feels cold on palpation

- The abdomen does not feel tense or hard on palpation

- Cold limbs

- Pale tongue

- Deep and Weak pulse

Key symptoms
Unformed stools. Deep and Weak pulse.

Treatment principle
Warm and tonify the Large Intestine.

Acupuncture points
Choose from: St 25, St 36, St 37, Sp 4, Ren 6 and UB 25.

Needle technique
Tonifying. Moxa is recommended.

Explanation

- St 25, St 36, St 37, Sp 4 and UB 25 warm and tonify the Large Intestine.

- Ren 6 warms and tonifies *yang*.

Herbal formula

- *Fu Zi Li Zhong Tang* (Warms and tonifies Spleen *yang*)

- *Zhen Ren Yang Zang Tang* (Warms and tonifies Kidney and Spleen *yang*, astringes and transforms Dampness from the Intestines)

Relevant advice
When there is Large Intestine *xu* Cold, it is beneficial to consume warm, cooked or baked food. It is advisable to eat foods that have a warming energy. Baked root vegetables, stews, soups, lamb, chicken, onions and leeks are all examples of warming food. Spices that will be beneficial are cloves, cinnamon, ginger, basil, rosemary and nutmeg.

Large Intestine *xu* Cold can be caused by the following patterns of imbalance

- Spleen *yang xu*

- Kidney *yang xu*

Large Intestine *xu* Cold can result in the following pattern of imbalance

- Damp-Cold in the Large Intestine

Stomach imbalances

The Stomach is the only *fu* organ directly involved in the production of *qi*, *xue* and *jinye*. This is because the Stomach is the organ that receives the food and liquids that have been ingested through the mouth that will be transformed into *gu qi* and *jinye*. The Stomach 'rots and ripens' the ingested food, preparing it for transformation by the Spleen. The Stomach also has the important function of sending *qi* downwards together with the impure residues that are left behind after the transformation process. The Spleen simultaneously sends its *qi* upwards together with the pure *qi* that has been extracted from the food and liquids. This *qi* mechanism is of great importance, not only for the movement of *qi* in the middle *jiao*, but also throughout the body, as all communication passes thorough this area. It is crucial for the entire production of vital substances in the body that the Stomach is capable of emptying and filling. If the Stomach cannot send the impure residue down to the Small Intestine, there will not be any space in the Stomach to receive new food or liquids. This will initially be experienced as a loss of appetite, nausea, bloating or a stuffed sensation in the epigastric region, because the Stomach and Spleen *qi ji* has ground to a halt and there is an accumulation of *qi*, food and liquids in the area. When the *qi* stagnates, it can also manifest with pain and discomfort. If the *qi* from the Stomach cannot descend, it can become rebellious and ascend upwards. This can give symptoms such as hiccups and belching, but it can also become so rebellious that there is vomiting. If the rebellious *qi* has arisen from a *xu* pattern, there will not be the explosive vomiting that characterises *shi* patterns, but instead involuntary regurgitation.

Disruption and disturbance of the Stomach's descending function can also manifest as constipation. This is because the Intestines are partly dependent on the downward dynamic of the Stomach *qi.*

If the disruption of the Stomach and Spleen *qi ji* becomes a chronic condition. It will affect the production of the vital substances and this will manifest with symptoms such as fatigue and weakness of the muscles.

Because the Stomach is the organ that receives all the food and liquids that have been consumed, what has been ingested will have a significant influence on the Stomach. The Stomach has a preference for moist, damp substances and is damaged by Dryness. This stands in contrast to the Spleen, which abhors Dampness. The Stomach is easily damaged by Heat and has a tendency to develop Heat patterns of imbalance. Again, the Spleen is the opposite. The Spleen is injured and burdened by Cold and prefers warmth. All of this means that the Stomach is harmed by food and beverages that are energetically hot and that its *yin* aspect is easily injured by spicy food, because this is often hot and because the spicy flavour itself can injure *yin*.

If there is an excess of Heat in the Stomach, as there is with Stomach Fire, the food will be 'burnt up' in the Stomach and the person will experience a gnawing or insatiable hunger because the Stomach is constantly empty. The Fire can be so intense that it begins to damage the organ itself. This will be perceived as a searing pain or burning sensation in the Stomach. Due to its inherent *yang* dynamic, Fire ascends upwards. This can cause Stomach *qi* to become rebellious and flow upwards. This will manifest as hiccups, acid reflux, heartburn and belching. Heat tends to make things become odorous, and this, combined with the ascending *qi* from the Heat, can manifest as bad breath.

Stomach *yin xu* Heat will not result in the same intense hunger as when there is Stomach Fire. When *yin xu* creates *xu* Heat, there will be an increased hunger but, unlike when there is Stomach Fire, the person will be quickly satiated. *Yin xu* will not cause the Stomach *qi* to becomes rebellious and there will not be the same burning pain in the abdomen. There can be more of a dull, stinging discomfort in the organ.

Heat will also make the person thirsty. If there is Stomach Fire, there will be an intense thirst with a desire to drink large quantities of cold beverages in large gulps. *Yin xu* Heat will also result in thirst, but in this case there will not be the same need to drink large gulps, more a preference for sipping water. Often there is only a dryness of the mouth and throat when there is Stomach *yin xu*, not because of the Heat but because the Stomach is the root of *yin* fluids. Stomach *yin xu* can therefore lead to dryness throughout the body. The dryness can also manifest with constipation, due to the stools being dry. Stomach Heat, both *xu* and *shi*, can similarly manifest with constipation.

Both *xu* and *shi* Heat can result in bleeding. Stomach Heat can often ascend up to the mouth, which is the sensory organ that is associated with the Earth Phase. The Stomach channel also traverses the gums. This means that bleeding gums and similar problems are often a sign of Stomach Heat and Stomach Fire. This problem can be further complicated if there is a concurrent condition of Spleen *qi xu*. Spleen *qi xu* can result in the Spleen not being able to hold *xue* inside the vessels. In addition to bleeding gums, Stomach Fire can cause blisters and mouth ulcers to form and Stomach Fire can be involved in dental problems such as paradentosis or tooth abscesses.

Despite the fact that the Stomach tends to have Heat and *yin xu* imbalances, it can also be negatively affected by exogenous Cold and cold food. This is because Cold can damage Spleen *yang*, thereby reducing the transformation of food in the Stomach, and also because Cold will stagnate and block Stomach *qi*. This disturbance of the Stomach *qi* will result not only in pain and discomfort in the Stomach, but also in nausea and vomiting. The difference between the vomiting that is experienced when there is Cold and when there is Heat is that vomit resulting from Cold conditions will be watery and contain undigested food matter. This is due to the food and liquid that have been ingested not being transformed due to the Cold. Heat, on the other hand, will manifest with vomit that is sour and sticky in consistency. Vomit resulting from *shi* conditions will usually alleviate nausea or pain and discomfort in the Stomach.

Xu and *shi* Cold in the Stomach will manifest with an attraction to warm food and hot drinks. The person will also have a marked aversion to ingesting anything that is cold in temperature, possibly also things that are energetically cold.

It is not only the energetics of the food consumed that can have an influence on a person, the Stomach is also disturbed by the amount of food eaten and the way it is eaten. Negative eating habits can result in food stagnation. Food stagnation can arise from eating meals too quickly, eating too much food at a time, eating food that is difficult to transform or eating food too late in the evening. The evening is also the *yin* period of the day. If a person eats too much in the evening, there will not be the same resources of *yang qi* available to transform the food. The transformation of the food stops at night. This means that if food is eaten late in the evening, it will tend to lie and rot in the Stomach overnight. In relation to the horary clock, the Stomach and Spleen are at their weakest between 7pm and 11pm, which is why the main meal should be eaten before noon. As well as blocking the *qi* mechanism, food stagnation will generate Dampness and Heat. The stagnation of *qi* will create distension and discomfort in the abdomen. Heat will also rise upwards from the stagnant food, agitating the Heart and *shen*. This, and the discomfort caused by the stagnation, will disturb the sleep and the person will wake frequently during the night, often with a sensation of Heat in the body or sweating profusely.

The Stomach should regularly fill and empty throughout the day. If a person constantly snacks, the Stomach will never have the opportunity to empty completely. This will lead to the stagnation of Stomach *qi* and create Food stagnation. Eating whilst working, driving, on the run and so on will stagnate Stomach *qi* and can lead to the Stomach *qi* becoming rebellious.

Patients with a history of anorexia and bulimia may have problems with their Stomach *qi*, because it has either been weakened by the lack of nourishment or become rebellious due to the repeated vomiting.

The Stomach is affected by the same emotions as the Spleen. Worry, speculation and vexation bind and thereby stagnate Stomach *qi*. Thinking too much and mental strain will also weaken the Stomach *qi*.

Frustration, irritation and unresolved emotions can stagnate Liver *qi*, which can then build up and 'invade' the Stomach, disrupting the descent of Stomach *qi*. Stagnant Liver *qi* can create Heat, which can invade the Stomach and create Heat in the Stomach.

General symptoms and signs of Stomach imbalances

- Pain or discomfort in the Stomach or epigastric region

- Poor or excessive appetite

- Belching, hiccups, or acid reflux

Shi patterns

Stomach Fire

Patterns of Stomach Fire can vary in intensity. There can be mild patterns of Stomach Heat and there can be intense patterns of Stomach Fire.

Aetiology

Like most Stomach and Spleen imbalances, Stomach Fire usually has its roots in dietary imbalances. Consuming food and beverages that have a hot energetic dynamic can create Stomach Fire. Alcohol, too much meat (especially lamb), fried food, grilled food and hot spices are among the most common factors contributing to Stomach Fire. Tobacco can also be factor, as it is Hot and affects both the Lung and the Stomach.

Food stagnation can be a cause of Stomach Fire. Therefore, eating too much at a time, eating too quickly, eating too late in the day and eating food that is difficult to transform can be an aspect of this pattern's aetiology.

Stress, repressed anger, frustration and irritation can generate Liver Fire, which can then invade the Stomach, creating Stomach Fire. Furthermore, prolonged anxiety and worry can stagnate Stomach *qi*, which can eventually generate Stomach Fire.

Symptoms and signs

- Searing, burning epigastric pain
- Insatiable or gnawing hunger
- Intense thirst, with a desire for cold beverages, the person will often drink in large gulps
- Acid reflux
- Constipation
- Nausea
- Vomiting of sour vomit
- Malodorous breath
- Blisters or ulcers in the mouth
- Bleeding gums
- Paradentosis
- Sour or bitter taste in the mouth
- Mental restlessness
- Dark urine

- Dry, parched lips

- The person may seem unsettled and restless

- The person may tend to be ebullient and talk quickly

- Red face

- Aversion to heat

- Redness in the middle of the tongue, with a dry, yellowish or brownish tongue coating

- Rapid and Full pulse, especially in the right *guan* and possibly *cun* positions

Key symptoms
Insatiable hunger, bad breath, thirst, acid reflux and redness in the middle of the tongue.

Treatment principle
Drain Stomach Fire.

Acupuncture points
Choose from: St 21, St 34, St 40, St 44, Ren 12, Ren 13, Sp 6, LI 11 and UB 21.

Needle technique
Draining, except for Sp 6, which should be tonified.

Explanation

- St 21, St 40, St 44, Ren 12, Ren 13 and UB 21 all drain the Stomach Fire and regulate Stomach *qi*.

- LI 11 drains Stomach Fire.

- St 34 drains Stomach Fire and stops bleeding from the gums.

- Sp 6 nourishes and protects Stomach *yin*.

Herbal formula

- *Qing Wei San* (Drains Stomach Fire, especially when it affects the teeth and gums)

- *Huang Lian Jie Du Pian* (Drains Fire from the middle *jiao*)

Relevant advice
When there is Stomach Fire the person should avoid all foods that are hot in their energy. They should eat cooling or neutral foods, especially boiled or steamed vegetables and foods that are moist or glutinous in their consistency, such as porridge.

This will help protect the Stomach's *yin* aspect. The ingestion of umeboshi plums will have a neutralising effect on Stomach Fire and can be used in acute conditions. If food stagnation is involved in the generation of Stomach Fire, it is important that the person follows the dietary advice for this pattern.

Stomach Fire can be caused by the following patterns of imbalance

- Stomach *qi* stagnation

- Liver Fire

- Food stagnation

Stomach Fire can result in the following patterns of imbalance

- Phlegm-heat

- Stomach *yin xu*

- *Xue* stagnation in the Stomach

Stomach *qi* stagnation

Stomach *qi* has a descending dynamic. If Stomach *qi* is disrupted by food stagnation, *xie qi* or imbalances in other organs, the Stomach will not be able to send its *qi* downwards. Initially, the stagnation of Stomach *qi* will cause pain, discomfort and bloating in the abdomen. With time, Stomach *qi* can become rebellious and ascend upwards, with symptoms such as belching, hiccups or vomiting as a consequence.

Aetiology

Eating too quickly, eating whilst stressed, working or eating whilst on the go will stagnate Stomach *qi*. Food, particularly spices, which have an ascendant dynamic, will disrupt the downward dynamic of Stomach *qi*.

Liver *qi* should support the Stomach in sending its *qi* in the correct direction. Stress, irritation, unresolved emotions, anger and so on can stagnate Liver *qi*. This will initially result in the Liver not supporting the descent of Stomach *qi*. Subsequently, Liver *qi* can invade and block the Stomach's *qi* mechanism.

Symptoms and signs

- Discomfort or pain in the Stomach or epigastric region

- Bloating

- The upper abdomen can feel tense or bloated on palpation

- Irritability

- Hiccups, belching or regurgitation

442

- Nausea

- The tongue can be a little red or swollen in the middle

- Wiry pulse on the right *guan* position

Key symptoms
Pain or discomfort in the epigastric region, belching and regurgitation.

Treatment principle
Regulate Stomach *qi*.

Acupuncture points
Choose from: St 21, St 34, St 36, Ren 11, Ren 12, Ren 13, Ren 22, SJ 6, Pe 6 and UB 21.

Needle technique
Draining.

Explanation

- St 21, St 34, St 36, Ren 11, Ren 12 and UB 21 regulate Stomach *qi*.

- Pe 6 and SJ 6 regulate *qi* in the middle *jiao*.

- Ren 13 and Ren 22 descend rebellious Stomach *qi*.

Herbal formula

- *Ban Xia Hou Po Tang* (Regulates Stomach *qi*)

Relevant advice
When there is Stomach *qi* stagnation, it is important that the person eats slowly, doesn't eat too much at a time and doesn't eat constantly. They should chew their food well and avoid foods that are difficult to transform. If stress and emotional frustrations, irritations and anger create Liver *qi* that invades the Stomach, the person should try and resolve these issues.

It is important that the person does not sit still for extended periods of time and that they do not sit in a slumped posture. Walking or stretching after meals is recommended. Physical exercise in general will be beneficial. Stroking downwards with the fingers from Ren 16 to Ren 8 will help Stomach *qi* to descend.

Stomach *qi* stagnation can be caused by the following patterns of imbalance

- Spleen *qi xu*

- Stomach *qi xu*

- Stomach *yin xu*

- Food stagnation

- Liver *qi* stagnation

Stomach *qi* stagnation can result in the following patterns of imbalance

- Food stagnation

- Stomach Fire

- Stomach *yin xu*

- Phlegm-Fire

- Stomach *xue* stagnation

Food stagnation

Food stagnation is often an overlooked aspect of a diagnostic picture, particularly in chronic and complex cases where there are many patterns intertwined with each other. Food stagnation, like Phlegm and *xue* stagnation, is often a cause and consequence of many chronic patterns of imbalance. This is because many patterns of imbalance can directly or indirectly disrupt the Stomach and Spleen's *qi* mechanism. Chronic food stagnation will also, in the long term, directly and indirectly lead to imbalances in many other places in the body. The foundation of food stagnation is often laid as early as the first year of a person's life. This will be the case if there was an improper diet and if the baby was repeatedly fed before the Stomach had been emptied of food.

There will often be vague and subtle signs of food stagnation rather than outright symptoms. Typically, the patient will have a slight sensation of fullness in the belly or bloating for some time after they have eaten, will burp or belch and will have discomfort in the epigastric region.

There can often be a vicious circle where food stagnation causes the creation of Stomach Heat, which results in a gnawing hunger. The person then eats constantly and the Stomach never completely empties, so even more stagnation of food in the Stomach will arise.

Aetiology

Food stagnation arises directly from eating too much at a time, eating too fast, not chewing the food properly, eating too late at night, constant snacking, eating whilst stressed or whilst working, eating whilst sitting in a twisted position and eating food that is difficult to transform.

If the Spleen and Stomach are also *qi xu*, food will not be transformed. If there is Damp and Phlegm, this will weaken the Spleen and block the Stomach and Spleen *qi* mechanism, so that the food stagnates. Liver *qi* stagnation can also disrupt the Stomach and Spleen *qi* mechanism, with food stagnation as a result. *Yang xu* can mean that there is not enough physiological heat to transform the food. *Yin xu* and

Heat can lead to the formation of Phlegm that will then block the Stomach and Spleen's *qi* mechanism.

Symptoms and signs

- Lack of appetite
- A full sensation in the epigastric region
- Epigastric discomfort
- Bad breath
- Belching that often tastes or smells of the food that has been eaten earlier
- Acid reflux
- Vomiting
- Abdominal bloating
- Discomfort when palpating on the upper abdomen
- Bloating and abdominal discomfort that is relieved by vomiting
- Insomnia or dream-disturbed sleep
- Feeling hot at night
- Loose stools or constipation
- The stools smell rotten or of sewage
- Odorous flatulence
- Thick and greasy tongue coating
- Slippery or Wiry pulse, especially in the right *guan* position

Key symptoms
Full sensation or discomfort in the epigastric region, belching that tastes of previously ingested food, thick, greasy tongue coating.

Treatment principle
Dissolve food stagnation, regulate Stomach *qi*.

Acupuncture points
Choose from: St 19, St 21, St 34, St 36, St 44, Sp 4, Ren 12, Ren 13 and Pe 6.

Needle technique
Draining.

Explanation

- St 19, St 21, St 34, St 36, Sp 4, Ren 12 and Ren 13 regulate Stomach *qi* and dissolve food stagnation.

- St 44 dissolves food stagnation, regulates the Stomach *qi* and drains Heat.

- Pe 6 regulates *qi* in the middle *jiao*.

Herbal formula

- *Bao He Wan* (Dissolves Food stagnation)

- *Jian Pi Wan* (Dissolves Food stagnation and tonifies Spleen *qi*)

Relevant advice

It is crucial that a person with food stagnation regulates the way they eat and what they eat. They should not eat too quickly or too much at a time. They should sit upright when eating and chew their food well. They should eat food that is easy to transform and they should not eat too late in the evening. Stroking downwards with the fingers from Ren 16 to Ren 8 will help Stomach *qi* and the ingested food to descend. Walking or stretching after meals is recommended. Physical exercise in general will be beneficial.

Food stagnation can be caused by the following patterns of imbalance

- Spleen *qi xu*

- Stomach *qi xu*

- Spleen *yang xu*

- Stomach *yin xu*

- Stomach *qi* stagnation

- Damp

- Phlegm

- Liver *qi* stagnation

Food stagnation can result in the following patterns of imbalance

- Spleen *qi xu*

- Stomach *qi xu*

- Stomach Fire

- Stomach *yin xu*

- Damp

- Damp-Heat

- Phlegm

- Phlegm-Fire

- Stomach *qi* stagnation

- Liver *qi* stagnation

Invasion of Cold in the Stomach

This will be an acute pattern resulting from climatic, dietary or pharmaceutical influences.

Aetiology

Exogenous Cold can invade the Stomach, either via the mouth or through the skin of the abdomen. If the invasion takes place through the mouth, it will be due to the consumption of food that has a very cold temperature or energy. This could, for example, be ice cream, ice water or other cold beverages, but it could also be due to the consumption of drugs or herbs that have a very cold energy.

Invasions of Cold via the skin will be due to contact with cold climatic influences, particularly if the abdomen is cooled down by wearing wet clothes.

Symptoms and signs

- Acute pain in the abdomen or epigastric region

- Vomiting of clear fluids

- Nausea

- Aversion to cold and cold beverages and food

- Hiccups

- The ingestion of cold substances will aggravate the symptoms

- Desire for warm food or beverages

- Pale urine

- The epigastric region feels cold when palpated

- Pale complexion

- Thick, white tongue coating

- Slow, Tight and Full pulse

Key symptoms

Acute abdominal pain, vomiting of clear fluids, thick and white tongue coating.

Treatment principle
Expel Cold from the Stomach, regulate Stomach *qi*.

Acupuncture points
Choose from: St 21, St 34, Sp 4, Ren 13 and Pe 6.

Needle technique
Draining. Moxa can be used with the needles.

Explanation

- St 21 and Ren 13 expel Cold from the Stomach and regulate Stomach *qi*.

- Sp 4 regulates Stomach *qi*.

- St 34 regulates Stomach *qi* and alleviates pain in the Stomach.

- Pe 6 regulates *qi* in the middle *jiao*.

Herbal formula

- *Da Jian Zhong Tang* (Warms the middle *jiao*, expels Cold, regulates *qi*)

Relevant advice
When there is an invasion of Cold in the Stomach, the person will benefit from eating and drinking food and beverages that have a warming and spicy dynamic and that are thermally hot, such as ginger tea. If the invasion is due to climatic influences or wet clothes, a ginger poultice on the abdomen can help to expel the Cold.

The person should avoid consuming food and beverages that are cold in their temperature and energy.

The upper abdomen should be kept warm and dry.

Invasion of exogenous Cold in the Stomach can be caused by the following patterns of imbalance
This is an acute disorder, therefore there will not usually have been a previous pattern. However, the following patterns can have predisposed the person to an invasion of exogenous Cold:

- Spleen *yang xu*

- Kidney *yang xu*

- *Wei qi xu*

Invasion of exogenous Cold in the Stomach can result in the following patterns of imbalance

- Stomach *qi* stagnation

- Damp

- Stomach *qi xu* and Cold

- *Xue* stagnation in the Stomach

Xue stagnation in the Stomach

This is always a chronic pattern that will have arisen from other Stomach imbalances.

Aetiology

The aetiology will depend on which patterns of imbalance are involved in the generation of *xue* stagnation.

Symptoms and signs

- Sharp, stabbing, piercing gastric pain

- Pain that is worse on palpation

- Pain that is aggravated by eating

- Vomiting of dark blood that looks like coffee grounds

- Dark blood in the stool

- Nausea

- The middle of the tongue or the entire tongue can be purple, the sub-lingual veins may be swollen and purple

- Choppy or Wiry pulse, especially in the right *guan* position

Key symptoms

Stabbing and piercing gastric pain, vomiting of dark blood, purple colour in the middle of the tongue.

Treatment principle

Invigorate *xue*, dissolve *xue* stagnation in the Stomach, regulate Stomach *qi*.

Acupuncture points

Choose from: St 21, St 34, St 36, Pe 6, Ren 10, Ren 12, Ren 13, Sp 4, Sp 10, UB 17 and UB 21.

Needle technique
Draining.

Explanation

- St 21, St 36, Ren 10, Ren 12, Ren 13 and UB 21 regulate Stomach *qi* and invigorate *xue* in the Stomach.

- St 34 invigorates *xue* in the Stomach and stops pain.

- UB 17 and Sp 10 invigorate *xue*.

- Sp 4 and Pe 6 together open *chong mai*, invigorate *xue* and regulate Stomach *qi*.

Herbal formula

- *Ge Xia Fu Zhu Yu Tang* (Invigorates *xue* below the diaphragm)

Relevant advice
This will depend on which imbalances underlie the *xue* stagnation in the Stomach.

Xue stagnation in the Stomach can be caused by the following patterns of imbalance

- Stomach *qi* stagnation

- Stomach Fire

- Phlegm-Fire

- Liver *qi* invading the Stomach

- Invasions of Cold in the Stomach

- Stomach *yin xu*

- Stomach *qi xu*

Xue stagnation in the Stomach can result in the following patterns of imbalance

- Stomach *qi* stagnation

- Food stagnation

Damp-Heat in the Stomach

This pattern is very similar to Damp-Heat in the Spleen and the two patterns are often closely related to each other. The difference between them is that when there is

Damp-Heat in the Stomach, there will be signs that Stomach *qi* is disrupted or that there is Heat in the Stomach channel.

Aetiology
Invasions by exogenous Damp-Heat, such as the ingestion of spoiled or infected food, living or working in warm and humid conditions and contact with viruses, bacteria, fungi and so on that have a Damp-Heat dynamic. Excessive consumption of foods that generate Damp-Heat, such as fried foods and alcohol.

Damp-Heat can often arise as a consequence of chronic Spleen *qi xu* and Damp conditions.

Symptoms and signs
- Heaviness and pain in the abdomen
- Nausea
- Vomiting
- Thirst with no desire to drink
- Sticky sensation in the mouth
- Heaviness in the arms and legs
- Sinusitis
- Jaw pain
- Nasal congestion
- Yellowish, sticky mucus in the nose and sinuses
- Yellowish complexion
- Yellow sclera
- Pimples, spots or sores around the mouth, on the forehead or on the cheeks, which are red with yellowish pus
- Dark, yellow urine
- Yellow, greasy tongue coating, the tongue may be red in the middle
- Fast and Slippery pulse

Key symptoms
Discomfort or pain in the abdomen, heaviness, yellow, greasy tongue coating.

Treatment principle
Drain Dampness and Heat, regulate Stomach *qi*.

Acupuncture points
Choose from: St 21, St 34, St 44, LI 11, Sp 6, Sp 9, Ren 9 and Ren 13.

Needle technique
Draining. No moxa.

Explanation

- St 21, St 34 and Ren 13 regulate Stomach *qi*.

- St 44 and LI 11 drain Damp-Heat.

- Sp 6, Sp 9 and Ren 9 drain Dampness.

Herbal formula

- *San Ren Tang* (Clears Heat and Drains Dampness)

- *Huang Lian Jie Du Tang* (Drains Damp-Heat)

Relevant advice
It is crucial that a person with chronic Damp-Heat in the Stomach avoids foods and beverages that create Heat, Dampness or Damp-Heat. Ideally, alcohol, fried foods, chocolate, hot spices such as chilli, dairy products, sugar and sweets should be avoided completely. The person should also consume a diet that tonifies the Spleen, which often is the root cause of the Damp.

Damp-Heat in the Stomach can be caused by the following patterns of imbalance

- Spleen *qi xu*

- Spleen *yang xu*

- Damp-Cold invading the Spleen

- Stomach Fire

Damp-Heat in the Stomach can result in the following patterns of imbalance

- Spleen *qi xu*

- Phlegm

- Phlegm-Fire

Xu imbalances

Stomach *yin xu*

It is important to remember that this pattern is often seen in combination with other patterns, such as Spleen *qi xu* or Spleen *yang xu*. This means that some of the symptoms and signs will not be as obvious because they are 'veiled' by the symptoms and signs of the other pattern and vice versa.

Aetiology

Eating irregularly, eating late in the evening and eating whilst working or stressed will all injure the Stomach *yin*. An excessive consumption of spicy food and food that is hot in its energy can harm the Stomach *yin*. Some medicines will also have an energy that injures the Stomach *yin*.

There may be a congenital tendency to have Stomach *yin xu*.

Invasions of exogenous *xie qi* can penetrate to *qi* level or create Heat in the *yangming* organs. This excess of Heat can injure Stomach *yin*.

Heat from the Liver can damage Stomach *yin* over time.

Symptoms and signs

- Poor appetite

- Constipation

- Dry mouth and throat, especially in the afternoon and evening

- Dry stool

- Dull pain, slight burning sensation or discomfort in the epigastric region

- Thin body

- Dry tongue, with cracks or lacking coating in the middle, the coating on the tongue can be rootless

- Fine, Empty or Superficial pulse in the right *guan* position

When there is Stomach *yin xu* Heat, there can also be:

- fever or a feeling of heat in the body in the evening and at night

- a hot sensation in the palms of the hands and soles of the feet

- restlessness at night

- night sweats

- bleeding gums

- a slight thirst with a desire to sip only small amounts at a time

- red and dry tongue or a tongue that is red in the middle, the tongue may lack coating and have cracks in the middle

- Rapid, Fine or Empty pulse, especially in the right *guan* position.

Key symptoms
Dry mouth and throat, dry stool, discomfort in the abdomen, dry tongue that lacks coating in the middle.

Treatment principle
Nourish Stomach *yin*.

Acupuncture points
Choose from: St 36, Sp 6, Ren 4, Ren 12, Kid 3, Kid 6, UB 20 and UB 21.

Needle technique
Tonifying.

Explanation

- St 36, Sp 6, Ren 12, UB 20 and UB 21 nourish Stomach *yin*.

- Ren 4, Kid 3 and Kid 6 nourish Kidney *yin*, thereby supporting Stomach *yin*.

Herbal formula

- *Sha Shen Mai Dong Tang* (Nourishes Stomach *yin*)

- *Shen Ling Bai Zhu Wan* (Tonifies Stomach *qi* and *yin*)

Relevant advice
When there is Stomach *yin xu*, it will be beneficial to eat foods that are wet and sticky. Things such as porridges, purées, soups and stews will therefore nourish Stomach *yin*. Foods that are dry in their consistency or in their energetic dynamic will do the opposite and have a negative effect on Stomach *yin*. Foods that are drying in their energy are those that are very spicy (the spicy taste disperses and dries) or have been baked in the oven for a long time. This means that a person with Stomach *yin xu* should try to avoid crackers, rice cakes, toast, baked vegetables and similar items.

Deep-fried and grilled foods have a very hot energy and this can also injure Stomach *yin*. Alcohol, too much meat (especially lamb) and spices such as chilli, garlic, pepper and so on all have a hot dynamic, which can damage Stomach *yin* in the long term.

Apart from being aware of what they eat, a person who is Stomach *yin xu* should pay close attention to how they eat. They should try to eat in as tranquil surroundings as possible, which means that they should not eat whilst working or driving, when they are stressed or whilst they are doing something else. They also need to rest and not exert themselves after they have eaten. They should not eat late in the evening and they should not eat too much at a time.

Stomach *yin xu* can be caused by the following patterns of imbalance

- Stomach *qi xu*

- Stomach Fire

- Liver Fire

Stomach *yin xu* can result in the following patterns of imbalance

- Kidney *yin xu*

- Spleen *yin xu*

- Heart *yin xu*

- Liver *yin xu*

- Lung *yin xu*

Stomach *qi xu*

This pattern is very similar to Spleen *qi xu*, both in its symptoms and in its aetiology. In fact, the two patterns often overlap and are commonly diagnosed together in clinical practice.

Aetiology

Eating too much at a time, eating too little, eating too often, eating whilst working or when stressed or eating irregularly are all factors that can weaken Stomach *qi*.

Stomach qi will be debilitated by prolonged overwork and stress. Chronic illnesses will particularly enfeeble both Stomach and Spleen *qi*.

Symptoms and signs

- Fatigue

- Discomfort in the abdominal area

- Loose stools

- Bloating after meals

- Fatigue after meals

- Pale face

- Poor sense of taste

- Poor appetite or no appetite in the morning

- Weak limbs or tiredness of the limbs

- Craving for the sweet flavour

- Tendency to gain weight

- Disinclination to speak and the voice lacks strength

- The person looks tired and emanates weariness

- Slumped posture

- Worries a lot or constantly speculates about things

- Pale, swollen tongue, possibly with teeth marks on the sides

- Weak pulse, especially in the right *guan* position

Key symptoms
Fatigue, loose stools, pale tongue with teeth marks and a Weak *guan* pulse.

Treatment principle
Tonify Stomach *qi*.

Acupuncture points
Choose from: St 36, Sp 3, Sp 6, Ren 12, UB 20 and UB 21.

Needle technique
Tonifying. Moxa can be used.

Explanation

- St 36, Sp 3, Sp 6, Ren 12, UB 20 and UB 21 tonify Stomach *qi*.

Herbal formula

- *Liu Jun Zi Tang* (Tonifies Stomach *qi*)

- *Shen Ling Bai Zhu Tang* (Tonifies Stomach *qi*)

Relevant advice
Dietary changes are alpha and omega in the treatment of Stomach *qi xu*. It is important that the person focuses on what and particularly how they eat. They should eat enough food and not fast or go on diets where they do not consume sufficient food. At the same time, they should not eat too much at a time, as this will result in food stagnation. Constant snacking will also weaken the Stomach *qi*.

The patient should try to eat as calmly as possible. This means that they should not eat whilst working or driving, when they are stressed or whilst they are doing something else. They should also ensure that they get enough rest and do not exert themselves after they have eaten. They should not eat too late at night. Walking around or lightly stretching the front of the body after eating will support the *qi* mechanism in the middle *jiao* and thereby support the Stomach *qi*.

The person will benefit from eating porridge in the morning, soups, mashed or puréed vegetables, stews, steamed or boiled vegetables, i.e. easily digestible food. The use of aromatic herbs in the diet will help to circulate *qi* and thereby help to prevent Food stagnation.

It is important that the person does not sit still for extended periods of time and that they do not sit in a slumped posture. Walking or stretching after meals is recommended. Physical exercise in general will be beneficial. Stroking downwards with the fingers from Ren 16 to Ren 8 will help Stomach *qi* to descend.

Stomach *qi xu* can be caused by the following pattern of imbalance

- Spleen *qi xu*

Spleen *qi xu* can result in the following patterns of imbalance

- Spleen *qi xu*
- Stomach *yin xu*
- Spleen *yang xu*
- Food stagnation
- Damp
- Phlegm
- *Xue* stagnation

Stomach *qi xu* and Cold

This is a sub-pattern of the Stomach *qi xu*. In these cases, there is both Stomach *qi xu* and an aspect of *yang xu*. In addition to Stomach *qi xu* symptoms, there will be signs that the transformation of food and liquids is not functioning optimally due to a lack of physiological heat.

Aetiology

In addition to the factors discussed under Stomach *qi xu*, there can also be an excessive consumption of food and beverages that have a cold energy or are physically cold. These can create Cold in the Stomach. Typical examples of these are things like ice cream, iced water, salads, raw vegetables and tropical fruits.

Invasions by exogenous Cold can damage Stomach *qi* when there have been repeated invasions or if the Cold has not been completely expelled.

Medicine that has a cold dynamic can also be involved in the generation of this pattern.

Symptoms and signs

- Watery vomit

- Preference for warm food and beverages

- Lack of thirst

- Cold and weak limbs

- Discomfort in the abdomen

- Fatigue

- Pale face

- Aversion to cold

- The epigastric region can feel cold when palpated

- The person may dress warmer than is normal for the season

- Pale, wet and swollen tongue

- Deep, Weak and Slow pulse, especially in the right *guan* position

Key symptoms
Cold limbs, a preference for warm food and beverages, fatigue and a pale tongue.

Treatment principle
Warm and tonify Stomach *qi*.

Acupuncture points
Choose from: St 36, Sp 6, Ren 6, Ren 12, UB 20 and UB 21.

Needle technique
Tonifying. Moxa is recommended.

Explanation

- St 36, Sp 6, Ren 12, UB 20 and UB 21 tonify Stomach *qi*.

- Ren 6 warms *yang*.

Herbal formula

- *Li Zhong Tang* (Warms and tonifies the middle *jiao*, expels Cold)

Relevant advice
In this pattern, it is advisable to consume food and beverages that are both nutritious and warming. The use of ginger is particularly recommended. The patient should

try to eat frequently and regularly. They should avoid eating too much at a time, so they don't create a stagnation of the food in the Stomach. Similarly, they should try not to snack constantly and nibble at food. They should also, as far as possible, avoid consuming food and beverages that are cold, both physically or energetically, such as ice cream, ice water and cold drinks, salad and raw vegetables, as well as too much fruit, especially tropical fruits.

Stomach *qi xu* and Cold can be caused by the following patterns of imbalance

- Stomach *qi xu*
- Spleen *qi xu*
- Spleen *yang xu*
- Invasions of exogenous Cold

Stomach *qi xu* and Cold can result in the following patterns of imbalance

- Spleen *yang xu*
- Stomach and Spleen *qi xu*
- Phlegm
- Food stagnation
- *Xue* stagnation

Combined patterns
Stomach and Spleen *qi xu*
This is discussed in the section on Spleen imbalance patterns below.

Liver *qi* invading the Stomach
This is discussed in the section on Liver imbalance patterns (page 590).

Spleen imbalances
The Spleen and its partner organ, the Stomach, are located in the middle of the body, both physically and energetically. Physically, the Spleen and Stomach occupy the middle *jiao*, which means that they are the central axle around which everything revolves. All movement of *qi*, *xue* and fluids and all communication between the body's lower and upper *jiao* have to pass through the middle *jiao*. The Spleen sends its *qi* upwards and the Stomach its *qi* downwards. If this mechanism is disrupted or gets blocked, it will have implications for the movement and communication of *qi*, *xue*

and fluids throughout the whole body. For example, the Small Intestine and Large Intestine are completely dependent on the Stomach and Spleen *qi* mechanism, and organs such as the Lung are also dependent on the Spleen sending *qi* and *jinye* up to it. If the Spleen is not able to perform its functions of transforming and transporting as it should, Dampness will arise. Initially the Dampness will accumulate and stagnate in the middle *jiao*. This will inhibit the movement of *qi* through the middle *jiao* and can thus interfere with the functioning of many other organs.

As well as their central role in the movement and transport of vital substances, the Stomach and Spleen, together with the Kidneys and Lung, are fundamental in the production of *qi*, *xue* and *jinye*.

The Spleen transforms the food and beverages that are ingested, separating the pure *qi* aspects from the impure. The Spleen then sends these pure aspects upwards to the upper *jiao*, whilst its partner organ, the Stomach, sends the remaining dregs downwards for further transformation and finally expulsion from the body. If the Spleen is weak, there will only be a limited production of *qi*, *xue* and *jinye*. This will affect the whole body and all the other organs, as well as the movement, transformation and transportation of these substances.

The aetiology of Spleen imbalances

It is said that 'the Spleen detests Dampness' and that it 'prefers dryness'. This means that the Spleen's *qi* mechanism is easily disrupted when there is Dampness. The Dampness can be exogenous or it can be internally generated. Invasions of exogenous Dampness are usually due to climatic influences, such as when a person spends time in a damp environment or is exposed to wet, humid weather. Invasions of exogenous Dampness have traditionally been a major aetiological factor in North-Western Europe, because this area has a cold and humid climate. In the old days, these aetiological factors were even more predominant, due to poorer standards of housing. At the same time, a greater proportion of the population was employed in occupations where they were more exposed to the elements. Exogenous Dampness is, however, still a problem, despite the improvement in housing and changes in the labour market. This is because the air is still generally quite damp and humid and people are exposed to the elements when cycling, walking, jogging and so on. It is therefore important that people are properly dressed and that they quickly change into dry clothes if they get wet. Dampness can enter the body through the legs' *yin* channels, so people, especially women, should ensure that they are adequately clothed on their legs and wear appropriate footwear when it is cold and damp.

Furthermore, living in buildings that have fungal infections such as dry rot can provoke or generate symptoms of Dampness in some clients. Mould and other fungi will therefore often be considered to be a form of exogenous Dampness.

Dampness can also be internally generated. This will occur because there is Spleen *qi xu* and the Spleen is unable to transform the food and liquids that have been consumed. The resulting Dampness will then in itself further burden the Spleen. Dampness can also arise from an excessive consumption of foods and beverages that have a Damp nature, such as dairy products, sweets, sugar, bananas, beer and wheat flour. One of the tasks that Spleen *yang* performs is that of transformation and transportation. If there is an excessive consumption of food and beverages that are cold, either in their energetic dynamic or in their temperature, this will strain the Spleen *yang*. Therefore, an immoderate consumption of raw vegetables, salad, fruit, cold water, ice cream and so on can have a negative effect on the Spleen. It is especially detrimental for the Spleen *yang* if cold water is drunk with meals.

In general, the diet and the way it is eaten is the single most important factor in the development of Spleen-related imbalances. People often eat and drink products that are too cold (both energetically and in their temperature), things that are too sweet or foods that in themselves create Dampness and Phlegm. They eat food that is too coarse and raw. They eat too quickly, too much at a time, late at night and food that is of poor quality. The tendency to have Spleen *qi xu* and Phlegm-Dampness is often initiated in the first years of a person's life. Giving a baby or a toddler the wrong diet or feeding them incorrectly can easily burden and weaken the Spleen, which is not fully developed and therefore vulnerable. This will create a fundamental tendency to have Spleen *qi xu* and for Dampness and Phlegm to form, which further compromises the Spleen *qi*, creating a vicious circle.

Although eating too much, too fast and too late are often cited as causes of Spleen and Stomach imbalances, it is important to remember that eating too little will also damage Spleen *qi*. Malnutrition due to starvation and hunger is not as big a problem in North-Western Europe as it was historically. Nevertheless, it is still a problem when someone has an eating disorder, eats a strict diet or eats a very one-sided diet. Furthermore, some people eat too much, but the food they eat is of very poor quality. All of these factors can lead to Spleen *qi xu*. Unfortunately, many people who are overweight and go on strict diets quickly put on weight when they start eating normally again. This is because the strict diet will have weakened their Stomach and Spleen *qi* and thereby led to the creation of Dampness and Phlegm. Patients who have a history of anorexia and bulimia will often have seriously damaged their Spleen and Stomach *qi*. This is due to the extreme malnutrition that is a consequence of their disorder fundamentally weakening their Spleen and Stomach *qi*, but also the repeated and forced vomiting will disrupt the Stomach and Spleen *qi* mechanism and these organs then have difficulty sending their *qi* in the right direction.

Some forms of pharmaceutical medicine, for example antibiotics, have a very cooling and Damp-producing energy. The use of these medicines can therefore injure Spleen *yang*.

Spleen *yang* is supported by Kidney *yang* and *mingmen*, but if these are weak Spleen *yang* will also become weakened and will not be able to fulfil its functions in relation to the transformation and transportation of *qi* and fluids in the body.

If the Spleen and Stomach *qi* mechanism is to function optimally, it is important physically that there is an open passage through which *qi* can be sent up and down from the middle *jiao*. If the person sits with a twisted midriff or sits slouched and slumped in a chair, it will physically block the movement of *qi*. Physical activity and exercise help to support the circulation of *qi* in the middle *jiao*. Therefore, a person who leads a very sedentary life will tend towards having a stagnation of *qi* in the middle *jiao*.

Worry, speculation, thinking too much and studying can 'bind' and stagnate the Spleen's *qi*. This can lead to a weakening of the Spleen *qi*. If a person reads, watches television, writes on the computer, surfs the internet and so on whilst they eat, it will weaken the Spleen *qi*. This is because the Spleen must use its *qi* to digest or separate the pure from the impure, both intellectually and physically. In general, studying and reading too much strains Spleen *qi* and can lead to Spleen *qi xu*.

Chronic illnesses, physical overexertion of the body and heavy bleeding or haemorrhaging can lead to Spleen *qi xu*. This is because the Spleen will have to overwork to create sufficient *gu qi* to replenish the chronic *xu* condition.

The pathology of Spleen imbalances

If the Spleen is not able to transform the food and fluids that are ingested adequately, the pure *qi* will not be separated from the impure dregs. This will result in pure *qi* being conveyed downwards along with the impure residue. This means that the person will lack *qi* and they will therefore feel tired and fatigued. When there is only a partial transformation of the consumed substances, Dampness will arise. This is because some of the impure residue that should have been separated from the pure *qi* will be sent upwards along with the pure *qi*, instead of being sent downwards to the Small Intestine. This can often be seen on the tongue, which develops a greasy or sticky coating.

Dampness can result in fatigue, because the Spleen is overburdened and thereby produces less *qi* and because the Dampness will inhibit the movement of *qi* in the body. When there is Dampness, the fatigue will often be most pronounced in the morning and after consuming Damp-producing foods. If there is Spleen *qi xu*, the fatigue becomes more pronounced as the day goes on. Both Dampness and Spleen *qi xu* can manifest with fatigue and sleepiness after meals. This is because the Spleen *qi* that is available is used to transform the food and because the Dampness that arises as a result of the inadequate transformation or was already present will block the pure *yang qi* from ascending up to the head. Furthermore, Damp-Phlegm can settle like a fog and block the *shen*.

If the transformation of the food has been incomplete or if there is Dampness, the stool can be loose and formless. If there is Spleen *yang xu* or if there has been an invasion of exogenous Damp-Cold that extinguishes the Spleen's physiological fire, the transformation of the ingested food and liquids will be so limited that the stools are watery and contain undigested food. If there is Damp-Heat, the Heat can cause the stool to become sticky and odorous. There may well be a stinging or burning sensation in the rectum. The Heat can be so intense that it agitates *xue* so much that it bursts the walls of the vessels, resulting in blood in the stool. Blood in the stool can also be seen when there is Spleen *qi xu*, because one of the Spleen's tasks is to hold *xue* inside the vessels. If there is Spleen *qi xu*, there can be bleeding in the Intestines, and in fact all forms of bleeding can be the result of Spleen *qi xu*. It is typical, for example, that mid-cycle spotting and prolonged or heavy menstrual bleeding in women can be a manifestation of Spleen *qi xu*. Furthermore, the inability to hold the *xue* inside the vessels can mean that Spleen *qi xu* manifests with easy bruising.

Spleen *qi* not only holds *xue* inside the vessels, it also lifts and holds organs in place. Thus, when there is Spleen *qi xu,* and particularly Spleen *yang xu,* it can manifest with organ prolapse, hernias, haemorrhoids and a sensation of heaviness or that everything is dragging downwards in the body.

If there is a reduction in the production of *gu qi,* it will not only result in fatigue, but it can also lead to *xue xu,* because *xue* is created from *gu qi.*

Furthermore, a poor production of *qi* and *xue* can cause the muscles, especially in the arms and legs, to feel weak or feeble, because the muscles lack nourishment. Dampness can manifest with a sensation of heaviness in the arms and legs. The limbs feel heavy because Dampness is a *yin* pathogen and because it inhibits the movement of *qi*. Damp-Heat, on the other hand, can make the muscles feel painful. If there is Spleen *yang xu,* the arms and legs can feel cold, because when there is *yang xu* there is not enough physiological heat in the body to warm the limbs. This lack of physiological heat is why the stool can be watery and contain undigested food. Watery stools and coldness of the limbs are key signs when differentiating Spleen *yang xu* in relation to Spleen *qi xu.*

When the Spleen and Stomach do not send their *qi* upwards and downwards respectively, it will stagnate in the middle *jiao*. This will manifest as abdominal bloating and distension. The distension and bloating will be most apparent after the ingestion of food. The *qi* stagnation in and around the Stomach and Spleen can also often manifest with a reduction in the appetite or nausea. Poor appetite is actually an interesting sign. In the Chinese textbooks, poor appetite is a key sign when diagnosing Spleen *qi xu*. Nevertheless, the majority of clients who are Spleen *qi xu* report that they have a healthy appetite. There can be several reasons why they respond in this way. First, there are several mechanisms that result in a person wanting or needing to eat. As well as ingesting food being a fundamental necessity in order to provide nourishment to the body, eating is a form of pleasure, a way of comforting the psyche and something to do when you are bored. Consequently, one or more of these mechanisms can result in a desire to put food into the mouth, even if the Stomach does not feel particularly hungry. Furthermore, many people with Spleen *qi xu* also have Heat in the Stomach. This means that they have an increased appetite. A useful question to ask patients is whether they have an appetite in the morning. Many people who are Spleen *qi xu* have no appetite in the morning and often skip breakfast. This is because the Spleen and Stomach are too weak to send their *qi* up and down, and the circulation of *qi* in and around the middle *qi* will only start functioning when there has been sufficient physical activity to activate it. This is even worse if there is Damp. Dampness tends to stagnate in and around the Stomach and Spleen when the person has been lying still all night, and this will block the already weakened movement of *qi.*

People who are Spleen *qi xu* will often have a craving to eat things that are sweet. This is because the sweet flavour tonifies the Spleen. Therefore, the Spleen being *qi xu* will cause the body to crave the sweet flavour in an attempt to tonify the Spleen. The problem is that most people react to this signal by consuming sweets, chocolates, cakes and other things that are very sweet. The sweet flavour here is very concentrated – so much so that the Spleen can have difficulty transforming it, resulting in Dampness and thereby a further weakening of the Spleen. This gives rise to a new craving for the sweet flavour to tonify the Spleen and a vicious cycle arises.

As well as the appetite being reduced when there are Spleen imbalances, the resultant Dampness means that there will be an increased amount of fluid, which can result in reduced thirst. The person can 'forget' to drink. The problem is that Dampness is a form of *xie qi*, and being *xie qi*, it has none of the moistening, lubricating and cooling qualities that *jinye* has. When there is Damp-Heat, the paradoxical situation can arise in which Heat causes the person to be thirsty but the Damp aspect means that the person does not feel like drinking.

Because Damp is a condensed form of body fluid, there can be a sticky sensation in the mouth. When there is Damp-Heat, there can also be a bitter taste in the mouth if the Heat aspect is intense.

If the Spleen is not able to perform its functions of transforming and transporting fluid in the body, oedema can arise. The oedema will be chronic and it will often be aggravated by consuming certain foods. Moreover, the oedema can also arise in the premenstrual period if stagnant Liver *qi* 'invades' the Spleen. Other symptoms and signs that Liver *qi* is invading the Spleen in the premenstrual period are abdominal bloating or distension, a craving for sweets and loose stools.

As stated, Dampness and Phlegm can arise as a consequence of Spleen *qi xu*. This can result in a tendency to put on weight. Dampness can manifest with the person developing a pear-shaped body, because Dampness seeps downwards to the lower *jiao* due to its *yin* nature. It is very typical for women to develop this type of body shape from the age of 35 years onwards, because when women enter the sixth *jing* cycle, *mingmen* decreases in intensity. At the same time, their Spleen *qi* is decreasing in strength because it has been working hard for 21 years to replenish the *xue* that has been lost through menstrual bleeding. Men do not start to gain weight due to the decrease in *mingmen* until they are 40 years old and enter their sixth *jing* cycle. Also, because men are more *yang*, the weight gain sits higher up around the belly.

Spleen *qi xu* does not necessarily lead to a gain in weight. Spleen *qi xu* can also be a cause of weight loss and a body that is too lean. The reduced production of *gu qi* that is a consequence of Spleen *qi xu* can lead to *qi xu* and *xue xu*, resulting in the muscles and tissues not receiving sufficient nutrition.

A person who is Spleen *qi xu* will often have a slightly pale face, because there can be a genuine lack of *xue*, due to the reduced production of *gu qi*, and not enough *qi* to carry *xue* up to the face. When there is Dampness, the face and possibly also the eyes can have a yellowish tinge or hue.

Constant worrying, speculating, ruminating and thinking too much in general will stagnate and bind, thereby ultimately weakening the Spleen *qi*. Conversely, if the Spleen is *qi xu*, this can manifest with a tendency to worry excessively or unnecessarily, the person also having difficulty in letting go of thoughts. This is because they are not able to transform information and extract the relevant from the irrelevant. Their *yi* stagnates and they start to think in rings. In extreme cases this can become obsessive, as in obsessive–compulsive disorder (OCD), or it can become a depressive condition. Spleen *qi xu* can also result in a person having difficulty studying and learning. This is especially noticeable if there is Damp-Phlegm, because it will cloud the *shen* and the person will have difficulty concentrating. It will feel as if their head is full of cotton wool or there is mental fog. Furthermore, the reduced production of *gu qi* can lead to *xue xu* and the brain not being nourished by Heart *xue*.

General symptoms and signs of a Spleen imbalance

- Fatigue, especially after meals
- Loose stools
- Poor appetite
- Tendency to gain weight

Shi patterns

Damp-Cold invading the Spleen

This pattern can be both acute and chronic. If it is an acute pattern, it will be due to an invasion of exogenous *xie qi*. It will, however, still be classified as an interior imbalance, because the *xie qi* is located in the interior.

Aetiology

Damp-Cold can invade the Spleen when a person has been living or working in a cold and humid environment, has been wearing wet clothes or has been consuming medicine, food or beverages that are cold and damp, in either their temperature or energy. Damp-Cold can also invade the body via the Spleen channel in the feet and legs, if the person has walked bare foot on cold and damp surfaces or has worn shoes that are not warm and dry enough.

Coming into contact with certain bacteria and viruses can result in Damp-Cold conditions. This can be anything from eating food that has gone off to cholera. This is because a pattern of imbalance is defined by its symptoms and signs. If the symptoms and signs are those that are seen in Damp-Cold, then that which has caused the imbalance will by definition be Damp-Cold in nature and will be treated accordingly.

Symptoms and signs

- Poor appetite

- Nausea

- Abdominal distension or sensation of fullness in the abdomen

- Loose stools or diarrhoea

- Sticky taste in the mouth

- Lack of thirst

- Loss or reduction in the sense of taste

- Heaviness of the arms and legs

- White, sticky vaginal discharge

- Oedema

- Cold sensation in abdomen

- Fatigue

- Heaviness in the body and head

- Brain fog, difficulty thinking clearly or a sensation that the head is full of cotton wool

- Dull, white complexion

- Thick, white and greasy tongue coating on a pale tongue, in chronic patterns the coating will not necessarily be as thick

- Slippery and Slow pulse, when there is an invasion of exogenous *xie qi*, the pulse will be fuller

Key symptoms
Loose stools, no appetite, no thirst, slippery pulse and white greasy tongue coating.

Treatment principle
Transform and drain Dampness and Cold.

Acupuncture points
Choose from: St 8, Sp 6, Sp 9, Ren 6, Ren 8, Ren 9, Ren 11 and UB 22.

- If there is also Spleen *qi xu*, add: Sp 3, St 36, Ren 12, UB 20 and UB 21.

Needle technique

Tonify St 36, Sp 3, Ren 12, UB 20 and UB 21. Draining or even technique on St 8, Sp 6, Sp 9 and UB 22. Moxa on Ren 6 and Ren 8; moxa can also be used on the other points.

Explanation

- St 8 drains Damp-Phlegm from the head.

- Ren 9, Sp 6, Sp 9 and UB 22 drain Dampness.

- Ren 6 and Ren 8 with moxa expel Damp-Cold from the middle *jiao*.

- Ren 11 regulates *qi* and drains Dampness from the middle *jiao*.

- St 36, Sp 3, UB 20 and UB 21 tonify Spleen *qi*, transform Dampness and regulate *qi* in the middle *jiao*.

Herbal formula

- *Hou Po Wen Zhong Tang* (Dispels Cold, transforms Dampness and regulates the Stomach and Spleen *qi*)

Relevant advice

A person with Damp-Cold invading the Spleen should avoid food and beverages that are cold, both energetically and in their temperature. They should also avoid consuming anything that produces Dampness. This means that dairy products, cold drinks, ice cream, sweets, cake, dried fruit, wheat, sugar, lettuce, cucumber, tomato, melon and tropical fruit should be avoided. They will benefit from consuming foods that are cooked, baked and roasted and have a warming energy. Ginger will be particularly good, as it is warming but also spicy and thereby expels exogenous *xie qi*.

Keeping the abdomen warm and dry is also vital in this pattern of imbalance.

Damp-Cold invading the Spleen can be caused by the following patterns of imbalance

- Spleen *qi xu*

- Spleen *yang xu*

Damp-Cold invading the Spleen can result in the following patterns of imbalance

- Spleen *yang xu*

- Phlegm-Dampness

- Damp-Heat

Damp-Heat invading the Spleen

The major difference between this and the previous pattern is the presence of Heat symptoms and signs. Like Damp-Cold invading the Spleen, this pattern can be both acute and chronic. An acute condition will occur when there is an invasion of exogenous *xie qi*, whereas a chronic condition is usually the result of Spleen *qi xu* creating Dampness or consuming food and beverages that create Dampness or Damp-Heat. Dampness, when it stagnates, will generate Heat and transform into Damp-Heat. This process is accelerated if there is already Heat present in the body. This will typically be Liver *qi* stagnation Heat.

This pattern is often characterised by there being a chronic condition of latent Damp-Heat, which flares up every time food or beverages are consumed that generate Damp, Heat or Damp-Heat.

In general, the symptoms will be milder and less pronounced when there is a chronic condition.

Aetiology

Invasions of exogenous Damp-Heat, such as the ingestion of contaminated food, living or working in hot and humid conditions and direct contact with viruses, bacteria and other pathogens that have a Damp-Heat nature. The excessive intake of foods that have Damp-Heat-generating energy can be both a root cause and an aggravating factor.

Damp-Heat can often arise as a consequence of chronic Spleen *qi* and Damp conditions.

Symptoms and signs

- Loose or sticky stools

- Odorous stools

- Burning or stinging sensation in the rectum when defecating

- Dark, scanty urine

- Oppressive or blocked sensation in the epigastric region or the lower part of the abdominal cavity

- Epigastric or abdominal pain

- Flatulence that is odorous

- Greasy or oily skin

- Smoky or dull yellowish sheen to the facial complexion

- Thirst with no desire to drink

- Poor appetite

- Nausea or vomiting

- Bitter taste or sticky sensation in the mouth

- Oily or sticky sweat

- Odorous sweat

- Slight fever or sensation of heat

- Aversion to heat or to hot, humid environments

- Red, itchy, inflamed or weeping skin diseases

- Oppressive headache or heaviness in the head

- Blurred sensation in the head as if the head is full of cotton wool

- Yellowish sclera

- Yellowish, sticky tongue coating possibly with red elevated papillae, the tongue may be red but it is often pale or normal coloured in chronic conditions where there is an underlying *xu* condition

- Rapid and Slippery pulse

Key symptoms
Sticky and odorous stools, yellowish sticky tongue coating and Slippery pulse.

Treatment principle
Drain Damp-Heat.

Acupuncture points
Choose from: St 25, St 28, St 44, LI 11, Sp 6, Sp 9 and UB 22.

- If there is also Spleen *qi xu*, add: Sp 3, St 36, Ren 12 and UB 20 and utilise a tonifying needle technique.

Needle technique
Draining.

Explanation

- St 25, St 28, St 44 and LI 11 drain Damp-Heat from the Stomach and Intestines.

- Sp 6, Sp 9 and UB 22 drain Dampness.

- St 36, Sp 3, UB 20 and Ren 12 tonify Spleen *qi*, transform Dampness and regulate *qi* in the middle *jiao*.

Herbal formula

- *San Ren Tang* (Clears Heat and Drains Dampness)

Relevant advice

It is essential that a person with chronic Damp-Heat invading the Spleen avoids, as far as possible, food and beverages that create Damp-Heat, Dampness or Heat. It is usually not enough to avoid sugar, sweets, cake and so on; they should also avoid dried fruits, stevia, artificial sweeteners and anything else that has a concentrated sweet flavour. Alcohol, hot spices including chilli, pepper, chocolate and garlic will also be problematic, as will dairy products. Whilst they should avoid things that create Damp-Heat, they should try to consume a diet that is beneficial for the Spleen.

Damp-Heat invading the Spleen can be caused by the following patterns of imbalance

- Spleen *qi xu*
- Spleen *yang xu*
- Damp-Cold invading the Spleen
- Stomach Fire

Damp-Heat invading the Spleen can result in the following patterns of imbalance

- Spleen *qi xu*
- Phlegm
- Phlegm-Fire

Xu imbalances

Spleen qi xu

Spleen *qi xu* is, alongside Liver *qi* stagnation, probably the most common pattern one meets in the clinic. This is mainly a consequence of the diet that many people consume and the way in which they eat their food, which often puts a great strain on the Spleen *qi*.

Most patterns of Spleen imbalances are simply variations of Spleen *qi xu*. Furthermore, Spleen *qi xu* is often central in the creation of patterns of imbalance in many other organs. Several of these combined patterns become self-generating, where one pattern results in the creation of the other and vice versa.

Aetiology

The primary cause of Spleen *qi xu* is consuming food and beverages that are cold (in both their temperature and energy), raw foods and food that is unrefined or Damp producing. Eating too much at a time, eating too quickly or not chewing the food enough will also burden the Spleen. Although eating several small meals is better for the Spleen, constantly snacking will also strain the Spleen because it will constantly have to transform the ingested food.

Spleen *qi* can also be weakened by excessive worrying, speculating, studying and ruminating.

Prolonged illness, excessive bleeding and overexertion are also a burden on the Spleen, because it has to replenish the *qi* and *xue* that have been consumed or lost.

Chronic Liver *qi* stagnation will often lead to a disturbance, and thereby a weakening, of Spleen *qi*.

Finally, living or working in a humid environment can strain the Spleen, because the Spleen abhors Dampness.

Symptoms and signs

- Fatigue

- Loose stools

- Abdominal bloating after meals

- Fatigue after meals

- Pale complexion

- Poor appetite or no appetite in the morning

- Weak limbs or tiredness in the limbs

- Craving for sweetness

- Tendency to gain weight

- Flatulence that is not odorous

- Disinclination to speak and the voice lacks strength

- The person emanates fatigue and a lack of energy

- Poor posture

- The skin or muscles may seem slightly doughy and lack tone

- Excessive worrying

- Pale, swollen tongue, possibly with teeth marks on the sides

- Weak pulse, especially in the right *guan* position

Key symptoms
Fatigue, loose stools, pale tongue with teeth marks and a Weak pulse.

Treatment principle
Tonify Spleen *qi*.

Acupuncture points
Choose from: St 36, Sp 3, Sp 6, Ren 12, UB 20 and UB 21.

Needle technique
Tonifying. Moxa can be used.

Explanation

• St 36, Sp 3, Sp 6, Ren 12, UB 20 and UB 21 tonify Spleen *qi*.

Herbal formula

• *Liu Jun Zi Tang* (Tonifies Spleen *qi* and transforms Phlegm-Dampness)

• *Bu Zhong Yi Qi Tang* (Tonifies and lifts Spleen *qi*)

Relevant advice
Dietary changes are alpha and omega in the treatment of Spleen *qi xu*. This encompasses both what is eaten and how it is eaten.

A person who is Spleen *qi xu* should eat as much prepared and warm food as possible. They should avoid raw vegetables, salads, food that is very coarse, cold drinks, ice cream and food that generates Dampness, such as sweets, dried fruit, artificial sweeteners, honey, stevia, dairy products, bananas, avocados and so on. They should avoid eating too quickly, too much at a time and whilst reading, watching television or working. They should chew their food well and avoid drinking too much at mealtimes. They will benefit from eating soups, mashed vegetables, purées, porridge in the morning, stews, steamed or boiled vegetables and baked vegetables, i.e. food that is easily digestible and, preferably, warm. The weaker their Spleen *qi* is, the more digestible their food should be, as long as it does not create Dampness.

Drinking a small cup of ginger tea at mealtimes will help to fortify Spleen *yang*, thereby assisting the Spleen in its transformation of the food. The use of herbs in the diet, especially aromatic spices like black pepper, ginger, cardamom, garlic, cumin, caraway and nutmeg, will also assist in circulating *qi*, dispersing Food stagnation and transforming Dampness, thereby alleviating the burden on the Spleen.

Foods that are particularly beneficial are: rice, oats, barley, most vegetables especially root vegetables, squash, sweet potatoes and those that are yellow or orange in colour, red lentils, tofu, chickpeas and chicken.

It is important that the person does not regularly sit still for extended periods of time and that they do not sit in a slumped posture. Walking or stretching after meals is recommended. Physical exercise in general will be beneficial, as long as the person does not overexert themselves. Stroking downwards with the fingers from Ren 16 to Ren 8 will help Stomach *qi* to descend.

Meditation is interesting in the context of Spleen *qi xu*. Often we recommend *yin* activities like meditation rather than physical activity when there are *qi xu* conditions. However, meditation where you sit still for long periods of time can burden the Spleen and excessive mental focus can consume Spleen *qi*. This does not, though, mean that meditation in itself is negative when there is Spleen *qi xu*, it just requires taking certain factors into consideration. If you are able to meditate with an empty mind then it will be beneficial. Meditation is also an excellent tool to reduce the tyranny of worry, speculation and repetitive thoughts. Walking meditation will generally be a better option for a person who is Spleen *qi xu*, as walking circulates *qi* in the middle *jiao*, while sitting still can cause *qi* to stagnate in the middle *jiao*.

Spleen *qi xu* can be caused by the following patterns of imbalance

- Liver *qi* stagnation

- Chronic *xue xu*

Spleen *qi xu* can result in the following patterns of imbalance

- Spleen *yang xu*

- Spleen *qi* sinking

- Spleen *qi* not holding *xue* inside the vessels

- Food stagnation

- Dampness

- Phlegm

- *Xue xu*

- Lung *qi xu*

- Heart *qi xu*

Spleen *yang xu*

Spleen *yang xu* is often a development of Spleen *qi xu*, but it can be the consequence of other imbalances. The symptoms and signs that define this pattern are very similar to those seen when there is Spleen *qi xu*. There will, though, also be signs of *xu* Cold in this pattern.

Aetiology

An excessive consumption of cold or cooling food and beverages (both in their temperature and energy), the consumption of antibiotics and repeated invasions of

Dampness and Cold in the middle *jiao* can all damage Spleen *yang*. Spleen *yang* will also be adversely affected by living or working in a cold and humid climate.

Spleen *yang xu* and Kidney *yang xu* are often seen together and one will often lead to the generation of the other. In the end, it becomes difficult to determine which is the root cause.

Symptoms and signs

- Fatigue

- Loose stools or watery stools containing undigested food

- Cold arms and legs

- Poor appetite

- Bloating after meals

- Craving sweet flavours

- Preference for warm food and beverages or a pronounced aversion to cold drinks and salads

- Pale face

- Desire to lie down

- Poor posture

- Aversion to cold

- Tendency to wrap their arms around themselves in an attempt to keep warm

- Can be dressed in warmer clothes than other people

- Cold limbs

- Weakness or fatigue in the arms and legs

- Oedema

- Tendency to put on weight

- Flatulence that is not odorous

- Pale, swollen and wet tongue, possibly with teeth marks on the sides

- Deep, Weak pulse, especially in the right *guan* position

Key symptoms
Fatigue, loose stools, aversion to cold, cold limbs and Weak pulse.

Treatment principle
Tonify and warm Spleen *yang*.

Acupuncture points
Choose from: St 36, Sp 3, Sp 6, Ren 6, Ren 12, UB 20 and UB 21.

Needle technique
Tonifying. Moxa is recommended.

Explanation

- St 36, Sp 3, Sp 6, Ren 6, Ren 12, UB 20 and UB 21 tonify Spleen *yang*.

Herbal formula

- *Li Zhong Tang* (Tonifies and warms Spleen *yang*)

Relevant advice
The advice given for Spleen *yang xu* is the same as that given for Spleen *qi xu*. When there is Spleen *yang xu*, it is even more important that the person avoids food, beverages and drugs that are cold in their energy or temperature, as well as consuming things that have a warming energy, such as cinnamon, ginger, cloves, lamb and so on.

Spleen *yang xu* can be caused by the following patterns of imbalance

- Spleen *qi xu*
- Kidney *yang xu*
- Invasions of Damp-Cold

Spleen *yang xu* can result in the following patterns of imbalance

- Spleen *qi* sinking
- Spleen *qi* not holding *xue* inside the vessels
- Kidney *yang xu*
- Food stagnation
- Damp
- Damp-Cold
- Phlegm
- *Xue xu*
- Lung *qi xu*

- Heart *qi xu*

- Heart *yang xu*

Spleen *qi* sinking

Spleen *qi* sinking is almost the same as Spleen *qi xu*. The difference between the two patterns is that when there is Spleen *qi* sinking, there are specific symptoms that relate to Spleen *qi* failing to carry out its function of lifting and holding organs and structures in the body in place. This can manifest in anything from a mild dragging sensation in the body to a prolapse of organs or structures, for example hernias and rectal prolapse. Spleen *qi* is also needed to hold a foetus in the Uterus during pregnancy. Spleen *qi* sinking can therefore also manifest with spontaneous miscarriages.

Aetiology

Apart from the relevance of the same aetiological factors that can result in Spleen *qi xu*, factors such as repetitive lifting of heavy objects will weaken Kidney *yang*, which supports the Spleen in its function of lifting and holding things in place in the body.

Symptoms and signs

- Organ prolapse – such as uterine prolapse, rectal prolapse, hernias, haemorrhoids and so on

- Dragging sensation as if the insides are about to fall out of the body

- Fatigue

- Loose stools

- Poor posture

- Difficulty sitting up straight

- Desire to lie down

- Limp muscles in the arms and legs

- Facial muscles appear weak so the cheeks are hanging

- Craving for sweetness

- Poor appetite

- Disinclination to speak

- Pale, swollen tongue with swollen sides and teeth marks

- Deep and weak pulse, especially in the right *guan* position

Key symptoms
Organ prolapse, dragging or sinking sensation, fatigue and weak pulse.

Treatment principle
Tonify and raise Spleen *qi*.

Acupuncture points
Choose from: St 36, Sp 3, Sp 6, Ren 6, Ren 12, Du 20, UB 20 and UB 21.

Needle technique
Tonifying. Moxa should be used on Ren 6 and Du 20.

Explanation

- St 36, Sp 3, Sp 6, Ren 12, UB 20 and UB 21 tonify Spleen *yang*.

- Ren 6 and Du 20 together raise and lift *qi* throughout the body when used with moxa.

Herbal formula

- *Bu Zhong Yi Qi Tang* (Tonifies and lifts Spleen *qi*)

Relevant advice
As well as following the advice that is recommended when there is Spleen *qi xu*, it is important that the patient avoids heavy lifting.

Spleen *qi* sinking can be caused by the following patterns of imbalance

- Spleen *qi xu*

- Spleen *yang xu*

- Kidney *yang xu*

Spleen *qi* sinking can result in the following patterns of imbalance

- Spleen *qi* not holding *xue* inside the vessels

- Kidney *yang xu*

Spleen *qi* not holding *xue* inside the vessels
This is again a variation of Spleen *qi xu*. In this pattern, the Spleen is not able to perform its function of keeping *xue* inside the vessels. This will manifest in bleeding and bruising. The bleeding can take many forms; it may be different kinds of menstrual disorders, such as mid-cycle spotting, heavy menstrual bleeding or prolonged menstrual bleeding, or there may be nosebleeds, blood in the urine or blood in the stools. It is, however, important to remember that 'Spleen *qi* not

holding *xue* inside the vessels' is just one of several patterns that can result in bleeding. Bleeding can also occur when there is *xu* or *shi* Heat and when there is *xue* stagnation. There will usually be a combination of more than one pattern at a time. Furthermore, it is important to remember that these patterns will lead to the development of *xue xu* over time.

Milder cases of Spleen *qi* not holding *xue* inside the vessels are seen in people who have a tendency to bruise easily.

Aetiology
The aetiology of this pattern is identical to that of Spleen *qi xu*.

Symptoms and signs

- Heavy or prolonged menstrual bleeding
- Spotting or bleeding in the middle of the menstrual cycle
- Blood in the urine
- Blood in the stool
- Nosebleeds
- A tendency to bruise easily
- Fatigue
- Loose stools
- Craving sweet flavours
- Weakness or fatigue in the limbs
- Pale complexion
- Pale tongue
- Weak or Fine pulse, especially in the right *guan* position

Key symptoms
Bleeding, fatigue, pale tongue and weak pulse.

Treatment principle
Tonify Spleen *qi* and astringe the vessels.

Acupuncture points
Choose from: St 36, Sp 1, Sp 3, Sp 6, Sp 10, Kid 8, Ren 12, UB 17, UB 20 and UB 21.

Needle technique
Tonifying. Moxa can be used on all points and must be used on Sp 1.

Explanation

- St 36, Sp 3, Sp 6, Ren 12, UB 20 and UB 21 tonify Spleen *qi*.

- Sp 10 stops bleeding.

- Sp 1 with moxa stops bleeding.

- Kid 8 stops uterine bleeding.

- UB 17 nourishes *xue*.

Herbal formula

- *Gui Pi Tang* (Tonifies Spleen *qi* and nourishes *xue*)

Relevant advice
The advice given in the section on Spleen *qi* is also relevant here.

Spleen *qi* not holding *xue* inside the vessels can be caused by the following patterns of imbalance

- Spleen *qi xu*

- Spleen *yang xu*

- Spleen *qi* sinking

- Kidney *yang xu*

Spleen *qi* not holding *xue* inside the vessels can result in following patterns of imbalance

- *Xue* stagnation

- *Xue xu*

- *Yin xu*

Spleen *yin xu*

Most modern textbooks refer to *yin xu* conditions in the Heart, Liver, Lung and Kidneys but not in the Spleen. Nevertheless, there have historically been discussions and disputes as to whether the Spleen also has a *yin xu* pattern. Many authors argue that the Spleen cannot be *yin xu* for the simple reason that the Spleen detests Dampness and prefers Dryness, while others believe that the Spleen *yin xu* is not only seen in practice but can also be justified theoretically.[23] Spleen *yin xu* will often be diagnosed as the combined pattern of Spleen *qi xu* and Stomach *yin xu*. From an acupuncture perspective, the differentiation between these two patterns and Spleen *yin xu* will only have academic interest, as the treatment will be largely the same.

Aetiology
Spleen *yin xu* can arise through chronic overexertion. An excessive consumption of hot, spicy food and medicines can injure the Spleen *yin*.

Spleen *yin xu* can be both a consequence and the root cause of *yin xu* in other organs. This is because the condition will impair the Spleen's transformation of the fluids that have been ingested and this is the first stage in the production of *jinye*.

Symptoms and signs
- Bloated abdomen after meals
- Easily sated and can only eat small meals
- Epigastric fullness
- No or poor sense of taste
- Dry lips
- Dry mouth
- Oral ulcers
- Thirst that is easily quenched
- Burning sensation in the stomach or the abdomen
- Matt complexion
- Weight loss or lean body
- Dry stools
- Weak or fatigued limbs
- Sensation of heat in the palms of the hands and soles of the feet
- Red and dry tongue that lacks coating, possibly red and peeled in the central area, there may be cracks on the tongue
- Fine and Rapid pulse

Key symptoms
Dry mouth and lips, easily sated, the central area of the tongue is red and lacks coating.

Treatment principle
Nourish Spleen *yin*.

Acupuncture points
Choose from: Sp 6, Ren 12, St 36 and UB 20.

Needle technique
Tonifying.

Explanation

- Sp 6, Ren 12, St 36 and UB 20 nourish Spleen *yin*.

Herbal formula

- *Yi Pi Tang* (Nourishes Spleen *yin*)

Relevant advice
A person who is Spleen *yin xu* should avoid eating food that is hot and spicy. They will benefit from eating food that has a slightly sweet flavour, but they must also be careful that they do not create Dampness. This is a fine balance because Spleen *yin* should be moistened and nourished, but as this is a Spleen *xu* condition, Dampness can easily arise.

Spleen *yin xu* can be caused by the following patterns of imbalance

- Stomach *yin xu*
- Stomach Fire
- Kidney *yin xu*
- Lung *yin xu*
- Heart *yin xu*
- Liver *yin xu*

Spleen *yin xu* can result in the following patterns of imbalance

- Stomach *yin xu*
- Kidney *yin xu*
- Liver *yin xu*
- Lung *yin xu*
- Heart *yin xu*
- Dampness
- Food stagnation

Combined patterns

Stomach and Spleen *qi xu*

Stomach and Spleen *qi xu* is extremely common; in fact, it is probably more common than a pure Spleen *qi xu* pattern.

Aetiology

The aetiology here is the same as that seen in Stomach *qi xu* and Spleen *qi xu*, i.e. consuming foods that are cold or uncooked, that create Dampness and that are unrefined. Eating too much at a time or too quickly will also put a strain on the Spleen and Stomach *qi*. Eating too little or eating a diet that lacks nutrients will weaken the Stomach and Spleen *qi*.

Although eating several small meals is beneficial for the Spleen, constantly snacking will place a strain on the Spleen *qi* because the Spleen will be constantly active.

Spleen *qi* and Stomach *qi* can also be weakened by worrying, constantly speculating, studying and thinking too much.

Prolonged illness, excessive bleeding and overexertion can weaken the Spleen *qi* and Stomach *qi*, as they will constantly have to replenish the *qi* and *xue* that has been consumed or lost.

Chronic Liver *qi* stagnation will often disrupt the functioning of and weaken the Stomach and Spleen *qi*.

Finally, working or living in a damp, humid climate or housing will burden the Spleen.

Symptoms and signs

- Fatigue
- Abdominal discomfort
- Loose stools
- Bloating after meals
- Fatigue after meals
- Pale complexion
- Deteriorated sense of taste
- Poor appetite or a lack of appetite in the mornings
- Weak or tired limbs
- Craving for sweetness
- Flatulence that is not odorous

- Tendency to put on weight

- Disinclination to speak and the voice lacks strength

- The person emanates a sense of tiredness and fatigue

- Poor posture

- A tendency to worry excessively or easily worry about things

- Pale, swollen tongue, possibly with teeth marks on the sides

- Weak pulse, especially in the right *guan* position

Key symptoms
Fatigue, loose stools, pale tongue with teeth marks and a Weak pulse.

Treatment principle
Tonify Stomach and Spleen *qi*.

Acupuncture points
Choose from: St 36, Sp 3, Sp 6, Ren 12, UB 20 and UB 21.

Needle technique
Tonifying. Moxa can be used.

Explanation

- St 36, Sp 3, Sp 6, Ren 12, UB 20 and UB 21 tonify Stomach and Spleen *qi*.

Herbal formula

- *Liu Jun Zi Tang* (Tonifies Stomach and Spleen *qi*)

- *Shen Ling Bai Zhu Tang* (Tonifies Stomach and Spleen *qi*)

Relevant advice
See Spleen *qi xu*.

Stomach and Spleen *qi xu* can be caused by the following patterns of imbalance

- Stomach *qi xu*

- Spleen *qi xu*

- Liver *qi* stagnation

- Food stagnation

Stomach and Spleen *qi xu* can result in the following patterns of imbalance

- Stomach *yin xu*

- Spleen *yang xu*

- Spleen *qi* sinking

- Spleen *qi* not holding *xue* inside the vessels

- Food stagnation

- Dampness

- Phlegm

- *Xue xu*

- Lung *qi xu*

- Heart *qi xu*

Spleen *qi xu* and Liver *xue xu*

These two patterns frequently occur together and Spleen *qi xu* will often be the underlying cause of Liver *xue xu*. It can therefore sometimes be appropriate to regard them as a common pattern.

Aetiology

Spleen *qi xu* often arises from the excessive consumption of cooling, Damp-producing or difficult-to-digest foods, such as dairy products, raw vegetables, wheat products, sugar, sweets and so on. Eating too much at a time or eating too little will weaken Spleen *qi*. Worrying or speculating excessively, as well as studying and thinking too much, will burden the Spleen.

Spleen *qi xu* will result in a poor production of *gu qi*. *Gu qi* is the post-heaven root of *xue*. This means that Spleen *qi xu* can lead directly to Liver *xue xu*. The situation is often further complicated by Liver *xue xu* being a contributing factor in the generation of Liver *qi* stagnation, which then invades and thereby weakens Spleen *qi*, and a vicious cycle arises.

A long-term condition of Liver *xue xu* can in itself also lead to Spleen *qi xu*, because the Spleen will be strained by constantly having to replenish the deficient *xue*.

Apart from Spleen *qi xu*, bleeding and a diet that does not contain sufficient *xue*-nourishing foods can also be root causes of Liver *xue xu*.

Symptoms and signs

- Fatigue

- Loose stools

- Fatigue after meals
- Dizziness, especially when getting up from sitting or lying down
- Difficulty focusing the eyes
- Visual disturbances such as floaters
- Dry eyes or a sensation of having grit in the eyes
- Pale, sallow complexion
- Pale, dry lips
- Poor appetite or no appetite in the mornings
- Craving sweet flavours
- The person emanates a sense of fatigue and tiredness
- Poor posture
- The skin may be dry and the flesh below may lack tone
- Weak muscles and fatigue in the arms and legs
- Depression, sadness or lack of vision in life
- Constant worrying or speculating over minor issues
- A tendency to be weepy and to be extra sensitive in the premenstrual phase
- Scanty or lack of menstrual bleeding
- Ridged fingernails or weak and fragile fingernails
- Pale, swollen tongue, possibly with teeth marks on the sides, the tongue may be dry, pale or orange sides to the tongue
- Fine, Weak or Choppy pulse, especially in both *guan* positions

Key symptoms
Fatigue, loose stools, pale complexion, dizziness, scanty menstruation, pale tongue.

Treatment principle
Tonify Spleen *qi* and nourish Liver *xue*.

Acupuncture points
Choose from: UB 17, UB 18, UB 20, UB 21, St 36, Sp 6, Liv 3, Liv 8, Ren 12 and Ren 4.

Needle technique
Tonifying. Moxa can be used on all the points and should be used on UB 17.

Explanation

- UB 17 nourishes *xue* in general.

- Liv 3, Liv 8, Sp 6 and UB 18 nourish Liver *xue*.

- Sp 6, St 36, Ren 12, UB 20 and UB 21 tonify Spleen *qi*.

- Ren 4 tonifies *yuan qi* and thereby increases production of *xue*.

Herbal formula

- *Gui Pi Tang* (Tonifies Spleen *qi* and nourishes *xue*)

Relevant advice

A person who is Spleen *qi xu* and Liver *xue xu* should eat a nutritious diet that includes a large proportion of green-leafed vegetables, beetroot, black beans, kidney beans, red meat, liver, bone marrow and other products that are rich in blood. The food should be well prepared and eaten hot. They should avoid dairy products, sugar, sweets and too many raw vegetables and salads.

Spleen *qi xu* and Liver *xue xu* can be caused by the following patterns of imbalance

- Liver *xue xu*

- Spleen *qi xu*

- Stomach *qi xu*

- Liver *qi* stagnation

- Food stagnation

Spleen *qi xu* and Liver *xue xu* can result in the following patterns of imbalance

- *Qi xu*

- *Xue xu*

- Spleen *qi xu*

- Spleen *yang xu*

- Liver *qi* stagnation

- Heart *xue xu*

- Liver *yin xu*

- Ascending Liver *yang*

- Kidney *jing xu*

Spleen and Lung *qi xu*
This pattern is discussed in the section on Lung imbalance patterns (page 393).

Spleen and Kidney *yang xu*
This pattern is discussed in the section on Kidney imbalance patterns (page 546).

Spleen *qi xu* and Heart *xue xu*
This pattern is discussed in the section on Heart imbalance patterns (page 487).

Liver *qi* invading the Spleen
This pattern is discussed in the section on Liver imbalance patterns (page 590).

Heart imbalances
The Heart is an interesting organ. In Western medicine, the heart and the brain are the two most important organs in the body. A person is declared dead when these organs are no longer functioning. The Western medicine heart and brain can be considered to be aspects of the same organ in Chinese medicine. Even though the brain is one of the six extraordinary *fu* organs and is created from Kidney *jing*, it is nourished by Heart *xue* and much of its functionality in Western medicine relates to the *shen*, which has its residence in the Heart. This makes the Heart the most important organ in the body in Chinese medicine. The Heart is described as being the Emperor in the body. The Heart is a true emperor – it does not do that much in the physical day-to-day functioning of the empire, but its balance and health are crucial for the functioning of the whole realm. If you look at the functions it performs, the Heart does very little compared with, for example, the Spleen. Yet it is the body's most important organ. Just like an emperor, *shen* is conscious of everything that is going on in the whole realm. Every detail is reported back to it. Events occur in the various organs and body parts, but it is *shen* that makes us aware that these have happened. For example, when we burn our finger, it is the tissue and skin of the fingers that are burnt, but it is our brain that perceives and interprets the signals that it receives from the nerve receptors in the fingers. In the same way, it is our *shen* that makes us conscious of the sensations our body experiences. This also happens on the emotional level. All emotional influences will have an impact, not only on the organs that these emotions resonate with, but also on the Heart. The Emperor has responsibility for the whole empire, therefore he must be omniscient so that he knows what needs to be done in all situations and at all times. It is his responsibility that the empire is harmonious and functions perfectly. Without his guiding hand, there would be chaos and rebellion in the empire. The whole empire would disintegrate. If the Emperor becomes weak or insane, he will not be able to rule his kingdom. The same is true of the Heart. If the Heart loses its stability, havoc will start to arise in the body. Therefore, there are many protective agencies around the Heart, including the Pericardium. It is important that an invasion does not penetrate into the Emperor's residence.

The aetiology of Heart imbalances

Due to its responsibility and importance, the Heart needs to be protected from attacks by exogenous *xie qi*. Heat that has been caused by invasions of exogenous *xie qi* can penetrate as deep as the Pericardium, which protects the Heart, but does not enter the Heart itself. This does not mean that the Heart cannot be disturbed by *xie qi* but that the *xie qi* that disrupts the Heart will be internally generated. The Heart is, for example, especially sensitive to all forms of internally generated Heat, both *xu* and *shi*. Due to its *yang* nature, Heat tends to rise upwards in the body and therefore it will often end up affecting the Heart, which is located in the upper *jiao*.

Invasions of exogenous Cold will not directly invade the Heart, but they can create a stagnation of Heart *xue*, which can affect the functioning of the Heart.

The Heart is particularly affected by feelings and emotions. Although the individual emotions affect specific organs, it is the *shen* that makes us conscious of these feelings and the effects that they have. Anger, for example, affects the Liver, but it is our *shen* that makes us aware that we are angry. When we are angry, the anger causes our Liver *qi* to ascend upwards and it can generate Heat in the Liver. When we are very angry, we are conscious of these changes, for example, the tension in the shoulders, neck and head due to the *qi* rushing upwards. We are also conscious of our emotional state. We are aware that we are angry. If anger affected only the Liver and not the Heart, these changes would take place without us being conscious of them. This means that any prolonged or extreme emotional influences will always have an impact on Heart *qi* and *shen*. The Heart itself is directly influenced by joy, and joy can be an aetiological factor that can be involved in the creation of Heart imbalances. It can seem strange that joy could be something that creates an imbalance in a person. Nevertheless, joy, or the lack of it, is a major aetiological factor in Heart imbalances. First, joy has a nourishing effect on the Heart and *shen*. A lack of joy in a person's life will lead to the creation of a *xu* condition of the Heart due to it being malnourished. This is also why several of the other emotions that are ascribed to other organs directly affect the Heart *qi*. Melancholy, sorrow, worry, fear and anger can all encompass an aspect of not being happy, of not being content. Second, there can also be too much joy. This does sound paradoxical, but joy not only nourishes the Heart, it also stimulates it. Too much stimulation of the Heart will dissipate and thereby weaken the Heart *qi*. This is typically seen when a person parties too much and is too ecstatic, especially if they consume stimulants and drugs or there is unbridled hedonism. This constant stimulation of the Heart's *yang* aspect, the *shen,* will exhaust Heart *qi* and, particularly, Heart *yin*.

Furthermore, several of the other emotions will have an indirect effect on the Heart by disrupting the functioning of their own organ. Anger, particularly when it is suppressed, i.e. frustration and irritation, can stagnate Liver *qi*. This can cause *qi* to stagnate in the chest and the Heart. Liver *qi* stagnation can also generate Fire in the Liver, which can rise up to the Heart and generate Heart Fire. Melancholy and sorrow will, apart from directly affecting the Heart, bind and weaken Lung *qi*. This can lead to *qi* stagnation, *qi xu* and the accumulation of Phlegm in the upper *jiao* and thereby in the Heart. Speculation and worry will bind and thereby weaken the Spleen *qi*. This can lead to *qi xu*, *xue xu* and Phlegm-Dampness, all of which will ultimately have an influence on the Heart. Fear weakens Kidney *qi* and can thus disrupt the cooperation and communication between the Kidneys and the Heart, as well as influencing the production of *qi* and *xue*.

Shock has a direct effect on the Heart. Shock dissipates and thereby significantly weakens Heart *qi*.

The Heart is nourished by joy in all its manifestations. These include love and affection. A lack of these, particularly in early childhood when the Heart, like other organs, is not stable, can lead to a person developing deep-rooted Heart imbalances that can affect them for the rest of their lives.

Stress is not an emotion in itself, but it is a condition that consists of several emotional aspects. The composition of stress and the relative amounts of these emotional aspects will be different from person to person and from stress situation to stress situation. Nevertheless, stress will always affect the *shen* and consume Heart *qi* and *yin*.

Dietary causes of Heart imbalances fall into two categories: those that affect the Heart directly and those that affect the Heart indirectly. Food, beverages and medicine that have a hot energy can directly create Heat in the Heart. Stimulants, such as recreational drugs, coffee and some types of pharmaceutical medicine drugs, can overstimulate the Heart, thereby spreading and consuming Heart *qi* and injuring the Heart *yin*. Foods, drinks and medicines that have a hot dynamic can, as well as creating Heat in other organs that will ascend upwards creating Heat in the Heart, lead to the formation of Phlegm. Phlegm can also arise through the excessive consumption of substances that in themselves produce Dampness and Phlegm.

Heat from food stagnation in the Stomach can also ascend and agitate the Heart. Food stagnation can arise when food is consumed that is difficult to transform because of eating too much, too quickly or too late in the evening.

The diet needs be nutritious enough to produce sufficient *qi* and *xue*; if it isn't, the Heart can become *qi xu* or *xue xu*.

Overworking, both mentally and physically, will weaken the Heart. Physical exertion and strain, such as working too much and too hard, illness, too much sex and so on, will weaken the *qi* and *yang* in the body. This can have both a direct and indirect impact on the Heart. Mental and emotional strain, such as studying, mental concentration, thinking a lot, working with a computer, excessive use of a smartphone and stress, will all consume Heart *yin* and *xue*.

Blood loss, such as heavy menstrual bleeding, childbirth and operations can lead to Heart *xue xu*. A significant loss of blood or fluids (such as extreme diarrhoea, vomiting or sweating) can weaken Heart *yang*.

Old age is characterised by a depletion of *qi*, *yin* and *yang*, as well as an increased accumulation of Phlegm and *xue* stagnation. These can all directly and indirectly affect the Heart.

Some Heart imbalances that manifest as mental-emotional disorders can be congenital, especially those that fall within the category of Phlegm blocking the *shen*.

There are several aetiological factors that by their nature are not traditionally described in Chinese medicine. Computers and televisions can have a debilitating effect on Heart *yin* because they overstimulate *shen* and consume Heart *xue*. This is compounded when they are used in the evening or at night as relaxation activities. The evening and night are the *yin* part of the day, when our *shen* should reduce its activity and become more passive and reflective. This means the use of things that stimulate and activate the *shen* will have a stronger negative impact when they are used in this period of the day. That we are so active and awake in the evening and at night is a modern challenge for our *yin*. Staying up and being mentally and physically active was not so much of an option before the advent of electricity and it has consequences for our *yin* aspects, particularly the Heart and Kidney *yin*.

The Heart has close relationships with several organs, and imbalances in these organs can lead to imbalances in the Heart. Liver *xue* and Heart *xue* are closely related and a *xu* condition of one of these will often result in a *xu* condition in the other. The same is true of Liver *qi* and Heart *qi*. A stagnation of one will often lead to a stagnation of the other. Gall Bladder *qi* and Heart *qi* do not have a close functional activity on the physical plane, but there is a relationship on the psychological level. A person who is Gall Bladder *qi xu* will also be Heart *qi xu*. Lung and Heart *qi* cooperate closely in relation to *zong qi*, and a *xu* condition in the Lung will affect the Heart and vice versa. The Heart and Kidneys have a *yin* and a *yang* relationship to each other. Kidney *yin* nourishes Heart *yin* and thus helps to control the Heart's fire aspect. The Heart's fire aspect helps to warm and activate Kidney *yang*, and Kidney *yang* supports Heart *yang*. Furthermore, *jing* is the material basis for *shen*. Heat from the Stomach can rise up to the Heart and create Heart Fire. Urinary Bladder imbalances can arise when there are Heart imbalances, even though these two organs do not have a direct connection, either physically or functionally. *Xie* Heat from the Heart can be transmitted via the Heart's partner organ, the Small Intestine, to the Urinary Bladder, which has a *taiyang* channel relationship to the Small Intestine. Furthermore, the Urinary Bladder divergent channel also connects to the Heart.

The pathology of Heart imbalances

When the Heart is imbalanced, this can manifest with changes in both its physical functions, such as the heartbeat, and how the *shen is* manifesting.

The Heart is the most *yang* organ in the body and the *shen* is the most *yang* aspect of the body's *qi*. This means that the Heart and in particular the *shen* are very sensitive to *xie* Heat due to its *yang* nature. On the physical level, Heat will over-activate the Heart, causing it to beat faster. This can manifest with palpitations and a rapid pulse. It is perhaps important to point out here that palpations in Chinese medicine means the subjective sensation that the physical heart is beating stronger and faster than normal. If the Heart is in balance, you are not aware of the heartbeat; it is not something you actually feel. Palpitations in Chinese medicine encompasses everything from being aware that the heartbeat is slightly more pronounced and is noticeable, on the one hand, to outright disorders such as atrial fibrillation, on the other. It is important to be conscious of this when interviewing a client, because many patients have a sensation of their heartbeat sometimes being slightly stronger, without them thinking of this as being palpitations. This is, nevertheless, an indication that there is a Heart imbalance in Chinese medicine, and it is an important sign.

Cold can also affect the Heart. The Heart as an organ cannot be directly invaded by exogenous Cold. Exogenous Cold can, however, stagnate Heart *xue* and Cold can therefore be a factor when there are Heart *xue* stagnation patterns. *Yang xu* conditions can also result in the Heart not performing its functions optimally. Like most Heart imbalances, Heart *yang xu* can manifest with palpitations. Where palpitations in Heat imbalances are the result of the Heart *qi* being agitated and over-activated, palpitations that are due to Heart *yang xu*, will be the result of Heart *yang* losing control of the rhythmical pumping function of the Heart. This is the same mechanism that results in palpitations when there is Heart *qi xu*. Heart *xue* and Heart *yin* should anchor the Heart's *yang* aspects, which include Heart *yang qi* and *shen*. If there is Heart *yin xu* or Heart *xue xu* they will not be able to anchor these *yang* aspects. This can, again, result in palpitations, due to the Heart no longer being able to control its rhythmic pumping, but this time there will also be a slight emotional unrest or anxiety that manifests concurrently with the palpitations, due to the *shen* not being anchored.

If there is a significant disruption of the physical functioning of the Heart, such as when there is Heart *xue* stagnation, there will not only be a disruption of the rhythm and strength of the heartbeat, but there will also be cardiac pain or pain in the thoracic region. The pain will be a fixed stabbing or piercing pain. If there is *qi* stagnation, there will not be the same sensation of pain but more of a sensation of chest oppression and tightness. It will feel as if there is an iron rim or a strong elastic stretched around the chest. Phlegm stagnation will manifest with a similar but different sensation. There will, again, be chest oppression, but Phlegm will manifest with a heavy, blocked sensation in the chest as if there is a great weight, such as a rock, lying on top of the thorax.

Because the Heart and the Lung have a very close relationship, a disturbance of the Heart *qi* will also manifest with the breathing being affected. Similarly, *zong qi* helps to drive *xue* through the vessels. If there is dysfunction in the Heart or if *zong qi* is weak or stagnated, *xue* will not reach out to the extremities. This can manifest in white, cold fingers and toes. This is typically seen when there is Heart *qi xu* and Heart *yang xu*. Purple fingernails are seen in conditions where there is *xue* stagnation, including Heart *xue* stagnation.

Shen encompasses the Western concepts of the mind and consciousness. When there are Heart imbalances, they will nearly always manifest with changes in the person's *shen*, which can be anything from almost unperceivable, subtle changes to severe personality disorders. *Shen* is nourished and anchored by Heart *yin* and

Heart *xue*. If these are weak, *shen* will lack nourishment and rooting. The person will be easily startled and unsettled, due to their *shen* lacking stability. Often, the lack of anchoring will also cause the person to have difficulty sleeping or be nervous, uneasy and restless. This will be more extreme if there is Heat due to *yin xu*. The agitation and restlessness will not only be mental, but it will also manifest physically with the person fidgeting and having nervous movements, especially when they are uneasy.

Shen is, in general, very sensitive to Heat. *Shi* Heat in particular agitates the *shen*. When the *shen* is agitated, the person will be mentally restless and feel uneasy. Their *shen* becomes too active. The difference between *xu* and *shi* Heat will often be seen in the intensity and severity of these manifestations. If there is *shi* Heat, the person will seem to be more stressed, their mental unrest will be more pronounced and they will be more irritable. If the Heat is intense, there will not only be mental unrest, but also actual mania.

As stated, a deficiency of Heart *yin* and Heart *xue* can manifest with insomnia, because the *shen* is not anchored at night, resulting in the person being awake and conscious. Excess Heat in the Heart, such as when there is Heart Fire or Phlegm-Heat, can also result in insomnia. In these situations, even though Heart *yin* and *xue* are not weak, they are not able to root the *shen* because it is being agitated by the *shi* Heat.

The Heart is responsible for and controls communication and contact with others. If there is an excess of Heat, the person can become too communicative. They will be too open. These are the people who share their whole life story with complete strangers, without the stranger even having shown any particular interest in hearing it. In the clinic, these clients can be difficult to interview, because they talk too much and give you far too many details, without you asking for them. They will usually also talk more quickly, because Heat over-activates the *shen*, resulting in a cascade of thoughts. The opposite of these patients are people who are uncommunicative and taciturn. They can also be difficult in a clinical setting, because it can be a problem drawing information out of them. This is usually a manifestation of the Heart *qi* stagnating or being blocked. Phlegm can also obscure the *shen* by enshrouding it in a blanket or lying like a mist around it. These people are not completely present. It can be difficult to create and maintain contact with them. Their communication can be a bit confused and their voice may sound slurred. If the Phlegm is very concentrated, the *shen* can become so obscured that they talk nonsense, saying one thing but meaning something completely different, or they are completely enclosed in their own world and talk to themselves. The blocking and shrouding of their *shen* will mean that their comprehension is impeded and they will also have difficulty concentrating.

The memory and concentration will also be affected by other Heart Imbalances. If *shen* lacks nourishment, for example if there is Heart *xue xu*, the memory and concentration will be poor. Heat can also result in poor concentration, although the dynamics are completely different. Heat will agitate *shen* so the mind is easily distracted, and there will be too many thoughts arising in the head making it difficult to maintain focus and concentrate on one thing at a time. The activity and agitation will also mean that their memory will often be poor because the information never had a chance to settle and thereby be stored. Phlegm blocking the *shen* will also result in difficulty concentrating. There is a mental fog and the person will have difficulty thinking clearly and comprehending what is going on around them.

Shen manifests in the eyes. This means that when the *shen* is affected it is possible to observe deviations here. Ideally, when the *shen* is in balance, the eyes will be clear and bright. There will be good eye contact between you and the patient. Heat agitates *shen* and can cause the person's eyes to dart about and they can have difficulty maintaining eye contact. When it is there, the eye contact will be clear and even intense. A person who is Heart *qi xu* will find it difficult to maintain eye contact, but this will be due to shyness or nervousness and their eyes will lack vitality and sparkle. Phlegm can cause the eyes to be dull and matt; the person's *shen* cannot shine through the mist. When there is Heart *qi* stagnation, it is as if the person's vision becomes introverted and does not extend outwards from their eyes. It is as if they lack vision and only look inwards towards themselves. When there is *shi* Heat, the opposite happens and the eyes can be very intense.

One of *shen*'s functions is to ensure that we conform to society around us and that our behaviour and responses are normal. If *shen* is agitated by Heat or blocked by Phlegm, this function is disturbed. This can result in a person saying and doing things that other people think are strange or weird. Their appearance may also seem peculiar to others. People whose *shen* is disturbed can often be recognised by their attire, their hair and their general appearance. Their clothes can be gaudy, discordant or just muddled. It is important, however, to remember that what seems abnormal to many people can be quite normal in a particular subculture; in this case the person's *shen* is in fine balance, they have just adopted different standards.

A person's *shen* is an individual refraction of the universal *shen*. If their *shen* is in harmony, they have a fundamental sense of belonging, a sense of tranquillity and security. When *shen* is agitated, blocked or undernourished, the person can lose this sensation and they can feel unease, anxiety or a fundamental loneliness.

A person who is Heart *qi xu* and whose *shen* is undernourished can have low self-esteem and lack self-confidence.

The tongue is controlled by the Heart. If there is Heart Fire, the tongue will not just be red, as is usual in Fire conditions, but there can also be ulcers and sores on the tongue. The difference between these ulcers and those seen in Stomach and Spleen imbalances is that when there is Heart Fire, the ulcers will be triggered or aggravated by stress or emotional pressure. When there are Stomach and Spleen imbalances, the ulcers are related to the diet. Furthermore, the ulcers will be more red and elevated when there is Heart Fire.

The tongue is also used in communication with others. As explained above, the Heart has a great influence on this communication and on our speech. Heart imbalances can also affect the tongue in other ways; stuttering and stammering can be due to the Heart *qi* being disrupted, meaning the Heart loses control of the tongue.

Heart Fire can manifest with a bitter or metallic taste[24] in the mouth in the morning. When there is Liver Fire, the bitter or metallic taste will be experienced throughout the day.

The Heart is nourished by and manifests with joy. If the Heart is *qi xu* or if there is *qi* stagnation, the person can seem doleful, unhappy and lacking in vitality.

The voice should also have vitality. This is not dissimilar to the tongue, pulse, skin and so on. These should have the quality of *shen*, i.e. a quality of vitality. The same is true of the voice, but there are not the same connotations. When there are *xu* conditions or stagnations in the Heart, the voice will lack a certain quality. This quality isn't volume and it isn't necessarily joy, but it is related more to movement. The voice should vary and change as they talk, especially as the subject area changes. This reflects the natural movement of the *shen*. The voice should not be stuck in a certain gear. No sound or emotion in the voice is wrong or inappropriate; it can only be inappropriate to what is being said or to the conversation in general. In the same way that the pulse should have *shen*, so should the voice. When the pulse is soft, yet firm and solid and is rhythmic in its beating, it tells us about the quality of the Heart. The voice should have an even flow and not be stuttering or confused, its tone should go up and down and it should have the sound of joy and happiness in it. If there is no joy, i.e. if Heart *qi* and *shen* are either blocked or undernourished, there will be a flatness and maybe even a tone of sadness in the voice. On the other hand, if there is too much Heat in the Heart, there can be too much of these qualities of joy and happiness. The voice can be unnaturally glad. This is the 'life and soul of the party' voice. Here, the voice will often be voluble and accompanied by too much laughter and the person can seem elated and unnaturally happy. Also, there will often be too many, and sometimes inappropriate, jokes. It may manifest with a constant need to create laughter by repeatedly telling funny stories and making jokes. All this indicates that there is too much Heat in the Heart. Heart *yin xu* Heat will, though, result in a voice that is not voluble and the person will have more of a nervous laugh or giggle while talking. There may be a short, nervous laugh that ends their sentences, like a sort of inappropriate punctuation mark.

Although the Heart has no direct influence on the physiology of fluids, it can nevertheless be involved in urinary imbalances. As well as urine becoming dark and odorous when there are Heat conditions in general, Heart Fire can drain down to the Urinary Bladder via its partner organ the Small Intestine. This can result in dark urine that may contain blood and a painful or burning sensation on urination.

General symptoms and signs of Heart imbalances

- Palpitations

- Restlessness and mental agitation

- Sleep disturbances

- *Shen* disturbances

- Mental-emotional symptoms

- Changes to the tip of the tongue

Shi patterns

Heart qi stagnation

Heart *qi* stagnation can be a distinct pattern of imbalance, but it is most often seen as a consequence of, and together with, Liver *qi* stagnation. The pattern arises almost exclusively from emotional causes.

Aetiology

Emotional imbalances where feelings are not expressed or where there is a prolonged presence of a particular emotion can lead to Heart *qi* stagnation.

Symptoms and signs

- Palpitations

- Tightness of the chest, chest oppression or the feeling that there is a tight band or rim around the chest

- Tension in and around the solar plexus

- Shortness of breath

- A need to yawn or sigh

- A sensation of there being a lump in the throat

- Poor appetite

- Disinclination to lie down

- Weak and cold hands

- Purple lips

- Insomnia

- Mental unrest

- Sadness

- Disinclination to speak

- The person is particularly uncommunicative and seems very closed and emotionally repressed

- The voice can be sad or flat

- Mood swings

- Depression

- Slightly purple or swollen edges on the front third of the tongue

- Wiry pulse in the left *cun* position, the pulse can be Knotted

Key symptoms
Palpitations, tightness of the chest, a need to sigh, the person gives the impression of being emotionally repressed.

Treatment principle
Spread Heart *qi* and open the chest. Activate *shen*.

Acupuncture points
Choose from: He 5, He 7, Pe 6, UB 14, UB 15, UB 17, Liv 14, Ren 17, Ren 14, Du 11 and St 40.

Needle technique
Spreading technique.

Explanation

- He 5, He 7, Pe 6, Ren 14, Du 11, UB 14 and UB 15 spread Heart *qi* and activate *shen*.

- Liv 14, Ren 17 and St 40 disperse *qi* in the chest.

Herbal formula

- *Ban Xia Hou Po Tang* (Disperses *qi* in the chest)

Relevant advice
Physical activity such as sport and exercise will help to circulate *qi* in the chest. Beating the chest with a loose fist or the upper back with a wooden spoon will help to invigorate the *qi* in the chest. Rolling the shoulders and swinging the arms can also be recommended. Due to the emotional aspects that are often at the root of this imbalance, it is important that the person addresses the underlying emotional issues.

Breathing exercises that involve slowly inhaling deeply and then quickly exhaling with force whilst making a loud noise will help to release stagnant *qi*.

Heart *qi* stagnation can be caused by the following patterns of imbalance

- Liver *qi* stagnation

- Heart *qi xu*

- Heart *xue* stagnation

- Heart *xue xu*

- Food stagnation

Heart *qi* stagnation can result in the following patterns of imbalance

- Liver *qi* stagnation

- Heart *xue* stagnation

- Heart *yin xu*

- Heart *xue xu*

- Phlegm

Heart *xue* stagnation

Heart *xue* stagnation is characterised by cardiac pain and pain in the chest. Only this pattern and 'Blocked Heart vessels' manifest with cardiac pain. Heart *qi* stagnation and Phlegm stagnation will manifest with a tight and a heavy, oppressed sensation in the chest respectively.

Heart *xue* stagnation can be a purely *shi* pattern and a combined *xu* and *shi* pattern, depending on the underlying pathology.

Aetiology

Heart *xue* stagnation can arise from chronic Heart imbalance patterns, especially *qi* stagnation, Cold and Phlegm. *Xu* patterns such as Heart *xue xu* or Heart *yang xu* can also be causes of Heart *xue* stagnation.

Symptoms and signs

- Piercing or stabbing chest pains or cardiac pain

- Tightness in the chest

- Palpitations

- Pain or tingling sensation in the left arm

- Cold hands

- Shortness of breath

- Matt and purple facial complexion, the face can be white when there is acute pain

- Blue or purple lips

- Purple tongue, purple or swollen sides on the front third of the tongue, swollen, purple sub-lingual veins

- Choppy or Wiry pulse, the pulse can be Knotted

Key symptoms
Cardiac pain, chest pain, blue or purple lips.

Treatment principle
Invigorate Heart *xue*.

Acupuncture points
Choose from: He 5, Pe 4, Pe 6, UB 14, UB 15, UB 17, Sp 10, Ren 17 and Ren 14.

Needle technique
Spreading or tonifying, depending on whether there is a *xu* or a *shi* condition. Moxa can be used.

Explanation

- He 5, Pe 4, Pe 6, Ren 14, UB 14 and UB 15 invigorate Heart *xue*.

- Sp 10 and UB 17 invigorate *xue*.

- Ren 17 invigorates *qi* and *xue* in the upper *jiao*.

Herbal formula

- *Xue Fu Zhu Yu Tang* (Invigorates *xue* in the Heart and the upper *jiao*)

Relevant advice
See the relevant advice in the sections dealing with the underlying patterns of imbalance.

Heart *xue* stagnation can be caused by the following patterns of imbalance

- Heart *xue xu*

- Heart *yang xu*

- Phlegm

- Heart *qi* stagnation

- Liver qi stagnation

Heart *xue* stagnation can result in the following pattern of imbalance

- Phlegm

Blocked Heart vessels

This is a combined pattern that will have its root in several patterns, with the common feature that they block *qi* and *xue* in and around the Heart. The most common patterns that are the cause of this imbalance are Heart *qi* stagnation, Heart *xue* stagnation, Cold and Phlegm.

Aetiology

Emotional stress and long-term emotional imbalances can stagnate Heart *qi* and eventually Heart *xue*. Overwork, too much sex and sweating whilst exposed to the cold will all weaken Heart *yang* and can thereby stagnate Heart *xue*.

Consuming Damp-producing foods can lead to the formation of Phlegm, which can block the movement of *qi* and *xue* in the Heart.

Symptoms and signs

- Piercing and stabbing cardiac pain, the pain is usually worse when the person is exposed to the cold

- Palpitations

- Shortness of breath

- Tight or heavy sensation in the chest

- Purple, matt or white and pale complexion

- Mental unrest or unease

- Depression

- Mental and physical fatigue with an oppressive feeling

- Dizziness

- Heavy headedness or headache

- Pulmonary sputum

- Cold hands

- Blue or purple lips

- Purple nails

- The tongue may be pale and swollen with a greasy coating, it can be purple in the front third

- Wiry, Choppy or Slippery pulse, the pulse can be Knotted

Key symptoms

Sharp or stabbing chest pain, purple lips and breathlessness.

Treatment principle

Invigorate Heart *qi* and *xue*, transform Phlegm, expel Cold and calm the *shen*.

Acupuncture points
Choose from: Pe 5, Pe 6, He 5, Ren 14, Ren 15, Ren 17, UB 14, UB 15, UB 17, Sp 10 and St 40.

Needle technique
Spreading technique.

Explanation

- He 5, Pe 6, Ren 14, Ren 15, UB 14 and UB 15 invigorate Heart *qi* and Heart *xue*.

- Sp 10 and UB 17 invigorate *xue*.

- Ren 17 circulate *qi* and *xue* in the upper *jiao*.

- Pe 5 and St 40 transform Phlegm and move *qi* in the chest.

Herbal formula

- *Dan Shen Yin* (Invigorates *xue* in the Heart and the upper *jiao*) combined with herbs relevant to the underlying pattern of imbalance

Relevant advice
Light physical activity will be beneficial, however it is important that the person does not overexert themselves if there is an underlying *xu* pattern. Beating the chest and the upper back with a loose fist or a wooden spoon or rolling the shoulders and swinging the arms can also be recommended. As well as getting adequate exercise, it is also important that they get sufficient rest and relaxation. They should avoid stress and overexerting themselves physically. If they play sports, it is important that they do not expose themselves to the cold when they sweat.

They should avoid foods that create Dampness and Phlegm.

Blocked Heart vessels can be caused by the following patterns of imbalance

- Heart *xue* stagnation
- Heart *qi* stagnation
- Phlegm
- Cold
- Liver *qi* stagnation
- Spleen *qi xu*
- Spleen *yang xu*
- Kidney *yang xu*

Blocked Heart vessels can result in the following patterns of imbalance

- Phlegm

- Heart *xue* stagnation

- *Qi xu*

- *Yang xu*

Phlegm obscuring the *shen*

Where the previous patterns manifest with both physical and mental symptoms and signs, this and the following patterns are much more mental-emotional in their manifestations.

Aetiology

Diet is often a major factor in the formation of Phlegm. This can also be the case here, where consuming Damp- and Phlegm-producing foods and foods that have a cold or hot energy can lead to the formation of Dampness or Phlegm. Chronic emotional imbalances can stagnate Heart *qi* and lead to Phlegm obscuring the *shen*.

Heat conditions can condense fluids and thereby create Phlegm. Chronic *yang xu* and *xue* stagnation can lead to fluids accumulating and forming Phlegm.

Certain medicines can create Phlegm that then obscures *shen*.

Phlegm obscuring *shen* may be a congenital pattern in children.

Symptoms and signs

- Mental confusion

- Slow thinking and comprehension

- Blurred, foggy sensation in the head, as if it is full of cotton wool

- Heavy sensation in the head

- Loss of consciousness

- Mental fatigue

- Difficulty concentrating

- Forgetfulness

- Depression

- Dull, matt eyes

- Inability to maintain eye contact

- The person seems absent and not fully present

- Incoherent speech, talks nonsense or has difficulty formulating sentences

- Muttering or talking to themselves

- The voice may be slurred

- Difficulty maintaining a structure in their lives

- Lack of motivation

- Increased need to sleep

- Nausea

- Heavy breathing or wheezing

- Rattling sound in the throat

- Vomit of sputum in extreme cases

- Swollen, flaccid tongue, possibly with a greasy coating

- Slippery pulse

Key symptoms
Mental confusion, foggy sensation in the head, difficulty concentrating, swollen tongue with greasy coating.

Treatment principle
Transform Phlegm, open the Heart.

Acupuncture points
Choose from: St 8, St 40, Du 20, Pe 5, St 36, Ren 12, Ren 14, UB 15 and UB 20. If there is loss of consciousness: He 9 and Du 26.

Needle technique
Draining, except on Ren 12, St 36 and UB 20.

Explanation
- St 8 and Du 20 drain Phlegm from the head and brighten the *shen*.

- Pe 5, St 40, Ren 14 and UB 15 transform Phlegm in the Heart and brighten the *shen*.

- St 36, Ren 12 and UB 20 transform Phlegm.

- Du 26 and He 9 revive consciousness.

Herbal formula
- *Di Tan Tang* (Resolves Phlegm and opens the Heart's orifices)

Relevant advice
The patient should avoid eating a diet that is Damp and Phlegm producing. They should ensure that they get a lot of fresh air and physical activity. As there is often a significant emotional aspect linked to this pattern, they should also try, whenever possible, to address the underlying emotional themes.

Phlegm obscuring the *shen* can be caused by the following patterns of imbalance

- Heart *qi* stagnation

- Spleen *qi xu*

- Damp

- Phlegm

- Heat conditions

- *Xue* stagnation

- *Yang xu*

Phlegm obscuring the *shen* can result in the following patterns of imbalance

- Phlegm-Heat in Heart

- Heart *xue* stagnation

- Spleen *qi xu*

Phlegm-Heat agitating the Heart

This pattern is similar in some ways to the previous one. The difference is that in this pattern Heat also agitates the *shen*. The Heat can have arisen due to the Phlegm stagnation itself or the Heat may have been one of the factors contributing to Phlegm being created.

Aetiology
The aetiology of Phlegm-Heat agitating the Heart is very similar to the aetiology of Phlegm obscuring *shen*. Diet will play a significant role, especially the consumption of food and beverages that have a hot dynamic, as well as those that directly generate Dampness and Phlegm. Emotional imbalances can create a stagnation of *qi* in the Liver and the Heart. Heat can simultaneously agitate the *shen* and lead to the creation of Phlegm. Phlegm stagnation can in itself lead to the generation of Heat.

Spleen *qi xu* or *yang xu* can also have contributed to the formation of Phlegm. This means that the aetiological factors that can lead to these conditions may also be involved in the evolution of this pattern.

Symptoms and signs

- Mental unrest and unease

- Mania

- Depression or mood swings

- Aggression, both verbal and physical

- Spontaneous and ill-considered actions

- Rapid body movements

- Difficulty sitting still and being settled

- Talking a lot and talking quickly

- Loud voice or shouting

- Incoherent speech, talking nonsense or having difficulty maintaining the structure of a conversation

- The voice may sound slurred

- Uncontrolled laughing or crying

- Laughing while talking

- Talking to themselves

- Inability to maintain eye contact

- Mental confusion

- The person may lack a sense of reality

- Red face

- Weird or peculiar attire or hair

- Palpitations

- Tightness, oppression or unrest in the chest

- Thirst

- Bitter or metallic taste in the mouth

- Insomnia

- Dream-disturbed sleep, possibly with nightmares

- Rattling sound in the throat

- Rapid breathing

- Dark urine

- Red tongue with red swollen tip, greasy yellowish coating, there can be a crack in the tip of the tongue

- Full, Rapid and Wiry or Full, Rapid and Slippery pulse

Key symptoms
Mania, talking quickly, mental restlessness, red tongue with yellow greasy coating and a Full pulse.

Treatment principle
Drain Phlegm-Heat, calm the *shen* and open the Heart.

Acupuncture points
Choose from: Pe 5, Pe 7, Pe 8, He 8, He 9, St 8, GB 13, St 40, Du 20, Du 24, Ren 15 and UB 15.

Needle technique
Draining.

Explanation

- St 8, GB 13, Du 20 and Du 24 drain Phlegm from the head and calm *shen*.

- Pe 5 and St 40 transform Phlegm and calm *shen*.

- Pe 7, Pe 8, He 8, Ren 15 and UB 15 drain Heat from the Heart and calm *shen*.

Herbal formula

- *Wen Dan Tang* (Transforms Phlegm, drains Heat and calms *shen*)

Relevant advice
The patient should avoid consuming anything that creates Heat, such as chilli, pepper, garlic, dark chocolate, alcohol, too much red meat especially lamb, fried food such as crisps, chips, falafel, and so on. They should also avoid Phlegm- and Damp-producing foods such as sweets, sugar, wheat, dairy products, bananas, avocados, dried fruit and so on.

It is important that the *shen* is not agitated further by stimulants such as coffee.

Phlegm-Heat agitating the Heart can be caused by the following patterns of imbalance

- Phlegm patterns

- Fire patterns

- Heart *qi* stagnation

- Liver *qi* stagnation

- Spleen *qi xu*

Phlegm-Heat agitating the Heart can result in the following patterns of imbalance

- Heart *xue* stagnation

- Spleen *qi xu*

- *Yin xu*

- *Xue* stagnation

- *Qi* stagnation

- *Qi xu*

Heart Fire

Shi Heat will agitate *shen* and this is reflected in the symptoms and signs, which will be pronounced. In this pattern *shen* is not blocked or smothered in the same manner as it is in 'Phlegm-Heat agitating the Heart', so there will not be the same mental confusion, blurred thinking and poor sense of reality.

It is also important to differentiate this pattern from Heart *yin xu* Heat; the symptoms of this pattern will be much more pronounced. When there is *shi* Heat, there will be mania and mental agitation rather than just mental restlessness. A Heart *yin xu* pulse will be weaker.

Heat from the Heart can drain downwards to the Urinary Bladder via the Small Intestine and create symptoms of Heat in the Urinary Bladder, such as burning pain when urinating and blood in the urine.

Aetiology

Excessive consumption of energetically hot food, medicine and beverages will generate Fire in the body, as will invasions of exogenous *xie qi*, *qi* stagnation and Phlegm stagnation.

Fire and Heat from other organs can rise up to the Heart due to the *yang* nature of Heat, agitating the Heart.

Long-term and powerful emotional imbalances can eventually lead to Heart *qi* stagnation that can create Heat in the Heart.

Symptoms and signs

- Insomnia

- Dream-disturbed sleep

- Red face

- Mental unrest and unease

- Mental and physical agitation

- Mania

- Aggression, both verbal and physical

- Irritability

- Rapid body movements

- Difficulty sitting still and being settled

- Talking a lot and talking quickly

- The person is very easy to connect with but has a tendency to give you too much and irrelevant information

- Palpitations

- Physical unease in the chest

- Tongue ulcers

- Dark urine or blood in the urine

- Burning pain on urination

- Uncontrolled laughing

- Laughs while talking

- Talks to themselves

- Difficulty maintaining eye contact because the eyes constantly dart about

- Thirst

- Bitter or metallic taste in the mouth

- Insomnia

- Rapid breathing

- Red tongue with red swollen tip, dry yellow tongue coating, there may be ulcers on the tongue

- The pulse can be Rapid and Flooding or Skipping

Key symptoms
Red face, palpitations, talks quickly, ebullience, thirst, bitter taste and red tongue.

Treatment principle
Drain Heart Fire and calm the *shen*.

Acupuncture points
Choose from: Pe 6, Pe 7, Pe 8, He 8, He 9, Ren 15, Du 14, Du 20, Du 24, UB 15 and Kid 1.

Needle technique
Draining technique. Even technique on Kid 1.

Explanation

- Pe 6, Pe 7, Pe 8, He 8, He 9, Ren 15 and UB 15 drain Fire from the Heart and calm the *shen*.

- Du 14 drains Heat.

- Du 20 and Du 24 calm *shen*.

- Kid 1 drains Fire downwards, tonifies Kidney Water and calms *shen*.

Herbal formula

- *Xie Xin Tang* (Drains Heart Fire)

Relevant advice
The patient should avoid all food and beverages that create Heat. This will include things such as alcohol, lamb, chilli and other hot spices, deep fried foods, dark chocolate, garlic and so on.

The Heart is already overstimulated in this pattern and therefore it should not be further stimulated. This means that coffee, black and green tea and anything that contains caffeine or other stimulants must be avoided.

Heart Fire can be caused by the following patterns of imbalance

- Heart *qi* stagnation

- Liver Fire

- Stomach Fire

- *Xue* Heat

Heart Fire can result in the following patterns of imbalance

- Phlegm-Heat agitating the Heart

- Heart *xue* stagnation

- Heart *yin xu*

- Kidney *yin xu*

- Liver Fire

- Stomach Fire

Xu imbalances

Heart *yin xu*

Where Kidney *yin xu* will often reflect and manifest with weakness of *jing*, Heart *yin xu* has a similar relationship with *shen*. The Heart's *yin* aspects nourish and anchor *shen*.

Aetiology

Heart *yin* is weakened by prolonged mental and emotional stress, anxiety, worry and fear. Lack of sleep, excessive thinking and use of the brain and general overexertion will all deplete Heart *yin*.

Heart *yin* is also depleted by the overuse of stimulants, such as coffee. Some medicines have a hot and spicy dynamic. This could injure Heart *yin*. An excessive consumption of food and beverages that have a hot or spicy dynamic, such as alcohol and chilli, will also injure *yin*.

Partying, too many late nights and too much exhilaration will consume Heart *yin*.

The use of computers and smartphones and watching television over-activate the mind and thereby consume Heart *yin*. This effect will be even more pronounced in the evening, when Heart *yin* should be tranquil.

Heat from Fire and *shi* Heat conditions in the body can rise up to the Heart and injure Heart *yin*. Heat and Fire conditions may be internally generated or the result of invasions of exogenous *xie qi*.

There can also be an inherent tendency to have Heart *yin xu*. Heart *yin xu* can also be a consequence of the ageing process and the general weakening of Kidney *yin*. In general, Kidney and Heart *yin* cooperate closely. Kidney *yin* should nourish Heart *yin*, ensuring that Heart Fire does not become excessive and uncontrollable. Kidney *yin xu* often results in Heart *yin xu*.

Yin xu in one or more of the other organs may eventually weaken *yin* generally in the body and thereby lead indirectly to Heart *yin xu*.

Symptoms and signs

- Insomnia

- Waking often at night and difficulty falling asleep due to restless thoughts

- Dream-disturbed sleep

- Palpitations

- Mental unease and restlessness
- Physical restlessness and agitation
- Anxiety
- Being easily startled
- Poor memory
- Dry mouth and throat
- Night sweats
- Hot at night
- Thin body
- Depression
- Dizziness
- Nervous voice or nervous chattering
- Nervous laugh while talking
- Dark urine
- Constipation or dry stools
- Red speckled tip or red tip of the tongue, crack in the tip of the tongue
- Empty or Fine pulse, especially in the left *cun* position

If there is Heart *yin xu* Heat, the following symptoms and signs may be seen:

- malar flush
- sensation of heat or fever late in the afternoon, the evening and at night
- hot sensation in the palms of the hands, soles of the feet and the chest
- mental restlessness and agitation
- talks a lot
- talks quickly
- thirst especially in the evening and at night, there is a need to sip small mouthfuls of water rather than to drink large gulps of cold water
- being easily stressed
- dark urine
- constipation or dry stools
- thin, red tongue with red tongue tip

- Empty or Fine and Rapid pulse, especially in the left *cun* position.

Key symptoms
Palpitations, insomnia, night sweats, mental unrest, being hot at night, being easily stressed.

Treatment principle
Nourish Heart *yin* and control Heat.

Acupuncture points
Choose from: He 6, He 7, Ren 14, Ren 4, UB 15, UB 23, Sp 6, Kid 6 and Kid 7.

Needle technique
Tonifying technique.

Explanation

- He 7, Ren 14 and UB 15 nourish Heart *yin*.

- He 6 and Kid 7 control night sweats and nourish Kidney and Heart *yin*.

- UB 23, Ren 4, Kid 6 and Sp 6 nourish Kidney *yin*.

Herbal formula

- *Tian Wang Bu Xin Dan* (Nourishes Heart and Kidney *yin*, calms *shen*)

Relevant advice
The patient should avoid stress, both in their work and emotionally. They should not work too much and they should get enough sleep and go to bed early. Coffee and other stimulants should be avoided, because they over-activate *shen* and thereby deplete Heart *yin*. Alcohol, hot spices and grilled and fried food should be avoided, as they can create Heat in the Heart and injure *yin*.

Using a computer or a smartphone and watching television in the evening is detrimental for Heart *yin*. This is because they activate *shen*, thereby consuming Heart *yin* at a time when *shen* and *yin* are supposed to be tranquil and dormant. If Heart *yin* is already weakened, it will be even harder for it to anchor and root *shen* in the evening.

The patient should try to create balance and harmony in their emotions and cultivate tranquillity and relaxation. Meditation can be a great help for these patients. The Heart is nourished and tonified by joy. The patient will benefit from doing or looking at things that make them happy. They can try to do something every day that gives them pleasure or to meditate, focusing on something that gives them joy. Too much stimulation of the senses and exhilaration, on the other hand, depletes Heart *yin*. Whilst looking at flowers, beautiful vistas or art nourishes Heart *yin*, going to nightclubs, partying, taking drugs or just being excited depletes Heart *yin*.

Heart *yin xu* can be caused by the following patterns of imbalance

- Kidney *yin xu*

- Liver *yin xu*

- Stomach *yin xu*

- Lung *yin xu*

- Heart *xue xu*

- Heart *qi* stagnation

- Fire

- *Shi* Heat

Heart *yin xu* can result in the following patterns of imbalance

- Heart *yin xu* Heat

- Liver *yin xu*

- Kidney *yin xu*

- Phlegm

Heart *xue xu*

The patterns of Heart *yin xu* and Heart *xue xu* are very similar in their symptoms and signs, because Heart *xue* is an aspect of Heart *yin*. The differentiation between the two patterns is based mainly on the presence or absence of *yin xu* or *xue xu* signs in the symptom picture. Otherwise, the symptoms and signs are very similar.

Aetiology

Xue xu arises for three main reasons: *xue* is lost either through bleeding or over-consumption, such as excessive physical training or excessive mental activity; there is a poor production of *xue*; the diet is not rich enough in food that directly nourishes *xue*.

Blood loss, such as in childbirth, heavy menstrual bleeding, bleeding disorders, operations and so on, may result in Heart *xue xu*. These factors can be relevant for a long time, in some cases several years after the loss of blood has occurred.

Excessive exercise, such as physical training, will consume *xue*. In some cases, excessive mental and emotional activity can also consume Heart *xue*.

A poor production of *xue* will be due to deficient conditions in the organs involved in the production of *xue*, in which case aetiological factors that weaken the Spleen and Kidneys will be involved. Even though the Spleen and Kidneys are in balance, Heart *xue xu* can arise if the person's diet is deficient in *xue*-nourishing foods.

Heart *xue xu* is often seen simultaneously with, or as a consequence of, Liver *xue xu*.

Symptoms and signs

- Insomnia

- Dream-disturbed sleep

- Palpitations

- Fatigue

- Dizziness

- Being easily startled

- Poor memory

- Being mentally absent

- Anxiety

- Sallow, pale face

- Pale, dry lips

- Pale, dry and thin tongue

- Fine or Choppy pulse, the pulse may be weakest in the left *cun* position

Key symptoms
Palpitations, insomnia, poor memory, pale lips and a pale tongue.

Treatment principle
Nourish Heart *xue*.

Acupuncture points
Choose from: He 7, Ren 14, Ren 15, Ren 4, UB 17, St 36, Sp 6, UB 15, UB 17 and UB 20.

Needle technique
Tonifying. Moxa can be used, particularly on UB 17.

Explanation

- He 7, Ren 14, Ren 15 and UB 15 nourish Heart *xue*.

- Ren 4, UB 17, St 36, Sp 6 and UB 20 nourish *xue*.

Herbal formula

- *Gui Pi Tang* (Nourishes Heart *xue* and Spleen *qi*, calms *shen*)

- *Ba Zhen Tang* (Nourishes *xue*)

Relevant advice

When there is Heart *xue xu*, it is important to eat a diet that nourishes *xue*. Things that nourish *xue* include green leafy vegetables, beetroot, seaweed, dates, kidney beans, black beans, aduki beans, red meat, bone marrow, blood sausages, heart and liver.

The patient should avoid sugar, stimulants such as coffee and too much alcohol. Nettle tea will be beneficial for them to drink.

The patient should not only eat a diet that is rich in *xue*-nutritious foods, but they should also eat a diet that is beneficial for their Spleen *qi*. This means eating warm, prepared food, such as soups, stews, baked vegetables and so on and avoiding salads, raw food and food and beverages that have a cold energy or produce Dampness.

The advice given in the section on Heart *yin xu* will also be relevant here.

Heart *xue xu* can be caused by the following patterns of imbalance

- Liver *xue xu*
- Spleen *qi xu*
- Spleen *yang xu*
- Heart *qi* stagnation

Heart *xue xu* can result in the following patterns of imbalance

- Heart *yin xu*
- Heart *xue* stagnation

Heart *qi xu*

This pattern has symptoms and signs that are specific to the Heart, such as palpitations, whilst also manifesting general *qi xu* symptoms and signs, such as fatigue. This pattern can be physical or mental-emotional, with the person lacking self-esteem, self-confidence or happiness.

There is a close relationship between the Heart and Lung in their functioning. This means that there will usually be tangible symptoms and signs of Lung *qi xu* when there is Heart *qi xu*. Heart *qi* will also be weakened by prolonged or excessive sorrow and melancholy, which also affects the Lung negatively because even though these emotions affect the Lung directly, *shen* and thereby the Heart will register and be conscious of these emotions and thereby also be affected by them. When a person experiences sorrow and melancholy, there is also a lack of joy. This means that Heart *qi* will lack nourishment. Heart *qi* in general is nourished by joy and love. A person whose life lacks joy, love and a sense of companionship and belonging will often become Heart *qi xu*. This can particularly be the case if the person did not experience enough love and attention or if they felt ostracised in childhood. In childhood the organs are not fully stable and their *qi* is more volatile. This means that the internal organs can be easily affected by aetiological factors such as the seven emotions. These factors will have a greater effect in childhood than they will in later life and can permanently influence the organ in question.

Aetiology

Blood loss, prolonged illness, physical strain and emotional imbalances. A lack of joy in life or loneliness can particularly lead to Heart *qi xu*. Shock scatters Heart *qi*, thereby weakening it.

The Heart controls sweating. Excessive sweating can deplete Heart *qi*.

The consumption of recreational drugs and some medicines can open the Heart and thereby spread Heart *qi*. This can weaken Heart *qi xu* over time.

Symptoms and signs

- Palpitations

- Slight shortness of breath

- Shallow breathing

- Pale complexion

- Mental, physical and/or emotional fatigue

- Spontaneous sweating

- Sadness, melancholy, lack of joy, feelings of loneliness, depression

- Low self-esteem or lack of self-confidence

- The person may seem very quiet, diffident or shy

- Speech impediments such as stammering

- The voice may sound flat and lack vitality or tone variation

- Lack of sparkle in the eyes

- Pale or normal-coloured tongue

- Deep and Weak, especially in the left *cun* position, the pulse may be Knotted

Key symptoms

Palpitations, fatigue, sadness, lack of self-confidence and a Weak pulse.

Treatment principle

Tonify Heart *qi*.

Acupuncture points

Choose from: He 5, He 7, UB 15, Ren 6, Ren 14, Ren 15, Ren 17 and St 36.

Needle technique
Tonifying. Moxa can be used.

Explanation

- He 5, He 7, Ren 14, Ren 15 and UB 15 tonify Heart *qi*.

- Ren 17 tonifies *qi* in the upper *jiao*.

- Ren 6 and St 36 tonify *qi*.

Herbal formula

- *Ding Zhi Wan* (Tonifies Heart *qi* and calms *shen*)

- *Sheng Mai San* (Tonifies Heart *qi* and *yin*)

Relevant advice
Heart *qi* is best tonified on the emotional level. It is important that the person cultivates joy in their life. Of course, this is easier said than done. As well as working with their emotions, the person can try to spend some time each day doing something that gives them genuine pleasure or they can sit and meditate on something that for them is beautiful.

Tonifying *qi* in general will also benefit the patient. This can be done through the diet, access to fresh air and breathing exercises, as well as getting enough rest and avoiding overexertion.

Heart *qi* can be depleted through excessive sweating. This means that the use of saunas and steam baths is not something that is recommended for these patients.

The patient should avoid the use of recreational drugs, medicines and experiences that spread Heart *qi*.

Heart *qi xu* can be caused by the following patterns of imbalance

- Spleen *qi xu*

- Lung *qi xu*

- Kidney *qi xu*

- Gall Bladder *qi xu*

- Heart *qi* stagnation

- *Xue xu*

Heart *qi xu* can result in the following patterns of imbalance

- Heart *yang xu*

- Heart *qi* stagnation

- Heart *yin xu*

- Heart *xue xu*

- Lung *qi xu*

Heart *yang xu*

Heart *yang xu* and Heart *qi xu* have a lot of symptoms and signs in common. Heart *yang xu* will, though, manifest with characteristic *yang xu* symptoms and signs. Heart *yang xu* can be a consequence of *yang xu* conditions in other organs, such as the Kidneys and the Spleen.

Aetiology

Heart *yang xu* can arise after a person has been sweating profusely. This will weaken the Heart's *yang* aspect. It can also arise when there have been other types of excessive fluid loss, such as severe diarrhoea, vomiting or bleeding.

Furthermore, aetiological factors that may lead to Spleen and Kidney *yang xu* can also be relevant. This could be things like overwork, too much sex, disease, old age, congenital weakness, an excessive intake of cold food, cold drinks and cold medicine.

Symptoms and signs

- Palpitations

- Slight shortness of breath

- Fatigue

- Depression

- Spontaneous sweating

- Chest oppression

- Cold hands

- Aversion to cold

- Pale or white face

- Slightly dark lips

- Lack of enthusiasm for life

- Mental lethargy

- Slow speech

- Poor posture

- Pale, wet, swollen tongue

- Slow, Deep pulse, the pulse may be Weak in the left *cun* position

Key symptoms
Palpitations, cold hands, Deep and Weak pulse.

Treatment principle
Warm and tonify Heart *yang*.

Acupuncture points
Choose from: He 5, He 7, UB 15, Ren 14, Ren 17, Ren 6, Du 4 and Du 14.

Needle technique
Tonifying technique. Moxa is recommended.

Explanation

- He 5, He 7, Ren 14 and UB 15 tonify Heart *yang*.

- Ren 17 tonifies *qi* and *yang* in the upper *jiao*.

- Ren 6, Du 4 and Du 14 tonify *yang*.

Herbal formula

- *Zhen Wu Tang Tang* (Tonifies and warms Kidney, Spleen and Heart *yang*)

Relevant advice
It is important that *yang* is protected and not further burdened when there is Heart *yang xu*. This means that the patient should avoid consuming food and beverages that have a cold energy or temperature. At the same time, they must not overexert themselves and men should avoid having too much sex.

Heart *yang* can be damaged by excessive sweating, therefore saunas and steam baths are something that is not recommended for these patients.

Heart *yang xu* can be caused by the following patterns of imbalance

- Heart *qi xu*

- Kidney *yang xu*

- Spleen *yang xu*

Heart *yang xu* can result in the following patterns of imbalance

- Heart *yang* collapse

- Phlegm obscuring the *shen*

- Heart *xue* stagnation

- *Qi* stagnation in the chest

- Kidney *yang xu*, overflowing Water

Heart *yang* collapse

Heart *yang* collapse is a more extreme and more serious condition than Heart *yang xu*. *Yang* is now too weak to move *xue* and body fluids. Heart *yang* collapse may be a consequence of Kidney *yang xu* or Heart *yang xu*.

Aetiology
The aetiology of Heart *yang* collapse will be the same as that described for Heart *yang xu*.

Symptoms and signs

- Palpitations

- Shortness of breath

- Shallow breathing

- Profuse sweating

- Cold limbs

- Blue or purple lips

- Grey or white complexion

- Possible loss of consciousness

- Pale or bluish tongue, the tongue may be short

- Deep, Weak or Hidden pulse

Key symptoms
Blue or purple lips, palpitations, Hidden pulse.

Treatment principle
Rescue Heart *yang*.

Acupuncture points
This is a severe and acute condition in which Western medical intervention is required. If this is not available, you can choose from: Ren 4, Ren 6, Ren 8, Du 4, Du 14, Du 20, UB 15, St 36 and Pe 6.

Needle technique
Tonifying, no retention of the needles. Moxa must be used. Direct moxa or moxa on ginger slices on Ren 4, Ren 6 and Ren 8 is necessary.

Explanation

- UB 15 tonifies Heart *yang*.

- Pe 6 circulates *qi* in the upper *jiao*.

- Du 4 and Du 14 tonify *yang*.

- Du 20 raises *yang*.

- St 36, Ren 4, Ren 6 and Ren 8 rescue *yang*.

Herbal formula

- *Zhen Fu Tang* (Rescues *yang*)

Relevant advice
This is usually an acute pattern, therefore lifestyle and dietary advice is not so relevant. It is important that the patient does not sweat, because this will further weaken Heart *yang*.

Heart *yang* collapse can be caused by the following patterns of imbalance

- Kidney *yang xu*

- Heart *yang xu*

Heart *yang* collapse can result in the following patterns of imbalance

- Collapse of *yang*

- Heart *xue* stagnation

Combined patterns
Heart *xue xu* and Spleen *qi xu*
This pattern is very common, especially in women. The pattern can arise from Heart *xue xu* or Spleen *qi xu*. One pattern can lead to the other and they will eventually become self-generating. Heart *xue xu* puts a strain on Spleen *qi*, because the Spleen has to work harder to constantly try and replenish *xue*. Spleen *qi xu* is the post-heaven root of *xue* and can therefore lead to Heart *xue xu*. The reason that this pattern is more common in women than men is that women lose *xue* through menstrual bleeding and childbirth and thus tend to be more *xue xu* in general.

Aetiology

This pattern can occur when there has been blood loss, such as through heavy menstrual bleeding, childbirth, surgery or physical trauma. The menorrhagia may in itself be due to Spleen *qi xu* when the Spleen is too weak to hold *xue* inside the vessels. The other causes of bleeding could be *xu* or *shi* Heat or *xue* stagnation. The aetiology of this pattern can therefore also include factors that lead to these conditions, and these patterns should be addressed in the treatment strategy, either immediately or in subsequent treatments.

Xue xu can also arise through excessive physical training where the need for *xue* to nourish the muscles exceeds the body's ability to produce *xue*. Excessive mental activity can also weaken Heart *xue* directly, as Heart *xue* nourishes the *shen* and the Brain.

The Spleen *qi xu* aspect can arise because the Spleen has to work extra hard to create more *gu qi* to replenish the lack of Heart *xue*. Spleen *qi xu* can also arise independently if the diet is of poor quality or if there is an excessive consumption of food and beverages that have a cold energy or temperature or that produce Dampness. If the diet lacks food that is directly *xue* nourishing, this in itself can lead to or worsen the Heart *xue xu* aspect of this pattern.

Spleen *qi xu* can also be a consequence of physical overexertion or disease. Worry, speculation, studying and thinking too much can not only bind Spleen *qi* and thereby weaken it, but also affect the Heart. Grief, sadness and anxiety will also be factors that can have a direct negative impact on the Heart.

Symptoms and signs

- Palpitations
- Fatigue
- Dizziness
- Poor memory
- Pale and sallow face
- Pale, dry lips
- Loose stools
- Poor appetite
- Being bloated immediately after eating
- Insomnia
- Dream-disturbed sleep
- Anxiety
- Being easily startled

- Scanty menstrual bleeding

- The person may be absentminded or not quite present

- Weak or low voice

- Pale tongue

- Choppy or Fine pulse

Key symptoms
Insomnia, palpitations, fatigue, loose stools and scanty menstrual bleeding.

Treatment principle
Tonify Spleen *qi*, nourish Heart *xue* and calm *shen*.

Acupuncture points
Choose from: He 7, St 36, Sp 3, Sp 6, Ren 12, Ren 14, UB 15, UB 17 and UB 20.

Needle technique
Tonifying. Moxa is recommended on UB 17 and St 36.

Explanation

- He 7, Ren 14 and UB 15 nourish the Heart *xue* and calm *shen*.

- St 36, Sp 3, Ren 12 and UB 20 tonify Spleen *qi*.

- Sp 6 tonifies Spleen *qi*, nourishes *xue* and calms *shen*.

- UB 17 nourishes *xue*.

Herbal formula

- *Gui Pi Tang* (Tonifies Spleen *qi*, nourishes the Heart *xue* and calms *shen*)

Relevant advice
If there is Spleen *qi xu* and Heart *xue xu*, a diet that is rich in food that both nourishes Heart *xue* and tonifies Spleen *qi* is recommended. This means that the person should eat a lot of green, leafy vegetables, beetroot, seaweed, dates, kidney beans, aduki beans, black beans, red meat, bone marrow, blood sausages, nettle tea, heart and liver. The food should be prepared, i.e. boiled, steamed, baked and so on, and it should be eaten warm. They should avoid raw vegetables, cold drinks, ice cream, sugar, stimulants such as coffee or too much alcohol. It is important that they chew their food slowly and thoroughly, and that they eat in calm surroundings, focusing on what they are eating.

Light exercise is beneficial, as it will help support the Spleen's *qi* mechanism. On the other hand, they should avoid sitting still for long periods of time or sitting with a slumped posture, especially after meals.

Profuse sweating should also be avoided, because it will weaken Heart *xue*.

Heart *xue xu* and Spleen *qi xu* can be caused by the following patterns of imbalance

- Spleen *qi xu*
- Heart *xue xu*
- Liver *xue xu*
- Heart *qi* stagnation
- Kidney *yang xu*
- Liver *qi* stagnation
- Damp
- Phlegm

Heart *xue xu* and Spleen *qi xu* can result in the following patterns of imbalance

- Spleen *yang xu*
- Kidney *yang xu*
- Kidney *yin xu*
- Lung *qi xu*
- Liver *qi* stagnation
- Liver *xue xu*
- Stomach *qi xu*
- Damp
- Phlegm
- Heart *yin xu*
- Heart *qi xu*
- Heart *xue* stagnation

Heart and Lung *qi xu*
This pattern is discussed in the section on Lung imbalance patterns (page 393).

Heart and Kidney *yin xu*
This pattern is discussed in the section on Kidney imbalance patterns (page 546).

Heart and Liver *xue xu*
This pattern is discussed in the section on Liver imbalance patterns (page 590).

Heart and Gall Bladder *qi xu*
This pattern is discussed in the section on Gall Bladder imbalance patterns (page 580).

Small Intestine imbalance
The main function of the Small Intestine is to receive the untransformed dross from the Stomach and separate the pure aspects that are still present from the impure waste. The pure fluids and *qi* that are extracted in the Small Intestine are transmitted upwards via the *san jiao*, and the impure fluids and solids are sent to the Urinary Bladder and the Large Intestine respectively. Although these processes take place in the Small Intestine, they do so under the influence and control of the Spleen and Kidney *yang*. This means that most signs of imbalance in the Small Intestine are viewed as being Spleen and Kidney imbalances and treated accordingly. For example, in the treatment of diarrhoea, Spleen and Stomach points will typically be used, not Small Intestine points. When the Small Intestine is treated in these situations, it is usually through the use of its lower *he*-sea point St 39.

Small Intestine imbalance patterns can arise when the Small Intestine is directly invaded from the exterior. This can occur through either the skin of the abdomen or the mouth and the Stomach. Cold can invade through the skin of the abdomen when this area has been exposed to the climate, for example when a person has worn too little or worn wet clothes. Damp-Heat, Damp-Cold or exogenous Cold can invade the Small Intestine via the mouth and Stomach when food that is contaminated or has gone off has been ingested or when food that is energetically very cold or hot, produces Dampness or has a very cold temperature has been ingested.

The long-term consumption of food and beverages that are energetically or physically cold will weaken Spleen *yang* and Kidney *yang*. Damp-Heat, Damp-Cold and *yang xu* can all disrupt the Spleen's ability to transform and transport. This can manifest with changes in the stool and/or pain in the abdomen. The consumption of energetically hot food, as well as emotional imbalances, can create Stomach Fire or Heart Fire, which can then be transmitted to the Small Intestine, creating Heat.

Parasitic worms are defined as aetiological factors that are 'neither exterior nor interior'. A person can have been infected through contact with contaminated food or dirt. Worms will enter the body through the mouth. The worms will block the movement of both *qi* and solids in the Small Intestine. By inhibiting the separation of the pure and the impure, worms will lead to malnutrition.

Qi stagnation in the Small Intestine can arise when *qi* stagnates in the middle and lower *jiao*. *Qi* stagnation in the Small Intestine could affect the stool and cause intestinal pain. There are several factors that can lead to *qi* stagnation here. Liver *qi* stagnation can arise due to emotional frustrations, stress, repressed anger and irritation. The stagnant Liver *qi* can accumulate and block the movement of *qi* through the Intestines. Worry, speculation and thinking too much will bind and thereby stagnate Spleen and Stomach *qi* so their *qi* mechanism grinds to a halt, with the result that *qi* movement through the Intestines is impaired. *Qi* stagnation in the Small Intestine can also be a consequence of too little exercise, poor posture and a general lack of physical movement. If a person spends too much time sitting still, especially if their posture is poor or they sit with a twisted midriff, it will physically prevent the movement of *qi* through the Intestines. This is a particular problem when a person eats whilst they are working on the computer.

Shi Heat can drain down to the Small Intestine from its partner organ, the Heart. This means that all of the aetiological factors that can lead to Heart Fire can be relevant here. Heat will disrupt the Small Intestine functions in relation to fluid physiology. The Heat can thereby be transmitted to the Urinary Bladder, resulting in symptoms such as painful or burning urination, dark urine and possibly blood in the urine.

In some cases, deafness can result from *xie qi*, for example Fire disrupting the flow of *qi* in the Small Intestine channel.

General symptoms and signs of a Small Intestine imbalance

- Abdominal pain
- Abdominal bloating
- Diarrhoea
- Constipation
- Borborygmi

Shi patterns
Shi Heat in the Small Intestine
Heat from the Heart or the Stomach can be transmitted to the Small Intestine. The Heat can then manifest with symptoms relating to the Small Intestine, and also to the Urinary Bladder, with which the Small Intestine has a functional and *taiyang* relationship.

Aetiology

Emotional imbalances and influences can create Heart Fire. The excessive consumption of food and beverages that are energetically hot, such as alcohol, fried and grilled food, lamb, hot spices and so on, can create Stomach and Heart Fire. The Fire in these organs can be transmitted to the Small Intestine.

Symptoms and signs

- Mental agitation or restlessness
- Insomnia
- Ulcers in the mouth and on the tongue
- Deafness
- Sore throat
- Turmoil in the chest
- Abdominal pain
- Thirst with a desire for cold drinks
- Dark, scanty urine with a burning sensation on urination
- Blood in the urine
- Red face
- The person talks quickly or talks a lot
- Red tongue with a red swollen tip and yellowish coating
- Fast, Flooding pulse, Wiry in the left hand *chi* position

Key symptoms

Abdominal pain, dark and painful urine, red tongue tip possibly with ulcers on the tongue.

Treatment principle

Drain Heat from the Heart and Small Intestine. Promote urination.

Acupuncture points

Choose from: SI 2, SI 5, He 5, He 8, St 39, Ren 3 and UB 28.

Needle technique

Draining.

Explanation

- SI 2, SI 5 and St 39 drain Heat from the Small Intestine.

- He 5 and He 8 drain Heart Fire.

- Ren 3 and UB 28 drain Heat from the Urinary Bladder.

Herbal formula

- *Dao Chi San* (Drains Heart Fire via the Small Intestine and the Urinary Bladder)

Relevant advice

Food and beverages that have a hot energy should be avoided.

Shi Heat in the Small Intestine can be caused by the following patterns of imbalance

- Heart Fire

- Stomach Fire

Shi Heat in the Small Intestine can result in the following patterns of imbalance

- Urinary Bladder Heat conditions

- Heart Fire

Small Intestine *qi* stagnation

The Small Intestine receives the untransformed residues from the Stomach. After further processing, the turbid fluids are sent to the Urinary Bladder and the impure dregs are sent down to the Large Intestine. Stagnation of *qi* in the Small Intestine can inhibit the descent of *qi* in the Small Intestine and thereby disrupt the transformation of fluids that takes place here, as well as causing pain and discomfort. This pattern is usually a pure *shi* pattern, but there can be a *xu* aspect as well when Spleen and Stomach *qi xu* result in stagnation in the Small Intestine.

Aetiology

Frustration, irritation, repressed anger, pent-up emotions and stress can all stagnate Liver *qi*. Stagnant Liver *qi* can then invade the Small Intestine and interfere with its *qi* mechanism. Worry, speculation and excessive thinking can bind Spleen *qi* and disrupt the Stomach and Spleen's *qi* mechanism. This can then disrupt the movement of *qi* and the functioning of the Small Intestine.

Excessive sitting and sitting in a twisted or slumped posture will physically block the movement and functioning of the Small Intestine *qi*.

An excessive consumption of food and beverages that are energetically and physically cold or that produce Dampness can weaken Stomach and Spleen *qi* and thereby the Small Intestine.

Symptoms and signs

- Abdominal bloating, discomfort at palpation of the abdomen
- Pain in the lower abdomen, which can radiate to the back, the pain is aggravated by pressure
- Discomfort when wearing tight clothing on the abdomen
- Borborygmi
- Flatulence
- Intestinal pain that is relieved by passing wind
- Constipation
- Testicular Pain
- There may be signs of Liver *qi* stagnation
- White tongue coating
- Wiry pulse, especially in *chi* positions

Key symptoms
Abdominal pain, borborygmi, Wiry pulse.

Treatment principle
Regulate and move *qi* in the Small Intestine, possibly regulate Liver *qi*.

Acupuncture points
Choose from: Ren 6, SJ 6, GB 34, Liv 3, Liv 13, St 27, St 29, Sp 4, Sp 6 and St 39.

Needle technique
Spreading. Moxa can be used.

Explanation

- Ren 6, SJ 6, St 27 and St 29 move and regulate *qi* in the Small Intestine.
- GB 34, Liv 3 and Liv 13 spread Liver *qi*.
- Sp 4 and Sp 6 tonify Spleen *qi* and regulate *qi* in the Small Intestine.

Herbal formula

- *Chai Hu Shu Gan Tang* (Spreads Liver *qi* and regulates Small Intestine *qi*)

Relevant advice
As well as addressing any emotional issues that may lie behind their *qi* stagnation, the patient must ensure that they get enough exercise. A short walk after eating is recommended. If this is not possible, stretching and light abdominal massage would be beneficial. Abdominal massage where the movement is in a clockwise direction will help circulate *qi* in the Intestines. Posture is important, especially when the person eats and immediately afterwards. Sitting straight and standing erect ensures that there is a free passage through the abdominal cavity.

Small Intestine *qi* stagnation can be caused by the following patterns of imbalance

- Liver *qi* stagnation
- Food stagnation
- Cold stagnation
- Stomach and Spleen *qi xu*

Small Intestine *qi* stagnation can result in the following patterns of imbalance

- Liver *qi* stagnation
- Stomach and Spleen *qi xu*

Small Intestine *qi* bound
This pattern is an acute pattern. Acute appendicitis will fall within this category.

The difference between this pattern and the previous one is that in this pattern there is not only a stagnation in the movement of *qi*, but also an actual blockage. When there is a stagnation of *qi*, the movement of *qi* is impeded, disrupted or irregular. When there is a blockage, there is no movement at all.

Aetiology
An invasion of exogenous Cold will block the movement of *qi* down through the Small Intestine. The Cold can have entered through the mouth, such as when food or beverages that are cold in their temperature or energy are ingested. The Cold can also have invaded through the skin of the abdomen or through the *yin* channels in the legs. This will happen if the person has been exposed to climatic cold or worn inadequate or wet clothing.

Symptoms and signs

- Abdominal bloating

- Acute and intense abdominal pain that is aggravated by pressure

- Constipation

- Vomiting

- Borborygmi

- Flatulence

- Painful facial expression

- Inhibited or limited body movements

- The pain is ameliorated by warmth

- Aversion to cold

- Cold abdominal skin

- Thick, white and greasy tongue coating

- Wiry pulse in the *chi* positions

Key symptoms
Intense abdominal pains, constipation, thick, white and greasy tongue coating.

Treatment principle
Expel Cold and disperse *qi* in the Small Intestine.

Acupuncture points
Choose from: Ren 6, SJ 6, GB 34, Liv 3, Liv 13, St 25, Sp 4, Sp 6, St 39 and *Lanweixue* (Ex-LE 7).

Needle technique
Draining. Moxa is recommended.

Explanation

- Ren 6, SJ 6, St 25 and St 39 invigorate and regulate *qi* in the Small Intestine.

- GB 34, Liv 3 and Liv 13 spread Liver *qi*.

- Sp 4 and Sp 6 tonify Spleen *qi* and regulate *qi* in the Small Intestine.

- *Lanweixue* is an empirical point for acute pain and blocking of the intestines.

Herbal formula

- *Tian Tai Wu Yao San* (Regulates *qi* and expels Cold from the Intestines)

Relevant advice
This is an acute pattern, therefore diet and lifestyle advice will have a limited effect. The person will benefit from eating or drinking things that are warm and spicy in their dynamic, such as ginger or turmeric.

Small Intestine *qi* bound can be caused by the following patterns of imbalance

- Liver *qi* stagnation

- Invasion of Cold in the Stomach

- Small Intestine *xu* Cold

Small Intestine *qi* bound can result in the following patterns of imbalance

- Liver *qi* stagnation

- Spleen *yang xu*

Worms in the Small Intestine
This pattern cannot be treated with acupuncture.

Aetiology
Ingestion of contaminated food, poor hygiene and inadequate cooking of food.

Symptoms and signs

- Abdominal pain

- Abdominal bloating

- Pale and sallow complexion

- Weight loss and poor growth in children

- Vomiting of worms

- Strange cravings

- Anal or nasal itching

- Insatiable hunger

Key symptoms
Weight loss, lack of growth in children, insatiable appetite.

Treatment principle
Kill and expel parasites.

Herbal formula

* *Li Zhong An Hui Tang* (Warms the middle *jiao* and kills worms)

* *Wu Mei Wan* (Drains Stomach Heat, warms the Intestines, tonifies *qi* and kills worms)

Relevant advice
Better hygiene and preparation of food.

Urinary Bladder imbalances

In Chinese physiology, the Urinary Bladder plays a wider role than it does in Western medicine physiology. In Western medicine, the Urinary Bladder stores and expels urine. It also does this in the Chinese medicine physiological model but here it has the additional function of helping to transform the impure body fluids that it receives from the Lung and Small Intestine.

For the Urinary Bladder to be able to fulfil these functions, it is dependent on Kidney *yang qi*. The Kidney *yang* warms and activates the Urinary Bladder and provides it with the necessary *qi* and warmth to be able to transform the impure fluids and transmit the pure fluids upwards through the *san jiao*, as well as enabling the Urinary Bladder to retain the urine until it is expelled out of the body. The expulsion of the urine from the Urinary Bladder is again dependent on the strength of the Kidney *yang qi*. This means that when the Urinary Bladder is incapable of performing its functions, it is not due to a *xu* condition in the Urinary Bladder but is because of either a deficiency of Kidney *yang* or the presence of *xie qi*.

If there is Kidney *yang xu*, the Urinary Bladder will lack the necessary *qi* and heat to be able to carry out its functions of transforming the impure fluids, sending pure fluids upwards and retaining and expelling urine. This will manifest with an increased volume of urine that is pale. There will be frequent voiding of copious amounts of clear and pale urine, because fluids that have not been transported will have seeped down to the lower *jiao*. The urine can also be cloudy due to the fluids not having been transformed.

Urination will also be more frequent and there may even be incontinence when there is Kidney *yang xu*, because Kidney *yang* will not be able to hold the urine inside the Urinary Bladder. On the other hand, there can also be problems voiding urine when there is Kidney *yang xu*. Kidney *yang* is the force behind this voiding function, expelling the urine from the Urinary Bladder. Kidney *yang xu* can therefore manifest with symptoms such as incomplete emptying of the Urinary Bladder, a weak stream of urine or post-urination dribbling. Although these symptoms are due to a dysfunction of the Urinary Bladder, the treatment will be aimed at tonifying Kidney *yang*, because this is where the root of the problem lies.

As well as a deficiency of Kidney *yang*, another cause of urinary disturbances is the *qi* mechanism of the Urinary Bladder being obstructed or disrupted by certain types of *xie qi*. Damp is often involved in *shi* patterns of imbalance in the Urinary Bladder, as it inhibits the movement of *qi* and can block the *qi* mechanism in the Urinary Bladder, which impedes the transformation and transportation of fluids and blocks the excretion of urine. The blockage will manifest in difficulty in urinating. There can be difficulty voiding the urine or in emptying the Urinary Bladder completely. The Dampness can also result in the urine becoming cloudy. In extreme cases, the accumulation of Dampness in the Urinary Bladder can lead to the formation of sand or stones in the Urinary Bladder. The lack of transformation and transporting of body fluids can result in an increased amount of urine in the Urinary Bladder, thus there may be more frequent or urgent urination with copious amounts of pale or cloudy urine.

The Dampness can be combined with Cold or Heat. If there is Cold present, it will further block the Urinary Bladder's *qi* mechanism and burden the Kidney's *yang* aspect, which will hamper the transformation and transportation of fluids. Due to its contracting nature, Cold can cause problems with voiding the urine, as well as difficulties in emptying the Urinary Bladder completely. The Dampness and the accumulation of fluids can result in the person having no thirst.

Heat can also combine with Dampness. When there is Heat, it can 'boil' the urine, so that the urine is dark, concentrated and odorous. In contrast to Cold, Heat has an expansive nature and creates over-activity. Heat can therefore force the urine out of the Urinary Bladder. There will then be a frequent urge to urinate, but because the Heat has evaporated and condensed the urine, there will only be small quantities of dark urine. This will be further exacerbated by the Dampness, which will in itself block the urination. Besides difficult and frequent urination, Heat will typically also manifest with a stinging and burning pain upon urination. The Heat can also cause the vessels to burst, so there can be visible blood in the urine. Heat can also result in fever and an increased thirst. Although there is thirst, the Damp aspect and the accumulation of fluids in the body can mean that there is no desire to drink. This is characteristic of Damp-Heat conditions.

Damp is *yin* in nature and seeps downwards. Therefore, when there is Dampness, there can be a heavy, sinking sensation in the lower *jiao*. This is most characteristic when there is Damp-Cold. The expansive nature of Heat means that Urinary Bladder Damp-Heat has a tendency to manifest with tension or distension in the lower *jiao*, especially in the area just above the pubic bone. This can be a subjective sensation or something that can be felt on palpation.

Damp can be both exogenous or internally generated. Internally generated Dampness is usually the result of Spleen and Kidney *xu* patterns or excessive consumption of food and beverages that produce Dampness. Exogenous Damp, like Cold, can invade the body when the person has been exposed to climatic cold and dampness. Dampness can invade directly through the skin, typically when the person has worn inadequate or wet clothing, for example a wet bathing costume. Damp and Cold can also enter the body via the *yin* channels in the legs.

Damp-Heat can arise in several ways. Damp-Cold will typically transform into Damp-Heat. This process is accelerated if there is already Heat present in the body. Damp-Heat can also be caused by the excessive consumption of food and beverages that directly create Damp-Heat, for example alcohol and fried food. Damp-Heat can invade the body from the exterior. This may be due to exogenous *xie qi* invading the body via the mucous membranes, i.e. bacterial infections in Western medicine terminology.

Heat can also be caused by emotional imbalances. There is a connection from the Heart via the Small Intestine channel to the Urinary Bladder. The Urinary Bladder also has a divergent channel that connects to the Heart. Heart Fire can therefore be transmitted to the Urinary Bladder, where it will combine with Dampness, resulting in Urinary Bladder Damp-Heat. Emotional imbalances that affect the Liver can also interfere with the Urinary Bladder. This is because the Liver channel passes around the urethra and the Urinary Bladder.

Invasions of exogenous *xie qi* can disrupt the functioning of the Lung so that it does not send fluids down to the Urinary Bladder. These fluids will accumulate in the body's tissue and there will be a lack of fluids in the Urinary Bladder. This will result in acute oedema and concurrent inhibited urination. This is not a Urinary Bladder pattern of imbalance but is discussed under Lung imbalances as 'Invasion of Wind-Water' (page 403).

In addition, all of the aetiological factors that deplete Kidney *yang* can be involved in Urinary Bladder imbalances due to the mechanisms described above.

General symptoms and signs of Urinary Bladder imbalances

- Urinary difficulties (problems with voiding, frequent or urgent urination, incontinence, painful urination)

- Cloudy, pale or dark urine

- Increased or decreased volume of urine

- Distension, tightness or pain in the area above the pubic bone

Shi patterns
Urinary Bladder Damp-Heat

Urinary Bladder Damp-Heat is typically an acute disorder. It can often develop into a chronic condition with acute episodes. Many women find that they suffer from recurrent urinary tract infections and that these infections increase in frequency. These infections are often treated with Western medication. Unfortunately, these pharmaceutical products often have a double negative effect. The Western medication clears the Heat aspect of the disorder, but does not address the Damp aspect. This means that there will remain a lingering Damp pathogen, which will start to generate Heat, resulting in symptoms of a new infection. Furthermore, due to its Cold nature, the medicine weakens Kidney and Spleen *yang*, resulting in additional Dampness that seeps down to the lower *jiao*, laying the foundation for a new Damp-Heat condition in the Urinary Bladder. This is again treated with Cold medication that does not drain the *xie qi* completely out of the Urinary Bladder but increases Dampness, and a vicious cycle is started.

Damp-Heat, as stated above, often arises when Damp-Cold transforms into Damp-Heat. This transformation will accelerate if there is already Heat present in the body. An excessive consumption of food and beverages that are energetically hot, stress and *qi* stagnation Heat are typical contributing factors.

Aetiology
Invasions of exogenous Damp, Cold and Heat. Dietary factors that produce Dampness and Damp-Heat, as well as the repeated use of medicines that are energetically cold. Stress, emotional frustrations, pent-up anger, hatred, jealousy and irritation can cause Liver *qi* stagnation Heat or Heart Fire, which can drain down to the Urinary Bladder.

Symptoms and signs

- Burning, stinging sensation during urination

- Frequent, urgent, but scanty urination

- Difficulty urinating or in fully voiding the Urinary Bladder

- Dark, yellowish, turbid and odorous urine

- Possibly blood in the urine

- Tightness and distension above the pubic bone

- Thirst with no desire to drink

- Fever or feeling of heat in the body

- Yellowish, greasy coating on the root of the tongue

- Raised, red papillae on the root of the tongue

- Rapid and Wiry or Rapid and Slippery pulse, the *chi* positions may be Full

Key symptoms
Burning sensation upon urination, urgent but scanty urination, dark and cloudy urine, greasy yellow coating on the root of the tongue.

Treatment principle
Drain Damp-Heat from the Urinary Bladder.

Acupuncture points
Choose from: Ren 2, Ren 3, Sp 6, Sp 9, LI 11, UB 22, UB 28 and UB 32.

Needle technique
Draining.

Explanation

- Ren 2, Ren 3, UB 28 and UB 32 drain Damp and Heat from the Urinary Bladder.

- Sp 6, Sp 9, UB 22 and LI 11 drain Damp-Heat.

Herbal formula

- *Ba Zheng Tang* (Drains Damp-Heat from the Urinary Bladder)
- *Bei Xie Fen Qing Yin II* (Drains Damp-Heat from the Urinary Bladder)

Relevant advice
When there is Urinary Bladder Damp-Heat, the person should avoid foods and beverages that generate Damp or Heat. They should avoid exposure to climatic influences that can result in Damp, Heat or Cold invading the body. They should also avoid stress and situations that can result in emotional frustrations.

Urinary Bladder Damp-Heat can be caused by the following patterns of imbalance

- Damp-Cold
- Damp
- Liver *qi* stagnation
- Liver *qi* stagnation and Urinary Bladder *qi* stagnation
- Heart Fire
- Kidney *yang xu*
- Spleen *qi xu*

Urinary Bladder Damp-Heat can result in the following patterns of imbalance

- Kidney *yin xu*

- Phlegm

- Urinary Bladder *xue* stagnation

- *Qi* stagnation

Urinary Bladder Damp-Cold

Urinary Bladder Damp-Cold will be either an acute condition or a chronic condition with acute episodes. It will typically alternate with, or develop into, Urinary Bladder Damp-Heat. It is a fundamental principle that *xie qi* takes on the characteristic of its host. The human body is *yang* and hot in relation to the environment around it. Our body temperature is 37 degrees Celsius. This means that *yin xie qi* will eventually turn into Heat. This is the same dynamic that happens when a person falls into the sea in winter or into boiling water: their body temperature will be influenced by their surroundings. Furthermore, the stagnation that Damp-Cold creates will itself generate Heat. Both Dampness and Cold will block the Urinary Bladder's *qi* mechanism.

Aetiology

Invasions of exogenous Damp and/or Cold. An excessive consumption of food and beverages or medicine that are energetically cold or damp, for example dairy products, raw foods, salads and ice cream.

Factors that weaken the Spleen or Kidney *yang* can also be involved, because Kidney *yang xu* and Spleen *yang xu* conditions can result in fluids not being optimally transformed and transported, giving rise to Dampness. Kidney *yang xu* will also result in the body being more vulnerable to invasions of exogenous Cold and Damp.

Symptoms and signs

- Difficult or painful urination

- Weak urinary flow

- Incomplete voiding of the Urinary Bladder

- Cloudy or oily urine

- Distension or tightness in the lower *jiao*

- Lumbar soreness

- Aversion to cold

- Pale tongue with thick, white, greasy coating on the root

- Slippery pulse

Key symptoms
Cloudy or oily urine, distension in the lower *jiao*, difficult urination, white, greasy tongue coating.

Treatment principle
Drain Damp-Cold from the Urinary Bladder.

Acupuncture points
Choose from: Ren 3, St 28, Sp 6, Sp 9, UB 22, UB 28 and UB 32.

Needle technique
Draining. Moxa is recommended.

Explanation

- Ren 3, St 28, UB 28 and UB 32 drain Dampness from the Urinary Bladder.

- Sp 6, Sp 9 and UB 22 drain Dampness from the Urinary Bladder.

Herbal formula

- *Bei Xie Fen Qing Yin I* (Warms and tonifies *yang*, drains Damp from the Urinary Bladder)

Relevant advice
A person with Urinary Bladder Damp-Cold should avoid food and beverages that can result in Cold or Dampness. They should avoid exposure to cold or damp environments and keep warm and dry, dressing appropriately for the weather. The person must be careful about what kinds of exercise and sports they practise. Swimming is not recommended and they should definitely remove their swimming costume immediately upon getting out of the water. Likewise, jogging or cycling in the rain is problematic, as are sports where the person sweats whilst they are exposed to the cold.

Urinary Bladder Damp-Cold can be caused by the following patterns of imbalance

- Spleen *yang xu*

- Kidney *yang xu*

- Damp

- Cold

Urinary Bladder Damp-Cold can result in the following patterns of imbalance

- Urinary Bladder Damp-Heat

- Kidney *yang xu*

Urinary Bladder *xue* stagnation

This is a chronic pattern that can arise from chronic patterns of imbalance in the Urinary Bladder. Chronic conditions of Dampness can impede the movement of *qi*, which can result in the stagnation of *xue* over time. Heat can condense *xue* so it becomes sticky and starts to stagnate. Stagnations of Liver *qi* can affect the *qi* mechanism in the Urinary Bladder, causing a stagnation of *qi*. When *qi* stagnates it can fail to circulate *xue*.

The stagnation of *xue* can also arise independently of other patterns, for example after surgery in the lower *jiao*.

Aetiology

Xue stagnation can be the result of physical trauma, surgery or medical investigations. Emotional issues such as frustration, irritation, repressed emotions and stress can lead to the stagnation of Liver *qi*, which can affect the movement of *qi* in the Urinary Bladder. Over time this can lead to the stagnation of *xue*. Heat that boils *xue* so it becomes sticky and stagnates can be due to emotional issues creating a stagnation of *qi* that generates Heat or dietary imbalances that lead to the generation of Heat or Dampness.

Symptoms and signs

- Difficult or painful urination

- Inhibited urinary flow

- Incomplete voiding of the Urinary Bladder

- There can be blood in the urine

- Tightness, pain or distension in the area above the pubic bone

- Small, visible, purple blood vessels or spider naevi

- Purple or dark spots on the root of the tongue, swollen, purple sub-lingual veins

- Choppy or Wiry pulse, especially in the left *chi* position

Key symptoms

Inhibited or difficult urination, distension in the lower *jiao*.

Treatment principle
Invigorate *xue* in the Urinary Bladder.

Acupuncture points
Choose from: Ren 3, Sp 6, Sp 10, St 28, UB 17, UB 28 and UB 32.

Needle technique
Draining.

Explanation

- Ren 3, St 28, UB 28 and UB 32 invigorate *xue* in the Urinary Bladder.

- Sp 6, Sp 10 and UB 17 invigorate *xue*.

Herbal formula

- *Shao Fu Shu Yu Tang* (Invigorates *xue* and removes stasis in the lower *jiao*)

Relevant advice
This will depend on the underlying pattern of imbalance. If there is Heat or Dampness, the patient should avoid consuming food and beverages that generate these. Any underlying emotional issues or stress should be addressed.

Physical exercise and movement will help to circulate *qi* and *xue*. It can be beneficial if the exercises focus on circulating *qi* in the lower jiao. Hula-hoops, sit-ups and rowing machines can help to do this. Massaging the lower *jiao* is also recommended.

Urinary Bladder *xue* stagnation can be caused by the following patterns of imbalance

- Urinary Bladder Damp-Heat

- Liver *qi* stagnation and Urinary Bladder *qi* stagnation

Urinary Bladder *xue* stagnation can result in the following pattern of imbalance

- Urinary Bladder stones

Urinary Bladder stones
This will be a chronic pattern that has arisen as a consequence of other chronic patterns of imbalance. Heat will usually be the precursor – 'boiling' the urine so it eventually forms small stones or sand.

Dampness can coagulate and form Phlegm, which can manifest as stones and sand in the urine.

Aetiology

Chronic patterns of Heat that usually underlie this pattern can be due to a residual pathogen. This will usually be due to the use of Western medication that has not fully cleared the pathogen. Both Dampness and Heat can lead to the formation of Phlegm. This means that aetiological factors, such as a diet that creates Heat or Dampness, can be involved. Likewise, emotional factors can lead to the creation of Heart Fire that can drain down to the Urinary Bladder and 'boil' the urinary fluids, resulting in stones.

Symptoms and signs

- Sudden or recurrent painful and blocked urination

- Inhibited urinary flow

- Incomplete voiding of the Urinary Bladder

- Piercing or cutting pain in the urethra that is better when urine flows freely

- Small stones or sand in the urine

- Tightness, pain or distension in the area above the pubic bone

- The tongue impression will depend on the underlying pattern of imbalance

- Wiry or Confined pulse in the left *chi* position

Key symptoms

Small stones or sand in the urine, painful urination.

Treatment principle

Expel stones and circulate *qi* in the Urinary Bladder.

Acupuncture points

Choose from: Ren 3, St 28, UB 28 and UB 32.

Needle technique

Draining. Electro-acupuncture is recommended.

Explanation

- Ren 3, St 28, UB 28 and UB 32 activate *qi* and expel stones from the Urinary Bladder.

Herbal formula

- *Shi Wei San* (Dissolves stones and promotes urination)

Relevant advice
This will depend on the underlying pattern of imbalance. If there is Heat or Dampness, the patient should avoid consuming food and beverages that generate these. Any underlying emotional issues or stress should be addressed.

Physical exercise and massage, where the focus is on circulating *qi* in the lower *jiao*, will be beneficial. Hula-hoops, sit-ups and rowing machines can help to do this.

Urinary Bladder stones can be caused by the following patterns of imbalance

- Urinary Bladder Damp-Heat
- Liver *qi* stagnation and Urinary Bladder *qi* stagnation
- Urinary Bladder *xue* stagnation

Urinary Bladder stones can result in the following pattern of imbalance

- Urinary *xue* stagnation

Xu patterns

Urinary Bladder *xu* Cold
If there is Kidney *yang xu*, the Kidneys may not be able to carry out their activities in relation to fluid physiology and the storage and expulsion of urine.

Urinary Bladder *xu* Cold is therefore Kidney *yang xu* with signs that there is a disturbance of the Urinary Bladder's functioning.

Aetiology
Kidney *yang* can be weakened by disease, as well as food, drinks and medicine that have a cold dynamic or temperature. Congenital weakness, old age, climatic cold, hard physical work, lifting heavy objects, standing for long periods of time and too much sex can weaken Kidney *yang*.

Symptoms and signs

- Frequent or urgent urination
- Copious amounts of pale, clear urine
- Nocturia or enuresis
- Incontinence
- Aversion to cold
- Cold limbs
- Shiny, white facial colour

- Pale, swollen, wet tongue with white coating

- Deep and Weak pulse

Key symptoms
Frequent urination, aversion to cold, pale swollen tongue.

Treatment principle
Warm Kidney *yang*, astringe the Urinary Bladder.

Acupuncture points
Choose from: Kid 3, Kid 7, Ren 3, Ren 4, Ren 6, UB 23, UB 28 and Du 4.

Needle technique
Tonifying. Moxa is recommended.

Explanation

- Kid 3, Kid 7, Ren 6, UB 23 and Du 4 tonify Kidney *yang*.

- Ren 3 and UB 28 drain Dampness from the Urinary Bladder.

Herbal formula

- *Suo Quan Wan* (Tonifies and warms Kidney *yang* and astringes the urine)

Relevant advice
See Kidney *yang xu*.

Urinary Bladder *xu* Cold can be caused by the following patterns of imbalance

- Kidney *yang xu*

- Spleen *yang xu*

- Spleen *qi xu*

- Cold

- Damp

Urinary Bladder *xu* Cold can result in the following patterns of imbalance

- Urinary Bladder Damp-Cold

- Urinary Bladder Damp-Heat

- Kidney *yang xu*

- Spleen *yang xu*

- Damp

Combined patterns

Liver *qi* stagnation and Urinary Bladder *qi* stagnation

This will usually be a recurrent chronic pattern with acute flare-ups that are triggered by stress and emotional issues, resulting in a stagnation of Liver *qi*. Instead of supporting the functioning of the Urinary Bladder by ensuring the free flow of *qi* in the body, stagnant Liver *qi* means that there is a general tendency to have *qi* stagnation in the body as a whole and it can specifically disrupt the *qi* mechanism in the Urinary Bladder, resulting in a disruption of the functioning of the Urinary Bladder. This is because the Liver channel traverses the external genitalia and the Urinary Bladder.

Aetiology

Liver *qi* stagnation often arises as a consequence of stress, irritation, emotional frustrations and pent-up emotions. Lack of exercise and physical movement can also be factors. Dietary factors or blood loss can result in Liver *xue xu*, which can be the underlying cause of Liver *qi* stagnation.

Symptoms and signs

- Inhibited or difficult urination
- Incomplete urination
- Urinary disturbances that are provoked or aggravated by stress or emotional factors
- Urinary disturbances that are worse or occur in the premenstrual period
- Tightness, pain or distension in the area above the pubic bone
- Hypochondriac tension
- Irregular menstrual cycle
- Premenstrual tension
- Cold hands and feet
- Slight swelling along the edge of the tongue
- Wiry pulse, especially in the left *guan* and *chi* positions

Key symptoms

Urinary disturbances that are aggravated by emotional factors or that manifest in the premenstrual period, Wiry pulse.

Treatment principle

Spread Liver *qi* and spread *qi* in the lower *jiao* and Urinary Bladder.

Acupuncture points
Choose from: Liv 3, LI 4, Ren 3, SJ 6, Sp 6, St 28, UB 18 and UB 28.

Needle technique
Spreading.

Explanation

- Liv 3, LI 4 and UB 18 spread Liver *qi*.

- Ren 3 and UB 28 spread *qi* in the Urinary Bladder.

- Sp 6, SJ 6 and St 28 circulate *qi* in the lower *jiao*.

Herbal formula

- *Tian Tai Wu Yao San* (Spreads Liver *qi* and expels Cold)

Relevant advice
When Liver *qi* stagnation is a significant aspect of the imbalance, it is important to address the underlying causes of this pattern. There will often be emotional issues involved in the generation of this pattern. If possible, the patient should try and address these issues.

If Liver *qi* stagnation is a consequence of Liver *xue xu*, the diet should be adjusted to address this aspect.

Physical exercise and movement will help to circulate *qi* in general. It will be especially beneficial if the exercises focus on circulating *qi* in the lower *jiao*. Hula-hoops, sit-ups and rowing machines can help to do this. Massaging the lower *jiao* is also recommended.

Liver *qi* stagnation and Urinary Bladder *qi* can be caused by the following patterns of imbalance

- Liver *qi* stagnation

- Liver *xue xu*

Liver *qi* stagnation and Urinary Bladder *qi* can result in the following patterns of imbalance

- Urinary Bladder *xue* stagnation

- Urinary Bladder Damp-Heat

- Urinary Bladder stones

Kidney imbalances

The aetiology of Kidney patterns of imbalance

The Kidneys encompass the most fundamental aspects of the body's *qi*. It is in the Kidneys that *jing* is stored and it is between the Kidneys that *mingmen* is located. In contrast to other organs, the Kidneys do not have any *shi* patterns of imbalance. This is because the Kidneys comprise the fundamental *yin* and *yang*, and these can only become *xu*. A *xu* condition in the Kidneys can easily result in the emergence of *shi* conditions elsewhere in the body, but the Kidneys themselves can only be *xu*. Because the Kidneys store *jing* and create *yuan qi*, they will be weakened when more *qi* is consumed than the body is capable of producing. This means that long-term illness, stress, working too much or too hard, a weakening of one of the other *qi*-producing organs and bleeding can all put a strain on the Kidneys. Working too hard physically will mainly weaken the Kidney's *yang* aspect, whereas stress, working too much mentally or working late in the evening or at night and sleeping too little will burden Kidney *yin*. *Yin* is replenished at night whilst we sleep and when we rest. A person who sleeps too little and works or parties at night weakens their *yin*.

The pre-heaven aspect of Kidney *jing* is inherited from the parents. This means that the health of the parents at the time of conception and the mother's health during pregnancy will have a significant effect on the quality of a person's *jing*. The age of the parent also plays a role. The older they are, the weaker their *jing* is and thereby the quality of the *jing* that they pass on to the child. In addition, there is a progressive weakening of Kidneys over the years as a person gets older. At the age of 40, half of a person's *yin* has been consumed. Old age is characterised by signs that the Kidneys are deficient. The hair turns grey or falls out, the teeth loosen, the bones are fragile, the hearing is poorer, the libido and fertility decrease, the memory fades, there is incontinence and so on.

Too much sex is an aetiological factor in many Kidney patterns of imbalance. This is because men lose *jing* and *yang* when they ejaculate. In fact, it is not only ejaculation that weakens the Kidneys, because when you become sexually aroused, *mingmen* flares up. This is why the cheeks, lips and nail beds become redder and you feel warmer. When *mingmen* flares up, it consumes *jing*. Some sources believe that all forms of desire activate *mingmen*. This means that desire will weaken the Kidneys in both men and women. Where men mainly lose *jing* through ejaculation, women lose *jing* through births, ovulation and menstruation. The eggs are *jing* and women therefore lose *jing* when eggs are released during ovulation. *Jing* is also used to nourish the foetus during pregnancy. Finally *tian gui* (heavenly water) or menstrual blood is *jing* that has been transformed by *mingmen* and Heart fire.

Standing and lifting weaken the Kidneys, especially Kidney *yang*. People whose work involves a lot of lifting or lifting heavy objects and people who stand for long periods of time will strain their Kidney *yang*.

Invasions of exogenous *xie qi* do not directly affect the Kidneys. On the other hand, repeated invasions of exogenous Cold will weaken Kidney *yang*. Invasions of exogenous *xie qi*, no matter whether they are Hot or Cold, can eventually lead to the generation of internal Heat. This will injure the Kidney *yin*, as will all Fire conditions. Chronic disease and recurrent illness will be a burden on the *zheng qi* and thereby also the Kidneys.

Emotionally, the Kidneys are affected by fear, anxiety and shock. If these emotions are very intense or are a chronic condition, they will weaken the Kidneys. This is often a vicious cycle: fear and anxiety weaken the Kidneys, but a person whose Kidneys are weak will often be excessively and unnecessarily fearful and anxious.

Treatment of disease can also weaken the Kidneys. This can happen if the medication used has a very hot or a cold dynamic. Improper or inadequate treatment can also draw exogenous *xie qi* deeper into the body or lock a remnant of the *xie qi* in the body. This can injure the Kidneys in the long term, either by generating Heat, which injures *yin*, or by weakening *qi* and *yang* in general.

Excessive consumption of an energetically hot or cold diet can burden Kidney *yin* and Kidney *yang* respectively.

Kidney *yin xu* and Kidney *yang xu* can both result in, and be the cause of, *yin xu* or *yang xu* conditions in other organs, because Kidney *yin* and Kidney *yang* are the root of *yin* and *yang* in the whole body. If they are weak, they will not nourish or support the *yin* and *yang* aspects of the other organs. On the other hand, if an organ is *yin xu* or *yang xu*, it will consume that aspect of the Kidneys so that it eventually also becomes weakened. Kidney *yin* has an especially close relationship with Liver, Heart, Lung and Stomach *yin*. Kidney *yang* has a similarly close relationship with Spleen, Lung and Heart *yang*.

The pathology of Kidney patterns of imbalance

If the Kidneys are out of balance, it will manifest with a weakening or dysfunction of one of the aspects or physiological functions that relate to the Kidneys. Kidney imbalances can be reduced or simplified to two main imbalances – Kidney *yin xu* and Kidney *yang xu*. Kidney *yin* encompasses Kidney *jing* and Kidney *yang* encompasses *mingmen* and Kidney *qi*.

Kidney *jing* is used to create bones, cartilage, teeth and hair. If there is a congenital *jing xu*, the person will often have a weak bone structure, weak teeth and thin hair. The growth and the transition to puberty, etc. are controlled by *jing. Jing xu* can be seen when there is slow development, poor growth, mental underdevelopment and a child enters puberty late or not at all. A girl who does not start menstruating or only starts menstruating late in puberty may well be *jing xu*.

Jing also manifests in the sperm and eggs. Infertility and low sperm counts can therefore be a manifestation of *jing xu*.

The brain is 'a flower blossoming on the spine' and it is created from *jing. Jing* therefore has an influence on the brain's activity and structure. Congenital problems that manifest with poor development of the mental faculties are often related to *jing xu*. In fact, most congenital problems and genetic defects have a *jing xu* aspect. If the brain is not nourished by Kidney *jing*, it can cause problems with the memory, concentration and dizziness. Kidney *yin* nourishes Heart *yin*, helping to anchor the *shen*. Kidney *yin xu* can therefore manifest with insomnia, as well as anxiety, mental restless and a sense of unease.

The Kidneys have a great influence on the bones, especially in the lumbar region and the knees. The bones are created and nourished by Kidney *jing*. Kidney *yang* in turn strengthens the bones and warms the lumbar and knees. This means that weakness, soreness and a cold sensation in the lower back and knees can be seen in Kidney imbalances.

Fluid physiology is dependent on the Kidneys. Kidney *yang* is used to transform and transport fluids in the body. When there is Kidney *yang xu*, the deficiency of *yang* will affect these processes, resulting in oedema or increased urination. The increased frequency and volume of urination that is characteristic of Kidney *yang xu* is due to this failure to transform and transport fluids optimally, as well as Kidney *yang* being used to hold urine in the Urinary Bladder. This means that incontinence, enuresis and nocturia can also be a manifestation of Kidney *yang xu*. Kidney *yang* is also the force behind the expulsion of urine out of the Urinary Bladder. Kidney *yang xu* can manifest with urinary difficulties, a weak stream of urine or dribbling when urinating.

The poor transformation and transport of fluids in the body when there is Kidney *yang xu* will result in the untransformed fluids seeping down to the lower *jiao* due to their *yin* nature. These fluids will accumulate in the Urinary Bladder, increasing the amount of urine and diluting it so that it is paler in colour. The urine will be a darker yellow colour and more scanty when there is Kidney *yin xu*, because there will be less fluid in the body, making the urine more concentrated. If there is *yin xu* Heat, the Heat will further concentrate the urine and make it even more dark and sparse.

Kidney *yang* also affects other aspects of fluid physiology. Kidney *yang* is the root of *wei qi*. If Kidney *yang* is weak or deficient, there may be problems controlling the pores in the skin. Spontaneous perspiration or sweating upon light activity can therefore be a sign of Kidney *yang xu*.

Kidney *yin xu* can also result in sweating disturbances. Night sweats are a classic manifestation of Kidney *yin xu*, because *yin* has become too weak to control Heat, especially at night, when *yin* should be more powerful than *yang*. The resultant *yang* Heat will expand upwards and outwards, driving fluids up to the surface of the skin. At night, *wei qi* circulates in the interior and therefore cannot keep the sweat inside the body.

The Kidneys controls the body's lower orifices. As discussed above, an impairment of the Kidney's functioning can result in urinary incontinence. It is not only the urinary system's orifice, though, that the Kidneys control the opening and closing of, Kidney *qi xu* can also result in increased discharge from the vagina. As it is a *yang xu* condition, the vaginal discharge will be watery and clear. In extreme cases, the Kidneys can be so weak that there will be faecal incontinence. This is seen in some elderly patients whose Kidney *qi* is weakened by old age.

Kidney *qi* is also used to hold the foetus inside the body and hold the Uterus closed during pregnancy. Kidney *qi xu*, can therefore manifest with spontaneous miscarriages. Kidney *jing xu* can also mean that the foetus does not develop as it should. This can be a factor when there is a history of recurrent miscarriages.

The Kidneys should also hold the sperm back and keep them inside the body. Both Kidney *yin xu* and the Kidney *yang xu* can manifest with premature ejaculation and nocturnal emissions. The mechanism is different when there is Kidney *yin xu* to when there is Kidney *yang xu*. When there is Kidney *yang xu*, the Kidney *yang* is not strong enough to hold the sperm back and when there is Kidney *yin xu*, the resultant Heat can drive the semen out of the body. As well as controlling and producing semen and sperm, the Kidneys have a significant influence on a person's libido. If Kidney *yang* is weakened, a person can lack sexual desire. Kidney *yang xu* can also manifest with impotence. This is because there can be a lack of sexual desire, but also because Kidney *yang* is necessary to create an erection. It is, however, important to remember that other organs also have an influence on potency and the libido, especially the Heart and Liver. When there is Kidney *yin xu* Heat, there can be an increased libido. If Heat is not controlled by *yin*, *mingmen* can flare up and there will be an increase in sexual desire.

Kidney *yang* receives and grasps the *qi* that is sent down from the Lung. Kidney *yang xu* and *qi xu* conditions can therefore result in dyspnoea and shortness of breath.

The Kidneys influence their sense organ, the ears. Kidney *jing xu* can manifest with ears that are very small or misshapen. Kidney *yin* and *jing* nourish the ears. If there is Kidney *jing xu* or Kidney *yin xu*, there can be hearing problems, such as tinnitus and deafness, especially if these are congenital or have developed gradually. Again, it is important to remember that other organs, such as the Liver, also affect the ears and thereby tinnitus.

Willpower, or *zhi* in Chinese, has its residence in the Kidneys. If the Kidneys are strong, a person has the willpower and determination to carry out the projects they have envisioned, i.e. that the Liver and *hun* have visualised. It is this willpower to grow that is seen in a seedling that has germinated. It is determined to grow up into the light, no matter what obstacles it meets. A person with weak Kidneys will sometimes lack the willpower and determination to complete projects. They will give up when they encounter resistance or become tired. The weak *zhi* can also result in depression, because the person loses the will to live.

Memory is also an aspect of the Chinese character *zhi*. This makes sense when we take into account that the brain is nourished by and created from *jing*.

As described, the Kidneys are the root of all *yin* and *yang* in the body. This means that when there are generalised *yin xu* and *yang xu* symptoms in the body, the Kidneys will usually be the focus of treatment.

General symptoms and signs of Kidney imbalances

- Knee problems

- Lumbar problems

- Tinnitus and hearing problems

- Urinary problems

- Problems with sexual function and libido

- Problems with fertility

- Hair loss

- Dyspnoea

- Oedema

- Weak pulse in the *chi* positions

- General *yin xu* and *yang xu* signs

Xu patterns

Kidney *yin xu*

Kidney *yin xu* is a weakening of *yin* at the deepest level. It could be caused by a chronic condition of *yin xu* in another organ or by the long-term overstraining of the body, mind or psyche. Because Kidney *yin* is such a deep and a fundamental aspect of the body, the imbalance will usually have built up gradually over time. Furthermore, because it is such a deep and fundamental deficiency and because Kidney *yin* also relates to *jing*, the treatment of this imbalance will also take longer than other imbalances that have a more superficial nature.

Aetiology

Long-term physical, emotional and mental overexertion, chronic stress, prolonged illness, working at night, using medications that are hot or spicy in their energy, excessive sex, a diet that includes an excess of food or drinks that are hot or spicy, too much coffee and other stimulants, congenital weakness and old age can all weaken *yin*.

Kidney *yin xu* will often occur as a consequence of chronic imbalances in the body. For example, a chronic *xue xu* condition will weaken *yin*. Similarly, prolonged or intense Fire conditions and febrile diseases can injure the fluids and thereby Kidney *yin*. Kidney *yin* is the root of all *yin* in the body. When Kidney *yin* is weakened, *yin xu* conditions in other organs can also arise.

Symptoms and signs

- Insomnia

- Dry mucous membranes

- Dry skin

- Dry mouth and throat

- Night sweats

- Poor memory

- Nocturnal emissions

- Premature ejaculation

- Infertility

- Tinnitus

- Poor hearing or deafness

- Dry eyes

- Weak or sore knees

- Lumbar weakness or soreness

- Thin or slender body

- Sparse and dark urine

- Dry stool or constipation

- Mild feeling of anxiety

- Depression

- Dizziness

- Thin, dry tongue that lacks coating and possibly has cracks in the surface of the tongue

- Fine or Empty pulse, the pulse may be relatively weak in the *chi* positions

Key symptoms
Night sweats, sore lower back, absent tongue coating.

Treatment principle
Nourish Kidney *yin*.

Acupuncture points
Choose from: UB 23, UB 52, Ren 4, Sp 6, Kid 3, Kid 6 and Lu 7.

Needle technique
Tonifying.

Explanation

- UB 23, UB 52, Ren 4, Kid 3 and Sp 6 nourish Kidney *yin*.

- Lu 7 and Kid 6 in combination open *ren mai* and *yin qiao mai* and thereby nourish Kidney *yin*.

Herbal formula

- *Liu Wei Di Huang Tang* (Nourishes Kidney *yin*)

- *Zou Gui Wan* (Nourishes Kidney *yin*)

Relevant advice

It is essential that a person who is Kidney *yin xu* gets enough rest and relaxation. This means that they must get ample sleep and go to bed early at night. They must not work too hard, neither should they spend too much time watching television and or staring at a computer screen. They should avoid stimulants, such as coffee, as these will stress their system. Alcohol is not good either, because it is both spreading and hot in its energy.

Sweating too much will mean that they lose body fluid. Therefore, a person who is Kidney *yin xu* should avoid saunas or steam baths.

Men, in particular, should limit how much sex they have, including masturbation, because *jing* is lost when ejaculating.

Shiatsu, massage and meditation are beneficial because they promote calmness and tranquillity in the body and mind, thereby nourishing *yin*.

Dynamic activities such as aerobics or action sports are not beneficial and should be discouraged, because they will further consume the person's *yin*. Lighter and more meditative activities such as qi gong, yoga and tai ji nourish *yin*, whilst activating *qi*.

Dietary advice includes avoiding food and beverages that are stimulating or hot in their dynamic. This includes coffee, black, green and white tea, alcohol, sugar and hot spices like chilli and garlic. The way food is prepared will affect its dynamic. Baked food, as well as being more warming in its dynamic, will be dynamically drier. The consumption of baked food should therefore be limited when there is a *yin xu* condition. Soups, stews and boiled vegetables, on the other hand, should be recommended. Concentrated proteins, green leafy vegetables, cereals and root vegetables nourish *yin* in general, as do things that are rich in minerals, such as seaweed. Oil and products that have a high oil content, for example nuts and seeds, will nourish and moisten *yin*. Foods that specifically nourish Kidney *yin* include: alfalfa sprouts, asparagus, potatoes, green beans, nettles, aduki beans, black beans, kidney beans, coconut milk, sesame seeds, walnuts, octopus, oysters, duck, kidneys, pork and egg yolks.

Kidney *yin xu* can be caused by the following patterns of imbalance

- Liver *yin xu*

- Heart *yin xu*

- Lung *yin xu*

- Stomach *yin xu*

- Liver *xue xu*

- Kidney *yang xu*

- Fire

- Heat

- *Xue xu*

Kidney *yin xu* can result in the following patterns of imbalance

- *Xu* Heat

- Liver *yin xu*

- Heart *yin xu*

- Lung *yin xu*

- Stomach *yin xu*

- Liver *xue xu*

- Kidney *yang xu*

- Kidney *jing xu*

- Phlegm

- *Xue* stagnation

Kidney *yin xu* Heat

In time, Kidney *yin xu* will develop into Kidney *yin xu* Heat. This will happen more quickly if there is already Heat present in the body. Symptoms will be the same as when there is Kidney *yin xu*, but there will also be more symptoms and signs of Heat.

Aetiology

See Kidney *yin xu*.

Symptoms and signs

- Insomnia

- Dry mucous membranes

- Dry skin

- Dry mouth and throat

- Thirst, particularly at night, with a desire to drink in small sips

- Night sweats

- Feeling hot in the evening and at night

- Sensation of heat in the palms of the hands, soles of the feet and chest
- Hot flushes
- Malar flush
- Tinnitus
- Poor hearing or deafness
- Dry eyes
- Weak or sore knees
- Lumbar weakness or soreness
- Thin or slender body
- Aching or pain in the bones
- Anxiety
- Constipation
- Dark, scanty urine
- Poor memory
- Nocturnal emissions
- Premature ejaculation
- Increased libido
- Mental anxiety and restlessness
- Restless or fidgeting body movements
- Talking quickly or talking a lot, but the voice is not loud
- Red, thin and dry tongue that lacks coating and possibly has cracks in the surface
- Rapid, Fine or Empty pulse, the pulse may be relatively weak in the *chi* positions

Key symptoms
Night sweats, hot at night, malar flush, red tongue without coating.

Treatment principle
Nourish Kidney *yin* and control Heat.

Acupuncture points
Choose from: UB 23, UB 52, Ren 4, Kid 1, Kid 2, Kid 3, Kid 6, Kid 7, Sp 6, He 6 and Lu 7.

Needle technique
Tonifying, except Kid 2, which can be drained.

Explanation

- UB 23, UB 52, Ren 4, Kid 3 and Sp 6 nourish Kidney *yin*.
- Kid 1 and Kid 2 control *yin xu* Heat.
- He 6 and Kid 7 control night sweats and nourish Kidney and Heart *yin*.
- Lu 7 and Kid 6 in combination open *ren mai* and *yin qiao mai* and thereby nourish Kidney *yin*.

Herbal formula

- *Zhi Bai Di Huang Tang* (Nourishes Kidney *yin* and controls *yin xu* Heat)
- *Da Bu Yin Wan* (Nourishes Kidney *yin* and controls *yin xu* Heat)

Relevant advice
See Kidney *yin xu*.

Kidney *yin xu* Heat can be caused by the following patterns of imbalance

- Kidney *yin xu*
- Fire
- Heat

Kidney *yin xu* Heat can result in the following patterns of imbalance

- Liver *yin xu*
- Heart *yin xu*
- Lung *yin xu*
- Stomach *yin xu*
- Liver *xue xu*
- Kidney *yang xu*
- Kidney *jing xu*
- Phlegm
- *Xue* stagnation

Kidney *yang xu*

In the same way that Kidney *yin xu* is a deficiency of the deepest aspect of *yin*, Kidney *yang xu* is a deficiency of the body's deepest *yang* aspect. The strength of Kidney *yang* is inextricably related to the strength of *mingmen*. When there is Kidney *yang xu*, *mingmen* will be weaker and thereby so will the production of *yuan qi*. This has implications for many of the body's physiological processes.

Aetiology

Kidney *yang* is weakened by food, beverages and medications that are cold in their energy or temperature, congenital weakness, chronic disease, old age, exogenous Cold, hard physical work and overexertion, lifting heavy objects, standing for long periods of time and too much sex. Kidney *yang* is also weakened by chronic *yang xu* conditions in other organs.

Symptoms and signs

- Soreness, weakness, fatigue or a sensation of cold in the lumbar region
- Sore, weak or cold knees
- Aversion to cold
- Cold limbs
- Frequent or urgent urination
- Copious amounts of pale-coloured urine
- Nocturia or enuresis
- Oedema
- Loose, watery stools
- Mental and physical fatigue
- Indifference and lack of vitality
- Wearing warmer clothing than others
- Tinnitus
- Dizziness
- Spontaneous sweating
- Infertility
- Poor sperm motility
- Pale complexion
- Slow and languid body movements

- Poor posture

- Weak libido

- Shortness of breath

- Lack of thirst

- Desire for hot drinks and hot food

- Pale, swollen and possibly wet tongue

- Deep and Weak pulse, the pulse may be relatively weak in the *chi* positions

Key symptoms
Sore or weak lumbar region, frequent urination or nocturia, aversion to cold. Pale tongue and Deep pulse.

Treatment principle
Warm and tonify Kidney *yang*.

Acupuncture points
Choose from: UB 23, Du 4, Ren 4, Ren 6, Kid 3 and Kid 7.

Needle technique
Tonifying. Moxa is strongly recommended.

Explanation

- UB 23, Du 4, Ren 4, Ren 6, Kid 3 and Kid 7 tonify and warm Kidney *yang*.

Herbal formula

- *Jin Gui Shen Qi Tang* (Tonifies and warms Kidney *yang*)

- *You Gui Wan* (Tonifies and warms Kidney *yang*)

Relevant advice
The patient should consume a diet that is warm in both its temperature and its energetic dynamic. They should completely avoid foods and beverages that have a cold dynamic and that are cold in their temperature, especially in winter. In practice, this means avoiding fruit unless it is boiled or baked, salad, raw vegetables and cold drinks. They should try to use more warming cooking methods when preparing food, such as oven-baked and grilled dishes, which are more warming than steamed and cooked dishes.

Hot spices such as chilli are not necessarily salutary because they will cause the person to sweat and thereby lose heat. Tonifying a *xu* condition is something that takes time and cannot be forced. The use of spices in general is helpful, though, as they can activate *yang*. Spices that warm and tonify Kidney *yang* are cinnamon, cloves, fennel, basil, sage, fenugreek, horseradish, rosemary and black pepper.

Foods that specifically tonify Kidney *yang* are oysters, smoked fish, salmon, tuna, lobster, trout, mussels, shrimp, lamb, venison, duck, roast pork, kidney, chestnut, walnuts, pistachio, black sesame seeds, quinoa, oats, buckwheat, millet, aduki beans, black beans, de Puy lentils, raspberry and cherry. Green tea is cooling, so black tea will be better. Otherwise, ginger tea, fennel tea, yogi tea and jasmine tea will all be good.

A person who is Kidney *yang xu* must ensure that they get enough exercise. Light exercise is beneficial when there is *yang xu* because it will activate *yang* and *qi*. They must, however, be careful that they do not train so intensely that they become fatigued or tired, because this will further drain their *yang*. It is a good idea to start the day with physical activities that can activate and circulate *qi*.

Keeping warm is important, especially in the lumbar region and the area below the navel. Wearing a belly-warmer or a woollen stomach scarf around the midriff and lumbar can be recommended. Protecting this area from drafts should be a priority. A ginger foot bath is also beneficial, as is drinking ginger tea.

Patients who are Kidney *yang xu* should avoid activities that weaken the Kidneys and *yang* in general. Besides the above advice, men should limit how much sex they have, including masturbation, as Kidney *yang* is expended upon ejaculation. Lifting heavy objects and standing weakens Kidney *yang* and should be avoided as much as possible.

Kidney *yang xu* can be caused by the following patterns of imbalance

- Spleen *yang xu*
- Kidney *yin xu*
- Damp
- Cold

Kidney *yang xu* can result in the following patterns of imbalance

- Spleen *yang xu*
- Kidney *yang xu*
- Heart *yang xu*
- Kidney *qi* not grasping Lung *qi*
- Kidney *yang xu*, overflowing water
- Damp
- Phlegm

- Cold

- *Xue* stagnation

- *Qi xu*

- *Xue xu*

Kidney *qi xu*

Kidney *qi xu* is similar in many ways to Kidney *yang xu*, because Kidney *qi* is an aspect of the Kidney *yang*. When there is Kidney *qi xu* there are symptoms that specifically relate to the functions of Kidney *qi*, such as the control of the lower orifices in the body and raising *qi* in the lower *jiao*. There will be fewer signs of *xu* Cold in this pattern.

Aetiology

In men Kidney *qi* is weakened by too much sex and in women it is weakened by giving birth and menstruation. Furthermore, hard physical work also weakens Kidney *qi*. Like other Kidney patterns of imbalance, Kidney *qi xu* is also a result of the ageing process.

Symptoms and signs

- Sore, weak or cold lumbar region

- Sore, weak or cold knees

- Aversion to cold

- Cold limbs

- Frequent urination

- Clear and copious urine

- Nocturia or enuresis

- Weak flow of urine

- Post-urination dripping

- Incontinence

- Watery or white vaginal discharge

- Nocturnal emissions

- Premature ejaculation

- Recurrent miscarriages

- Uterine prolapse

- Distension in the lower *jiao*

- Mental and physical fatigue

- Slow and languid body movements

- Poor posture

- Pale tongue

- Deep and Weak pulse in the *chi* positions

Key symptoms
Weak stream of urine, post-urination dripping, watery or whitish vagina discharge and a sore lower back.

Treatment principle
Stabilise and tonify Kidney *qi*, raise Kidney *yang*.

Acupuncture points
Choose from: Ren 4, Ren 6, Du 4, Du 20, Kid 3, Kid 7, Kid 13, UB 23 and UB 32.

Needle technique
Tonifying. Moxa is recommended and is necessary on Ren 6 and Du 20.

Explanation

- UB 23, Du 4, Ren 4, Kid 3 and Kid 7 tonify Kidney *qi*.

- Kid 13 and UB 32 stabilise Kidney *qi* and the Urinary Bladder.

- Ren 6 and Du 20 raise *yang*.

Herbal formula

- *Jin Gui Shen Qi Tang* (Warms and tonifies Kidney *yang*)

- *You Gui Wan* (Warms and tonifies Kidney *yang*)

Relevant advice
Men should avoid ejaculating and women should avoid becoming pregnant. The patient should avoid lifting heavy objects and working too hard or placing a physical strain on the body. They should eat a diet that strengthens Kidney *yang*.

Kidney *qi xu* can be caused by the following patterns of imbalance

- Spleen *yang xu*

- Kidney *yang xu*

Kidney *qi xu* can result in the following pattern of imbalance

- Kidney *yang xu*

Kidney *qi* not grasping Lung *qi*

The Kidneys are responsible for grasping the *qi* that the Lung sends down. If Kidney *qi* or Kidney *yang* is weak, the Kidneys will not be able to grasp and hold down the Lung *qi*. This will disrupt the functioning of the Lung and there will be dyspnoea.

Aetiology

There may be a congenital weakness of the Kidneys and Lung. Working too hard physically, lifting and standing for long periods of time weaken the Kidney *qi*. Too much sex, chronic illness and old age are also possible factors.

Symptoms and signs

- Shortness of breath

- Shallow, superficial breathing

- Difficulty inhaling

- Spontaneous sweating

- Lumbar weakness, fatigue or soreness

- Sore or weak knees

- Dizziness

- Pale complexion

- Fatigue, both mental and physical

- Disinclination to speak

- Puffy face or puffiness around the eyes

- Pale tongue

- Deep and Weak pulse, especially in the *chi* positions

Key symptoms

Dyspnoea, lumbar soreness, deep and weak pulse in the *chi* positions.

Treatment principle

Tonify and warm the Kidneys, strengthen the Kidneys' ability to grasp *qi*, regulate Lung *qi*.

Acupuncture points
Choose from: Kid 3, Kid 4, Kid 7, Kid 25, Ren 4, Ren 6, Ren 17, Du 4, Lu 7, Lu 9, UB 13 and UB 23.

Needle technique
Tonifying. Moxa is recommended.

Explanation

- UB 23, Du 4, Ren 4, Ren 6, Kid 3 and Kid 7 tonify Kidney *qi*.

- Kid 4 tonifies the Kidney's ability to grasp Lung *qi*.

- Kid 25, Ren 17, Lu 7, Lu 9 and UB 13 regulate Lung *qi*.

Herbal formula

- *Su Zi Jiang Qi Tang* (Regulates Lung *qi*, transforms Phlegm and warms Kidney *yang*)

Relevant advice
Men should avoid having too many ejaculations and women should avoid becoming pregnant. Both sexes should avoid lifting heavy objects and overworking. Light physical exercise is okay, but the patient should avoid training excessively and exhausting physical activity. Fresh air and breathing exercises will be beneficial. The patient should eat foods that tonify Kidney *yang* (see the section on Kidney *yang xu* on page 556).

Kidney *qi* not grasping Lung *qi* can be caused by the following patterns of imbalance

- Spleen *qi xu*

- Spleen *yang xu*

- Lung *qi xu*

- Kidney *yang xu*

Kidney *qi* not grasping Lung *qi* can result in the following patterns of imbalance

- Lung *qi xu*

- Phlegm

- Stagnation of *qi* in the upper *jiao*

Kidney *yang xu*, overflowing water

When there is a significant Kidney *yang xu*, it may result in the transformation and transportation of fluids becoming so poor that fluids accumulate in the flesh under the skin. In some situations, the imbalance is not limited to the Kidneys and will also affect the Heart or the Lung. If the Heart is involved, there can also be palpitations and cold hands. If the Lung is involved, there will be watery, foamy sputum, coughing and/or difficulty breathing.

Aetiology

Kidney *yang xu*, overflowing water can arise when there is a deficiency in one or more of the following organs: Kidneys, Spleen, Lung and Heart. Kidney *yang* is weakened by disease, cold food, congenital weakness, old age, exogenous Cold, overwork, lifting heavy objects, standing for long periods of time and too much sex. Spleen *yang* is particularly weakened by food that is cold in its energy and temperature and cold medicine. Heart *yang xu* can have been influenced by emotional imbalances and Lung *yang* can be weakened by invasions of exogenous Cold.

Symptoms and signs

- Oedema, especially in the legs
- Abdominal bloating and oppression in the lower part of the abdominal cavity
- Aversion to cold
- Lumbar soreness, weakness or fatigue
- Sore or weak knees
- Puffy eyelids
- Cold limbs
- Pale or white face
- Sparse but pale-coloured urine
- Swollen, pale and wet tongue
- Deep, Weak and Slow pulse, the pulse may be relatively weak in the *chi* positions

If there is overflowing water that affects the Lung, there can also be:

- clear, watery, frothy sputum
- difficulty breathing
- shortness of breath
- cough with loose, thin sputum.

If there is overflowing water that affects the Heart, there can also be:

- palpitations

- shortness of breath

- cold hands.

Key symptoms
Oedema, sparse, but clear and pale urine, swollen, pale and wet tongue, Deep and Weak pulse.

- If the Lung is affected: watery sputum.

- If the Heart is affected: palpitations

Treatment principle
Tonify and warm Kidney *yang*, transform and drain fluids. Possibly tonify the Heart or the Lung.

Acupuncture points
Choose from: Kid 3, Kid 7, Ren 4, Ren 6, Ren 9, Du 4, UB 20, UB 22, UB 23, Sp 6, Sp 9, St 28 and St 36.

- If there is overflowing water that affects the Lung, add: Lu 7, UB 13 and Du 12.

- If there is overflowing water that affects the Heart, add: Du 14, UB 15, Du 11 and Ren 17.

Needle technique
Tonifying, except on Ren 9, St 28, Sp 6 and Sp 9, which should be drained. Moxa is recommended.

Explanation

- UB 23, Du 4, Ren 4, Ren 6 and Kid 3 tonify and warm Kidney *yang*.

- Kid 7 tonifies and warms Kidney *yang* and regulates the water passages.

- Ren 9 and St 28 regulate the water passages and drain Dampness.

- UB 20 and St 36 tonify Spleen *yang*.

- Sp 6 and Sp 9 drain Dampness.

- Lu 7, UB 13 and Du 12 regulate Lung *qi* and open the water passages.

- Du 14 tonifies *yang*.

- UB 15, Du 11 and Ren 17 regulate Heart *qi* and open the water passages.

Herbal formula

- *Zhen Wu Tang Tang* (Warms *yang* and drains water)

Relevant advice

The person should avoid eating foods and drinks that have a cold energy or temperature. They will benefit from drinking ginger tea or using ginger and cinnamon in their cooking. They should avoid lifting heavy objects, standing too much and physical strain. Men should avoid having too many ejaculations.

Kidney *yang xu*, overflowing water can caused by the following patterns of imbalance

- Spleen *yang xu*

- Kidney *yang xu*

- Lung *qi xu*

- Heart *yang xu*

- Heart *qi xu*

- Damp

- Cold

Kidney *yang xu*, overflowing water can result in the following patterns of imbalance

- Heart *yang xu*

- Lung *qi xu*

- Phlegm

- *Xue* stagnation

- Damp

- Spleen *yang xu*

- *Qi xu*

Kidney *jing xu*

Kidney *jing* is an aspect of Kidney *yin*, but it is also a distinct imbalance with specific symptoms and signs. Because Kidney *jing* is such a fundamental and basic aspect of the body's constitution, and is in part a form of *qi* that is inherited from the parents, a *jing xu* condition is an imbalance that is difficult to rectify. Some believe that you cannot replenish deficient *jing*, only improve the quality of remaining *jing*.

Aetiology

Kidney *jing* is partially inherited from the parents. This means that their age and health at the time of conception have crucial implications for the quality of a person's *jing*. *Jing* can also be weakened by chronic diseases, chronic stress, mental and physical overexertion, excessive sex, births, pregnancies and old age.

Symptoms and signs

- Frail constitution
- Weak teeth
- Porous or fragile bones
- Slender or thin body
- Mental or physical underdevelopment in children
- Deafness
- Tinnitus
- Dizziness
- Poor memory
- Delayed or absent development of secondary sexual characteristics in puberty
- Prematurely grey or white hair
- Infertility
- Lumbar weakness
- Weak knees
- Amenorrhoea
- Poor concentration
- Weakened mental capacity
- Hollow, depressed area in the root of the tongue
- Weak pulse in the *chi* positions

Key symptoms

Frail constitution, weak teeth and bones, infertility, depressed area on the root of the tongue.

Treatment principle

Nourish Kidney *jing*.

Acupuncture points
Choose from: Kid 3, Kid 6, Kid 13, Ren 4, UB 23, UB 52, UB 11 and GB 39.

Needle technique
Tonifying.

Explanation

- Kid 3, Kid 6, Ren 4, UB 23 and UB 52 tonify Kidney *jing*.

- UB 11 and GB 39 tonify the bones.

Herbal formula

- *Zou Gui Wan* (Nourishes Kidney *jing*)

Relevant advice
A person who is Kidney *jing xu* must ensure that they get enough rest and relaxation and they should not drive themselves too hard mentally or physically. Men who are *jing xu* should avoid having too much sex. Pregnancy and childbirth will further weaken the *jing* in a woman who is *jing xu*. They should avoid stimulants, especially coffee and caffeine. Foods that are attributed *jing*-nourishing qualities are royal jelly, eggs, roe/caviar, seeds, nuts, propolis/pollen, bone marrow, brain, kidney, oysters, seaweed and algae, artichokes, raw milk, nettles and oats.

Kidney *jing xu* can be caused by the following patterns of imbalance

- Kidney *yin xu*

- Kidney *yang xu*

- *Qi xu*

- *Xue xu*

Kidney *jing xu* can result in the following patterns of imbalance

- Kidney *yin xu*

- Kidney *yang xu*

- *Qi xu*

- *Xue xu*

Combined patterns

There can be combined patterns that do not just manifest simultaneously but in fact have become a joint pattern. This is particularly relevant with regards to Kidney imbalances, as Kidney *yin* and Kidney *yang* are the foundation of *yin* and *yang* in the whole body. When Kidney *yin* and Kidney *yang* are out of balance, the imbalance will usually encompass other organs. When there is a chronic imbalance in another organ, it will often end up affecting the Kidneys.

Kidney *yin xu* and Kidney *yang xu*

As discussed in the introduction, unlike other organs, the Kidneys do not have any *shi* patterns of imbalance and can quite easily be *yin xu* and *yang xu* concurrently.

Kidney *yin xu* and Kidney *yang xu* often arise as a consequence of each other, because they are mutually dependent and, in reality, are just aspects of each other. This means that when one aspect is *xu*, the other aspect will also become *xu* over time. One of the aspects, however, will always be more *xu* than the other. This aspect will therefore be the primary focus of the treatment, but the other aspect will also be treated at the same time. The patient will manifest with a combination of both Kidney *yin xu* and Kidney *yang xu* symptoms and signs. The tongue and pulse will be crucial factors that determine which imbalance is the most dominant. The treatment of Kidney *yin xu* and Kidney *yang xu* with needles is relatively straightforward, as the points used are generally the same, but the major difference is the use of moxa when there is Kidney *yang xu*. When employing herbs or pre-prepared pills, the situation is slightly more complex. It is important to determine which aspect is to be the primary focus of the treatment. One approach that can be utilised when treating with pre-prepared pills is to prescribe more of one type of pills than the other. For example, if Kidney *yin xu* is more pronounced than Kidney *yang xu*, the patient could be prescribed six *Liu Wei Di Huang* pills and two *Jin Gui Shen Qi* pills three times a day. Another approach is to administer the pills to treat Kidney *yang xu* in the morning and the pills to treat Kidney *yin xu* in the evening. It is, of course, possible to combine both these two approaches.

The aetiology, symptoms and treatment of the two patterns are described above in the sections discussing Kidney *yin xu* and Kidney *yang xu*.

Kidney *yin xu* and Liver *yin xu*

Kidney *yin* and Liver *yin* have a common root, which means that a *xu* condition in one can easily lead to a *xu* condition in the other.

Aetiology

Kidney and Liver *yin xu* can result from ageing, mental and physical overexertion, chronic illness, too little sleep, emotional stress and problems, frustrations and pent-up emotions, too much sex, too much coffee, dietary factors and medicines that are warming or spreading in their energy, long-term *xue xu* or Heat conditions and chronic *yin xu* conditions in other organs.

Symptoms and signs

- Dry eyes
- Blurred vision

- Night blindness

- Nagging headache

- Dizziness

- Insomnia

- Night sweats

- Numbness or tingling in the limbs

- Leg cramps in the evening and at night

- Thin body

- Poor hearing

- Dry mouth and throat

- Dry mucous membranes

- Dry hair and skin

- Dry stools

- Sparse or absent menstrual bleeding

- Infertility

- Thin tongue with a lack of coating, possibly cracks in the surface of the tongue

- Fine or Empty pulse, the pulse may be relatively weak in the left *chi* and *guan* positions

If Liver and Kidney *yin xu* have resulted in *xu* Heat, there can also be:

- hot flushes

- heat in the evening and at night

- a hot sensation in the palms of the hands, soles of the feet and centre of the chest

- a thirst with a desire to drink in small sips

- a red and dry tongue that lacks coating, possibly with cracks in the surface

- Fine and Rapid pulse, and possibly a Superficial pulse.

Key symptoms
Dry eyes and throat, insomnia, night sweats, lack of tongue coating, being warm in the evening or hot at night. If there is *xu* Heat, there can be hot flushes.

Treatment principle
Nourish Kidney and Liver *yin*, possibly control *xu* Heat.

Acupuncture points
Choose from: Kid 3, Kid 6, Kid 13, Sp 6, Liv 3 inserted through to Kid 1, Liv 8, Ren 4, UB 18, UB 23 and UB 52.

Needle technique
Tonifying.

Explanation

- Kid 1, Kid 3, Kid 6, Kid 13, Ren 4, UB 23 and UB 52 nourish Kidney *yin*.

- Sp 6 nourishes Kidney and Liver *yin*.

- Liv 3 and UB 18 nourish Liver *yin*.

Herbal formula

- *Liu Wei Di Huang Tang* (Nourishes Kidney and Liver *yin*)

- *Qi Ju Di Huang Tang* (Nourishes Kidney and Liver *yin* and controls Liver *yang*)

- *Zou Gui Wan* (Nourishes Kidney and Liver *yin*)

Relevant advice
See Kidney *yin xu* and Liver *yin xu*.

Kidney *yin xu* and Liver *yin xu* can be caused by the following patterns of imbalance

- Kidney *yin xu*

- Liver *xue xu*

Kidney *yin xu* and Liver *yin xu* can result in the following patterns of imbalance

- *Yin xu* Heat

- Ascending Liver *yang*

- Kidney *yang xu*

Kidney *yin xu* and Heart *yin xu*

This pattern is also known as 'Kidney and Heart not harmonised', because it reflects a disharmony in the fundamental balance between Fire and Water that these two organs are a resonance of. Water, in the form of Kidney *yin*, should nourish Heart *yin* and thereby control the Heart's *yang* fire aspect. If Kidney and Heart *yin* are weak, there will be an imbalance between Fire and Water. As it is a *xu* condition, there will not be the same intense and aggressive signs that *shen* is disturbed as when there is Heart Fire. When there is *yin xu*, *shen* will be more unsettled than agitated.

Aetiology

Heart and Kidney *yin xu* can arise from the following aetiological factors: ageing, mental and physical overexertion, chronic illness, too little sleep, emotional stress, anxiety, shock, depression, sadness, too much sex, too much coffee, dietary factors and medicine that are hot or spreading in their energy, chronic *xue xu* or Heat conditions and chronic *yin xu* conditions in other organs.

Symptoms and signs

- Insomnia
- Mental unrest
- Dream-disturbed sleep
- Anxiety
- Poor memory
- The person talks quickly and a lot
- Restlessness
- Restless or nervous movements
- Dizziness
- Tinnitus
- Poor hearing
- Palpitations
- Lumbar soreness or weakness
- Weak or sore knees
- Hot flushes
- Feeling of heat in the evening and at night
- Night sweats
- Hot sensation in the palms of the hands, soles of the feet and chest
- Malar flush
- Dark urine and scanty urination
- Premature ejaculation
- Nocturnal emissions

- Dry stools

- Thin body

- Thin, red tongue that lacks coating, red tongue tip, possibly cracked in the surface of the tongue

- The pulse is Fine or Empty, the left *chi* and *cun* positions may be weaker than the rest of the pulse, the pulse may be Rapid.

Key symptoms
Insomnia, palpitations, restlessness, night sweats, red tongue tip and malar flush.

Treatment principle
Nourish Kidney and Heart *yin*. Control Heat and calm the *shen*.

Acupuncture points
Choose from: Kid 3, Kid 6, Kid 7, Kid 9, Ren 4, Ren 15, He 5, He 6, He 7, UB 15, UB 23 and UB 52.

Needle technique
Tonifying.

Explanation

- Kid 3, Kid 6, Kid 7, Kid 9, Ren 4, UB 23 and UB 52 nourish Kidney *yin*.

- Ren 15, He 5, He 6, He 7 and UB 15 nourish Heart *yin*.

Herbal formula

- *Tian Wang Bu Xin Dan* (Nourish Heart and Kidney *yin*, calms *shen*)

Relevant advice
See Kidney *yin xu* and Heart *yin xu*.

Kidney *yin xu* and Heart *yin xu* can be caused by the following patterns of imbalance

- Kidney *yin xu*

- Heart *yin xu*

Kidney *yin xu* and Heart *yin xu* can result in the following patterns of imbalance

- *Xue* Heat

- Liver *yin xu*

- Phlegm

Kidney *yin xu* and Lung *yin xu*

The Lung is the 'delicate organ'. It is the only *yin* organ that is in direct contact with the environment outside of the body, which makes the Lung vulnerable to invasions of exogenous *xie qi*. The consequence of this is that Dryness and Heat can damage Lung *yin*. The Lung and the Kidneys cooperate closely with regards to the physiology of fluids in the body. One of the functions of the Kidneys is to moisten the Lung. This means that Kidney *yin xu* can injure Lung *yin*, and a chronic Lung *yin xu* will place a strain on Kidney *yin*.

Aetiology

Kidney and Lung *yin xu* can be a consequence of respiratory diseases, poor indoor climate with dry air, tobacco smoke, air pollution, ageing, mental and physical overexertion, chronic illness, stress, worry, unresolved or prolonged sorrow, too little sleep, too much sex, too much coffee, dietary factors and medicines that are hot or spreading in their energy, chronic *xue xu* or Heat conditions and chronic *yin xu* conditions in other organs.

Symptoms and signs

- Dry or tickling cough that is worse in the evening and at night or when the person is tired, the cough is weak

- Dry throat

- Ticklish sensation in the throat

- Shortness of breath on exertion

- Dry skin

- Lumbar soreness

- Sore knees

- Insomnia

- Night sweats

- Tinnitus

- Dizziness

- Dark and scanty urine

- Poor hearing

- Thin body

- Thin tongue with a lack of coating. There may be two small diagonal cracks in the front portion of the tongue

- Fine or Empty pulse, the pulse may be relatively weak in the right *cun* and left *chi* positions

Key symptoms
Dry cough, dry throat, lack of tongue coating.

Treatment principle
Nourish Kidney and Lung *yin*.

Acupuncture points
Choose from: Kid 3, Kid 6, Kid 7, Kid 9, Ren 4, Ren 17, Lu 1, Lu 9, UB 13, UB 23 and UB 52.

Needle technique
Tonifying.

Explanation

- Kid 3, Kid 6, Kid 7, Kid 9, Ren 4, UB 23 and UB 52 nourish Kidney *yin*.

- Lu 1, Lu 9 and UB 13 nourish Lung *yin* and regulate Lung *qi*.

Herbal formula

- *Mai Wei Di Huang Tang* (Nourishes Lung and Kidney *yin*)

Relevant advice
See Kidney *yin xu* and Lung *yin xu*.

Kidney *yin xu* and Lung *yin xu* can be caused by the following patterns of imbalance

- Kidney *yin xu*

- Lung *yin xu*

- Lung dryness

- Lung Heat

- Phlegm-Heat in the Lung

Kidney *yin xu* and Lung *yin xu* can result in the following patterns of imbalance

- Phlegm

- Liver *yin xu*

Kidney *yang xu* and Spleen *yang xu*

Spleen *yang* is reliant on heat from Kidney *yang* and *mingmen* to transform and transport the food and liquids that are consumed. If Spleen *yang* is weakened by the consumption of cold or raw foods, cold drinks or cold medicine, or if the Spleen is affected by the accumulation of Dampness, the weakening of the Spleen will place a burden on Kidney *yang*. This is because Kidney *yang* will have to work harder to heat and support Spleen *yang*. Conversely, a weak Kidney *yang* will not support Spleen *yang* and this will place a greater demand on the Spleen *yang*, thereby weakening it.

Aetiology

Spleen and Kidney *yang* are weakened by the following factors: Cold- or Damp-creating foods, raw food, cold drinks, cold medicine, physical overexertion, standing for long periods of time, lifting heavy objects, too much sex, invasions of exogenous Cold, ageing and congenital weakness.

Symptoms and signs

- Diarrhoea or watery stools that contain undigested food
- Watery stools early in the morning
- Frequent urination with large amount of clear, pale-coloured urine
- Nocturia or enuresis
- Aversion to cold
- Cold limbs
- Oedema
- Lack of thirst
- Lumbar soreness
- Cold lumbar region
- Sore, weak or cold knees
- Impotence
- Low libido
- Poor sperm quality
- Infertility
- Watery vaginal discharge
- Mental and physical fatigue
- Depression

- Indifference and indolence

- Poor appetite

- Disinclination for cold drinks or foods

- Pale complexion

- Dressing warmer than is normal for the season

- Pale, swollen and wet tongue with a white coating

- Deep and Weak pulse, right *guan* and *chi* positions may be relatively weak

Key symptoms
Watery stools containing undigested food, frequent urination with clear and copious amounts of urine, aversion to cold, sore lower back, sore knees and a Deep, Weak pulse.

Treatment principle
Warm and tonify Kidney and Spleen *yang*.

Acupuncture points
Choose from: Kid 3, Kid 7, Sp 3, St 25, St 36, St 37, Ren 4, Ren 6, Ren 8, Ren 12, UB 20, UB 21, UB 23 and Du 4.

Needle technique
Tonifying. Moxa is strongly recommended.

Explanation

- Kid 3, Kid 7, Ren 4, Du 4 and UB 23 tonify Kidney *yang*.

- Sp 3, St 36, Ren 12, UB 20 and UB 21 tonify Spleen *yang*.

- St 25 and St 37 tonify Spleen *qi* and regulate the Intestines.

- Ren 6 tonifies *yang*.

- Ren 8 warms the middle *jiao*.

Herbal formula

- *Li Zhong Tang* (Warms and tonifies Spleen *yang*)

- *Jin Gui Shen Qi Tang* (Warms and tonifies Kidney *yang*)

Relevant advice
See Kidney *yang xu* and Spleen *yang xu*.

Kidney *yang xu* and Spleen *yang xu* can be caused by the following patterns of imbalance

- Kidney *yang xu*
- Spleen *yang xu*
- Spleen *qi xu*
- Cold
- Damp

Kidney *yang xu* and Spleen *yang xu* can result in the following patterns of imbalance

- Spleen *qi xu*
- Kidney *yang xu*, overflowing water
- Kidney *qi* not grasping Lung *qi*
- Damp
- Phlegm
- *Xue* stagnation
- *Qi* stagnation
- *Qi xu*

Pericardium and *san jiao* imbalances

There is often no description of *san jiao* patterns of imbalance in textbooks, apart from in those that use the diagnostic model 'diagnosis according to *san jiao*'. The only Pericardium pattern of imbalance that is usually discussed is Pericardium Heat in the diagnostic models 'diagnosis according to the Four Levels' and 'diagnosis according to *san jiao*'. This is because most authors consider the Pericardium and Heart to be very closely integrated, so they only differentiate Heart imbalance patterns.

Maciocia (2005) lists six specific Pericardium patterns of imbalance, one of which is the aforementioned Pericardium Heat. Maciocia argues that if there are symptoms and signs that can be related to the Pericardium channel and its connections and relationship with the chest, i.e. the Lung channel and the Liver channel, and not only to Heart organ symptoms and signs, you should diagnose a Pericardium pattern of imbalance (Maciocia 2005, p.487).

I have chosen to discuss only the pattern of Pericardium Heat. This is because the other patterns are so similar to the patterns already differentiated in the section on Heart imbalances in terms of their symptoms, aetiology and treatment, I feel that further differentiating these patterns has only academic rather than practical interest. I will only discuss the aetiology and pathology that is relevant to Pericardium Heat. For a more detailed discussion of the aetiology and pathology that is relevant to the other Heart and Pericardium patterns, the reader is referred to the section on Heart patterns of imbalance (page 487).

San jiao diagnosis is discussed in Section 9, 'Diagnosis According to the Six Stages, Four Levels and *San Jiao*'.

Shi patterns

Heat blocking the Pericardium

This is not something that you would normally meet in an ordinary clinical setting. When Heat has penetrated down to this level, the patient will usually be treated with Western medicine and will probably be hospitalised.

If the body is invaded by exogenous Heat, the Heat will initially affect the *wei* level or the *qi* level. In some cases, *xie* Heat can penetrate to the *ying* level. The *ying* level is the superficial aspect of *xue*. When the disease has penetrated this far down down to the *ying* level, it is deeper and more serious than when the disease was at the *qi* level. *Xie* Heat can penetrate to the *ying* level if *xie qi* is sufficiently virulent or if it is treated incorrectly or inadequately. Furthermore, *xie qi* can penetrate directly from the *wei* level to the *ying* level, because the Lung and Pericardium both have their residence in the upper *jiao*. *Xie qi* will, therefore, be able to transmit directly from Lung *wei qi* for Pericardium *ying qi*.

Ying qi is the *qi* aspect of *xue*. *Xue* Heat will agitate the *shen*, which has its residence in the Heart. This will result in restlessness and insomnia. The Heat can be so intense that it creates Phlegm. The Phlegm and the Heat will block and agitate the *shen* so the person may be delirious or raving or they may lose consciousness.

The Heat will also injure *yin*. This is why the tongue lacks coating, the pulse is Fine and the symptoms are worse at night.

There can be a rash or petechiae because the Heat has agitated *xue*, rupturing the walls of the vessels.

Normally, the hands and feet would feel hot when there is so much Heat present. This is not the case in this pattern, as the extremities are cold because *xie* Heat blocks the body's physiological heat from reaching the extremities. This is called 'True Heat, False Cold'.

Even though there is intense Heat, there is no thirst. This is because the Heat is so intense that it forces fluids upwards in the body to the mouth.

Aetiology

The pattern will be due to an invasion of exogenous *xie qi*.

Symptoms and signs

- High fever that is worse at night

- Insomnia

- Mental and physical restlessness

- No thirst

- Petechiae

- Red or purple skin rashes (erythema and purpura)

- Delirium

- Unconsciousness or coma

- The skin feels hot when palpated

- Cold hands and feet

- Dark red, dry tongue without coating

- Rapid and Fine pulse

Key symptoms
Dry mouth and no thirst, high fever but cold hands, unconsciousness, red tongue without coating.

Treatment principle
Drain Heat from the Pericardium.

Acupuncture points
Choose from: Pe 3, Pe 8, Pe 9, Sp 10, UB 40, LI 11, Du 14 and Du 26.

Needle technique
Draining. Bleed Pe 3, Pe 9, UB 40 and Du 14.

Explanation

- Pe 3, Pe 8 and Pe 9 drain Heat from the Pericardium.

- UB 40, LI 11, Du 14 and Sp 10 drain *xue* Heat.

- Du 26 revives consciousness.

Herbal formula

- *Qing Ying Tang* (Drains *ying* level Heat)

Relevant advice

This is an acute pattern, therefore advice regarding diet or lifestyle is not relevant. The patient must be seen by a Western doctor.

Heat blocking the Pericardium can be caused by the following patterns of imbalance

- *Wei qi*-level Heat

- *Qi*-level Heat

Heat blocking the Pericardium can result in the following pattern of imbalance

- *Xue*-level Heat

Gall Bladder imbalances

The Gall Bladder is an interesting organ. It is a regular *fu* organ but is also one of the six extraordinary *fu* organs. It differs from other *fu* organs in that it does not receive and excrete impure products but stores bile, which is regarded as a pure substance. However, it is on the mental-emotional level that the main difference lies. The Gall Bladder plays a major role in decision making. It is the Gall Bladder that enables us to make a decision and at the same time it gives us the courage to carry out the decisions we have taken. It cooperates closely with its partner organ, the Liver, which controls making plans and strategies. It is not enough to have a vision and to define a strategy, there must also be the determination and the courage to take the decision and carry it out. The Gall Bladder is the only *fu* organ with a pattern of imbalance that manifests primarily on the mental-emotional level. If there is Gall Bladder and Heart *qi xu*, the person will be timid and nervous and have difficulty making decisions. They will lack the courage to pursue their dreams. The Chinese say that a person who is brave has a 'big gall bladder' whilst a person with a 'small gall bladder', is a person who is cowardly and lacking in courage.

Apart from collaborating in making plans and taking decisions, the Liver and Gall Bladder cooperate closely in relation to bile. The Gall Bladder receives bile that it stores and later secretes when it is used for the digestive process. This secretion of bile is dependent on Liver *qi* and its free movement.

The Gall Bladder and the Liver have such a close relationship that they can almost be seen as being each other's *yin* and *yang* aspects. This means that many of the *shi* patterns that are seen in the Liver manifest with symptoms in the Gall Bladder channel.

The Gall Bladder is affected negatively when Dampness and Damp-Heat block the free movement of *qi* and bile. The Dampness and Heat can be exogenous in the form of climatic factors or can be due to the diet if there is an excessive consumption of food and beverages that create Damp and Damp-Heat, typically fried food and food with a high fat content. Dampness and Damp-Heat can also be generated internally when there is imbalance in other *zangfu* organs. Jaundice may be a sign of Damp or Damp-Heat in the Gall Bladder. Yellowing of the skin, yellow sclera, etc. are always a sign of the presence of Damp or Damp-Heat. In this situation, Damp blocks the free movement of *qi* and bile from the Gall Bladder. Because there is stagnation of *qi*, there will often be pain in the region and the Damp will also give rise to a sensation of heaviness. Damp will often manifest with a sticky sensation in the mouth. The person can also have a bitter taste if there is also Heat.

When there is Damp-Heat, the Heat aspect will result in the person being thirsty, but the Damp aspect will mean that they do not want to drink anything.

Damp can also manifest with a heavy headache and difficulty in thinking clearly. The urine can be cloudy due to Dampness, but also dark and sparse due to the presence of Heat. The stools can be either loose or constipated, depending on whether Dampness or Heat is the dominant form of *xie qi*. When Dampness blocks the *qi ji* or *qi* mechanism in the middle *jiao*, there can be symptoms such as nausea, vomiting or lack of appetite.

The combination of Dampness, Heat and *qi* stagnation can lead to the formation of Phlegm in the Gall Bladder. This will result in the formation of gallstones, which will then further block the free movement of the bile and *qi* in the Gall Bladder.

Emotionally, the Gall Bladder is affected by the same factors as the Liver, i.e. anger, frustration, irritation and unresolved emotions. This is because these emotions can lead to the stagnation of Liver *qi*, on which the Gall Bladder depends to carry out its duties. The stagnation of *qi* can also generate Heat in the Gall Bladder. The pattern Gall Bladder and Heart *qi xu* will often be a congenital pattern or a pattern that has arisen in early childhood. It is often a consequence of a shock in utero or in childhood, a lack of love, attention or recognition or bullying or prolonged fear. Small children are particularly vulnerable because their organs are still developing and their *qi* is not stable. Children are *yang* and lack the stability of *yin*. This means that the Heart and Gall Bladder *qi* can easily be dissipated or depleted. Adults who have been subjected to an extreme shock or violent experiences may also develop a similar pattern. Post-traumatic stress syndrome is an aspect of this pattern. This person will also be afraid and anxious and have difficulty making decisions.

General symptoms and signs of Gall Bladder imbalances

- Digestive problems
- Difficulty making decisions
- One-sided coating on the tongue
- Hypochondriac tension

Gall Bladder Damp-Cold

This pattern and Gall Bladder Damp-Heat are very similar in their aetiology and pathology. There can also be a progression from the one to the other. The tongue and pulse will be some of the most crucial factors in differentiating between these two patterns.

Aetiology

Dampness in the Gall Bladder can arise when there has been an excessive consumption of fried food or food with a high fat content such as dairy products, fatty meat and so on. Exogenous Damp can also invade the body and disrupt the functioning of the Gall Bladder.

Damp can be internally generated when there is Spleen *qi xu*. If there is Liver *qi* stagnation, this will exacerbate the stagnation that is caused by the Dampness.

Symptoms and signs

- Yellowish coloured skin

- Yellowish sclera

- Hypochondriac tension

- Costal pain or distension

- Abdominal bloating

- Nausea or vomiting, especially after intake of fatty food

- Sensation of heaviness in the body

- Heavy headache

- Sticky sensation in the mouth

- Lack of thirst

- Cloudy or oily urine

- Loose or putty-like stools that may be clay coloured or very pale

- Thick, greasy or sticky tongue coating that is either one-sided or has a wide stripe of coating on each side of the tongue

- Slippery and Wiry pulse

Key symptoms

Yellow skin and eyes, tightness, pain or distension below the ribs, sticky, white tongue coating.

Treatment principle
Drain Dampness from the Gall Bladder and spread *qi*.

Acupuncture points
Choose from: GB 24, GB 34, GB 41, Sp 6, Sp 9, SJ 5, SJ 6, Liv 14, *Dannangxue* (Ex-LE 6), UB 18, UB 19, UB 22 and Du 9.

Needle technique
Draining.

Explanation

- GB 24, GB 34, Du 9 and UB 19 drain Dampness from the Gall Bladder and spread Gall Bladder *qi*.

- GB 41 and SJ 5 open *dai mai* and drain Dampness from the Gall Bladder.

- UB 22, Sp 6 and Sp 9 drain Dampness.

- Liv 14 and UB 18 spread Liver *qi*.

- SJ 6 circulates *qi* in all three *jiao.*

- *Dannangxue* is an empirical point for the treatment of Gall Bladder disorders.

Herbal formula

- *Yin Chen Zhu Fu Yu Tang* (Transforms Dampness and warms and tonifies the Spleen *yang*)

Relevant advice
It is important to avoid consuming foods that produce Dampness, especially foods that are rich in fat and oil. Gall Bladder Damp-Cold can be negatively affected by climatic influences. This means that the person should ensure that they are properly dressed and do not live or work in damp places. If Spleen *qi xu* or Liver *qi* stagnation is part of the picture, the relevant advice for these imbalances should also be followed.

Gall Bladder Damp-Cold can be caused by the following patterns of imbalance

- Invasions of Damp and Cold

- Spleen *qi xu*

- Liver *qi* stagnation

Gall Bladder Damp-Cold can result in the following patterns of imbalance

- Gall Bladder Damp-Heat

- Liver *qi* stagnation

- Phlegm

- *Xue* stagnation

Gall Bladder Damp-Heat

As described above, Gall Bladder Damp-Cold and Gall Bladder Damp-Heat appear to be very similar in their aetiology, pathology and symptoms. The difference in this pattern is signs of Heat that were not apparent in Gall Bladder Damp-Cold.

Aetiology

The aetiology is the same as described in the previous pattern, as well as the consumption of food and beverages that directly generate Damp-Heat, such as alcohol and fried food. Factors such as stress, repressed anger and unresolved emotions can create a stagnation of Heat or Fire in the Liver, which can then generate Heat in the Gall Bladder.

Symptoms and signs

- Yellowish skin

- Yellowish sclera

- Hypochondriac tension, bloating or pain below the costal

- Costal pain or distension

- Nausea or vomiting, especially after consuming greasy food

- Sense of heaviness in the body

- Heavy headache

- Bitter taste in the mouth

- Thirst without a desire to drink

- Dark or scanty urine

- Constipation or sticky stools that may be clay coloured

- Irritability and anger

- Dizziness

- Thick, yellowish, greasy or sticky tongue coating that is either one-sided or has two stripes of coating on each side of the tongue

- Slippery, Wiry and Rapid pulse

Key symptoms
Yellow skin and eyes, hypochondriac tightness, pain or bloating, sticky yellow tongue coating, Rapid, Wiry or Slippery pulse.

Treatment principle
Drain Dampness and Heat from the Gall Bladder and spread *qi*.

Acupuncture points
Choose from: GB 24, GB 34, GB 41, GB 43, Sp 6, Sp 9, SJ 5, SJ 6, Liv 14, *Dannangxue* (Ex-LE 6), UB 18, UB 19, UB 22, LI 11 and Du 9.

Needle technique
Draining.

Explanation

- GB 24, GB 34, GB 43, Du 9 and UB 19 drain Damp-Heat from the Gall Bladder and spread Gall Bladder *qi*.

- GB 41 and SJ 5 open *dai mai* and drain Damp-Heat from the Gall Bladder.

- UB 22, Sp 6 and Sp 9 drain Damp-Heat.

- Liv 14 and UB 18 spread Liver *qi*.

- SJ 6 circulates *qi* and drains Heat in all three *jiao*.

- LI 11 drains Damp-Heat.

- *Dannangxue* is an empirical point for the treatment of Gall Bladder disorders.

Herbal formula

- *Long Dan Xie Gan Tang* (Drains Heat and drains Liver and Gall Bladder Damp-Heat)

Relevant advice
The patient should avoid consuming alcohol and foods that generate Dampness and Heat, especially foods that are rich in fat. Damp-Heat in the Gall Bladder can be affected negatively by climatic influences. The patient should therefore avoid living and working in humid conditions. If Spleen *qi xu* or Liver *qi* stagnation are part of the picture, the relevant advice for these imbalances should also be followed.

Gall Bladder Damp-Heat can be caused by the following patterns of imbalance

- Gall Bladder Damp-Cold

- Invasions of Damp and Heat

- Spleen *qi xu*

- Liver *qi* stagnation Heat

- Liver Fire

Gall Bladder Damp-Heat can result in the following patterns of imbalance

- Liver *qi* stagnation

- Phlegm

- *Xue* stagnation

Combined patterns

Liver and Gall Bladder Damp-Heat

When there is Damp-Heat in the Liver and Gall Bladder, there will be symptoms and signs of both Damp-Heat in the Liver and Gall Bladder Damp-Heat.

Aetiology

The consumption of food and medicine that create Dampness or are hot in their energy.

Emotional imbalances that weaken the Spleen, such as worry and pensiveness, or emotions such as frustration, pent-up anger and irritation that stagnate Liver *qi*, thereby generating Heat in the Liver.

There can also be direct invasions of exogenous Damp-Heat, especially in tropical climates.

Symptoms and signs

- Fever or aversion to heat

- Blocked or stuffy sensation in the chest and below the ribs

- Sensation of heaviness and fatigue in the body

- Yellow skin colour and yellowish sclera

- Red and weeping skin disorders, rashes and sores

- Itching, burning or stinging skin, sores or rashes

- Genitals ulcers or ulcers around the mouth

- Copious, yellowish, sticky discharge from the vagina that is odorous

- Swollen or red and painful genitals

- Irregular menstrual cycle or spotting

- Yellow, sticky sweat

- Bitter or sticky taste in the mouth

- Dark and sparse urine, the urine may be odorous

- Burning sensation on urination

- Lack of appetite

- Nausea or vomiting, especially after consuming greasy food

- Headache

- Constipation or sticky stools that may be clay coloured

- Irritability and anger

- Thirst without a desire to drink

- Red tongue with even redder sides, greasy, yellowish coating possibly only on one side or two bilateral yellow stripes

- Fast, Slippery and/or Wiry pulse, a Wiry pulse in the left *guan* position

Key symptoms
Sensations of heaviness and fatigue, bitter or sticky taste, nausea, yellow skin, dark urine and yellow greasy tongue coating.

Treatment principle
Drain Damp-Heat from the Liver and Gall Bladder.

Acupuncture points
Choose from: Liv 2, Liv 14, UB 18, UB 19, GB 24, GB 34, GB 41, SJ 5, *Dannangxue* (Ex-LE 6), LI 11, Sp 6 and Du 9.

Needle technique
Draining.

Explanation

- Liv 2, Liv 14, GB 24, GB 34, UB 18, UB 19 and Du 9 drain Damp-Heat from the Liver and Gall Bladder.

- GB 41 and SJ 5 together open *dai mai* and drain Damp-Heat.

- Sp 6 and Sp 9 drain Dampness.

- LI 11 drains the Damp-Heat.

- *Dannangxue* is an empirical point for the treatment of Gall Bladder disorders.

Herbal formula

- *Long Dan Xie Gan Tang* (Drains Damp-Heat from the Liver and Gall Bladder)

Relevant advice

When there is Damp-Heat in the Liver and Gall Bladder, the patient should avoid consuming substances that create Heat or Dampness, especially if these substances have an affinity with the Liver. Alcohol, hot spices, fried food and too much red meat should particularly be avoided, as well as foods such as dairy products, sugar, sweets, nuts, bananas and avocados. A Liver that is burdened by pharmaceutical medicine, alcohol, chemicals, heavy metals and other pollutants will have difficulty carrying out its metabolic functions, so caution should be exercised and the consumption of all kinds of medicine, including dietary supplements and herbal remedies, should be limited as much as possible.

Stress and pent-up emotions, especially anger and frustration, can create Heat in the Liver. A person with Damp-Heat in the Liver and the Gall bladder should try and address these emotional issues. Exercise, sport and physical training will be beneficial, as physical activity will help to circulate and spread stagnant Liver *qi*, which is often involved in the creation of Heat in the Liver.

Liver and Gall Bladder Damp-Heat can be caused by the following patterns of imbalance

- Spleen *qi xu*
- Damp-Heat
- Liver *qi* stagnation Heat
- Invasions of exogenous *xie qi*
- Gall Bladder Damp-Cold

Liver and Gall Bladder Damp-Heat can result in the following patterns of imbalance

- Liver Fire
- Phlegm
- Liver *xue* stagnation

Heart and Gall Bladder *qi xu*

Heart and Gall Bladder *qi xu* arises because a person is born with an unstable *shen* or their *shen* has been disturbed and unsettled by a significant shock or prolonged anxiety. The person's mother may have been exposed to shock, excessive sadness, anxiety or other emotional influences during the pregnancy and this might have affected foetal *qi*. The person may also have grown up in a family or an environment where there has been a lack of love or there has been outright neglect. Severe shock, fright and fear in adults can spread the Heart *qi* and weaken Gall Bladder *qi*. This can be seen in post-traumatic stress syndrome.

The unsettled and unstable *shen* will mean that the person is anxious, skittish and easily frightened. The weak Gall Bladder *qi* will also mean that they are nervous and have difficulty making decisions.

When it is congenital, the person will have always been very shy and easily frightened.

Aetiology
Powerful shock, anxiety, lack of love in childhood or congenital character traits.

Symptoms and signs

- Easily startled, nervous and lacks courage

- Frequent anxiety attacks

- Shyness

- Indecision

- Palpitations, mainly caused by shock, fright, anxiety and nervousness

- Wakes up early in the morning

- Frequent nightmares, waking with anxiety

- Dream-disturbed sleep

- Spontaneous sweating

- Fatigue

- Slight breathlessness

- Possibly a thin crack on the tip of the tongue

- Deep, Weak pulse, especially on the left-hand side

Key symptoms
Nervousness, shyness, lack of determination.

Treatment principle
Tonify Heart and Gall Bladder *qi*.

Acupuncture points
Choose from: UB 15, UB 19, Ren 15, *yintang* (Ex-HN 3), GB 40 and He 7.

Needle technique
Tonifying.

Explanation

- UB 19 and GB 40 tonify Gall Bladder *qi*.

- UB 15 and He 7 tonify Heart qi and calm *shen*.

- Ren 15 and *yintang* calm *shen*.

Herbal formula

- *Gan Mai Da Zao Tang* (Nourishes the Heart and calms the *shen*)

Relevant advice
Psychotherapy may be relevant, since much of the aetiology of this pattern lies on the psycho-emotional level and probably dates from early childhood. Some clients may feel that they will benefit from healing or similar therapies.

It is important that a person with Heart and Gall Bladder *qi xu* avoids shock or stressful situations.

Meditation, yoga and mindfulness will be beneficial.

Heart and Gall Bladder *qi xu* can be caused by the following patterns of imbalance
This is more a constitutional pattern so there will not necessarily be any previous patterns.

Heart and Gall Bladder *qi xu* can result in the following patterns of imbalance

- Heart *qi xu*

- Heart *yin xu*

Liver imbalances
The Liver is not directly involved in the production of *qi*, *xue* or *jinye*, so there are very few Liver *xu* patterns of imbalance. The Liver has the important function of ensuring that *qi* flows freely and unhindered throughout the whole body. This means that the Liver has a determining influence on the movement of *qi* and *xue* in the body, and Liver imbalances will often be involved in imbalances in other organs. There is often a focus on Liver *qi* stagnation when analysing pathological conditions and the way in which Liver *qi* disrupts and blocks other organ's *qi ji* or *qi* mechanisms. It is, however, important to remember that this is a pathological condition. When the Liver is in balance, it has the important function of supporting the other organ's *qi ji* and the movement of *qi* and *xue* in the body in general.

The Liver is also a reservoir for *xue*. This means that *xue* imbalances often affect the Liver and *xue* can be affected by Liver imbalances.

The Liver is the General, whose task it is to plan and create strategies. This task is closely related to the Liver's *shen* aspect, the *hun*. One of the aspects of the *hun* is that it enables us to have vision, to imagine something in the future that has not happened yet. This is what we utilise when we lay out plans and strategies. We have a vision of how the future might be. People with a strong *hun* have a clear idea of what they want. They have goals and they pursue them, whatever the cost.

The Liver also defines our boundaries. If the Wood Phase is strong, a person can set their boundaries in relation to others. If the Liver is weak, a person often gets stepped on and they have difficulty saying 'no' or 'stop' to others. If the Liver is *xu*, the person lacks a strong vision of what they want for themselves or they lack the courage to pursue their goals. When they meet someone with a more powerful *hun*, they get brushed aside by this person's momentum, or they give up when somebody criticises them or has a different meaning. On the other hand, if a person has an over-active Liver, they do not respect other people's boundaries. Their needs come first, because they have a vision of what they want. They do not care about other people's visions if they conflict with theirs. Liver *qi* should ideally be flexible like a young tree. It should have the strength to grow upwards and outwards to fulfil its potential but at the same time be flexible enough to be able to bend and withstand pressure when the wind blows or when there are physical obstacles in its way. It should not be stiff and brittle as this will eventually cause it to snap, but it should not be weak and limp, letting itself be overshadowed and crowded out by others. As humans, we are social beings and we should be flexible enough to accommodate the visions and needs of others, not just steamroller everyone and everything that stands in our path, but we should also be determined enough to accomplish our own dreams and visions.

Most politicians and business leaders have a strong *hun*. They have a clear vision of how they think things should be and a strategy to achieve these aims. They have no problem sacrificing other people if it helps them achieve their own goals. On the other hand, their Liver *qi* stagnates violently when there is someone or something that blocks them from achieving what they want. Artists are another group that have a strong *hun*. They can look at a lump of clay or a blank canvas and see a piece of art, which they are then able to bring forth. Many athletes also have a strong *hun*. This is what enables them to be able to push themselves beyond their physical limits. They are able to overcome both fatigue and pain in order to achieve their goals. This tendency can be recognised in some clients. They push themselves harder than their bodies (i.e. *qi* and *jing*) are able to sustain in the long run. These people often develop Kidney *xu* imbalances because they consume more *qi* than they can produce. It is often these Kidney *xu* symptoms that are the reason that they seek treatment.

The aetiology of Liver patterns of imbalance

Due to its dynamic ascendant and expansive energy, the Liver is adversely affected by limitations. This is particularly evident on the mental-emotional level. All kinds of frustration, irritation and suppressed or unresolved emotions will stagnate Liver *qi*.

It is the ability of the Liver and the *hun* to have a vision and a goal whilst also having the dynamic to move towards this goal, which is the Liver's strength. Unfortunately, it is also its weak point. Frustration, and thereby Liver *qi* stagnation, arises every time you are prevented from doing what you want to and every time you are forced to do something you do not want to or do not like, i.e. each time the *hun* is prevented from fulfilling its vision. When we live in a society with other people, we will constantly be impinged upon by other people's visions and ideas. This means that you will, to a greater or lesser degree, have to make compromises and not do what you would ideally like to.

Every movement in life is either towards what you want or want to do or away from what you don't want or don't want to do. It may be that you are trying to achieve some goal or it may be that you are trying to avoid something unpleasant. Each time you are blocked in this movement towards pleasure and satisfaction, or away from suffering or pain, it will stagnate the Liver *qi*. There is a significant difference between how much your vision or ideal of yourself and your life is obstructed and how much you will be subjected to other people's visions and how much you can determine your own life or the number and size of the compromises that you have to make. It can be anything from having to live with a tyrannical husband or having a boss who humiliates and harasses you, to having to spend Sunday afternoon with your in-laws, do the washing-up or just stand in a queue. Anything that prevents you from doing or being what you want or being where you want to be will stagnate Liver *qi*. The extent to which these things stagnate a person's Liver *qi* is also determined by how good they are at accepting the circumstances of their life. Two people faced with the same intransigent situation will have different degrees of dissatisfaction, depending on their ability to accept the reality they are confronted with.

This is important to remember when treating chronically ill patients. Being ill and not being able to live life as they would like, whilst having physical or emotional pain, will stagnate a person's Liver *qi*. This means that even though Liver *qi* stagnation was not necessarily a part of their diagnostic picture in the beginning, it will often have become an element of their imbalance dynamic by the time that we meet them in the clinic.

Anger, which is the feeling or emotion that has a resonance with Liver and the Wood Phase, can affect the Liver negatively in two ways. Anger has a very strong *yang* dynamic. Anger causes Liver *qi* to ascend upwards. This means that anger can aggravate and trigger conditions caused by ascending Liver *yang* or Liver Fire. On the other hand, because anger is so dynamic and powerful in its energy, it will have an equally powerful stagnating effect on the Liver *qi* if it is not expressed.

As well as consuming *qi* and *yin*, stress can have a stagnating effect on Liver *qi*. This is because stress can be extremely frustrating. It is said that stress does not arise from all the things that you have to do but from all the things that you don't have time to do. Frustration at not achieving your objectives and goals, as well as feeling inefficacious, will stagnate Liver *qi*. Stagnation of Liver *qi*, combined with the consumption of the Kidney and Heart *yin*, which is often another consequence of stress, can lead to the generation of Heat in the body.

The Liver organ is not particularly vulnerable to invasions of exogenous *xie qi*, yet climatic wind, which resonates with the Wood Phase, can have an effect on the Liver. Exposure to the wind can cause the eyes, which are controlled by the Liver, to water. People with Liver imbalances can be more irritable when there are strong winds. Some even claim that the rate of homicide rises when the sirocco wind blows in Spain. The resonance between wind and the Liver can be seen in the Liver imbalances that can result in internally generated Wind. Here, the Wind can be a symptom that the Liver is out of balance as opposed to an aetiological factor.

Even though the Liver organ is not particularly vulnerable to exogenous invasions of *xie qi*, the Liver channel can be invaded by Dampness and Cold. This can happen if a person has walked around barefoot on cold and damp surfaces or has worn insufficient clothing or shoes on their legs and feet.

Although it is the sour taste that resonates with the Liver, food and beverages that are energetically hot are most often an aetiological factor in Liver imbalances. Unfortunately, many people with Liver imbalances are often attracted to things such as alcohol and hot spices, because their spicy flavour will spread stagnant Liver *qi*. The problem is that they also have a hot energy and this will create Heat in the Liver. Alcohol is particularly bad, because as well as being energetically hot, it often has a sour flavour that will lead the Heat directly to the Liver. This is seen, for example, when red wine triggers a migraine in people who have a tendency to have ascending Liver *yang* or Liver Fire. It is also why people can get a loud, resonant voice or become aggressive when they drink alcohol.

Consuming food that produces Dampness, especially if it is also warm or hot in its energy, can create Damp-Heat in the Liver. The diet can also result in *xu* imbalances in the Liver. This is seen if the diet does not contain sufficient *xue*-nourishing foods, resulting in the person becoming Liver *xue xu*.

Liver *xue* will also be weakened when blood is lost through heavy menstrual bleeding, childbirth, surgery and physical trauma.

The Liver has, by virtue of its *qi*-spreading function, an important influence on other organs in the body. Liver *qi* stagnation can often be an aetiological factor in the generation of other imbalances in other organs, but the Liver is also negatively affected by imbalances in other organs. A vicious cycle can arise where imbalances in the various organs eventually become self-generating. For example, Liver *qi* stagnation can disrupt the Spleen in its functioning. This can result in a diminished production of *xue*, leading to the Liver becoming *xue xu*. Liver *xue xu* can then result in the Liver becoming stiff and rigid and thereby leading to a stagnation of Liver *qi*, which then disrupts the Spleen. The Spleen then produces less *xue*, which makes the Liver *xue xu* and so on.

Heat in the body can create *xue* Heat. Because *xue* is stored in the Liver, *xue* Heat can create Heat in the Liver.

The Liver and Heart cooperate closely in relation to *xue*, and Liver *xue xu* and Heart *xue xu* usually manifest together. The *hun* and *shen* also have a close relationship, following each other in their 'entering and exiting'.

The Lung and Liver collaborate in relation to *qi*: The Lung descends *qi* and spreads *qi* through the channels and vessels, whilst the Liver ensures the free movement of *qi* in the whole body. Kidney *yin* and Liver *yin* have a common root, which means that if there is Kidney *yin xu*, Liver *yin xu* will often develop as a consequence and vice versa.

The pathology of Liver imbalances

Anger in all its forms affects the Liver and when the Liver is imbalanced it often manifests with the person being irascible and easily angered. Anger is extremely *yang* in nature. It rises to the head and it is explosive. People with Liver *shi* imbalances can have a short fuse and be bad tempered. When there is Liver *qi* stagnation, the person can internalise their anger and frustration for a long time. When they do finally release their anger, it is often the wrong people who bear the brunt. The more Heat that there is, the more irritable the person will be and the shorter their fuse. Due to its ascendant dynamic, anger can aggravate or trigger symptoms that are manifestations of ascending Liver *yang* or Liver Fire. This will typically be things like headaches, pain behind or in the eyes, tinnitus or vertigo.

Stagnation of Liver *qi* can also manifest with the person being irascible or bad tempered. When there is Liver *qi* stagnation, the person will easily feel frustrated and they will often be impatient. There will frequently be mood swings when the Liver *qi* is not flowing freely and unhindered as it should do when the Liver is harmonious.

If the *hun* is blocked, as can be the case when there is Liver *qi* stagnation or Liver *xue* stagnation, or if the *hun* lacks nourishment, such as when there is Liver *yin xu* or Liver *xue xu*, it can result in depression, with the person having difficulty seeing a future for themselves. This can be seen in the eyes. It is as if they do not look outwards and instead their vision is turned inwards. This is because Liver *qi* stagnation prevents the *hun* from being able to 'exit and enter' freely.

At night the *hun* returns to the Liver. If the *hun* is not anchored by Liver *yin* and Liver *xue* or is agitated by Heat, it will create visions or dreams. A person mainly dreams in rapid eye movement (REM) sleep. In REM sleep the *hun* is active, which can be seen in the characteristic rapid movements of the eyes whilst the person is sleeping. When the *hun* is not anchored by Liver *xue*, the person can dream a lot and suffer from insomnia. If there is Heat in the Liver, it will agitate the *hun* at night and the person will sleep restlessly. They will have many, and sometimes violent, dreams or nightmares. Heat in the Liver, particularly Heat from Liver *qi* stagnation, can cause the person to wake early and have difficulty falling asleep again.

The sound in the voice that is a manifestation of the Liver is shouting, which can be heard when a person is angry. This can also be a more permanent quality in some people's voices. The harshness will not be as extreme as when a person is angry, but there will be a slight hardness and resonance in the voice. This will usually indicate a *shi* pattern of imbalance in the Liver. If there is Liver *qi* stagnation, the person can have a staccato voice that sounds a bit like a machine gun. This type of voice arises through the combination of the hardness in the voice that is characteristic of Liver *shi* imbalances and the unevenness and juddering that is the result of the Liver *qi* not flowing freely. When there are *xu* conditions in the Liver, the voice will lack the shouting quality; it will be too soft and lack clout. This will be especially noticeable in situations where the person is angry or when the voice is raised.

Liver *shi* imbalances will often manifest with symptoms and signs in the Liver's partner channel, the Gall Bladder channel. In these cases, the symptoms and signs will typically be hemilateral. Migraines or throbbing headaches are a typical example of this. Another characteristic of Liver *shi* symptoms is that they are triggered or aggravated by stress, anger, frustration and similar emotional influences and often manifest in the premenstrual period in women.

In general, symptoms and signs that have a close relationship with the menstrual cycle can indicate that there is a Liver imbalance. Whereas Liver *shi* symptoms typically manifest in the premenstrual period, Liver *xue xu* and Liver *yin xu* signs and symptoms can be more pronounced immediately after or towards the end of menstrual bleeding.

The Liver has a significant influence on the menstrual cycle. This is due to the Liver's close relationship with the movement of *qi* and *xue*, and because the Liver is a reservoir for *xue* and supplies the *chong mai* with *xue*, thereby enabling menstrual bleeding. If there is Liver *xue xu*, there can be too little *xue* to create menstrual bleeding. This will result in either amenorrhoea, scanty menstrual bleeding or a long menstrual cycle. The cycle can also be longer when there is a stagnation of Liver *xue*. In these cases, the stagnation of *xue* will not only delay the menstrual bleeding, but also the menstruation will be painful with a sharp, stabbing pain that is constant and fixed in its location. The menstrual blood will be dark and clotted, and the passing of clots will often ameliorate the pain. Dysmenorrhoea can also be a manifestation of Liver *qi* stagnation. In these cases, the pain will be more spasmodic and cramping in nature. The cycle can be irregular when there is Liver *qi* stagnation. This is due to *qi* and *xue* not flowing smoothly and rhythmically. The stagnation of *qi* in the Liver channel can result in the breasts being tender or swollen. Mood swings in the premenstrual period are another classic sign of Liver *qi* stagnation, especially if the woman is more irritable than normal. Liver *xue xu* can manifest with a woman being weepy and sensitive during this period. The stagnation of Liver *qi* in the premenstrual period can also disrupt the functioning of the Spleen and the Stomach. This means that there can be abdominal bloating, irregular or loose stools, oedema and an increased craving for sweets during the premenstrual phase. Stagnated Liver *qi* can become rebellious and 'invade' the organs in the middle *jiao*, disrupting their *qi* dynamic. If the Liver *qi* is stagnated or if the Stomach and/or Spleen *qi* is weak, the Liver can 'invade' these organs. This will lead to symptoms such as abdominal pain or bloating, alternating constipation and loose stools or belching. Liver Fire can invade the Lung, resulting in a cough with yellowish or bloody sputum, dyspnoea and chest oppression.

Bloating, distension and pressure are some of the main characteristics of Liver *qi* stagnation. When *qi* stagnates, it creates a greater tension or pressure in the area. This can give a sensation of being distended or bloated, and it is this sensation that is critical, not whether there is actual physical bloating. If the area is bloated or swollen, this will just be a confirmation that there is a stagnation of *qi* in the area. As well as disrupting the middle *jiao*, Liver *qi* stagnation can cause costal pain or chest oppression, where there will be a sensation of the chest being bound by a strong elastic or a metal rim. The stagnation of *qi* in the upper *jiao* can result in difficulty with breathing deeply.

The Liver is physically located just below the costal margin. The Liver and Gall Bladder channels traverse this area. This means that when Liver *qi* stagnates, there can be tension in the hypochondriac region. This is interesting because it is a defining sign of Liver *qi* stagnation in Chinese medicine textbooks, however not many Western patients report it. If, on the other hand, you ask Western patients whether they have tension in the diaphragm and the solar plexus, they will often say yes when there is Liver *qi* stagnation.

Liver *qi* stagnation will often, over time, generate Heat in the Liver. This can ultimately lead to Liver Fire, but in milder cases it will just result in the emergence of Heat signs such as thirst, a rapid pulse, red sides of the tongue, irritability and so on.

Heat conditions in the Liver can also manifest with redness of the eyes. This is because the eyes are the Liver's sense organ, and the Gall Bladder channel starts its course in the corner of the eyes and Liver *shi* conditions tend to manifest themselves in the Gall Bladder channel.

The eyes are nourished and moistened by Liver *xue* and Liver *yin*. If there is Liver *xue xu*, the lack of nourishment of the eyes can cause the person to have trouble focusing or there may be floaters or spots in the field of vision. If there is Liver *yin xu*, the eyes can be dry and feel gritty because they are not moistened by Liver *yin*. Ascending Liver *yang* or Liver Fire can increase the pressure inside the eye and this will cause pain inside or behind the eyes.

When there is Liver *qi* stagnation, the body will often try to disperse the stagnation by yawning or sighing. When the body inhales a large amount of air, as you do when you yawn or sigh, it will increase the strength of the *zong qi*. This will help to increase the force behind the *qi* in the channels and vessels and thereby spread the stagnant *qi*.

When Liver *qi* stagnates, it can lead to the accumulation of Phlegm in the throat. This will give the characteristic sensation of having a lump in the throat that cannot be swallowed. The sensation may not be constant but will typically be influenced by the person's emotions. The Chinese describe this sensation as feeling as if there is a plum stone stuck in the throat and call it 'plumstone *qi*'.

Headaches and dizziness can arise when there is too much *qi* ascending to the head, which is typical in Liver *shi* conditions, or when there is too little *xue* ascending to the head, which is a consequence of Liver *xue xu*.

The Liver channel passes around the genitals. If the Liver is invaded by exogenous Cold or if there is stagnation of *qi* in the Liver channel, the person can have pain or tension in or around the genitals. That is also why Liver *qi* stagnation can result in impotence in men. Damp-Heat in the Liver can also mean that there may be red, weeping sores on or around the genitals. Damp-Heat in the Liver can manifest with red and suppurating ulcers elsewhere along the Liver channel.

Liver *xue* nourishes the tendons. This means that the tendons, sinews and joints in general can become stiff when there is Liver *xue xu*. The nails are a type of tendon in Chinese medicine anatomy. A classic sign of Liver *xue xu* is fingernails that are soft or brittle or break easily. The fingernails are often ridged and can be very dry when there is Liver *xue xu*. The lack of nutrition from Liver *xue* may mean that the muscles in general lack strength and suppleness, whereas Liver *qi* stagnation will manifest with muscles that are stiff and tense. When there is Liver *xue xu*, there can also be a tingling sensation or numbness in the arms and legs. This is because the muscles and tendons lack nourishment. *Xue* returns to the Liver and leaves the muscles when they are inactive and at night. This means that some people who are Liver *xue xu* or *yin xu* experience unrest and cramping in their legs in the evening and at night.

When the Liver generates internal Wind, it will make the muscles extremely stiff and rigid or they will spasm and cramp. This can be seen when there are fever cramps in small children or a rigid neck muscle in meningitis, but it could also just be tics in the facial muscles.

Heat in the Liver, like Heat elsewhere in the body, can injure fluids and desiccate the body. When there is Liver *qi* stagnation Heat or Liver Fire, there can be tangible signs that the fluids are being consumed by Heat such as thirst, dark urine and dry stools. Furthermore, there will often be a bitter taste in the mouth when there is Liver Fire.

General symptoms and signs of Liver imbalances

- Menstrual disorders

- Mood swings

- Irritability

- Bloating or tension

- Hypochondriac tension

Shi patterns

Liver qi stagnation

Liver *qi* stagnation is rarely seen as a distinct pattern but usually occurs in conjunction with other patterns, where it is either the precipitating pattern or the consequence of another pattern of imbalance. Often the two patterns become mutually generating.

Liver *qi* stagnation is usually a consequence of the way we live. It is almost endemic in society. Everybody has some degree of Liver *qi* stagnation, but the important issue is how great a degree of stagnation there is and how it manifests. Modern society, with all the demands, stress factors and expectations that it presents us with or, perhaps correctly, that we place on ourselves, together with all the compromises and conformance that are necessary when coexisting with other people, will inevitably create varying degrees of Liver *qi* stagnation. Every time we are prevented from doing or being exactly what we want, our Liver *qi* will stagnate. Not being able to be or do exactly what you want is a consequence of social interaction. There is, though, a difference in how much a person accepts these limitations and how much they are frustrated by them. Unfortunately, the more Liver *qi* stagnation that there is, the more easily a person is frustrated and they thereby have more difficulty accepting limitations. This creates a vicious cycle.

The stagnation will be greatest in a person who is *shi* and *yang* in their energy. This means that Liver *qi* stagnation is more explicit in men. In men, Liver *qi* stagnation manifests as aggressiveness and irascibility. If the person is more *xu*, the Liver *qi* stagnation will not be expressed as much, but this can be more destructive and disruptive because it is not released as outbursts of anger, but is internalised, thereby disrupting the functioning of other organs.

Aetiology

The main cause of Liver *qi* stagnation is frustration, irritation, accumulated anger, pent-up emotions, stress and a person's boundaries not being respected. There can often be an underlying Liver *xue xu* in women when there is Liver *qi* stagnation, because the Liver is not lubricated and moistened by *xue* and therefore becomes stiff and inflexible. Stagnation of *qi*, *xue*, Phlegm or food can impede the free movement of *qi* in the body and thereby block the spreading function that Liver *qi* has.

Symptoms and signs

- Cold hands and feet, the buttocks and tip of the nose can also be cold

- Abdominal distension or tightness

- Chest oppression or difficulty breathing deeply

- Hypochondriac tension or tension in the solar plexus area

- Mood swings

- Depression

- Irritability

- Irregular menstrual cycle

- Menstrual pain

- Premenstrual syndrome (PMS)

- Breast tenderness in the premenstrual period

- Frequent yawning or sighing

- Sensation of having a lump in the throat

- Alternating constipation and loose stools

- Incomplete defecation

- Pebble-like stools that look like goat droppings

- Lack of movement in the facial muscles

- Stiffness and lack of movement in the body when the person is talking

- Hard or staccato voice

- The person may seem inflexible or rigid in their attitude

- The person can be difficult to engage when being interviewed

- Lack of energy or tiredness, especially in the morning and if they have been inactive

- Grumpiness in the mornings

- There are often no changes in the tongue when there is Liver *qi* stagnation but there may be slightly swollen edges on the sides of the tongue; if the stagnation of Liver *qi* has generated Heat, the sides of the tongue could be red or red speckled; the tongue can sometimes have a slightly mauve tinge

- Wiry pulse, especially in the left *guan* position

Key symptoms
Wiry pulse, mood swings, bloating, irritability, PMS, irregular or painful periods.

Treatment principle
Spread Liver *qi*.

Acupuncture points
Choose from: Liv 3, Liv 13, Liv 14, UB 18, GB 34, LI 4 and Pe 6.

Needle technique
Draining.

Explanation

- Liv 3, particularly in combination with LI 4 spreads Liver *qi*.

- Liv 13 spreads Liver *qi* in the middle *jiao*, especially when it invades the Spleen.

- Liv 14 spreads Liver *qi* in the middle and upper *jiao*, especially when it invades the Stomach or when *qi* stagnates in the upper *jiao*.

- GB 34 spreads Liver *qi*, especially when it affects the muscles and tendons.

- UB 18 spreads Liver *qi*.

- Pe 6 calms *shen* and spreads Liver *qi*, especially in the middle and upper *jiao*.

Herbal formula

- *Chai Hu Shu Gan Tang* (Spreads Liver *qi*)

- *Xiao Yao San* (Spreads Liver *qi*, nourishes Liver *xue* and tonifies the Spleen)

Relevant advice

When there is Liver *qi* stagnation, it is best, whenever possible, to address and work with any mental-emotional factors that can lead to the Liver *qi* stagnating. Stress should be avoided.

Physical activity is beneficial because it circulates *qi* and thereby spreads Liver *qi*. People whose Liver *qi* stagnates often train a lot or work out. This is a form of self-medication where they consciously or subconsciously try to relieve or prevent their symptoms. The danger is, though, that some people begin to train excessively and damage their *xue* and *yin* as a consequence. A person whose Liver *qi* stagnates should possibly be wary of playing competitive sports, because the competition aspect may aggravate their condition when they lose or when their teammates do not do what they think they should. Dancing, aerobics, running, swimming or cycling are good options, because they can dynamically activate and circulate *qi*. Gentler forms of movement such as tai ji, qi gong and yoga are also salutary because they help *qi* to flow, but these can be perceived as being too slow and boring for people when there is Liver *qi* stagnation. The resulting frustration and impatience can aggravate their Liver *qi* stagnation. More dynamic activities are therefore often a better idea, at least in the beginning. Dancing will be a particularly good way to physically activate Liver *qi*, because it is usually a pleasurable activity and will therefore simultaneously nourish the Heart. It is very important that the activities in which the person engages do not feel like things that have to be done, thereby becoming a source of frustration and further stagnating the person's Liver *qi*. Shouting or singing are good ways to spread Liver *qi*, especially because singing is pleasurable and thereby also nourishes Heart *qi*.

It can be a good idea to incorporate physical activity into the daily routine, for example by cycling or walking to work instead of driving, taking the stairs instead of the elevator or getting off the bus a stop earlier and walking the last part of the journey.

Breathing exercises that involve slowly inhaling deeply and then quickly exhaling with force whilst making a loud noise will help to release stagnant *qi*.

A person whose Liver *qi* stagnates should try to avoid eating too much at one time or eating rich food, especially concentrated proteins such as meat, dairy products, nuts and food that has a high oil content, because this will create further stagnation. Aromatic spices, herbs and foods that are slightly spicy will move *qi*, care must be taken if these also have a warm or hot energy because *qi* stagnations tend to create Heat. Unfortunately, people with Liver *qi* stagnation are often attracted to alcohol and spices, such as chilli, precisely because their spicy flavour spreads the stagnant *qi*. Unfortunately, this often results in the generation of Heat.

Going for a walk after eating will help to circulate *qi* in the body.

A teaspoon of vinegar or lemon juice and a teaspoon of honey in a glass of warm water will help to temporarily relieve Liver *qi* stagnation.

Liver *qi* stagnation can be caused by the following patterns of imbalance

- Liver *xue xu*
- Liver *yin xu*
- Stagnation conditions elsewhere in the body

Liver *qi* stagnation can result in the following patterns of imbalance

- Liver *qi* stagnation Heat
- Liver *qi* invading the Spleen
- Liver *qi* invading the Stomach
- Stagnation of *qi* in the upper *jiao*
- Heart *qi* stagnation
- Liver *xue* stagnation
- Liver Fire

Liver *qi* stagnation Heat
Liver *qi* stagnation Heat occurs when stagnant Liver *qi* starts to generate Heat in the Liver.

Aetiology
The aetiology here is the same as that of Liver *qi* stagnation. Drinking alcohol and eating spicy food, fried food and food that is warming in its energy can be contributing factors.

Symptoms and signs

The symptoms and signs are the same as those seen in Liver *qi* stagnation, with the difference that there will also be Heat signs, for example thirst, dark urine, a red face and restlessness. Several of the symptoms and signs described for Liver *qi* stagnation will be more pronounced. Where Liver *qi* stagnation can result in a person internalising their emotions, a person with Liver *qi* stagnation Heat will be more irascible and irritable and have a quick temper. The Heat will often also result in them being impatient. Their face may be red. The sides of the tongue will be red or there will be red speckles on the sides.

Key symptoms

These are the same as for Liver *qi* stagnation, plus red sides of the tongue, thirst, a quick temper and irritability.

Treatment principle

Spread Liver *qi* and drain Heat from the Liver.

Acupuncture points

Choose from: Liv 2, Liv 3, Liv 13, Liv 14, UB 18, GB 34, LI 4 and Pe 6.

Needle technique

Draining.

Explanation

- Liv 2 drains Heat from the Liver and spreads Liver *qi*.

- Liv 3, particularly in combination with LI 4, spreads Liver *qi* in general.

- Liv 13 spreads Liver *qi* in the middle *jiao*, especially when it invades the Spleen.

- Liv 14 spreads Liver *qi* the middle and upper *jiao*, especially when it invades the Stomach or when *qi* stagnates in the upper *jiao*.

- GB 34 spreads Liver *qi*, especially when it affects the muscles and tendons.

- UB 18 spreads Liver *qi* and clears Heat from the Liver.

- Pe 6 calms *shen* and spreads Liver *qi*, especially in the middle and upper *jiao*.

Herbal formula

- *Chai Hu Shu Gan Tang* (Spreads Liver *qi*)

- *Jia Wei Xiao Yao Wan* (Drains Liver Heat, spreads Liver *qi*, nourishes Liver *xue* and tonifies the Spleen)

Relevant advice
The advice that was given for Liver *qi* stagnation is applicable, as well as advising the client to avoid foods and beverages that have a warming energy, especially alcohol.

Liver *qi* stagnation Heat can be caused by the following pattern of imbalance

- Liver *qi* stagnation

Liver *qi* stagnation Heat can result in the following patterns of imbalance

- Liver *qi* invading the Spleen
- Liver *qi* invading the Stomach
- Liver *yin xu*
- Liver *xue* stagnation
- Liver Fire
- Heart *qi* stagnation
- Stagnation of *qi* in the upper *jiao*
- Phlegm

Liver *xue* stagnation

The Liver has a significant influence on the movement of *xue* in the body. This is because the Liver is responsible for the free flow of *qi* and thereby *xue* in the body and because the Liver is a reservoir where *xue* is stored.

Aetiology
Qi invigorates *xue* and the Liver ensures the free flow of *qi* in the body. This means that chronic Liver *qi* stagnation can develop into Liver *xue* stagnation. Liver *xue* stagnation will always be a more chronic and more serious condition than Liver *qi* stagnation. The aetiological factors that can lead to Liver *qi* stagnation will be relevant here. In addition, Cold and Heat conditions in the body can lead to the stagnation of *xue*, so aetiological factors that result in Heat and Cold can also be relevant.

Symptoms and signs

- Dysmenorrhoea, the pain is piercing or stabbing
- Dark, clotted menstrual blood
- Irregular menstrual bleeding
- Abdominal pain

- Lumps in the abdominal cavity

- Vomiting of blood

- Costal pain

- Hypochondriac pain

- Purple nails

- Purple lips

- Dark complexion

- Purple and swollen sub-lingual veins

- Purple tongue or purple sides on the tongue, possibly purple spots on the side of the tongue

- Wiry or Choppy pulse

Key symptoms
Swollen, purple, sub-lingual veins, dark and clotted menstrual blood, piercing or stabbing menstrual pain, Wiry or Choppy pulse.

Treatment principle
Spread Liver *qi* and invigorate *xue*.

Acupuncture points
Choose from: Liv 3, Sp 6, Sp 10, UB 17, UB 18, GB 34, Pe 6 and Sp 4.

Needle technique
Draining.

Explanation

- Liv 3 and GB 34 spread Liver *qi* and thereby invigorate Liver *xue*.

- Sp 6 spreads Liver *qi* and invigorates *xue*.

- Sp 10 and UB 17 invigorate *xue* throughout the body.

- UB 18 spreads Liver *qi* and invigorates Liver *xue*.

- Pe 6 and Sp 4 together open *chong mai*. *Chong mai* regulates the movement of *xue* in the small *luo* vessels. It is supplied with *xue* from the Liver, and it sends *xue* down to the Uterus (*bao*).

Herbal formula

- *Ge Xia Zhu Yu Wan* (Invigorates *xue* below the diaphragm)

- *Yan Hu Suo San* (Invigorates *qi* and *xue* in the Uterus)

Relevant advice

Physical activity is important when there is Liver *xue* stagnation. This is because the physical movement will activate *qi* and *xue* and promote their circulation. If the underlying pattern is Liver *qi* stagnation, the advice given for this pattern should be followed. If Cold or Heat are the root cause, the advice given for these patterns should be followed.

Liver *xue* stagnation can be caused by the following patterns of imbalance

- Liver *qi* stagnation

- Heat

- Cold

Liver *xue* stagnation can result in the following patterns of imbalance

- Phlegm

- *Qi* stagnation

Ascending Liver *yang*

Liver *qi* is very *yang* in its dynamic and therefore already has a tendency to ascend. If there is a deficiency of *yin* or an excess of *yang* in the Liver, its *qi* will rise upwards. *Yang qi* has an expansive nature. This means that symptoms of ascending Liver *yang* are often distending or throbbing in nature. The symptoms will typically occur suddenly and they will often be related to factors such as stress and emotional influences.

Wind is an aspect of Liver *yang* so there will be an overlap between Liver Wind symptoms and signs and those seen when there is ascending Liver *yang*. There is also a marked similarity between ascending Liver *yang* and Liver Fire, with many of the symptoms and signs being the same. The difference between these two patterns is the presence of Heat. The treatment of these two patterns with acupuncture is largely the same, but the herbal treatment will be different.

Aetiology

Ascending Liver *yang* is never seen alone, but it will always be combined with other Liver patterns of imbalance. It is correct to say that ascending Liver *yang* has its root in a Liver *yin xu* condition where the deficient Liver *yin* is unable to control and anchor Liver *yang*. It is important to keep in mind that Liver *xue* is an aspect of Liver *yin*. Therefore, the aetiological factors that are relevant for both Liver *yin xu* and Liver *xue xu* can have relevance here. Liver *yin xu* evolving from a purely *xu* pattern to a *xu/shi* pattern will require the presence of other factors that can cause Liver *yang* to ascend, such as the consumption of substances that are warming or ascending in their energy, for example alcohol and strong spices. Anger causes *qi* to rise upwards and can therefore be a relevant factor. Accumulation of stagnant *qi* in the Liver, as is the case in Liver *qi* stagnation, can force the Liver *yang* to rise. This means that aetiological factors such as frustration, irritation and repressed emotions can also have relevance here. Stress is frustrating and can cause *qi* to stagnate. At the same time, being stressed is something that consumes Kidney *yin* and thereby also Liver *yin*. A vicious cycle can soon develop. When Liver *yang* is excessive, it will consume and injure Liver *yin*. The more deficient Liver *yin* is, the less able it will be to control Liver *yang*, which then becomes excessive.

There is a big difference in how ascending Liver *yang* imbalances manifest themselves, which depends on how *xu* Liver *yin* is and how *shi* Liver *yang* is. For some clients, their Liver *yin* is just too weak to anchor the Liver *yang*. In others, Liver *yang* is so excessive that it will require a very robust Liver *yin* aspect to anchor it. There will usually be a clear dominance of ascending Liver *yang* in younger clients due to their *yin* still being relatively strong and their Liver *yang* becoming excessive due to their lifestyle and diet. Older people, on the other hand, tend to be more *yin xu*, so there will be a greater *xu* aspect in their ascending Liver *yang* condition.

The difference between how much *xu* and *shi* there is will influence the treatment strategy. The more Liver *yin xu* there is, the more focus there will be in the treatment on nourishing Liver *yin*. Conversely, if ascending Liver *yang* is the dominant aspect, there will be more focus on draining and controlling Liver *yang*.

Symptoms and signs

- Hemilateral headache that is throbbing in nature

- Pain behind the eyes, the pain will be throbbing or distending

- Dizziness

- Tinnitus and deafness

- Irritability, aggression, quick temper and anger

- Insomnia

- The voice can have a shouting quality or have a harsh tone

- The muscles can be hard or tense

- The eyes may appear fixed and staring

- The tongue may have swollen sides, red sides or red speckling along the sides

- Wiry pulse, especially in the left *guan* position

Key symptoms
Headache, irritability and a Wiry pulse.

Treatment principle
Descend and control ascendant Liver *yang*.

Acupuncture points
Choose from: Liv 3, SJ 5, LI 4, GB 20, GB 21, GB 38, GB 43, Du 20 and UB 18.

Needle technique
Draining.

Explanation

- Liv 3 descends Liver *yang* and nourishes Liver *yin*.

- LI 4 in combination with Liv 3 spreads Liver *qi* and thereby soothes the Liver.

- SJ 5 drains Liver *yang*, especially when symptoms are manifested in the *shaoyang* channels.

- GB 38 and GB 43 drain Liver *yang* from the head, especially when the symptoms manifest in the Gall Bladder channel.

- GB 20 drains Liver *yang* from the head and calms Liver Wind.

- GB 21 sends Liver *yang* downwards.

- Du 20 descends *yang* from the head.

- UB 18 calms the Liver.

Herbal formula

- *Tian Ma Gou Teng Yin* (Controls ascending Liver *yang* and Liver Wind)

Relevant advice
The advice given for Liver *yin xu* is also relevant here. It will be advisable for the person to avoid consuming substances that create Heat in the Liver or cause the Liver *yang* to rise. Alcohol will frequently have a negative impact, in particular red wine, as the sour taste will channel its effect directly to the Liver.

Anger causes *qi* to rise, so the person must try to avoid getting into situations where they can become angry. As described above, stress will also have a negative effect.

Exercise and dynamic activities will activate and spread Liver *qi*. This will reduce the 'pressure' in the Liver, which may have helped to force Liver *yang* upwards.

Ascending Liver *yang* can be caused by the following patterns of imbalance

- Liver *yin xu*

- Kidney *yin xu*

- Liver *qi* stagnation

- Liver *xue xu*

Ascending Liver *yang* can result in the following patterns of imbalance

- Liver *yin xu*

- Liver Fire

- Liver Wind

Liver Fire

Liver Fire and ascending Liver *yang* are very similar in their aetiology and pathology. The difference between them is that in Liver Fire there are signs of Heat and Liver *qi* stagnation or dietary reasons are more likely to be the root cause of the imbalance.

Aetiology

Prolonged emotional imbalances can lead to the stagnation of Liver *qi*. In time, the stagnant Liver *qi* will generate Fire in the Liver. Unfortunately, many people use alcohol as a way to loosen their stagnated Liver *qi*. The alcohol will quickly dissipate stagnant Liver *qi*, but it will also generate Heat in the Liver. Strong spices such as chilli have a similar effect. Consuming foods that have a hot energy can either directly generate Heat in the Liver or indirectly create Heat in the Liver by creating Fire in the Stomach or *xue* Heat that then transmits to the Liver and creates Heat there.

Symptoms and signs

- Thirst

- Bitter taste in the mouth

- Red face

- Red eyes

- Red ears

- Sensation of heat in the head

- Aversion to, or discomfort from, heat

- Constipation

- Dark urine

- Bleeding

- Quick body movements

- Hemilateral headache that is throbbing in nature

- Throbbing pain or distension behind the eyes

- Dizziness and vertigo

- Tinnitus and deafness

- Irritability, aggressiveness, a quick temper and anger

- Impatience

- Insomnia

- The voice can have a shouting quality or have a hard tone

- The eyes may be fixed and staring

- Red tongue with even redder sides and a yellowish dry coating

- Wiry and Rapid pulse

Key symptoms
Headache, irritability, red sides of the tongue, bitter taste and Wiry and Rapid pulse.

Treatment principle
Drain Liver Fire and calm the Liver.

Acupuncture points
Choose from: Liv 2, GB 20, GB 43, Du 14, UB 18 and Pe 7.

Needle technique
Draining.

Explanation

- Liv 2 and GB 43 drain Liver Fire.

- Du 14 drains the Fire and Heat.

- Pe 7 drains *jueyin* Heat.

- GB 20 drains *yang qi* from the head.

- UB 18 calms the Liver.

Herbal formula

- *Long Dan Xie Gan Tang* (Drains Liver Fire)

Relevant advice
The patient should avoid consuming substances that create Heat in the Liver. In particular, alcohol, hot spices, fried food and too much red meat should be avoided.

Stress and pent-up emotions, especially anger and frustration, create Heat in the Liver. When there is Liver Fire it is advisable to try to resolve these emotions.

Physical activity, such as sport, running, swimming or dancing will be beneficial, because it will disperse stagnant Liver *qi*, which is often involved in the creation of Liver Fire.

Liver Fire can be caused by the following patterns of imbalance

- Liver *yin xu*
- Kidney *yin xu*
- Liver *qi* stagnation
- Stomach Fire
- *Xue* Heat

Liver Fire can result in the following patterns of imbalance

- Liver *yin xu*
- Liver Wind
- Phlegm
- Heart Fire
- Stomach Fire
- Lung Heat
- *Xue* Heat

Liver Wind

Liver Wind can arise as a consequence of four different imbalances: extreme Heat in the whole body, for example when a fever creates *xue* Heat, which then creates Heat in the Liver; chronic ascendant Liver *yang*, which will often be the cause of Liver Wind in elderly patients; Liver *xue xu*, where Liver *xue*, which is an aspect of Liver *yin*, is not able to anchor Liver Wind, which is an aspect of Liver *yang*; Liver Fire, where the Fire burns so intensely that it generates Wind.

I will describe the symptoms and treatment of these four patterns separately.

Wind in the body is similar to climatic wind in several ways and it can be just as destructive. It can be as mild as a light breeze and cause only mild symptoms such as tics or a slight dizziness or it can be as wild as a hurricane and cause paralysis, spasms and a cerebrovascular accident, particularly when Wind is created by Heat. It can be very destructive and sometimes even fatal. One of the dangerous aspects of Wind is that it can stir up Phlegm, swirl the Phlegm up to the head and block the 'orifices'. This will cause the person to lose consciousness and the ability to talk and make the tongue stiff. Phlegm can also block the channels so the person becomes paralysed. Some of the disorders in Western medicine caused by internally generated Wind are meningitis, tetanus, febrile convulsions, epilepsy and a stroke.

Wind can create a gentle movement like a flag fluttering gently back and forth on a summer day, but it can also make the same flag stand rigid and stiff in the air, moving to neither one side nor the other, as in an autumn storm. In both cases it is characteristic that the movements are involuntary, and this is also the case in the body, with all involuntary movement of the muscles, twitches, cramps and spasms being due to Wind.

EXTREME HEAT GENERATING LIVER WIND

If there is extreme Heat in the body, such as when there is an invasion of exogenous *xie qi* for example, the *xie qi* can generate so much Heat that it affects the Liver, with the Heat in the Liver generating Wind. This is comparable to a forest fire: when there is a forest fire, the hot air will rise upwards, the vacuum this creates will draw in the air in from the surrounding area and this creates a strong wind that rushes upwards.

The symptoms of this imbalance will be acute and they will often be extreme. In Western medicine, diseases such as febrile seizures, tetanus and meningitis fall within this category.

Aetiology

Exposure to exogenous *xie qi* is the main cause of this pattern. If there is already Heat present in the body or the person is *yin xu*, this pattern will arise quickly. This is typical in babies, as they are relatively *yang*, with a warm constitution but their *yin* is weak. They therefore have a greater tendency to develop febrile seizures than adults when there are invasions of exogenous *xie qi*. This means that they are very vulnerable when there are epidemic diseases.

Symptoms and signs

- High fever

- Extreme thirst

- Red face

- The skin feels quite hot when palpated

- Dry, red lips

- Seizures

- Muscle spasms

- Extreme stiffness in the neck and back, the back can be stretched and bent like a bow

- Involuntary clenching of the hands and toes

- Shaking or involuntary movements of the limbs, such as in epilepsy

- The jaw may be locked

- In extreme cases, coma

- The eyes may be closed, staring or upwardly staring

- Extremely red tongue that is stiff and motionless, possibly veering to one side, there will be a dry and yellowish or black coating

- Rapid and Wiry pulse

Key symptoms
Tremors, spasms, high fever and a Rapid, Wiry pulse.

Treatment principle
Calm Liver Wind and drain Heat.

Acupuncture points
Choose from: Liv 2, Liv 3, *Shixuan* (Ex-UE 11), *jing*-well points, Du 8, Du 14, Du 16, Du 20, GB 20 and LI 11.

Needle technique
Draining. *Shixuan* (Ex-UE 11) and *jing*-well points should be bled.

Explanation

- Liv 2, Liv 3 and Du 8 calm the Liver and extinguish Liver Wind.

- *Shixuan* (Ex-UE 11) and *jing*-well points drain *xue* Heat and extinguish internally generated Wind.

- Du 14 drains the Fire and extinguishes internally generated Wind.

- Du 16, GB 20 and Du 20 extinguish internally generated Wind, especially when the symptoms affect the head.

- LI 11 drains Heat.

Herbal formula

- *Ling Jiao Gou Teng Yin* (Drains Heat from the Liver and extinguishes Wind)

Relevant advice
This is an acute condition that is caused by an invasion of exogenous *xie qi* that has penetrated to the *xue* level. Dietary and lifestyle advice are therefore of less relevance.

Extreme Heat generating Liver Wind can be caused by the following pattern of imbalance

- Invasion of exogenous *xie qi*

Extreme Heat generating Liver Wind can result in the following pattern of imbalance

- Phlegm-Wind

LIVER FIRE GENERATING LIVER WIND

The extreme Heat generated by Liver Fire can be so intense that it can generate Wind.

Aetiology

The aetiology is the same as for Liver Fire.

Symptoms and signs

- Dizziness

- Tremors

- Muscle spasms

- Hemilateral throbbing headache

- Red eyes

- Irritability

- Irascibility and anger

- Tinnitus

- Acute deafness

- Thirst

- Bitter taste

- Dark urine

- Constipation

- Bleeding

- Violent dreams and nightmares

- Restless sleep

- Fixed and staring eyes

- Shouting quality to the voice, loud voice
- Red tongue that is stiff and motionless, possibly veering to one side, the tongue will have a dry and yellowish coating
- Rapid, Wiry pulse

Key symptoms
Tremors and spasms, hemilateral throbbing headache, irritability, bitter taste, Rapid and Wiry pulse.

Treatment principle
Calm Liver Wind and drain Liver Fire.

Acupuncture points
Choose from: Liv 2, Liv 3, Du 8, Du 14, Du 16, Du 20, GB 20 and GB 43.

Needle technique
Draining.

Explanation
- Liv 2, Liv 3 and Du 8 calm the Liver, drain Heat from the Liver and extinguish Liver Wind.
- Du 14 drains Fire and extinguishes internally generated Wind.
- Du 16, GB 20 and Du 20 extinguish internally generated Wind, especially when the symptoms manifest in the head.
- GB 43 drains Liver Fire.

Herbal formula
- *Ling Jiao Gou Teng Yin* (Drains Heat from the Liver and extinguishes Wind)

Relevant advice
See Liver Fire.

Liver Fire generating Liver Wind can be caused by the following pattern of imbalance
- Liver Fire

Liver Fire generating Liver Wind can result in the following pattern of imbalance
- Phlegm-Wind

ASCENDING LIVER *YANG* GENERATING LIVER WIND

This pattern will always have its root in either Liver *yin xu* or Liver *xue xu*. There will be minor variations in some of the symptoms depending on whether it is Liver *yin xu* or Liver *xue xu* that is the underlying cause. Furthermore, there are differences between Liver *xue xu* leading to the pattern 'Ascending Liver *yang* generating Wind' and the next pattern 'Liver *xue xu* generating Wind'. The former is a combination of a *xu* and a *shi* pattern, whereas the latter is an exclusively *xu* pattern. This means that the symptoms will be milder and less extreme when it is a purely *xu* pattern.

Aetiology

The aetiology is the same as for the pattern Ascending Liver *yang*.

Symptoms and signs

- Dizziness

- Tremors

- Hemilateral throbbing headache

- Irritability

- Tics

- Tinnitus

- Dry eyes

- Dry skin

- Insomnia

- Poor memory

- Thin and dry tongue

If the condition is due to Liver *yin xu* or Liver and Kidney *yin xu*, there can also be:

- deafness

- dry mouth and throat

- malar flush

- night sweats

- feeling hot at night

- dark urine

- lumbar soreness or fatigue

- restlessness

- thin tongue that lacks coating, the tongue may be red
- Wiry or Fine pulse.

If the condition is due to Liver *xue xu*, there can also be:

- dry lips
- pale complexion
- difficulty focusing the eyes
- spots or floaters in the visual field
- scanty menstrual bleeding
- numbness in the arms and legs
- tingling sensation in the arms and legs
- weak, frayed or ridged fingernails
- pale and thin tongue
- Choppy, Fine or Wiry pulse.

Key symptoms
Dizziness, tremors, insomnia, dry eyes.

Treatment principle
Calm Liver Wind and nourish Liver *yin* and *xue*.

Acupuncture points
Choose from: Liv 3, Liv 8, Du 16, Du 20, GB 20, UB 18 and Sp 6.

- If there is Liver *yin xu*, add: Kid 3, Kid 6, Ren 4 and UB 23.
- If there is Liver *xue xu*, add: St 36, Ren 12 and UB 17.

Needle technique
Draining technique on Du 16, Du 20 and GB 20, even technique on Liv 3 and UB 18 and tonifying technique on the rest of the points.

Explanation

- Liv 3 and UB 18 nourish Liver *yin* and Liver *xue* and extinguish Liver Wind.
- Liv 8 and Sp 6 nourish Liver *yin* and Liver *xue*.
- Du 16, GB 20 and Du 20 extinguish internally generated Wind, especially when the symptoms affect the head.
- Kid 3, Kid 6, Ren 4 and UB 23 nourish Kidney *yin*. Kidney *yin* and Liver *yin* have a common root.

- St 36 and Ren 12 together with Sp 6 tonify the Spleen and thereby the production of *xue*.
- UB 17 nourishes *xue*.

Herbal formula

- *Zhen Gan Xi Feng Tang* (Calms Liver Wind and nourishes Kidney and Liver *yin*)
- *Da Ding Feng Zhu* (Nourishes Liver *xue* and extinguishes Wind)

Relevant advice

See Ascending Liver *yang*, as well as Liver *yin xu* and Liver *xue xu*.

Ascending Liver *yang* generating Liver Wind can be caused by the following pattern of imbalance

- Ascending Liver *yang*
- Liver *yin xu*
- Liver *xue xu*
- Liver *qi* stagnation

Ascending Liver *yang* generating Liver Wind can result in the following pattern of imbalance

- Phlegm-Wind

LIVER *XUE XU* GENERATING LIVER WIND

This condition will arise when Liver *xue*, which is an aspect of the Liver *yin*, is too weak to anchor Liver Wind, which is an aspect of Liver *yang*. When there is *xue xu* it is as if *xue* does not completely fill the vessels, so a vacuum in the vessels arises through which Wind can move. This is similar to the gusts of wind that blow thorough underground railway tunnels, where the vacuum created by the train in the tunnel draws in air that then rushes around the tunnels. Similarly, Wind can rush around the vessels and channels when there is a vacuum created by *xue xu*.

Aetiology

The aetiology is the same as for Liver *xue xu*.

Symptoms and signs

- Dizziness
- Tremors

- Muscle spasms

- Tics

- Tingling sensation or numbness in the limbs

- Difficulty focusing the vision

- Floaters or spots in the visual field

- Insomnia

- Poor memory

- Sparse or no menstrual bleeding

- Pale lips

- Dry lips

- Pale and sallow complexion

- Weak, hesitant voice that lacks resonance

- Pale, thin and dry tongue with pale sides

- Choppy or Fine pulse

Key symptoms
Dizziness, flickering in front of the eyes, shaking, pale sides of the tongue.

Treatment principle
Nourish Liver *xue* and calm Liver Wind.

Acupuncture points
Choose from: Liv 3, Liv 8, UB 17, UB 18, Sp 6, St 36, LI 4, Du 16, Du 20 and GB 20.

Needle technique
Tonifying except on LI 4, Du 16, GB 20 and Du 20, which are drained.

Explanation

- Liv 3 and UB 18 nourish Liver *xue* and extinguish internally generated Wind.

- Liv 8, UB 17, St 36 and Sp 6 nourish *xue*.

- Du 16, GB 20 and Du 20 extinguish internally generated Wind, especially when the symptoms affect the head.

- LI 4 calms *yang* and thereby internally generated Wind.

Herbal formula

- *E Jiao Ji Zi Huang Tang* (Nourishes Liver *xue* and extinguishes Wind)

Relevant advice
See Liver *xue xu*.

Liver *xue xu* generating Liver Wind can be caused by the following pattern of imbalance

- Liver *xue xu*

Liver *xue xu* generating Liver Wind can result in the following pattern of imbalance

- Phlegm-Wind

Damp-Heat in the Liver
When there is Damp-Heat in the Liver, there are signs and symptoms of a generalised Damp-Heat condition, as well as specific Liver symptoms and signs. It is important to note that Damp-Heat in the Liver can be a relatively serious condition. It is often seen when the liver in Western medicine physiology is not able to break down and excrete bilirubin as it should. Symptoms of Damp-Heat in the Liver can indicate that there has been a significant reduction in the liver function due to some form of liver failure.

Aetiology
Excessive consumption of food and medicine that are hot in their energy or produce Dampness.

Emotional imbalances that weaken the Spleen or stagnate Liver *qi* and thereby generate Heat in the Liver. This could be worries and speculation that bind and thereby weaken Spleen *qi* or unresolved emotions, frustration, repressed anger, irritation and so on that stagnate Liver *qi*.

Exogenous Dampness can invade the Liver channel in the legs and be transmitted via the channel to the Liver organ. There can also be direct invasions of exogenous Damp-Heat, especially in tropical climates.

The condition can also arise when there is latent heat from an unresolved pathogen in the Liver. This can lead to chronic conditions such as hepatitis in Western medicine.

Symptoms and signs

- Fever or aversion to heat

- Chest oppression

- Costal tension or pain

- Hypochondriac tension

- Sense of heaviness and fatigue in the body

- Yellow skin colour and yellowish sclera

- Red and suppurating skin diseases, rashes and sores

- Itching, burning or stinging skin, sores or rashes

- Genital sores or sores around the mouth

- Copious, odorous, yellow, sticky vaginal discharge

- Swollen or red and painful genitals

- Irregular menstrual bleeding, spotting

- Yellow, sticky sweat

- Bitter taste or sticky sensation in the mouth

- Dark and scanty urine, the urine may be odorous

- Burning urination

- Poor appetite

- Nausea

- Thirst with no desire to drink

- Red tongue with even redder sides, greasy, yellow tongue coating

- Rapid, Slippery and/or Wiry pulse, Wiry pulse in the left *guan* position

Key symptoms
Feelings of heaviness and fatigue, bitter or sticky taste, nausea, yellow skin and sclera, dark urine and yellow greasy tongue coating.

Treatment principle
Drain Damp-Heat from the Liver.

Acupuncture points
Choose from: Liv 2, Liv 5, Liv 8, Liv 14, UB 18, UB 22, GB 34, GB 41, SJ 5, Sp 6 and Du 9.

Needle technique
Draining.

Explanation

- Liv 2, Liv 14, GB 34 and UB 18 drain Damp-Heat from the Liver.

- Liv 5 and Liv 8 drain Damp-Heat from the lower *jiao*, especially the genitals.

- GB 41 and SJ 5 open *dai mai* and drain Damp-Heat.

- UB 22, Sp 6 and Du 9 drain Damp-Heat.

Herbal formula

- *Long Dan Xie Gan Tang* (Drains Damp-Heat from the Liver)

Relevant advice

When there is Damp-Heat in the Liver, the person should avoid consuming substances that create Heat or Dampness, especially if these substances have an affinity with the Liver. Alcohol, hot spices, fried food and too much red meat should be avoided. Foods such as dairy products, sugar, sweets, nuts, bananas and other Damp-producing foods should be also avoided. A Liver that is burdened by medication, alcohol poisoning and so on will have difficulty metabolising chemicals, therefore caution should be exercised in the consumption of all kinds of medicine, including dietary supplements and herbal remedies.

Stress and pent-up emotions, especially anger and frustration, create Heat in the Liver. It is therefore important to address these emotions when possible.

Physical activity, such as sport and fitness, tai ji, yoga or qi gong, will be beneficial because it will help to disperse stagnant Liver *qi*, which is often involved in the creation of Damp-Heat in the Liver.

Damp-Heat in the Liver can be caused by the following patterns of imbalance

- Spleen *qi xu*

- Damp-Heat

- Liver *qi* stagnation Heat

- Invasions of *xie qi*

Damp-Heat in the Liver can result in the following patterns of imbalance

- Liver Fire

- Phlegm

- Liver *xue* stagnation

Stagnation of Cold in the Liver channel

The *yin* channels in the legs are vulnerable to invasions of Dampness and Cold and this imbalance will often arise when the person has been wearing too little or wet clothing on the legs and feet. The condition will usually be acute.

Aetiology
Invasions by exogenous *xie qi.*

Symptoms and signs
- Distension, tightness or pain in the groin or around the bladder
- Pain or shrinkage of the genitalia
- Distension, tightness or pain in the area above the pubic bone in the hypochondriac region
- Pain that is ameliorated by heat
- Aversion to cold
- Cold hands and feet
- Headache at the vertex
- Nausea
- Explosive, watery vomiting
- Wet and white tongue coating
- Slow, Deep and Confined or Tight pulse, especially in the left *guan* and *chi* positions

Key symptoms
Pain above the pubic bone and around the genitals, aversion to cold, Wiry and Slow pulse.

Treatment principle
Expel Cold and course *qi* in the Liver channel.

Acupuncture points
Choose from: Ren 1, Ren 2 and Ren 3, Liv 1, Liv 3, Liv 5 and LI 4.

Needle technique
Draining. Moxa is recommended.

Explanation

- Ren 1, Ren 2 and Ren 3 drain Dampness from the lower *jiao* and resolve stagnations of *qi* in and around the genitals.

- Liv 1, Liv 3 and Liv 5 circulate *qi* in the Liver channel.

- LI 4 expels Cold.

Herbal formula

Tian Tai Wu Yao San (Regulates Liver *qi*, warms and expels Cold from the Liver channel, stops pain)

Relevant advice

If the stagnation of Cold in the Liver channel is a chronic or recurring pattern, the person must make sure that they wear adequate and appropriate clothing and footwear. They should avoid exposure to the cold and damp.

Stagnation of Cold in the Liver channel can be caused by the following patterns of imbalance

- Invasion of exogenous *xie qi*

- Liver *qi* stagnation

Stagnation of Cold in the Liver channel can result in the following patterns of imbalance

- *Qi* stagnation in the lower *jiao*

- *Xue* stagnation in the lower *jiao*

Xu patterns

Liver *xue xu*

The Liver has a very close relationship with *xue*. Liver *qi* helps to ensure that there is free movement of *xue* in the body and it is in the Liver that *xue* is stored. The Liver constantly ensures that the correct amount of *xue* is circulating in the body at any given time. During physical activity *xue* is sent out into the body and when the body is resting *xue* returns to the Liver. At night *xue* is mainly gathered in the Liver, where it helps to anchor the *hun*.

Xue, for its part, helps to nourish and moisten the Liver. Therefore it is essential that there is sufficient Liver *xue* to keep the Liver soft and flexible, otherwise Liver *qi* will have a tendency to stagnate.

Liver *xue* is an aspect of Liver *yin*, so there will be an overlap of symptoms and signs between these two patterns but there are also important differences.

Due to menstruation and childbirth, women have a greater tendency to be Liver *xue xu* than men.

Aetiology

The are three main causes of Liver *xue xu*: poor production of *xue*; insufficient consumption of food that nourishes *xue*; loss of *xue* through bleeding. Excessive physical training can also consume *xue* meaning that *xue xu* arises.

Blood loss during childbirth, heavy menstrual bleeding, bleeding disorders, operations, physical trauma and so on can lead to Liver *xue xu*. The condition can still be present a long time after the blood loss; in some cases this can be years later.

Excessive physical activity, especially in women who train hard, can lead to Liver *xue xu*. This does not only affect professional sportswomen or dancers, but can also affect women who train to run marathons, triathlons or Ironman events, because the excessive training consumes *xue*, which is used to nourish the muscles. This is why many women who play sport, dance and train at a high level stop menstruating.

Poor production of *xue* will be due to weakness of the organs involved in *xue* production. This will be due to aetiological factors that weaken the Spleen and Kidneys and will eventually lead to Liver *xue xu*.

Even if the Spleen and Kidneys are strong enough, Liver *xue xu* can still arise if the person's diet is deficient in foods that directly nourish *xue*.

Symptoms and signs

- Dizziness, especially when getting up from a seated or lying position
- Spots or floaters in the vision
- Difficulty focusing the vision
- Dry eyes or a sensation of grit in the eyes
- Eyes that water in the wind
- Sensitivity to bright light
- Poor night vision
- Insomnia
- Pale and sallow complexion
- Pale and dry lips
- Dry skin
- Ridged fingernails or weak and frayed fingernails
- Dry hair
- Hair loss

- Numbness or tingling in the limbs

- Weak muscles

- Leg cramps or restless legs, especially in the evening and at night

- Amenorrhoea or scanty menstrual bleeding

- Depression, sadness or lack of vision in life

- Tendency to be weepy and very sensitive during the premenstrual phase

- Indecisiveness

- The voice may lack resonance and be hesitant

- The voice may lack resonance even when they are angry

- Thin, pale and dry tongue, pale or orange sides of the tongue

- Fine or Choppy pulse

Key symptoms
Dizziness, floaters in the vision, scanty menstrual bleeding, ridged or weak fingernails and pale sides of the tongue.

Treatment principle
Nourish Liver *xue*.

Acupuncture points
Choose from: UB 17, UB 18, UB 20, UB 21, St 36, Sp 6, Liv 3, Liv 8 and Ren 4.

Needle technique
Tonifying. Moxa can be used and should be used on UB 17.

Explanation

- UB 17 nourishes *xue*.

- Liv 3, Liv 8, Sp 6 and UB 18 nourish Liver *xue*.

- Sp 6, St 36, UB 20 and UB 21 tonify Spleen *qi* and thereby the production of *xue*.

- Ren 4 tonifies *yuan qi* and thereby the production of *xue*.

Herbal formula

- *Bu Gan Tang* (Nourishes Liver *xue*)

Relevant advice

It is important that a person who is Liver *xue xu* eats a diet that nourishes *xue*. They will benefit from eating red meat, bone marrow and blood sausages. Eating organic liver[25] will be especially salutary, because it nourishes both *xue* and the Liver directly. Green-leafed vegetables will also be beneficial, because they have a high iron content and because their green colour has a resonance with the Liver. Other foods that nourish *xue* are beetroot, seaweed, dates, kidney beans, black beans, aduki beans, goji berries, angelica and nettle tea. A person who is Liver *xue xu* should avoid sugar, stimulants such as coffee and too much alcohol.

The patient should eat a diet that not only directly nourishes Liver *xue*, but also tonifies Spleen *qi*, i.e. warm, prepared food that is not cold in its energy and does not produce Dampness.

Lying down for 20 minutes in the middle of the day is recommended, as it enables *xue* to return to the Liver.

Excessive training should be discouraged.

Liver *xue xu* can be caused by the following patterns of imbalance

- *Xue xu*

- Spleen *qi xu*

- Spleen *yang xu*

- Kidney *yin xu*

Liver *xue xu* can result in the following patterns of imbalance

- Spleen *qi xu*

- Liver *qi* stagnation

- Heart *xue xu*

- Liver *yin xu*

- Ascending Liver *yang*

- Kidney *jing xu*

Liver *yin xu*

It is rare to see this pattern alone. It will usually be a consequence of, or result in, Kidney *yin xu*, so there will usually be a combined pattern of Liver and Kidney *yin xu*. Liver *yin xu* is also frequently an aspect of other Liver patterns such as ascending Liver *yang* and Liver Wind.

Liver *yin* encompasses Liver *xue*. This means that there will be similar symptoms and signs as those that are present in Liver *xue xu*, but there will also be specific *yin xu* signs. Liver *xue xu* is often a precursor of this pattern.

Aetiology

The aetiology will be the same as for Liver *xue xu*, especially since Liver *xue xu* can often be a precursor of Liver *yin xu*. Furthermore, factors that weaken Kidney *yin* and *yin* in general can be contributing factors. Chronic illness, stress, physical, emotional and mental overexertion, drugs, excessive sex, working at night, too little sleep, a diet that is hot or drying in its dynamics, too much coffee and other stimulants, congenital weakness and old age can all weaken *yin*. Kidney *yin xu* will often arise as a consequence of chronic imbalances in the body.

Chronic Liver Fire can injure Liver *yin*.

Symptoms and signs

- Dizziness
- Dry eyes
- Difficulty focusing the vision
- Matt, pale face with red cheeks
- Insomnia
- Dry skin
- Dry hair
- Dry or weak fingernails
- Cramps or restless legs in the evening and at night
- Tingling or numbness in the arms and legs
- Sparse menstrual bleeding or amenorrhoea
- The person may appear to be slightly restless
- Depression or lack of initiative
- The person may seem indecisive and cannot figure out what they want
- Thin, dry tongue without coating and possibly with cracks.
- Empty or Fine pulse

If Liver *yin xu* has led to *xu* Heat there can also be:

- night sweats
- feeling hot in the evening and at night
- a sensation of heat in the palms of the hands and soles of the feet
- malar flush

- anxiety

- thirst with a desire to sip water

- dry mouth and throat

- menorrhagia or metrorrhagia

- a red, thin tongue that lacks coating

- a Rapid and Fine or Empty pulse.

Key symptoms
Dry eyes, dry skin, lack of tongue coating and a Fine pulse.

Treatment principle
Nourish Liver *yin*.

Acupuncture points
Choose from: UB 18, UB 23, UB 52, Liv 3, Liv 8, Ren 4, Sp 6, Kid 3 and Kid 6.

Needle technique
Tonifying.

Explanation

- Liv 3, Liv 8, UB 18 and Sp 6 nourish Liver *yin*.

- UB 23, UB 52, Ren 4, Kid 3 and Kid 6 nourish Kidney *yin*, which is the root of Liver *yin*.

Herbal formula

- *Liu Wei Di Huang Tang* (Nourishes Kidney and Liver *yin*)

- *Zhi Bai Di Huang Tang* (Nourishes Kidney and Liver *yin* and clears *xu* Heat)

Relevant advice
It is essential that a person who is Liver *yin xu* gets enough rest and relaxation. This means that they must have ample sleep and go to bed early at night. They must not work too hard nor spend too much time watching television and staring at computer screens. They should avoid stimulants such as coffee, which would stress their system. Alcohol is not good for them because it is both spreading and warming in its energy and creates Heat in the Liver, which can injure Liver *yin*.

Dynamic activities such as aerobics or action sports will be detrimental and should be discouraged, because they will further consume *yin*. The person should instead cultivate gentler and more meditative forms of motion such as qi gong, yoga and tai ji. Massage and meditation are especially beneficial because they increase peace and tranquillity in the body and thereby benefit *yin*.

The client should try to avoid foods that are stimulating and warming. This includes coffee, alcohol, dark chocolate and hot spices like chilli. Generally, concentrated proteins, cereals and root vegetables nourish *yin*. Green, leafy vegetables will be especially good, because the green colour will resonate with the Liver and thereby directly tonify Liver *yin*.

Using a lot of water in the preparation of food, especially soups and stews, is preferable to baking things in the oven, which is more drying. Oil and products that have a high oil content, such as nuts and seeds, will nourish and moisten *yin*. Foods that specifically nourish Liver *yin* are: artichokes, beetroot, tomato, avocado, seaweed, dates, grapes, lemon, nettles, olive oil, lima beans, mung beans, kidney beans, pine nuts, sesame seeds, tahini, crab, oysters, beef, liver and rabbit.

Liver *yin xu* can be caused by the following patterns of imbalance

- Liver *xue xu*

- Kidney *yin xu*

- Liver Fire

Liver *yin xu* can result in the following patterns of imbalance

- Kidney *yin xu*

- Heart *yin xu*

- Ascending Liver *yang*

- Liver *qi* stagnation

Combined patterns

Liver *qi* invading the Spleen

When there is pronounced and chronic Liver *qi* stagnation, Liver *qi* can 'invade' the Stomach and the Spleen. In these situations the Liver *qi* will no longer support the Stomach and Spleen *qi ji* and instead will block it. This will often lead to symptoms such as rebellious *qi* in the Stomach. The Intestines and the abdomen can become bloated due to the stagnation of *qi*. Crucial to diagnosing Liver *qi* stagnation in these cases is whether the symptoms get worse or are triggered by emotional factors or stress and whether the symptoms are worse during the premenstrual phase rather than being triggered by the ingestion of certain foods.

This is a combined *xu/shi* pattern. Therefore, it is important to establish, both in this and in the subsequent pattern, whether Liver *qi* stagnation is the dominant aspect or the Spleen or Stomach are weak and have let themselves be invaded.

Aetiology

Some of the most common reasons that Liver *qi* stagnates are frustration, irritation, accumulated anger, pent-up emotions and stress. Women can often have an underlying condition of Liver *xue xu*, which means that the Liver is not moistened sufficiently and becomes stiff and inflexible. Food stagnation and Dampness can prevent the free movement of *qi* in the body and thereby block the Liver's function of spreading *qi*.

Another important aspect of this pattern will be factors that weaken the Spleen, such as the consumption of food and liquids that are cold or have a cooling energy and foods that are difficult to digest because they are too coarse or are raw. Eating irregularly and eating whilst working or when stressed can also often be contributing factors.

Symptoms and signs

- Abdominal bloating, especially if the bloating is affected by stress or emotional influences

- Hypochondriac tension or tightness in the solar plexus region

- Alternating constipation and loose stools – if Liver *qi* stagnation is the dominant aspect, there will be increased tendency to have constipation; conversely, if Spleen *qi xu* is dominant, there will be a tendency to have loose stools

- Flatulence

- Fatigue

- Craving for the sweet flavour

- Poor appetite in the mornings

- Nausea

- Cold hands and feet, the buttocks and tip of the nose may also be cold

- Irritability

- Mood swings

- Tendency to worry and think in circles

- The person may have a hard or staccato voice

- Pale, swollen tongue with teeth marks, the sides of the tongue may be red or red speckled

- Wiry pulse in the left *guan* position and Weak pulse in the right *guan* position, sometimes the pulse is also Wiry in the right *guan* position

Key symptoms
Abdominal bloating, alternating stools, Wiry pulse.

Treatment principle
Harmonise the Liver and Spleen by spreading Liver *qi* and tonifying Spleen *qi*.

Acupuncture points
Choose from: Sp 3, Sp 6, St 36, Ren 6, Ren 12, Liv 3, Liv 13, Liv 14, Pe 6, GB 34, UB 18 and UB 20.

Needle technique
Draining technique on Liv 3, Liv 14, UB 18, Pe 6 and GB 34. Tonifying technique on Sp 6, St 36, Ren 12 and UB 20. Even technique on Liv 13.

Explanation

- Sp 3, Sp 6, St 36, Ren 12 and UB 20 tonify Spleen *qi*.

- Liv 3, Liv 14, UB 18, Pe 6 and GB 34 spread stagnated Liver *qi* and soothe the Liver.

- Liv 13 regulates *qi* in the middle *jiao* and harmonises the Spleen and Liver.

- Ren 6 regulates *qi* in the middle *jiao*.

Herbal formula

- *Xiao Yao Wan* (Harmonises the Liver and Spleen)

Relevant advice
A person with Liver *qi* stagnation should, where possible, try and resolve any emotional causes of their Liver *qi* stagnation. They should avoid stress.

Physical activity is beneficial because it circulates Liver *qi*. People with Liver *qi* stagnation may train a lot, which can be a conscious or subconscious form of self-medication. There is a risk that people with Liver *qi* stagnation train excessively and end up weakening their *xue* and *yin*.

It is important that the activities in which the person engages do not become chores that they 'have to do', as this will further stagnate their Liver *qi*.

They should eat a diet that tonifies and does not weaken the Spleen. This entails eating warm, prepared food. They should avoid too much salad, raw vegetables and fruit. They should also avoid sweets, sugar, honey and artificial sweeteners. Dairy products create Dampness and thereby burden the Spleen, so they should be avoided. A person whose Liver *qi* stagnates should try to avoid eating too much at a time or eating rich food, especially concentrated proteins such as meat, dairy products, nuts and food that has a high oil content, because this will create further stagnation. Aromatic spices, herbs and foods that are slightly spicy will move *qi*, but they must be careful if these also have a warm or hot energy, because *qi* stagnations tend to create Heat. Unfortunately, people with Liver *qi* stagnation are often attracted to alcohol and spices such as chilli, precisely because their spicy flavour spreads the stagnant *qi*, but this often results in the generation of Heat.

It is not only what is eaten that is important, but also how the food is eaten. It is detrimental to eat when in a rush, whilst working or whilst discussing issues that can stagnate Liver *qi*. The person should preferably sit straight and upright whilst they eat and get some light movement, go for a walk or stretch after meals to support the Spleen's *qi* dynamic. Alternatively, they can lightly massage their abdomen to circulate *qi*.

Liver *qi* invading the Spleen can be caused by the following patterns of imbalance

- Liver *qi* stagnation
- Spleen *qi xu*
- Spleen *yang xu*
- Food stagnation

Liver *qi* invading the Spleen can result in the following patterns of imbalance

- Spleen *qi xu*
- *Xue xu*
- Damp
- Phlegm
- Food stagnation

Liver *qi* invading the Stomach

This pattern is very similar to the previous pattern in its pathological mechanisms and aetiology. There will also be an overlap between the two patterns and both patterns can be seen in the same patient.

Aetiology

The difference between this pattern and the previous one is that in this pattern the Stomach will be more influenced by foods that are hot and ascending in their energy and will be less affected by food that is physically cold or has a cooling energy. Food can stagnate in the Stomach if it is too difficult to transform, if too much is eaten at a time or if it is eaten too quickly or too late in the evening. This will create food stagnation and thereby Heat in the Stomach, which may cause the Stomach *qi* to become rebellious. Otherwise, the aetiology will be the same as in Liver *qi* invading the Spleen.

Symptoms and signs

- Abdominal bloating and abdominal pain that occur or are exacerbated by stress and emotional influences

- Hypochondriac tension or tightness in the solar plexus region

- Cold hands and feet, the buttocks and tip of the nose may also be cold

- Nausea

- Acid regurgitation or heartburn

- Vomiting

- Burping

- Hiccups

- Irritability

- Mood swings

- The person may have a hard or staccato voice

- Pale tongue with red sides or red speckled sides

- Wiry pulse in the left *guan* position and Weak pulse in the right *guan* position, sometimes the pulse is Wiry in the right *guan* position

Key symptoms
Abdominal bloating, cold hands and feet, belching and a Wiry pulse.

Treatment principle
Harmonise the Stomach and Liver by tonifying Stomach *qi* and spreading Liver *qi*.

Acupuncture points
Choose from: St 21, St 36, Ren 10, Ren 11, Ren 12, Ren 13, Liv 3, Liv 14, Pe 6, GB 34, UB 18 and UB 21.

Needle technique
Draining technique on Liv 3, Liv 14, Pe 6, GB 34, Ren 13, St 21 and UB 18. Tonifying technique on St 36, Ren 10, Ren 11, Ren 12 and UB 21.

Explanation

- Liv 3, UB 18 and GB 34 spread stagnant Liver *qi*.

- Pe 6 and Liv 14 spread Liver *qi* and regulate *qi* in the middle *jiao*.

- Ren 13 and St 21 regulate rebellious Stomach *qi*.

- St 36, Ren 10, Ren 11, Ren 12 and UB 21 tonify and regulate Stomach *qi*.

Herbal formula

- *Ban Xia Hou Po Tang* (Regulates Liver *qi* and Stomach *qi*)

Relevant advice
The advice that was given for the pattern Liver *qi* invading the Spleen is relevant here.

The person should also avoid food that has an ascending dynamic, for example chilli. They should also avoid eating food that creates food stagnation, eating too late at night, eating too quickly or eating too much at a time.

Stroking the fingers down the Ren channel from Ren 15 down to Ren 9 after a meal can help descend Stomach *qi*.

Liver *qi* invading the Stomach patterns can be caused by the following patterns of imbalance

- Stomach *qi xu*
- Liver *qi* stagnation
- Spleen *qi xu*
- Food stagnation
- Damp

Liver *qi* invading the Stomach patterns can result in the following patterns of imbalance

- Stomach Fire
- Stomach *yin xu*
- Spleen *qi xu*
- Food stagnation
- Damp
- Phlegm

Liver Fire invading the Lung

The Liver is anatomically immediately below the Lung. This means that if there is Liver Fire, the Fire can rise upwards and invade the Lung. This will create Heat in the Lung and interfere with the Lung's descending of *qi*. In this pattern there will be symptoms and signs of Liver Fire, as well as symptoms and signs indicating that the functioning of the Lung is disturbed.

Aetiology

Foods and beverages that have a hot energy can also create Liver Fire, including alcohol, fried foods, too much red meat, especially lamb, and spices such as chilli and pepper.

Chronic emotional imbalances can create Liver *qi* stagnation, which is often a root cause of Liver Fire. *Xue* Heat can also be an underlying cause, because the Liver is a reservoir for *xue* and the Heat from the *xue* can cause the Liver itself to become hot.

Symptoms and signs

- Shortness of breath or difficulty breathing

- Chest oppression

- Hypochondriac tension

- Cough with yellowish or bloody sputum

- Constipation

- Bitter taste in the mouth

- Throbbing headache

- Dizziness

- Red eyes

- Anger, irritability and anger

- Intense, slightly staring eyes

- Appears to be stiff or slightly distended in the chest region

- Sparse, dark urine

- Red face

- Quick body movements

- Burning urination

- Thirst

- Red tongue with even redder sides and red front. Dry yellowish tongue coating

- Rapid and Wiry pulse

Key symptoms

Cough with yellow sputum, dyspnoea, hypochondriac tension, headache, Rapid and Wiry pulse.

Treatment principle
Drain Liver Fire, regulate Lung *qi*.

Acupuncture points
Choose from: Liv 2, Liv 14, Ren 17, Ren 22, Lu 5, Lu 7, Pe 6 and LI 11.

Needle technique
Draining.

Explanation

- Liv 2 drains Liver Fire.

- Liv 14 and Pe 6 spread Liver *qi* and regulate *qi* in the chest.

- Ren 17 and Ren 22 regulate *qi* in the upper *jiao*.

- Lu 5 drains Heat from the Lung and regulates Lung *qi*.

- Lu 7 regulates Lung *qi*.

- LI 11 drains Heat.

Herbal formula

- *Long Dan Xie Gan Wan* (Drains Liver Fire)

Relevant advice
Because Liver Fire is the root cause of this imbalance, the person must avoid consuming substances that create Heat in the Liver. In particular, alcohol, hot spices, fried food and too much red meat should be avoided. Stress and pent-up emotions, especially anger and frustration, create Heat in the Liver. A person with Liver Fire should therefore try to resolve these issues or, if this is not possible, try and reach an acceptance of the situation. Physical exercise is recommended, because it will help spread and disperse stagnant Liver *qi*, which is often involved in the creation of Liver Fire.

Liver Fire invading the Lung can be caused by the following patterns of imbalance

- Liver Fire

- Liver *qi* stagnation Heat

Liver Fire invading the Lung can result in the following patterns of imbalance

- Lung Phlegm-Heat

- Phlegm-Heat

- Lung *yin xu*

- *Xue* stagnation

- Heart Fire

Liver and Heart *xue xu*

When there is Liver *xue xu*, it will often lead to Heart *xue xu*, because the Liver and Heart have a very close relationship to *xue*. The Liver stores *xue* and the Heart governs *xue*. Furthermore, the Liver *xue* anchors and nourishes the *hun*, whilst the Heart *xue* anchors and nourishes the *shen*. The *hun* is 'that which follows the *shen* in its entering and exiting'. Insomnia will be an important sign of Liver and Heart *xue xu*.

Aetiology

There are three main causes of Liver and Heart *xue xu*: poor production of *xue*; insufficient consumption of food that nourishes *xue*; the loss of *xue* through bleeding or the consumption of *xue* through excessive physical training and excessive mental activity.

Poor production of *xue* will be due to weakness of the organs involved in *xue* production. This is will be due to aetiological factors that weaken the Spleen and Kidneys and will eventually lead to Liver and Heart *xue xu*.

Even if the Spleen and Kidneys are strong enough, Liver and Heart *xue xu* can still arise if the person's diet is deficient in foods that directly nourish *xue*.

Blood loss during childbirth, heavy menstrual bleeding, bleeding disorders, operations, physical trauma and so on can lead to Liver and Heart *xue xu*. The condition can still be present a long time after the blood loss; in some cases this can be years later.

Excessive physical activity, especially in women who train hard, can lead to Liver *xue xu*. This does not only affect professional sportswomen or dancers, but can also affect women who train to run marathons, triathlons or Ironman events, because the excessive training consumes *xue*, which is used to nourish the muscles. This is why many women who play sport, dance and train at a high level stop menstruating.

Symptoms and signs

- Palpitations

- Dizziness, especially when getting up from a sitting or lying position

- Floaters in the eyes

- Difficulty in focusing the eyes

- Dry eyes or a feeling that there is grit in the eyes

- Sensitivity to bright light

- Poor night vision

- Poor memory

- Poor concentration

- Being easily startled

- Insomnia

- Dream-disturbed sleep

- Anxiety

- Nervousness

- Pale and sallow complexion

- Pale lips

- Dry skin

- Ridged fingernails or weak and frayed fingernails

- Dry hair

- Hair loss

- Numbness or tingling in the limbs

- Weak muscles

- Cramps or restless legs, especially in the evening and at night

- Scanty menstrual bleeding or amenorrhoea

- Depression, sadness or lack of vision in life

- A tendency to be weepy and extra sensitive during the premenstrual phase

- Indecisiveness

- Lack of charisma

- Excessively apologetic or self-deprecating

- The voice can lack resonance and have a hesitant quality

- Thin, pale and dry tongue, Pale or orange sides of the tongue

- Fine or Choppy pulse

Key symptoms
Palpitations, insomnia, dizziness, floaters, sallow complexion, scanty menstrual bleeding and pale sides of the tongue.

Treatment principle
Nourish Liver and Heart *xue*.

Acupuncture points
Choose from: UB 15, UB 17, UB 18, UB 20, UB 21, Ren 14, He 7, St 36, Sp 6, Liv 3, Liv 8 and Ren 4.

Needle technique
Tonifying. Moxa can be used and should be used on UB 17.

Explanation

- UB 17 nourishes *xue*.

- Liv 3, Liv 8, Sp 6 and UB 18 nourish Liver *xue*.

- He 7, Ren 14 and UB 15 nourish the Heart *xue*.

- Sp 6, St 36, UB 20 and UB 21 tonify Spleen *qi* and thereby the production of *xue*.

- Ren 4 tonifies *yuan qi* and thereby the production of *xue*.

Herbal formula

- *Gui Pi Tang* (Nourish Heart *xue* and Spleen *qi*)

Relevant advice
It is important that a person who is Liver and Heart *xue xu* eats a diet that nourishes *xue*. They will benefit from eating red meat, bone marrow and blood sausages. Eating organic liver[26] will be especially salutary because it nourishes both *xue* and the Liver directly. Green-leafed vegetables will also be beneficial, because they have a high iron content and because their green colour has a resonance with the Liver. Other foods that nourish *xue* are beetroot, seaweed, dates, kidney beans, black beans, aduki beans, goji berries, angelica and nettle tea. A person who is Liver and Heart *xue xu* should avoid stimulants such as coffee and alcohol.

As well as eating a diet that directly nourishes Liver *xue*, the patient should eat a diet that tonifies Spleen *qi*, i.e. warm, prepared food that is not cold in its energy and does not produce Dampness.

Lying down for 20 minutes in the middle of the day is recommended so *xue* can return to the Liver.

Meditation is recommended as it can tonify the Heart.

Excessive training should be discouraged.

Liver and Heart *xue xu* can be caused by the following patterns of imbalance

- Liver *xue xu*
- Heart *xue xu*
- Spleen *qi xu*

Liver and Heart *xue xu* can result in the following patterns of imbalance

- Liver *yin xu*
- Heart *yin xu*
- Kidney *yin xu*

Heart and Kidney *yin xu*

This is discussed in the section on Kidney patterns of imbalance (page 546).

DIAGNOSIS ACCORDING TO THE SIX STAGES, FOUR LEVELS AND *SAN JIAO*

The three diagnostic theories: diagnosis according to the Six Stages; diagnosis according to the Four Levels and diagnosis according to *san jiao* are three separate theories that explain how diseases arise and develop after the body has been invaded by exogenous *xie qi*. The three theories explain both the mechanisms of the disease, and at the same time they are used as a template to determine the level and location in the body where the *xie qi* is present.

The theories are used to analyse the relative strength of the *xie qi* (pathogenic *qi*) in relation to the body's *zheng qi* (anti–pathogenic *qi*), as well as giving an idea of the direction the disease is moving in, whether there is an improvement or deterioration in the condition. Disease is a dynamic process. It is something which is constantly changing and developing. This means that the treatment strategy must also be something that is being constantly adapted to the match the situation, taking into account the current situation and in which direction the disease is developing.

The three theories are not contradictory and are used in different situations, depending on amongst other things, the character of the *xie qi*. The theories can sometimes also be used alongside each other or consecutively, depending on how the situation develops. It requires flexibility in one's mindset and the ability to let go of Western medicine's either/or mentality.

Historical overview

Even though the three diagnostic approaches of 'The Six Stages, Four Levels and *san jiao*' all chart the development of imbalances resulting from the invasion of exogenous *xie qi*, the first approach is more than 1,500 years older than the other two theories. The oldest theory, which still has great relevance to this day, is the theory of the Six Stages. This theory was formulated by one of Chinese medicine's most important figures Zhang Zhong Jing in 220 CE in the classical text *Shang Han Lun* (Discussion on Cold-induced Diseases). This book is still one of the cornerstones of Chinese medical education in China. The herbal formulas from this book are still some of the most used prescriptions today. Zhang Zhong Jing analysed how the initial symptoms of an invasion manifest and how the symptoms develop depending on the relative strengths and relationship between the body's *zheng qi* and the *xie qi*. He described how disease can develop when exogenous *xie qi* penetrates via the energetic aspects of the body, that are defined by the six great channels and their corresponding organs. *Taiyang* being the most superficial and exterior aspect and *jueyin* the deepest. Zhang Zhong Jing explained the body's febrile reactions and the corresponding Heat signs, as the result of the struggle between *zheng qi* and *xie qi*.

What had been the catalyst in the development of Zhang's work was that within 10 years, two–thirds of the inhabitants of his village had died in epidemics, especially cholera. This made it both imperative to find cures, but it also provided a rich basis for observing how diseases evolved, how the symptoms changed from day to day and observing whether various treatment strategies worked in practice.

Even though the treatment approach set forth in the *Shang Han Lun* was very effective, there were however also holes in the theory and this became more and more apparent, especially around 14–1500 CE when China was plagued by several epidemics including the bubonic plague. Zhang Zhong Jing's theories assumed that the body had been exposed to climatic influences, especially Cold. His theories could not explain how people could infect each other just by their mere proximity to each other. It could also not satisfactorily explain how symptoms manifested with Heat from the very beginning.

Ye Tian Shi (1667–1746 CE) devoted his life to studying febrile diseases. His theories were published after his death in the classic text *Wen Re Lun* (The Classic of Heat Diseases). In this model, disease is differentiated in relation to four energetic levels, the deeper the level, the more severe the condition. It introduces for the first time the concept that exogenous *xie qi* can be transmitted from person to person and that exogenous *xie qi* can invade the body via the mucous membranes in the mouth, nose and genitals. The invading *xie qi* will be energetically hot from the beginning, which means that the symptoms manifest as Heat and rapidly injure the fluids in the body and injure *yin*.

The theories in *Wen Re Lun* were further developed in the book *Wen Bing Tiao Bian* (The Text on Differentiation and Treatment of Heat Disorders) written by Wu Ju Tong in 1798 CE. In this work, Heat disorders and their development are analysed in relation to a *san jiao* model instead of four energetic levels.

Diagnosis according to the Six Stages

In the theory of the Six Stages the body is divided into six energetic levels that can be affected by exogenous *xie qi*. The deeper the level that exogenous *xie qi* has penetrated to, the more serious the condition is. The relationship between the strength of the invading *xie qi* and the body's *zheng qi* will have an influence on how deep the *xie qi* penetrates.

The six energetic stages are:

- *taiyang* – Urinary Bladder and Small Intestine

- *shaoyang* – Gall Bladder and *san jiao*

- *yangming* – Stomach and Large Intestine

- *taiyin* – Lung and Spleen

- *shaoyin* – Kidney and Heart

- *jueyin* – Liver and Pericardium.

Taiyang is the most superficial aspect and *jueyin* is the deepest. Exogenous *xie qi* can penetrate deeper into the body in the following ways:

- by continuing sequentially through the various stages

- by skipping over one or more stages

- by penetrating from the channel down to its internal organ or its partner's channel organ.

There may be overlapping patterns where there are symptoms and signs of two stages simultaneously.

If is there already a *xu* condition in an organ or an aspect, *xie qi* will more easily penetrate to this level. For example, if there is Kidney *yang xu* and the person is invaded by Wind-Cold in the *taiyang* aspect, the Cold can penetrate directly to the *shaoyin* aspect due to the *yin yang* relationship between the Urinary Bladder (*taiyang*) and the Kidneys (*shaoyin*).

In the Six Stages model, it is Cold that has invaded the body and created imbalances. Heat can, though, arise when Cold penetrates deeper into the body.

When there are apparent Heat symptoms and signs without any preceding Cold signs, this is explained as being being a consequence of 'latent Heat'. Latent Heat can arise when Cold invades the body in the winter. The Cold will be inactive and can later transform and turn into Heat. In spring *yang* will begin to rise upwards and outwards. This movement of *yang* will result in the latent Heat being driven upwards and outwards to the exterior, where it will activate the body's defence mechanisms. There will therefore be signs of Heat without the person having been exposed to *xie qi*. Signs and symptoms of Heat can also quickly manifest in an invasion of Wind-Cold if there is Heat already present in the body.

Diagnosis in relation to the Six Stages analyses the relative strengths of *zheng qi* and *xie qi*, whether the disease is advancing or retreating. Distinction is made between Heat and Cold, *xu* and *shi*, and whether *xie qi* is located in the interior and the exterior. This determines the treatment, for example whether *xie qi* should be drained or expelled, or whether *zheng qi* should be tonified.

The Six Stages diagnosis differentiates the following:

- **Where the disease is**: Whether the disease is in the interior or the exterior and if it is only on the channel level or the *zangfu* organs are affected. In relation to an Eight Principles diagnosis, the *taiyang* stage is an exterior imbalance; *shaoyang* stage is half interior, half exterior; and the rest are interior imbalances.

- **What the nature of the disease is**: Whether the disorder is *xu* or *shi*, Hot or Cold. When *zheng qi* is strong, there will be a *shi* condition. In general, it is a *shi* condition when the disorder is in the *taiyang* and *yangming* stages and a *xu* condition when the disorder is in one of the three *yin* stages. *Shaoyang* stage is often a combined *xu/shi* condition. *Taiyang* stage is usually characterised as being Cold. When *xie qi* is in the *yangming* aspect, there is Heat; *shaoyang* can be either a Hot condition or a combination of Heat and Cold. The *yin* stages can be either Hot or Cold, depending on whether it is *yin* or *yang* that is injured.

- **How the disease is developing**: Disease development is a dynamic process that is in a process of constant change, especially in the initial stages. The theory of the Six Stages can be used to determine if the disease is improving or deteriorating. It does this by assessing the relative strength of *zheng qi* and *xie qi* and in which direction the disease is moving. If it is penetrating downwards from one of the exterior aspects, this is a negative sign. Conversely, if the symptoms change and the pattern changes from one of the deeper stages to one of the more exterior stages, it is a positive sign.

- **The treatment principle**: The Six Stage diagnosis determines the nature of a disorder. This then dictates the way in which the disorder should be treated. For example, if *xie qi* has invaded the *taiyang* aspect, this is a *shi* condition and the treatment principle will be to 'open to the exterior and expel *xie qi*' using a draining needle technique on points that expel Wind-Cold. Conversely, if there is a *yang xu* condition in the *taiyin* aspect, Spleen *yang* should be 'tonified and warmed' using a tonifying needle technique and preferably moxa on points that tonify Spleen *qi* and *yang*.

In the three *yang* stages, it is the *yang* organs and channels that are affected. The symptoms and signs generally reflect that is a *shi* condition. The three *yin* stages are more *xu* in nature because in the preliminary stages *zheng qi* is relatively strong, and this will result in more powerful symptoms due to the struggle between a strong *zheng qi* and the *xie qi*. When *xie qi* penetrates to the *yin* stages, *zheng qi* will have become weakened and is no longer able to withstand the *xie qi*.

It is important to keep in mind that even though the interior *xu* patterns in the Six Stages are ostensibly the same as *zangfu* patterns of diagnosis, such as Spleen *yang xu* for example, the disorder in the Six Stages has primarily arisen due to an invasion of exogenous *xie qi* and not necessarily due to diet and lifestyle. They may well be involved, but they are not the primary reasons for the imbalance.

Taiyang stage

This is the most superficial aspect of the Six Stages and the invasion at this stage is relatively superficial. There are four main patterns that can be differentiated at this stage. Two of them are channel-level imbalances and are therefore pure exterior imbalances, but there are also two *fu* organ imbalances, where the exogenous *xie qi* has penetrated into the interior. In one of these imbalances there will still be clear signs that the *xie qi* is present in the exterior aspect.

The two channel-level imbalances are the *taiyang* patterns most often seen in the clinic and in everyday life. Zhang Zhong Jing distinguished between an invasion of Wind-Cold in the *taiyang* aspect where Cold is the dominant *xie qi* and an invasion of Wind-Cold where Wind is dominant. The difference between the two situations is essentially that in the first scenario it is a pure *shi* condition, whereas when Wind is dominant there is a *xu/shi* condition.

The key symptoms that characterise the *taiyang* stage are a Superficial pulse, headache and stiffness in the neck and shoulders and an aversion to wind and cold.

The *taiyang* channels helps to govern and control *wei qi*. *Wei qi*, as well as protecting the body against exogenous *xie qi*, warms the skin and controls the sweat pores. This has significant implications for how many of the symptoms manifest themselves.

In the *taiyang* stage, exogenous *xie qi* has invaded the body by penetrating the *wei qi*. It is usually Wind and Cold that have invaded the body. Cold by itself can have difficultly penetrating through the *wei qi*. This is because the Cold has a *yin*, contracting dynamic and this will cause the pores in the skin to close. Wind, though, has a *yang* and a very scattering dynamic. Wind can therefore scatter *wei qi* and open the pores. Wind is therefore termed the spearhead that leads other forms of *xie qi* into the body.

Exogenous *xie qi* can succeed in overcoming and breaking through the body's *wei qi* in three ways.

- If *wei qi* is very powerful it will not require long-term exposure to the *xie qi* before it can invade the body. This could, for example, be when a person has fallen through the ice and has been strongly chilled by the cold water. Although it is only a short-term exposure to the cold, the cold is so powerful that it is able to pierce through the *wei qi*, even in a person whose *wei qi* is strong and powerful.

- Exogenous *xie qi* can also penetrate the *wei qi* if there is a prolonged exposure to the *xie qi*. In this case the *xie qi* does not need to be as intense as in the first case, but because there is a continued and persistent influence, the *xie qi* will over time break through. An example of this could be a person who has cycled home in the rain and sleet and been thoroughly drenched and cooled down. If they cycled two kilometres and then changed into dry clothes afterwards they would not become ill. If, on the other hand, they cycled 15 kilometres and did not have the opportunity to change into dry clothes afterwards, they may well catch a cold.

- The final scenario where *xie qi* can invade the *taiyang* stage is when *wei qi* is deficient. This will typically be a person who is *qi xu*. This could be an elderly person, a very small child, a person who has just been ill or a person who is physically run down. In these situations, the *xie qi* does not need to be very strong for it to be able to overcome the *wei qi*. The *wei qi* is simply too weak to protect the body. If a person with a strong *wei qi* goes for a walk for 15 minutes without a jacket on in the winter, their *wei qi* is strong enough to withstand the cold. But if a person who is very *qi xu* did the same, they may well catch a cold or fall ill. This is why elderly people have to wear more clothes than young people and are generally more sensitive to draughts and open windows.

Even if a person has strong *wei qi*, *xie qi* can easily invade the body if the person sweats whilst they are exposed to wind and cold. This is because the pores will be open, which allows exogenous *xie qi* to enter. That is why it is very important that people cover themselves with warm clothes after they have, for example, been running or done other forms of physical activity that have caused them to sweat. It is also the reason people catch colds when there is air-conditioning.

The *taiyang* stage can be differentiated into two channel patterns, one that is *shi* and one that is *xu*. In addition, there are two *fu* patterns.

Invasion of Wind-Cold in the *taiyang* aspect – Cold is dominant

In this pattern, *xie qi* has been so virulent that it has been strong enough to penetrate the body's *wei qi*. *Zheng qi* is relatively strong. This means that the symptoms and signs will be more pronounced than in the pattern 'Invasion of Wind-Cold in the *taiyang* aspect – Wind is dominant'.

The symptoms are characterised by *xie qi* inhibiting the spreading and circulation of *wei qi*. It means that there is a very pronounced aversion to cold. This is because *xie qi* is blocking the circulation of *wei qi* so that it cannot warm the skin. This aversion to cold is different to that which is experienced when there is *yang xu*. When there is *yang xu* the person is not capable of generating warmth in the body. This means that if a person who is *yang xu* wraps themselves up in warm clothes and blankets, they can get warm and maintain their sensation of warmth. When Cold has invaded the body, the person is capable of generating warmth, but *wei qi* is simply not able to circulate the heat out to the skin and the muscles. This means that even if the person wraps themselves up in warm clothes and packs themselves under quilts, they still do not feel warm.

The stagnation of Cold will also prevent the pores in the skin from opening, due to the contracting nature of Cold. At the same time, Cold will block *wei qi*, which opens and closes the pores. This means that a defining sign in this pattern is the inability to sweat. A priority in the treatment principle is therefore to 'open to the exterior', which in this context means to induce a sweat, thereby expelling the invasion of exogenous *xie qi*.

The headache, joint pain and stiffness of the shoulders and the neck is due to *xie qi* blocking the circulation of *qi* in the *taiyang* channels. The stagnation of *qi* causes pain and discomfort: '*Bu tong ze tong, tong ze bu tong*' ('Where there is no flow, there is pain. Where there is free flow, there is no pain'). The headache will feel tight in character.

Wei qi is an aspect of the Lung and it is the Lung that spreads *wei qi* throughout the body. When *xie qi* blocks *wei qi*, it will also disrupt the functioning of the Lung. This can be observed when there are signs that the Lung's descending and spreading function of *qi* is disturbed and there is coughing and sneezing. This disruption of the Lung's functioning can also be seen when fluids are not spread as they should be. There will initially be a slight oedema of the face, especially a puffiness around the eyes. This is in fact one of the reasons that people can immediately see that someone has a cold or is 'under the weather'. The fluids will accumulate in the Lung or they will rise upwards along with the rebellious Lung *qi* to the nose, resulting in a runny nose with clear watery mucus or with eyes watering.

There may be a slight fever that is the result of the struggle between *zheng qi* and *xie qi*.

The pulse will be Superficial. This is because the struggle is taking place in the exterior aspect of the body. The pulse will have a tight quality due to Cold blocking the flow of *qi*.

Aetiology
Exposure to wind and cold.

Symptoms and signs

- Acute headaches that are tight, the headache will be located in the neck and along the Urinary Bladder channel

- Stiffness of the neck, shoulders and upper back

- Skin and muscle aches

- Aching joints

- Aversion to cold and difficulty keeping warm

- Aversion to cold, wind and draughts

- Lack of sweating (this is a key symptom when differentiating between a *xu* and *shi* condition)

- Runny nose and watering eyes

- Facial oedema or puffiness around the eyes

- Possible low-grade fever

- Thin, white and wet tongue coating

- Superficial and Tight pulse

Key symptoms
Aversion to cold, headache and stiffness in the shoulder and neck, lack of sweating, aching muscles and joints, Superficial and Tight pulse.

Treatment principle
Expel Wind-Cold, activate *wei qi*.

Acupuncture points
Choose from: SI 3, UB 10, UB 12, UB 62, LI 4, Lu 7, Du 14 and GB 20.

Needle technique
Draining. Cupping and moxa is recommended.

Explanation

- SI 3 and UB 62 open the *taiyang* channel, activate *wei qi* and expel Wind and Cold.

- UB 10 and GB 20 expel Wind and Cold.

- LI 4, Lu 7 and UB 12 activate *wei qi*, expel Wind and Cold and regulate Lung *qi*.

- Du 14 activates *wei qi*.

Herbal formula

- *Ma Huang Tang* (Expels Wind-Cold)

- *Ge Gen Tang* (Expels Wind-Cold)

Relevant advice
When a person has been invaded by Wind-Cold in the *taiyang* channels, they should avoid eating rich food and should preferably only eat soup. They will benefit from drinking hot, spicy drinks such as a whisky toddy, hot ginger tea or an infusion of garlic, cayenne pepper and ginger. They should then wrap themselves up in blankets or quilts to induce a sweat.

Invasion of Wind-Cold in the *taiyang* aspect – Cold is dominant can be caused by the following pattern of imbalance

- No previous pattern

Invasion of Wind-Cold in *taiyang* – Cold is dominant can result in the following patterns of imbalance

- *Taiyang fu* pattern

- *Yangming* stage pattern

- *Shaoyang* stage pattern

- *Taiyin* stage pattern
- *Shaoyin* stage pattern

Invasion of Wind-Cold in the *taiyang* aspect – Wind is dominant

In this pattern there is *wei qi xu*. This means that *xie qi* does not need to be so potent to be able to invade the body, and the symptoms and signs will not be as pronounced as in the previous *taiyang shi* pattern. Because the person is *wei qi xu*, they will often have a strong aversion to sitting in a draught and being exposed to the wind.

A key symptom that can differentiate this from the previous pattern is that in this pattern the person will sweat spontaneously, but the sweating will not relieve the condition. The person sweats spontaneously because the deficient *wei qi* is not able to control the pores and is not strong enough to expel the *xie qi*.

The pulse will be weaker in this pattern and it will not be Tight, because the deficiency of *qi* means that there is less stagnation. The mechanisms behind the other symptoms and signs are the same as in the previous pattern.

Aetiology
Exposure to wind and cold.

Symptoms and signs

- Acute headache
- Stiffness in the neck, shoulders and upper back
- Aversion to cold and especially wind and draughts
- Spontaneous sweating, but without it relieving the symptoms
- Sneezing and coughing
- Runny nose and watery eyes
- Facial oedema or puffiness around the eyes
- Possible low-grade fever
- Aching in the muscles and joints
- Thin, white and wet tongue coating
- Superficial and Slow pulse

Key symptoms
Aversion to wind, spontaneous sweating, Superficial pulse.

Treatment principle
Expel Wind-Cold, activate *wei qi*, tonify *wei qi*.

Acupuncture points
Choose from: SI 3, UB 10, UB 12, UB 62, LI 4, Lu 7, Lu 9, St 36, Sp 6, Ren 12 Du 14 and GB 20.

Needle technique
Tonifying technique on Lu 9, St 36, Sp 6 and Ren 12, draining technique on the rest of the points. Moxa is recommended.

Explanation
- St 36, Sp 6, Ren 12 and Lu 9 tonify post-heaven *qi* and thereby *wei qi*.
- SI 3 and UB 62 open the *taiyang* channel, activate *wei qi* and expel Wind-Cold.
- UB 10 and GB 20 expel Wind-Cold.
- LI 4, Lu 7 and UB 12 activate *wei qi*, expel Wind-Cold and regulate Lung *qi*.
- Du 14 activates *wei qi*.

Herbal formula
- *Gui Zhi Tang* (Expels Wind-Cold, harmonises *ying* and *wei*)

Relevant advice
When a person has been invaded by Wind-Cold in the *taiyang* channels, they should avoid eating rich food and should preferably only eat soup. They will benefit from drinking hot, spicy drinks such as a whisky toddy, hot ginger tea or an infusion of garlic, cayenne pepper, ginger and honey. They should then wrap themselves up in blankets or quilts to induce a sweat. They should avoid exposure to draughts and they should make sure that they are suitably clothed when they are outdoors. They should preferably rest and stay indoors until they are healthy again.

An invasion of Wind-Cold in the *taiyang* aspect – Wind is dominant can be caused by the following patterns of imbalance
- *Qi xu*

An invasion of Wind-Cold in the *taiyang* aspect – Wind is dominant can result in the following patterns of imbalance
- *Taiyang fu* pattern
- *Yangming* stage pattern
- *Shaoyang* stage pattern
- *Taiyin* stage pattern
- *Shaoyin* stage pattern

Taiyang Cold syndrome	*Taiyang* Wind syndrome
No sweating	Sweating that does not alleviate the symptoms
Extreme aversion to cold	Less aversion to cold, extreme aversion to wind and draughts
Severe headache and stiff neck	Milder headache and stiff neck
Tight pulse	The pulse is not Tight

Taiyang fu – accumulation of Water

This is one of the two organ patterns that Zhang Zhong Jing differentiated in the *taiyang* stage. *Xie qi* can sometimes transmit directly from the channel level to the *fu* organ. There will, though, still be signs that there is an invasion of the exterior aspect of the body.

Wei qi, which circulates in the exterior aspect of the body, is disrupted, meaning that the person will have an aversion to cold and the pulse will be Superficial.

The Urinary Bladder, and to some extent the Small Intestine, will have been disturbed by the presence of exogenous *xie qi*. This can be seen in the fact that their functions are disrupted. There can be a retention of urine, painful urination, acute oedema and watery vomiting after consumption of fluids, because the exogenous Cold blocks the transformation and transport of fluids in the body.

Cold can transform into Heat. This can result in signs such as fever, thirst and a Rapid pulse.

Aetiology
Invasion of Wind and Cold.

Symptoms and signs

- Acute oedema

- Aversion to cold

- Slight fever

- Slight thirst

- Watery vomiting after consuming fluids

- Painful urination

- Retention of urine

- Irritability

- Superficial and Rapid pulse

Key symptoms
Acute oedema, retention of urine, aversion to cold, Superficial pulse.

Treatment principle
Expel Wind-Cold, regulate the Urinary Bladder, drain fluids.

Acupuncture points
Choose from: Ren 3, Ren 9, Lu 7, Sp 9, UB 22 and UB 39.

Needle technique
Draining.

Explanation

- Ren 3, Ren 9, Sp 9, UB 22 and UB 39 regulate the water passages and drain fluids.

- Lu 7 regulates the water passages and expels Wind-Cold.

Herbal formula

- *Wu Ling San* (Promotes sweating, warms *yang* and drains water)

Relevant advice
When there is an invasion of Wind-Cold affecting the *taiyang fu*, the person should drink hot, spicy drinks such as a whisky toddy, hot ginger tea or an infusion of garlic, cayenne pepper, ginger and honey. They should then wrap themselves up in blankets or quilts to induce a sweat. They should avoid eating heavy meals.

Taiyang fu – accumulation of water can be caused by the following pattern of imbalance

- *Taiyang* channel invasion patterns

Taiyang fu – accumulation of water can result in the following pattern of imbalance

- *Taiyang fu* – accumulation of *xue*

Taiyang fu – accumulation of *xue*

This is the second of the two organ patterns that were differentiated by Zhang Zhong Jing in the *taiyang* stage. The combination of Heat and the stagnation resulting from the presence of exogenous *xie qi* can result in *xue* stagnating in the lower *jiao* and specifically in the Urinary Bladder. This is a deeper level than the previous pattern. The previous pattern will correspond to a *qi*-level pattern in diagnosis according to the Four Levels, whereas this pattern will correspond to a *xue*-level pattern.

Xue stagnation will manifest with pain and discomfort in the area above the pubic bone. There will be difficult and painful urination. Heat can result in urgent urination. Both *xue* stagnation and Heat can result in blood in the urine.

Heat can also ascend to the Heart, making the person restless and irritable.

The presence of Heat and *xue* stagnation will also be evident in the person's tongue and pulse.

Aetiology
Invasion of Wind and Cold.

Symptoms and signs

- Painful, urgent and difficult urination

- Blood in the urine

- Pain and discomfort in the area above the pubic bone

- Mental restlessness

- Purple-red tongue that lacks coating

- Rapid and Choppy pulse

Key symptoms
Painful, urgent and difficult urination with blood in the urine, purple tongue.

Treatment principle
Spread *qi* and *xue* in the Urinary Bladder, drain Heat from the Urinary Bladder.

Acupuncture points
Choose from: Ren 3, Ren 9, Liv 3, Sp 6, Sp 10, UB 17, UB 22 and UB 39.

Needle technique
Draining.

Explanation

- Ren 3 and Sp 6 move *xue* and drain Dampness from the Urinary Bladder.

- Ren 9, UB 22 and UB 39 regulate the water passages and drain fluids.

- Sp 10 and UB 17 move *xue*.

- Liv 3 regulates *qi* in the Urinary Bladder.

Herbal formula

- *Tao He Cheng Qi Tang* (Breaks up *xue* stasis and eliminates Heat)

Relevant advice
The person should avoid consuming substances that are hot in their energy, as these will create further Heat.

Taiyang fu – accumulation of *xue* can be caused by the following pattern of imbalance

- *Taiyang* channel invasions

Taiyang fu – accumulation of *xue* can result in the following pattern of imbalance

- *Taiyang fu* accumulation of water

There are also combined *taiyang* patterns. The most important of these are Invasion of Wind-Cold combined with internal Heat and Invasion of Wind-Cold combined with internal Phlegm-Fluids blocking the Lung. In both cases there will be visible symptoms and signs of both patterns simultaneously.

Yangming stage

If exogenous *xie qi* is not expelled from the *taiyang* aspect or if it has been treated improperly or inadequately, *xie qi* will penetrate into one of the deeper aspects. The *xie qi* will usually penetrate into the *yangming* aspect. When *xie qi* is in the *yangming* aspect, the disease is no longer in the exterior. This means that many of the signs and symptoms that characterise the *taiyang* stage will not be present here. This is because the clash between *zheng qi* and *xie qi* is no longer between the superficial *wei qi* and *xie qi* but is taking place deeper in the body. The body's *zheng qi* is still strong, which means that the struggle, and thereby the resulting symptoms and signs, will be strong. This is a pure *shi* condition.

The struggle between *zheng qi* and *xie qi* will generate a lot of Heat. *Yangming* is 'rich in *qi* and *xue*'. This means that the symptoms in this stage will be especially ferocious. When *xie qi* has penetrated into the *yangming* aspect, the symptom picture is characterised by the four 'greats': a great (high) fever; a great thirst; great (profuse) sweating; and a great (Flooding) pulse.

The Heat generated by the struggle will cause the person's body temperature to rise. At the same time, the intense heat will send *qi* upwards and outwards in the body. This rapid, expansive movement of *qi* will drive fluids to the surface of the body and out through the pores in the skin, which is why there is profuse sweating in the initial stages. The intense Heat and sweating will injure the fluids and the person will therefore develop a great thirst with a desire for cold drinks. The presence of intense Heat will be reflected in the pulse, which is Flooding and Rapid. The face will usually be red in colour and the person will feel hot when palpated, especially on the forehead. The Heat can also affect their *shen* and cause them to be physically and mentally restless, have difficulty sleeping and be irritable. If the Heat is very intense, they may lose consciousness or be delirious and raving. Heat can also agitate *qi* in the chest, causing the person to have a sensation of turmoil in the chest.

Heat will also be visible on the tongue, which will be red with a dry yellowish coating.

Zhang Zhong Jing mainly differentiated between *xie qi* located in the channel and in the organ aspects. The main difference between the two patterns is whether there is constipation or not. Heat in the Stomach and Large Intestine organs will desiccate fluids in the organs, resulting in constipation and abdominal pain.

Yangming channel syndrome

The channel pattern is characterised by formless *xie* Heat that spreads throughout the body, driving fluids up to the skin.

An important difference between the *yangming* and *taiyang* stages is that there is no aversion to cold in the *yangming* stage, but there will instead be an aversion to heat. Whilst *xie* Cold in the *taiyang* aspect will have resulted in the person packing themselves under blankets and quilts in an attempt to warm the skin and muscles, the person will now kick off the bedding in attempt to cool down. This is because in the *taiyang* stage the Wind and Cold will have blocked *wei qi* so that it cannot warm the skin and muscles. In this stage the struggle between *zheng qi* and *xie qi* is generating so much Heat that the body is overheating.

Aetiology

Insufficient or incorrect treatment of exogenous *xie qi* in the *taiyang* stage or *xie qi* is strong enough to penetrate deeper. If the person already has a Heat condition, or if they are a '*shi*' person, the symptoms will be more extreme.

Symptoms and signs

- Strong fever but no aversion to cold

- Profuse sweating

- Great thirst with a desire for cold drinks

- Irritability

- Delirium

- Turmoil in the chest

- Red face

- The skin feels hot

- Mental and physical restlessness

- Dark urine

- Red tongue, yellow and dry tongue coating

- Rapid, Flooding and Full pulse

Key symptoms
High fever and no aversion to cold, thirst, profuse sweating, constipation, Rapid and Flooding pulse.

Treatment principle
Drain Heat from the *yangming* aspect.

Acupuncture points
Choose from: LI 11, St 44, St 43, Ren 12 and Du 14.

Needle technique
Draining.

Explanation

- LI 11, St 44, St 43 and Ren 12 drain *yangming* Heat.

- Du 14 drains *shi* Heat.

Herbal formula

- *Bai Hu Tang* (Drains *yangming* Heat)

Relevant advice
The patient should eat foods that are cooling and moistening. They should avoid foods and beverages that have a hot energy.

Yangming channel pattern can be caused by the following pattern of imbalance

- *Taiyang* stage invasion of exogenous *xie qi*

Yangming channel pattern can result in the following patterns of imbalance

- *Yangming* organ stage

- *Shaoyang* stage

- *Taiyin* stage

- *Shaoyin* stage

- *Jueyin* stage

Yangming organ stage

The *yangming* channel stage can develop into the *yangming* organ or *fu* stage when *shi* Heat has injured the fluids in the Stomach and Large Intestine. This can result in *xie qi* binding and developing 'form'.

The struggle between *xie qi* and *zheng qi* has decreased, so the symptoms are less intense than those seen in the *yangming* channel or *jing* stage.

Aetiology

Insufficient or incorrect treatment of exogenous *xie qi* in the *taiyang* stage or when *xie qi* is strong enough to penetrate deeper. If the person already has a Heat condition or if they are a '*shi*' person, the symptoms will be more extreme.

Symptoms and signs

- Strong fever, but no aversion to cold
- Profuse sweating
- Great thirst with a desire for cold drinks
- Abdominal bloating and pain that is worse with pressure
- Constipation
- Irritability
- Delirium
- Turmoil in the chest
- Red face
- The skin feels hot
- Mental and physical restlessness
- Dark urine
- Red tongue, yellow and dry tongue coating
- Rapid, Flooding and Full pulse

Key symptoms

High fever and no aversion to cold, constipation, thirst, profuse sweating, Rapid and Flooding pulse.

Treatment principle

Drain Heat from the *yangming* organs, activate and moisten the Intestines.

Acupuncture points

Choose from: LI 11, St 44, St 43, St 25, St 37, Sp 15, Du 14, SJ 6 and Ren 12.

Needle technique

Draining.

Explanation

- LI 11, St 44, St 43 and Ren 12 drain *yangming* Heat.

- St 25, St 37 and SJ 6 drain Heat from the Large Intestine organ and activate *qi* in the Large Intestine.

- Sp 15 spreads *qi* in the Intestines.

- Du 14 drains *shi* Heat.

Herbal formula

- *Da Cheng Qi Tang* (Purges Heat and moves *qi* in the *yangming* organs)

Relevant advice

The patient should eat foods that are cooling and moistening, such as spinach and cabbage. They should avoid foods and beverages that have a hot energy.

Yangming channel pattern can be caused by the following patterns of imbalance

- *Taiyang* stage invasion of exogenous *xie qi*

- *Yangming* channel stage

Yangming channel pattern can result in the following patterns of imbalance

- *Yangming* organ stage

- *Shaoyang* stage

- *Taiyin* stage

- *Shaoyin* stage

- *Jueyin* stage

- *Yangming* organs stage syndrome can easily develop into *xue* Heat generating Wind in small children. This will manifest with febrile convulsions or meningitis.

- The *yangming* and *taiyin* aspects are internally and externally connected. If *yangming* Heat is not drained out of the body it can combine with *taiyin* Dampness resulting in Damp-Heat. This Damp-Heat can disrupt the functioning of the Liver and Gall Bladder and lead to Liver and Gall Bladder Damp-Heat (i.e. jaundice).

Shaoyang stage

The *shaoyang* is the pivot or hinge between the interior and the exterior. *Xie qi* can get stuck here in its movement in or out of the body. *Shaoyang*-stage syndromes usually develop from *taiyang* or *yangming*-stage syndrome. It can also arise directly. When *xie qi* gets stuck here, it is because the *xie qi* is not strong enough to penetrate deeper into the body, but *zheng qi* is not strong enough to drive it out and up, which results in a stalemate situation. This type of pattern can be seen in some patients with chronic fatigue or a state of malaise or illness that they just can't seem to shake off. There will typically be an alternation between symptoms and signs that typify the *taiyang* and *yangming* stages, because *xie qi* is locked in between these two stages and will move up and down between them.

One of the defining symptoms of the *shaoyang* stage is the alternation between fever and feeling cold. When exogenous *xie qi* is in the exterior aspect of the body, there is usually a fever with a concurrent aversion to cold. When there is a *shaoyang* pattern, the fever and chills are not concurrent but alternate with each other. The alternating fever and chills arise from the struggle between *xie qi* and *zheng qi* and indicate which of the two are dominant at that time.

The patient can experience a bitter taste in the mouth due to extreme Heat in the Gall Bladder. The Heat can also cause the throat to feel dry and can manifest with irritability and dizziness.

There can be tension and tightness of the ribcage and chest when *xie qi* blocks the flow of *qi* in the *shaoyang* channels. The stagnation of *qi* can also affect the Stomach, giving rise to nausea, poor appetite or vomiting.

Shaoyang-stage patterns can often be combined with *taiyang* and *yangming* stage patterns, in which case there will be symptoms and signs of both patterns.

Aetiology

Insufficient or incorrect treatment of *xie qi* in one of the other stages. It is often a consequence of the person not having rested enough whilst they were ill or having started working again before they were fully fit. This can result in *xie qi* being retained because the person's *zheng qi* is not strong enough to expel the *xie qi* completely. Vaccinations can also cause *xie qi* to get locked in the *shaoyang* aspect.

Symptoms and signs

- Alternating fever and chills
- Bitter taste
- Tension or tightness in the thorax or costal region
- Poor appetite
- Nausea
- Dry throat

- Headache

- Dizziness

- Irritability

- Turmoil in the chest

- The tongue may have a yellowish coating on only one side

- Wiry pulse on the left wrist

Key symptoms
Alternating chills and fever, bitter taste in the mouth, no appetite, Wiry pulse on the left wrist.

Treatment principle
Harmonise *shaoyang* and expel *xie qi*.

Acupuncture points
Choose from: GB 34, GB 41, SJ 5, Du 14, St 36, Sp 3 and Ren 12.

Needle technique
Draining on GB 34, GB 41, Du 14 and SJ 5. Tonifying on St 36, Sp 3 and Ren 12.

Explanation

- SJ 5, GB 34 and GB 41 expel *xie qi* from the *shaoyang* aspect.

- St 36, Sp 3 and Ren 12 tonify *zheng qi* so that it can expel *xie qi* from the *shaoyang* aspect.

- Du 14 activates *wei qi* and drains Heat.

Herbal formula

- *Xiao Chai Hu Tang* (Harmonises *shaoyang*)

Relevant advice
The patient must avoid overexerting themselves and they must try to avoid new invasions of *xie qi*.

The *shaoyang* pattern can be caused by the following patterns of imbalance

- *Taiyang* stage

- *Yangming* stage

- *Taiyin* stage

- *Shaoyin* stage

- *Jueyin* stage

The *shaoyang* pattern can result in the following patterns of imbalance

- *Taiyang* stage
- *Yangming* stage
- *Taiyin* stage
- *Shaoyin* stage
- *Jueyin* stage

Taiyin stage

This is the first of the *yin* stages and the disease is not life threatening. If properly treated, the prognosis is good.

When *xie* Cold invades the *taiyin* aspect, it will damage the Spleen *yang*. The functions of Spleen *yang* include the transformation of the food and fluids that are ingested. When the Spleen *yang* aspect is compromised, the Spleen has difficulty performing its functions. This dysfunction of Spleen *yang* combined with the presence of Damp-Cold will result in a blockage of the *qi ji* or *qi* mechanism in the middle *jiao*. This will characterise the diagnostic picture, with symptoms and signs such as watery diarrhoea containing undigested food, watery vomiting, nausea, a poor appetite, abdominal bloating and fatigue. The person will lack thirst due to the accumulation of Dampness and stagnant fluids. They will have an aversion to cold and their skin will feel cold when palpated, because they are *yang xu*. Because it is a *yang xu* condition, they will be able to get warm if they wear sufficient clothes or lie beneath a blanket. This differentiates the pattern from a *taiyang* stage pattern, where the person cannot get warm, despite wearing warm clothes or lying beneath thick blankets.

Aetiology

The *taiyin*-stage pattern can arise because exogenous *xie qi* has directly invaded the interior in a person who is Spleen *yang xu* or when exogenous *xie qi* that has been in the outer aspects penetrates deeper. *Xie qi* can penetrate inwards when *zheng qi* starts to become deficient or exhausted. *Taiyin*-stage patterns can also arise due to medical treatment. This will typically be due to the use of antibiotics, which are cold in their dynamic and can draw the *xie qi* inwards and downwards.

This pattern can also combine with patterns from the other stages, for example *taiyang* patterns. In these situations, there will be symptoms and signs from both patterns.

Symptoms and signs

- Abdominal bloating
- Loss of appetite
- Nausea

- Watery vomit

- Watery diarrhoea

- Lack of thirst

- Cold limbs

- The skin feels cold, especially on the abdomen

- Pale complexion

- The person has difficulty keeping warm

- The person is dressed in warm clothing

- The person sits with their arms around themselves or lies curled up

- Fatigue

- Pale tongue with moist, white coating

- Slow, Weak and Deep pulse

Key symptoms
Watery diarrhoea, bloated abdomen, nausea, pale tongue with white, moist coating.

Treatment principle
Tonify Spleen *yang*.

Acupuncture points
Choose from: Ren 8, Ren 12, St 36, Lu 9, Sp 3, Sp 9, St 21, UB 20 and UB 21.

Needle technique
Tonifying on all points except on Sp 9 and St 21. Moxa must be used.

Explanation

- Ren 8 with moxa expels cold from the middle *jiao*.

- Ren 12, St 36, Sp 3, UB 20 and UB 21 tonify Spleen *yang*.

- Lu 9 tonifies *taiyin*.

- Sp 9 drains Damp-Cold.

- St 21 regulates Stomach and Spleen *qi*.

Herbal formula

- *Li Zhong Tang* (Warms Spleen *yang* and expels Cold)

Relevant advice

The patient should eat foods that are warm, both in their temperature and energetic dynamic, for example ginger and other spices. They should eat cooked food and avoid food and drinks that are cold in their temperature and energy. They must keep the abdomen warm and avoid getting cold. Because they are *qi xu*, they must get enough rest and not overexert themselves.

The *taiyin* pattern can be caused by the following patterns of imbalance

- *Taiyang* stage

- *Yangming* stage

- Spleen *yang xu*

The *taiyin* pattern can result in the following patterns of imbalance

- *Shaoyin* pattern

- *Jueyin* pattern

- *Shaoyang* pattern

- Spleen *yang xu*

Shaoyin stage

The *shaoyin* stage is more critical than the previous stages. When *xie qi* has penetrated this far down, it has started to injure the Heart and Kidneys. These organ's *yang* or *yin* aspects are weakened and *zheng qi* is not able to resist *xie qi*. The *shaoyin*-stage pattern can occur because exogenous *xie qi* has penetrated to this depth from one of the other stages or when exogenous *xie qi* directly invades the *shaoyin* aspect. A direct invasion can occur if a person who is *yang xu* or *qi xu* sweats profusely whilst being exposed to the cold.

The symptoms and signs that define the *shaoyin* Cold and *shaoyin* Heat patterns are dependent on the nature of the *xie qi* and on which aspect of the Kidneys are deficient.

Shaoyin Cold stage

The symptoms and signs in this pattern reflect that Kidney *yang* is burdened and weakened. This will be seen in the fact that many of the functions that *yang* performs will be compromised. Kidney *yang* supports Spleen *yang* in its function of transforming the food and fluids that have been ingested. This means that there can be watery diarrhoea containing undigested food when there is *shaoyin* Cold. The diarrhoea will typically occur early in the morning, just after the person has woken up. It can, in fact, often be the reason that the person wakes up very early in the morning.

The depletion of *yang* will weaken the production of *qi*, resulting in fatigue.

Kidney *yang* is the fundamental driving force in all fluid physiology. When there is Kidney *yang xu*, there will be visible oedema, a lack of thirst and frequent urination with copious amounts of clear urine. Sometimes the urination and diarrhoea will be so frequent and copious that the person, instead of lacking thirst, will have a pronounced thirst due to dehydration.

Yang xu will also be evident in that the person will feel cold, will have an aversion to cold and will dress warmly. Their arms and legs will feel especially cold. They will sleep in a curled-up position beneath a thick quilt. The person will have a preference for warm food and drinks, and they will have an aversion to cold food and drinks, because the ingestion of cold substances will aggravate their symptoms.

The Heart *yang xu* aspect will manifest with a lack of motivation, lethargy and indolence.

Aetiology

The *shaoyin* Cold syndrome can develop from multiple aetiologies. There can be a direct invasion of Cold into this aspect of the body, especially if the person is already Heart *yang xu* or *qi xu* and is invaded by exogenous Wind and Cold whilst sweating.

Cold *xie qi* can sometimes be so powerful that it quickly overcomes the resistance of the body's *zheng qi* and penetrates into the interior aspects of the body. Because the *xie qi* is cold in nature, it will damage the body's *yang* aspects. If the person is Kidney or Heart *yang xu*, this process will be quicker.

There can also have been repeated invasions of exogenous Cold, which eventually weaken Kidney *yang*. This is particularly relevant if the person does not rest enough during and after an illness.

Symptoms and signs

- Aversion to cold

- Sleeps in a curled-up position

- Cold limbs

- Diarrhoea containing undigested food

- Watery vomit

- Nausea

- Loss of appetite

- Fatigue

- Mental lethargy

- Copious amounts of clear urine

- Frequent urination

- Lack of thirst with a preference for hot drinks; there can, though, sometimes be a profuse thirst if severe diarrhoea has damaged fluids

- White or pale face

- Preference for hot drinks and food

- Pale and wet tongue with white coating

- Deep, Weak and Slow pulse

Key symptoms
Aversion to cold, frequent urination, Deep Slow and Weak pulse.

Treatment principle
Warm and tonify Kidney and Heart *yang*.

Acupuncture points
Choose from: Kid 3, Kid 7, He 5, UB 15, UB 23, Du 4, Ren 4 and Ren 6.

Needle technique
Tonifying. Moxa is necessary.

Explanation

- Kid 3, Kid 7 and UB 23 tonify Kidney *yang*.

- Du 4, Ren 4 and Ren 6 tonify Kidney *yang* and *yuan qi*.

- He 5 and UB 15 tonify Heart *yang*.

Herbal formula

- *Si Ni Tang* (Warms and tonifies Kidney *yang*)

Relevant advice
The patient will benefit from eating and drinking things that are warming in their energy and temperature, whilst avoiding things that are cooling. Ginger, garlic and cinnamon will be particularly beneficial. They should ensure that they keep warm and avoid getting cold. It is important that they rest and do not overexert themselves.

The *shaoyin* Cold pattern can be caused by the following patterns of imbalance

- *Taiyang* stage

- *Taiyin* stage

- Kidney *yang xu*

- Heart *yang xu*

- Spleen *yang xu*

The *shaoyin* Cold pattern can result in the following patterns of imbalance

- *Jueyin* pattern

- *Taiyin* pattern

- Kidney *yang xu*

- Heart *yang xu*

- Spleen *yang xu*

Shaoyin Heat stage

When the exogenous Cold penetrates deeper into the body, it usually transforms into Heat. The Heat is especially virulent in the *yangming* stage. The Heat can be so intense that it damages *yin*. *Yin* can be damaged by a single episode of very intense *xie* Heat or by repeated invasions of *xie qi*, which transform into Heat and injure *yin*. This process will be further accelerated if the person is already *yin xu*.

The Kidney is the root of all *yin* in the body. This means that if *yin* is injured, it will weaken the Kidney's *yin* aspect. When the Kidneys are *yin xu*, *xu* Heat can arise. Both *yin xu* Heat and *shi* Heat due to *xie qi* can damage Heart *yin* and agitate *shen*. Kidney *yin* should also nourish Heart *yin* and control Heart Fire. This is the fundamental axis of Water and Fire in the body.

When there is Heat in the Heart, both the physical and *shen* aspects of the Heart become agitated. This will manifest with insomnia, irritability and palpitations.

Yin xu can be evident in night sweats, a malar flush, feeling hot in the evening and at night, a red tongue that lacks coating and a Rapid, Fine pulse.

Aetiology
Invasion of Wind-Cold that has transformed into Heat and damaged *yin*.

Symptoms and signs

- Irritability

- Insomnia

- Night sweats

- Mental restlessness

- Palpitations

- Malar flush

- Night fever

- Dryness of the mouth, especially at night

- Dark and scanty urine

- Red tongue without coating, the tip of the tongue is even more red

- Rapid, Fine pulse

Key symptoms
Night sweats, insomnia, dry mouth, red tongue without coating.

Treatment principle
Nourish Heart and Kidney *yin*.

Acupuncture points
Choose from: He 6, Kid 3, Kid 6, Kid 7, Ren 4, Ren 14, UB 15, UB 23 and UB 52.

Needle technique
Tonifying.

Explanation

- He 6 and Kid 7 nourish Heart and Kidney *yin* and control night sweats.

- Kid 3, Kid 6, Ren 4, UB 23 and UB 52 nourish Kidney *yin*.

- Ren 14 and UB 15 nourish Heart *yin*.

Herbal formula

- *Huang Lian E Jiao Tang* (Nourishes *yin* and descends Fire)

Relevant advice
The patient should avoid overexerting themselves and they must ensure that they get enough sleep and go to bed early. Coffee and other stimulants or substances containing caffeine should be avoided because they over-activate the Heart and thereby consume *yin*. Alcohol, hot spices and grilled and fried food will all generate Heat and further injure *yin*, so they should be avoided.

**The *shaoyin* Heat pattern can be caused by
the following pattern of imbalance**

- *Yangming* stage

The *shaoyin* Heat pattern can cause the following pattern of imbalance

- *Jueyin* stage

Jueyin stage

This is the deepest level that *xie qi* can reach. It is very critical when *xie qi* has reached this stage. There is an extreme *zheng qi xu* and the regulation of *yin* and *yang* has become chaotic. At this point *yin* and *yang* can start to separate. This will often manifest with symptoms of extreme Heat or Cold or a violent alternation between the two. There will often be a symptom of Heat and Cold simultaneously. The Heat can, for example, manifest in the upper part of the body and the Cold in the lower part. There may be extreme Heat symptoms in the torso but extreme Cold symptoms in the extremities.

The Heat will injure the fluids, there can be a strong thirst and the person's skin and flesh can be wizened. Ascending *yang* will manifest with a sensation of heat, turmoil, and pain in the chest.

The presence of Heat and Cold simultaneously can manifest with a gnawing hunger but no desire to eat. There may be vomiting and diarrhoea.

A more harmless variant of this pattern is observed, however, when there are intestinal worms.

Aetiology

Exogenous *xie qi* that has penetrated into the body's deepest level and fundamentally damaged *yin* or *yang*. Ingestion of contaminated food.

Symptoms and signs

- Restlessness and turmoil in the chest
- Extreme thirst
- Pain and burning sensation in the cardiac region
- Hunger with no desire to eat
- Cold limbs
- Diarrhoea
- Vomiting
- Vomiting of worms
- Wiry pulse

Key symptoms

Restlessness and heat in the cardiac region, cold limbs, hunger with no desire to eat, persistent thirst.

Treatment principle

Drain Heat from above and Cold from below, harmonise *yin* and *yang*.

Acupuncture points
Choose from: St 36, Ren 12, Liv 3, Pe 6 and Du 20.

Needle technique
Tonify St 36 and Ren 12, even technique on Liv 3 and Pe 6 and drain Du 20.

Explanation

- Liv 3 harmonises the Liver channel.

- Pe 6 harmonises the Pericardium.

- St 36 and Ren 12 harmonise the Stomach.

- Du 20 lowers rebellious *yang qi*.

Herbal formula

- *Wu Mei Wan* (Drains the internal organs, tonifies *qi* and expels parasites)

- *Wu Zhu Yu Tang* (Warms and tonifies the Liver and Stomach, drains Heat and descends rebellious Stomach *qi*)

Relevant advice
This will depend on how much Heat and Cold is present. It is important that the patient gets adequate rest and does not overexert themselves.

If there are worms, the person should take medication that kills the worms and avoid further contact with sources of infection.

The *jueyin* pattern can be caused by the following patterns of imbalance

- *Taiyin* stage

- *Shaoyin* stage

The *jueyin* pattern can result in the following patterns of imbalance

- *Taiyin* stage

- *Shaoyin* stage

Diagnosis according to the Four Levels
In this diagnostic approach, the patterns are differentiated in relation to four energetic levels rather than six channels. The deeper the level, the more severe the condition. This diagnostic analysis for the first time introduced the concept that exogenous *xie qi*, and thereby disease, can be transmitted from person to person and that exogenous *xie qi* can invade the body via the mouth, the nose and the genitals. In this analysis the exogenous *xie qi* is energetically hot from the very beginning,

hence the term *wen bing* or Heat diseases. In Heat diseases the symptoms will reflect the presence of Heat and the *yin* aspects of the body will be rapidly injured. Because Heat is a *yang* form of *xie qi*, it is very dynamic and the symptom picture can rapidly change. A person can go from being healthy to seriously ill in a very short period of time. The pathogen's *yang* nature can also be seen in the fact that even strong and healthy people can become ill after being in contact with exogenous *xie* Heat. Many highly contagious diseases and epidemics, such as the bubonic plague, ebola, influenza, measles and so on, are examples of *wen bing* or Heat diseases.

Wen bing theories differentiate not only between four energetic levels (*wei, qi, ying* and *xue*) but also between different types of Heat, for example Wind-Heat or Damp-Heat in the *wei* level and Lung Heat or Stomach Heat, etc. in the *qi* level.

Diagnosis according to the Four Levels determines the following:

- The disease location: If the *xie qi* is in the interior or exterior in relation to the Eight Principles and how deep an aspect of the interior it is that is affected.

- What the nature of the disorder is: Whether it is *xu* or *shi*. When *zheng qi* is strong, the condition will be defined as being *shi*. In general, when exogenous *xie qi* is in the *wei* and *qi* levels, it is a *shi* condition. When the *ying* and *xue* levels are affected, it is usually a *xu* condition. In contrast to the Six Stages, all the patterns of imbalance are Heat imbalances.

- About how the disease develops: Disease development is a dynamic process that is constantly changing, especially in the beginning. As with the Six Stages, this diagnosis model is used to assess the relative strength of *zheng qi* and exogenous *xie qi* in relation to each other. It can also be used to gauge the direction in which the disease is moving. If the disease is penetrating downwards, it is a negative sign. If, on the other hand, the symptoms change from one of the deeper levels to symptoms of one of the more superficial levels, it is a positive sign.

- The treatment principle: The nature of the disorder determines how it should be treated. If there is Heat in the *wei* level it must be expelled outwards. If it is deeper down, it must be drained. If there is a *xu* condition, that which is *xu* needs to be supported and so on.

Wei level

Wei level is the most superficial level and is very similar to the *taiyang* stage of the Six Stages. It is the first level that is attacked by an infectious disease. Many of the symptoms and signs are indications that *wei qi* has been disrupted in its functions and activities. Many of the symptoms and signs are the same as those seen in the *taiyang* stage, but in this level there is Heat and this means that there are also differences in the symptom picture.

Differentiation is made between invasions of different types of *xie* Heat: Wind-Heat, Damp-Heat, Dry-Heat and Summer-Heat. Wind-Heat is the most common and most important differentiation, especially for acupuncturists.

Wind-Heat

At first glance, Wind-Heat appears to be very similar to an invasion of Wind-Cold in the *taiyang* stage of the Six Stages, but when there is Wind-Heat, there is less aversion to cold.

Even though there is less aversion to cold, there is still an aversion to wind and cold. This is because the invading *xie qi* blocks the circulation of the warming *wei qi*. The disruption of *wei qi* can also be seen in the fact that there is often little or no sweating.

There can also be a headache, but where the headache in the *taiyang* stage was tight in nature, the headache seen in Wind-Heat imbalances is more pounding or throbbing. This is due to the expansive dynamic that Heat has.

Heat will cause the person to have a fever or feel feverish without necessarily having an elevated body temperature. The Heat will often be palpable on the person's forehead, which will feel warm to the touch.

Heat will damage the fluids and make the person thirsty. Their pulse will be Rapid.

Wind-Heat can disturb the functioning of the Lung, resulting in a cough or sore throat.

Aetiology

Contact with exogenous *xie* Heat.

Symptoms and signs

- Acute fever with mild aversion to wind and cold

- No or little sweating

- Throbbing headache

- Thirst

- Sore throat

- Red, swollen throat

- Cough

- Irritability

- Restlessness

- Yellowish or dried mucus in the nose

- The forehead may feel warm when touched

- The tip of the tongue may be red and there may be a thin, yellowish coating on the front of the tongue

- Rapid and Superficial pulse

Key symptoms
Fever and aversion to cold, Rapid and Superficial pulse.

Treatment principle
Expel Wind-Heat, activate *wei qi*.

Acupuncture points
Choose from: Du 14, LI 4, LI 11, Lu 7, Lu 10, Lu 11, UB 12, UB 13 and GB 20.

Needle technique
Draining. Cupping is recommended.

Explanation

- Du 14 activates *wei qi* and drains Heat.

- LI 4, LI 11, Lu 7, UB 12 and UB 13 expel Wind and Heat.

- Lu 10 and Lu 11 drain Heat from the Lung and throat.

- GB 20 expels Wind and drains *yang* from the head.

Herbal formula

- *Yin Qiao San* (Expels Wind-Heat)

- *Sang Ju Yin* (Expels Wind-Heat)

Relevant advice
When there is an invasion of Wind-Heat, it is best not to eat or to only eat light food. The person should drink tea that is both cooling and spicy, for example elderflower, chrysanthemum or mint tea.

An invasion of Wind-Heat can be caused by the following pattern of imbalance

- No previous pattern

An invasion of Wind-Heat can result in the following patterns of imbalance

- *Qi*-level Heat

- *Ying*-level Heat

Damp-Heat

In this pattern there is an invasion of Damp-Heat in the *wei* level. This is equivalent to an invasion of Damp-Heat in the upper *jiao* in diagnosis according to *san jiao*.

Damp-Heat is heavier and more obstructive than Wind-Heat. This will result in aching and heaviness of the limbs. Dampness can block the sweat pores so there is no sweating or the Heat can make the sweat sticky in consistency.

Because there is impure *yin* in the head and a lack of pure *yang*, the headache in this pattern will feel heavier than the one felt in a Wind-Heat pattern and the person will have difficultly thinking clearly.

Damp-Heat can also block and disturb the movement of *qi* inside the body, resulting in poor appetite, nausea and chest oppression. There may be diarrhoea or constipation, depending on whether Dampness or Heat is the dominant aspect.

Aetiology
Exposure to Damp-Heat *xie qi*.

Symptoms and signs

- Fever that is worse in the afternoon

- Nausea

- Aversion to cold

- Heavy and aching limbs

- Poor appetite

- Abdominal bloating

- Heavy headache

- Chest oppression

- Lack of sweating or sticky sweat

- Fatigue

- Diarrhoea or constipation

- Greasy, yellow tongue coating

- Fast and Slippery pulse

Key symptoms
Heavy headache, heaviness of the limbs, Rapid and Slippery pulse.

Treatment principle
Expel and drain Damp-Heat, activate *wei qi*.

Acupuncture points
Choose from: Du 14, LI 4, LI 11, Lu 7, Sp 3, Sp 9, Ren 12 and Pe 6.

Needle technique
Draining.

Explanation

- Du 14 drains Heat and activates *wei qi*.

- LI 4 and Lu 7 activate *wei qi* and expel exogenous *xie qi*.

- LI 11 expels exogenous *xie qi* and drains Damp-Heat.

- Sp 3 and Sp 9 drain Damp-Heat.

- Ren 12 and Pe 6 regulate the *qi ji* in the middle and upper *jiao*.

Herbal formula

- *Huo Po Xia Ling Tang* (Expels Damp-Heat from the exterior)

Relevant advice
The person should avoid consuming food and beverages that create Damp-Heat. In general, it is best not to eat or to only eat light meals when there are invasions of exogenous *xie qi* in the exterior.

An invasion of Damp-Heat can be caused by the following patterns of imbalance

- No previous pattern

- Damp-Heat

An invasion of Damp-Heat can result in the following patterns of imbalance

- *Qi*-level Heat

- *Ying*-level Heat

- Damp-Heat

- Spleen *qi xu*

Dry-Heat

This pattern has traditionally been prevalent in the autumn in China, when the climate is extremely dry. In North-Western Europe this pattern can arise due to living or working in buildings with a very dry indoor climate. An invasion of Dry-Heat can disrupt not only the functioning of *wei qi*, but also the Lung, because the Lung is easily damaged by Dryness. The disruption of *wei qi* can be seen in an aversion to wind and cold, because the *wei qi* is no longer able to protect the body against them. There may be a slight sweat due to the Heat aspect. The presence of Heat and the struggle between *xie qi* and *zheng qi* will result in a slight fever or fever sensation.

The disruption of the Lung's descending and spreading function can result in coughing and possibly chest pain due to the stagnation of *qi*. The Heat will evaporate fluids in the body, so that rubbery, yellowish sputum is formed.

The Dryness and Heat will injure fluids and lead to the dryness of the nose and throat, the person will be thirsty and the tongue dry.

Aetiology
Exposure to Dry-Heat *xie qi*.

Symptoms and signs

- Dry nose and throat
- Fever
- Slight aversion to cold and wind
- Light sweat
- Cough with sticky or rubbery sputum
- The cough can cause chest pain
- Headache
- Thirst
- Dry tongue coating
- Rapid and Superficial pulse

Key symptoms
Dry nose and throat, fever with aversion to wind and cold. Rapid and Superficial pulse.

Treatment principle
Expel Wind-Heat, activate *wei qi*.

Acupuncture points
Choose from: Du 14, LI 4, LI 11, Lu 9, Lu 10, UB 12, UB 13, Kid 6 and Sp 6.

Needle technique
Draining.

Explanation

- Du 14 and LI 11 drain Heat and activate *wei qi*.
- LI 4, UB 12 and UB 13 activate *wei qi* and expel exogenous *xie qi*.
- LI 11 expels exogenous *xie qi* and drains Heat.
- Kid 6, Sp 6 and Lu 9 moisten the Lung.

Herbal formula

- *Sang Xing Tang* (Expels Wind-Heat and Dryness)

Relevant advice

The person should avoid places where the air is very dry.

An invasion of Dry-Heat may be caused by the following pattern of imbalance

- No previous pattern

An invasion of Dry-Heat can result in the following patterns of imbalance

- *Qi*-level Heat
- *Ying*-level Heat
- Lung *yin xu*

Qi level

Qi-level Heat can arise because there has been a direct invasion of exogenous *xie qi* in the *qi* level or because exogenous *xie qi* has penetrated deeper from the *wei* level. Exogenous *xie qi* can penetrate deeper to the next level if it is strong enough or if the previous level has been treated incorrectly or inadequately. This pattern will develop more rapidly and the symptoms will be stronger in a person who already has a *shi* Heat condition.

When there is a *qi*-level disorder, both *xie qi* and *zheng qi* are strong. This will result in pronounced *shi* Heat symptoms. *Qi*-level disorders are differentiated according to which organ is affected. There are many subcategories, which mainly have relevance when using herbal medicine. The most relevant patterns for acupuncturists are described below.

The *xie* Heat will itself disturb the *qi ji* in the interior and the Heat will drive *yang qi* upwards and outwards. This is further reinforced by the extreme Heat that arises as a consequence of the struggle between *zheng qi* and *xie qi*. This results in the generalised symptoms and signs that are seen in this level. These are very similar to the symptoms and signs that are seen in the *yangming* stage of the Six Stages and these two stages and levels are also overlapping. *Shaoyang*-stage symptoms can also be differentiated as *qi*-level Heat.

The generalised symptoms and signs of this level are fever with an aversion to heat but not to cold. There is no aversion to cold because the *xie qi* no longer disrupts the functioning of *wei qi*. On the other hand, there is so much heat in the body that the person has an aversion to heat.

Heat injures fluids and this results in a great thirst with a desire for cold drinks. The urine will be dark.

There may be profuse sweating due to the Heat, but there can also be a lack of sweating because the fluids are exhausted. The extreme Heat can ascend to the Heart and agitate the *shen*. This can be seen when the person is restless and irritable.

There is a bitter taste in the mouth and a thick, dry, yellow coating on the tongue. The pulse will be Rapid and Full.

Qi-level Heat should be further differentiated with regard to which organ is affected. Each organ pattern will manifest with specific symptoms and signs that reflect the disturbance of its functions.

Heat can easily injure *yin*. This will manifest with symptoms and signs of *yin xu*.

There can also be simultaneous *wei*- and *qi*-level Heat, with a resultant mixture of symptoms and signs from both levels.

Aetiology
Invasions of exogenous Heat that have not been expelled from the *wei* level or that have been treated incorrectly or inadequately. Direct invasions of Heat to the *qi* level after being exposed to exogenous *xie qi*.

Symptoms and signs

- High fever with no aversion to cold

- Profuse sweating (or no sweating if the Heat has damaged fluids)

- Extreme thirst with a desire for cold drinks

- Red face

- Restlessness and irritability

- The skin may feel warm to the touch

- Restless sleep with violent dreams

- Red tongue with dry, yellow coating

- Rapid, Full, Flooding pulse

Key symptoms
High fever with no aversion to cold, profuse sweating and thirst, Rapid and Flooding pulse.

Treatment principle
Drain Heat.

Acupuncture points
Choose from: LI 11 and Du 14.

Needle technique
Draining. Bleed Du 14.

Explanation

- LI 11 and Du 14 drain Heat from the *qi* level.

Herbal formula

- *Qin Qi Hua Tan Tang* (Drains Phlegm-Heat from the Lung)
- *Xie Bai San* (Drains Heat from the Lung)
- *Bai Hu Tang* (Drains *yangming* Heat)
- *Da Cheng Tang* (Drains Heat from the *yangming* organs)
- *Da Chai Hu Tang* (Drains *shaoyang* Heat)
- *Zhi Zi Dou Chi Tang* (Drains Heat from the chest and diaphragm)

Relevant advice
The person should avoid consuming food and beverages that will create additional heat in the body.

Qi-level Heat can be caused by the following pattern of imbalance

- *Wei*-level Heat

Qi-level Heat can result in the following patterns of imbalance

- *Ying*-level Heat
- *Xue*-level Heat

The treatment will be most effective if it is possible to differentiate where in the *qi* level the Heat is. The Heat can be located in one or more *zangfu* organs, in which case there will be symptoms and signs that are specific to these organs. The treatment will then be focused on draining Heat from these organs. The most relevant patterns are discussed below.

Lung Heat

In addition to the symptoms and signs described above, Heat will have damaged fluids in the Lung and disrupted the Lung's *qi ji*. This will result in a loud, barking cough, because it is a *shi* condition. There will be sticky, yellowish sputum that is difficult to expectorate. Breathing will be impaired because *xie qi* is blocking the Lung's ability to descend and spread *qi*. The blockage of *qi* will also result in chest pains.

Aetiology

Exposure to exogenous *xie qi* that has either invaded the Lung directly or penetrated down from the *wei* level.

Symptoms and signs

- Fever or feeling of heat with no aversion to cold
- Cough with yellow, sticky sputum that is difficult to expectorate
- Profuse sweating
- Thirst
- Chest pain
- Dyspnoea
- Red face
- Restlessness
- Restless sleep
- Red tongue with yellow coating
- Rapid pulse

Key symptoms

Fever, cough with yellow sticky sputum, thirst, Rapid pulse.

Treatment principle

Drain Heat from the Lung, regulate Lung *qi*.

Acupuncture points

Choose from: Lu 1, Lu 5, Lu 10, Lu 11, LI 11, Du 14 and UB 13.

Needle technique

Draining. Possibly bleed Du 14.

Explanation

- Lu 1, Lu 5 and UB 13 drain Heat from the Lung and regulate Lung *qi*.

- Lu 10 and Lu 11 drain Heat from the Lung.

- Du 14 and LI 11 drain *qi*-level Heat.

Herbal formula

- *Qin Qi Hua Tan Tang* (Drains Phlegm-Heat from the Lung)

- *Xie Bai San* (Drains Heat from the Lung)

Relevant advice

The person should avoid consuming food and beverages that will create additional Heat in the body. Cigarette smoking is not recommended, because it will create Heat and Phlegm in the Lung.

Lung Heat can be caused by the following pattern of imbalance

- *Wei*-level Heat

Lung Heat can result in the following patterns of imbalance

- *Ying*-level Heat

- *Xue*-level Heat

- Phlegm-Heat in the Lung

- Lung *yin xu*

Heat in the chest and diaphragm

In addition to the symptoms and signs discussed under *qi*-level Heat, there will be signs and symptoms resulting from the accumulation of Heat in the chest and diaphragm. The Heat will disrupt and agitate *qi* in the upper *jiao*. This will result in a sense of turmoil in the chest. Heat will agitate the *shen*, resulting in irritability, restlessness and insomnia. The Heat can ascend to the throat resulting in a sore throat. By damaging fluids, the Heat can manifest with an intense thirst, dry mouth and dry lips, as well as constipation.

Aetiology

Exposure to exogenous *xie qi* that has either invaded the *qi* level directly or penetrated down from the *wei* level.

Symptoms and signs

- Persistent fever, no aversion to cold

- Restlessness

- Burning sensation and/or a sensation of turmoil in the chest and diaphragm

- Insomnia

- Irritability

- Constipation

- Sore throat

- Dry and chapped lips

- Dry mouth and throat

- Thirst

- Sweats

- The skin may feel hot to the touch

- Red face

- The tongue may be dry in the central area with a yellow, dry coating

- Rapid, Full pulse

Key symptoms
Restlessness, pain or turmoil in the chest and diaphragm, fever and irritability.

Treatment principle
Drain Heat from the upper *jiao*.

Acupuncture points
Choose from: Du 14, SJ 6, SJ 5, LI 11, Ren 15, Ren 17, UB 16, UB 17, Pe 6 and Pe 8.

Needle technique
Draining.

Explanation

- Du 14, SJ 6, SJ 5 and LI 11 drain Heat.

- Ren 15, Ren 17, UB 16 and UB 17 drain Heat from the chest and diaphragm.

- Pe 6 and Pe 8 drain Heat from the Pericardium.

Herbal formula

- *Zhi Zi Dou Chi Tang* (Drains Heat from the chest and diaphragm)

- *Qing Qi Hua Tan Tang* (Drains Phlegm-Heat from the Lung and chest)

Relevant advice
The person should avoid consuming food and beverages that will create additional Heat in the body.

Heat in the chest and diaphragm can be caused by the following pattern of imbalance

- *Wei*-level Heat

Heat in the chest and diaphragm can result in the following patterns of imbalance

- *Ying*-level Heat

- *Xue*-level Heat

- Heart Fire

Heat in the Stomach and Intestines

This pattern is basically the same as the *yangming* stage in the Six Stages, and the pathomechanisms will be the same. The reader is therefore referred to this section (page 654) for more details.

Aetiology
Exposure to exogenous *xie qi*, which has either invaded the *qi* level directly or penetrated down from the *wei* level.

Symptoms and signs

- Constipation or green watery diarrhoea (false diarrhoea caused by a blockage in the Intestines)

- Abdominal bloating and distension, the pain is aggravated by pressure

- Fever, especially in the afternoon, but no aversion to cold

- Profuse sweating

- Mental confusion

- Restlessness

- Frontal headache

- Bleeding gums

- Red face

- Red tongue with a dry and yellowish coating

- Rapid, Full, Flooding pulse

Key symptoms
Constipation, bloated abdomen, fever, Rapid and Flooding pulse.

Treatment principle
Drain Heat from the Stomach and Large Intestine.

Acupuncture points
Choose from: LI 11, SJ 6, St 25, St 34, St 37, St 44, UB 21, UB 25 and Du 14.

Needle technique
Draining. Du 14 can be bled.

Explanation

- LI 11, SJ 6, St 25, St 37 and UB 25 drain Heat from the Stomach and Large Intestine and activate *qi* in the Intestines.

- St 34, St 44 and UB 21 drain Heat from the Stomach.

- Du 14 drains the *qi*-level Heat.

Herbal formula

- *Da Cheng Qi Tang* (Purges Heat and moves *qi* in the Intestines)

Relevant advice
A person with Stomach and Large Intestine Heat should eat foods that are cooling and moistening. They should avoid foods and beverages that have a hot energy.

**Stomach and Large Intestine Heat can be caused
by the following pattern of imbalance**

- *Wei*-level Heat

**Stomach and Large Intestine Heat can result in
the following patterns of imbalance**

- *Ying*-level Heat

- *Xue*-level Heat

- Stomach *yin xu*

Damp-Heat

Dampness and Heat can bind together and are difficult to separate. Invasions of Damp-Heat often occur in the summer when the weather is rainy and in humid and hot climates. There is often an underlying Spleen Dampness. It is also mainly the functioning of the Stomach and Spleen that is disturbed when there are invasions of Damp-Heat.

The way that the symptoms manifest will be influenced by whether it is Dampness or Heat that is the predominant pathogen.

There can be a fever that is most noticeable in the afternoon. This is explained by Dampness being a *yin* form of *xie qi* and *yin* is on the increase after noon. When the *yin* Dampness contains *xie* Heat, the *xie* Heat will increase together with *yin* in the afternoon. The Heat will often cause the person to sweat. This will temporarily relieve the fever, but the fever will soon return. The person will often find that the fever comes in waves.

Dampness blocks the movement of *qi* creating a sensation of heaviness. This will be most apparent in the limbs. The Heat aspect will make the muscles feel sore and ache.

The Stomach and Spleen *qi* mechanism will be blocked by the Dampness. This can result in nausea and a loss of appetite. There will also be diarrhoea that is odorous and sticky. The Heat can cause a stinging or burning sensation in the rectum during and after bowel movements.

Dampness can also block *qi* in the upper *jiao*, resulting in chest oppression.

The Heat's *yang* dynamic can ascend the *yin* Dampness to the head. At the same time, Dampness can itself block the ascent of clear *yang* to the head. This will result in a heavy headache and difficulty in thinking clearly. The Heat will cause the headache to be pounding or throbbing in nature.

Damp-Heat will be seen in the complexion, which can be yellowish. The skin and the sweat can be oily.

Restlessness and irritability will arise if the Heat aspect agitates the *shen*.

Aetiology
Exposure to exogenous *xie qi* that has either invaded the *qi* level directly or penetrated down from the *wei* level.

Symptoms and signs

- Fever that is reduced by sweating, but soon rises again

- Fever that is worse in the afternoon and comes in waves

- Heavy and aching muscles, especially in the limbs

- Nausea

- Poor appetite

- Loose, sticky, odorous stools

- Chest oppression

- Heavy and possibly pounding headache

- Difficulty in thinking clearly

- Oily skin

- Yellowish complexion

- Restlessness or irritability

- Red tongue with yellow, sticky coating

- Rapid and Slippery pulse

Key symptoms
Odorous diarrhoea, fever, yellowish, greasy tongue coating, Rapid and Slippery pulse.

Treatment principle
Drain Damp-Heat.

Acupuncture points
Choose from: Du 14, LI 11, St 25, St 44, Sp 9, Sp 6 and Ren 12.

Needle technique
Draining.

Explanation

- Du 14 and LI 11 drain *qi*-level Heat.

- St 25 and St 44 drain Damp-Heat from the Intestines.

- Sp 6 and Sp 9 drain Damp-Heat.

- Ren 12 drains Dampness from the middle *jiao*.

Herbal formula

- *San Ren Tang* (Drains Damp-Heat)

Relevant advice
The person must avoid consuming foods that produce Dampness or Heat.

Damp-Heat can be caused by the following pattern of imbalance

- *Wei*-level Heat

Damp-Heat can result in the following patterns of imbalance

- *Ying*-level Heat

- *Xue*-level Heat

- Spleen *qi xu*

Gall Bladder Heat

This pattern is virtually the same as the *shaoyang* stage in the Six Stages. The reader is referred to this section for an explanation of the pathomechanisms of the symptoms and signs (page 659). The only real difference between the *shaoyang* stage and *qi*-level Gall Bladder Heat, is that the latter has more Heat and Dampness signs.

Aetiology
Exposure to exogenous *xie qi* that has either invaded the *qi* level directly or penetrated down from the *wei* level.

Symptoms and signs

- Alternating fever and chills
- Bitter taste in the mouth
- Costal and hypochondriac distension or pain
- No appetite
- Nausea
- Dry throat
- Headache
- Dizziness
- Irritability
- Sensation of turmoil in the chest
- The tongue may have a yellowish coating on one side and a white coating on the other side
- Wiry pulse, especially on one of the wrists, Rapid pulse

Key symptoms
Alternating fever and chills, bitter taste in the mouth, Rapid and Wiry pulse.

Treatment principle
Drain Gall Bladder Heat.

Acupuncture points
Choose from: GB 34, GB 41, SJ 5 and Du 14.

Needle technique
Draining.

Explanation

- SJ 5, GB 34 and GB 41 drain Heat from the Gall Bladder.

- Du 14 activates *wei qi* and drains Heat.

Herbal formula

- *Da Chai Hu Tang* (Drains *shaoyang* Heat)

Relevant advice

A person with Gall Bladder Heat must ensure that they do not overexert themselves and they must be very careful to avoid new invasions of exogenous *xie qi*. They should avoid eating food that creates Heat.

Gall Bladder Heat can be caused by the following pattern of imbalance

- *Wei*-level Heat

Gall Bladder Heat can result in the following patterns of imbalance

- *Ying*-level Heat

- *Xue*-level Heat

Ying level

The *ying* level is the upper level of *xue*. It is the *qi* aspect of *xue*. When *xie qi* has penetrated down to the *ying* level, it is a deeper and more serious disorder than when *xie qi* was in the *qi* level.

Xie qi can penetrate to the *ying* level if *xie qi* is sufficiently virulent or if the invasion of the *qi* level has been treated improperly or inadequately. Furthermore, *xie qi* can jump directly from the *wei* level to the *ying* level. This is because both the Lung and the Pericardium have their residence in the upper *jiao*. This means that exogenous *xie qi* can be transmitted directly from Lung *wei qi* to Pericardium *ying qi*.

The Heart and Pericardium are easily influenced by *xue* imbalances, especially *xue* Heat. Because *xie* Heat is affecting an aspect of *xue*, there will be signs that the person's *shen* is affected. This is because *xue* is the residence of *shen*. These signs could be insomnia or restlessness. The Heat can also have created Phlegm, which can block the orifices of the Heart. This could mean that the person talks incomprehensibly, and there can be delirium and even a loss of consciousness or a coma.

The Heat in the Pericardium will also mean that there may be palpitations and a sensation of turmoil in the chest.

The Heat can agitate *xue* so much that the walls of the blood vessels rupture. This can manifest as petechiae. There can also be red skin rashes.

When *xie qi* penetrates from the *qi* level to the *ying* level, there will be a dramatic change in the symptom picture. At first glance it could appear to be a positive sign that the high fever, severe sweating and overflowing pulse that characterises the *qi* level have abated, but it is not. This is because the changes that arise are indications that *xie qi* is starting to injure the body's *yin* aspect. The high fever that the person had is now replaced by a fever that is only present in the evenings and at night. The pulse is no longer Rapid, Full and Flooding, which was a consequence of the fierce struggle between *xie qi* and *zheng qi*. Now the pulse is Deep, Rapid and Fine, which indicates that the *zheng qi* is weak and that there is now *yin xu* Heat, rather than *shi* Heat. The sweating is no longer profuse, because there is now *yin xu* Heat rather than *shi* Heat and fluids are exhausted and have dried out.

An interesting sign is that the person has a lack of thirst, despite the intense Heat. This is because the Heat will have driven the fluids upwards in the body to the mouth so that the person, despite the lack of fluids, does not feel the need to drink. This is, again, a crucial difference to the symptoms and signs of the *qi* level.

Observation of the tongue is important when differentiating between *xie* Heat in the *qi* level and the *ying* level. This is because the tongue will show that the extreme Heat has damaged *yin*. The thick and yellowish coating, which is characteristic of *qi*-level Heat has vanished and the tongue body proper is much more red in colour.

There can be signs of 'false Cold'. This will manifest with icy extremities, while the person's torso is burning hot. This is due to the extreme Heat 'binding' *qi*, so it does not reach the hands and feet.

Aetiology
Exposure to exogenous *xie qi* that has penetrated down to the *ying* level from the *wei* or *qi* level.

Symptoms and signs

- Fever that worsens at night

- Insomnia

- Restlessness

- Dry mouth but no thirst

- Petechiae

- Red skin rashes

- Unconsciousness or coma

- Delirium

- Raving

- The skin on the torso feels hot, but the hands and feet are icy cold
- Dark, red tongue without coating
- Fast, Deep, Fine pulse

Key symptoms
Fever that is worst at night, dry mouth but no thirst, red tongue without coating, Rapid and Fine pulse.

Treatment principle
Drain Heat from the *ying* Level and nourish *yin*. Possibly restore consciousness.

Acupuncture points
Choose from: Pe 3, Pe 8, Pe 9, Du 14, Du 26, Kid 6, Sp 10 and UB 40.

Needle technique
Draining. Micro-bleed Pe 9, Du 26 and UB 40.

Explanation

- Pe 3, Pe 8 and Pe 9 drain Heat from the Pericardium.
- Du 26 restores consciousness.
- Du 14 drains Heat.
- UB 40 and Sp 10 drain *xue* Heat.
- Kid 6 nourishes *yin*.

Herbal formula

- *Qing Ying Tang* (Clears *ying*-level Heat)
- *An Gong Niu Huang Wan* (Clears *ying* Heat and restores consciousness)

Relevant advice
Patients with these conditions will probably be in treatment with Western medicine.

Ying-level Heat can be caused by the following patterns of imbalance

- *Wei*-level Heat
- *Qi*-level Heat

Ying-level Heat can result in the following pattern of imbalance

- *Xue*-level Heat

Xue level

In these patterns, *xie qi* has penetrated down to the deepest level of *xue*. This is the final stage in a disease development. The symptoms are serious and complex and remission is difficult. This is because it is the body's most fundamental substances, *xue* and *yin*, that are injured.

It is mainly the Liver, Heart and Kidneys that are affected. The Liver and Heart are affected because they have a relationship with *xue* and the Kidneys because *yin* is seriously injured. The extreme Heat can generate Wind that disrupts the movement of *xue* and further injures *yin*.

Xue-level patterns are included for the sake of completeness. It is unlikely that you will see these in an ordinary clinical setting. Patients with these symptoms will usually be admitted to an intensive care unit of a hospital.

Xue Heat agitating *xue*

The Heat causes *xue* to become chaotic in its movement and *xue* is so agitated that it ruptures the walls of the vessels. The Heat and deficient *yin* will mean that the *shen* is not rooted at night and there will be extreme restlessness and insomnia. The agitation of *shen* by the Heat can be so extreme that there is mania or delirium.

Because *yin* is injured, there can also be classic *yin xu* signs such as hot palms of the hands and soles of the feet, night fever, a Rapid but Fine pulse and a red tongue without coating.

Aetiology
Xie qi that has penetrated from the *qi* or *ying* level.

Symptoms and signs

- Bleeding of dark red blood from the mouth, nose, lungs, anus, vagina, under the skin, etc.

- High fever that is worse at night

- Insomnia

- Restlessness

- Delirium or raving

- Mania

- The palms of the hands and soles of the feet are very hot

- Very red tongue with elevated papillae and no tongue coating

- Very Rapid and Fine pulse

Key symptoms
Bleeding from body's orifices, night fever, very red tongue and a Rapid, Fine pulse.

Treatment principle
Drain *xue* Heat and stop bleeding.

Acupuncture points
Choose from: *Jing*-well points, *shixuan* (Ex-UE 11), UB 17, UB 40, Sp 1, Sp 10, LI 11, Liv 1, Liv 2, Pe 3 and Du 26.

Needle technique
Draining. Bleed Pe 3, UB 40, *jing*-well and *shixuan* points.

Explanation

- Du 26, *jing*-well and *shixuan* points drain Heat and restore consciousness.

- Sp 1 and Liv 1 stop bleeding.

- UB 17, UB 40, Sp 10, Liv 2, Pe 3 and LI 11 drain *xue* Heat.

Herbal formula

- *Xi Jiao Di Huang Tang* (Drains Heat from the *xue* level)

Relevant advice
The person will probably be in intensive medical care.

Xue Heat agitating *xue* can be caused by the following patterns of imbalance

- *Qi*-level Heat

- *Ying*-level Heat

Xue Heat agitating *xue* can result in the following pattern of imbalance

- *Yin* and *xue xu*

Xue Heat generating Wind
The extreme Heat and injuring of *yin* and *xue* in the Liver can result in the Liver causing Wind to begin to stir. This can manifest as febrile convulsions, muscle spasms and tremors, dizziness and neck stiffness. The ascending Heat from the Liver can cause headaches, red eyes, upwardly staring eyes, the person grinding their teeth and irritability. The Heat will also result in fever and thirst.

Aetiology
Xie qi that has penetrated from the *qi* or *ying* level.

Symptoms and signs

- Convulsions

- Stiffness of the neck

- Muscle spasms and tremors

- Grinding teeth

- Headache

- Dizziness

- Red eyes

- The eyes may stare upwards

- Irritability

- Mania

- Fever

- Thirst

- Dark red tongue without coating

- Rapid, Fine or Wiry pulse

Key symptoms
Fever cramps, stiffness in the neck, dark, red tongue and Rapid pulse.

Treatment principle
Drain *xue* Heat and calm Wind.

Acupuncture points
The person will probably be in intensive medical care. If this is not possible, or whilst waiting, you can choose from the following points: *Jing*-well points, *shixuan* (Ex-UE 11) points, UB 62, SI 3, Sp 10, LI 11, Liv 2, Liv 3, GB 20, Du 16 and Du 20.

Needle technique
Draining. Bleed *jing*-well and *shixuan* points.

Explanation

- *Jing*-well, *shixuan* points and LI 11 drain Heat.

- Liv 2 and Liv 3 drain Heat from the Liver and calm Wind.

- GB 20, Du 16 and Du 20 descend *yang* and calm Wind.

Herbal formula

- *Da Ding Feng Zhu* (Extinguishes Wind and nourishes *yin* and *xue*)

Relevant advice
The person will probably be in intensive medical care.

**Xue Heat generating Wind can be caused by
the following patterns of imbalance**

- *Qi*-level Heat

- *Ying*-level Heat

Xue Heat generating Wind can result in the following pattern of imbalance

- *Yin* and *xue xu*

Xue Heat injuring *yin*

In this pattern, the extreme Heat injures *yin*. There will be classic *yin xu* symptoms and signs, but they will be very extreme and the condition will have arisen as a consequence of an invasion of exogenous *xie qi*. There may well be an underlying *yin xu* condition, which means that when there is Heat, *yin* has greater difficulty controlling it and is more easily injured by the Heat.

Aetiology
Xie qi that has penetrated from the *qi* or *ying* level.

Symptoms and signs

- Fever that is higher in the evening and at night

- No sweating when the fever has fallen

- Red face

- Sensation of heat in the palms of the hands, soles of the feet and chest ('five palm heat')

- Dry mouth

- Weakness of the body

- Wizened body

- Deafness

- Irritability

- Restlessness

- Red tongue without coating

- Rapid and Fine pulse

Key symptoms
Fever that is worse at night, 'five palm heat', wizened body, Rapid and Fine pulse.

Treatment principle
Rescue *yin*.

Acupuncture points
Choose from: *Jing*-well points, UB 40, Sp 10, LI 11, Kid 1, Kid 3, Kid 6 and Ren 4.

Needle technique
Draining on UB 40, Sp 10 and LI 11. Tonifying on Kid 1, Kid 3, Kid 6 and Ren 4.

Explanation

- *Jing*-well points UB 40, Sp 10 and LI 11 drain *xue* Heat.

- Kid 1, Kid 3, Kid 6 and Ren 4 rescue *yin*.

Herbal formula

- *Da Bu Yin* (Rescues *yin*)

Relevant advice
The person will probably be in intensive medical care.

Xue Heat injuring _yin_ can be caused by the following patterns of imbalance

- *Qi*-level Heat

- *Ying*-level Heat

Xue Heat injuring _yin_ can result in the following pattern of imbalance

- *Yin* and *xue xu*

Yin expiring and extreme dehydration

The extreme Heat from the invasion of exogenous *xie qi* has damaged *yin* and *jinye*. This will cause the body to shrink and wither. The extremities are cold, because there is 'false Cold' due to *yin* having collapsed and the extreme Heat has bound *qi* in the body.

Aetiology
Xie qi that has penetrated from the *qi* or *ying* level.

Symptoms and signs

- Withered limbs

- Withered lips and tongue

- Dry gums

- Sunken eyes

- Unconsciousness

- Cold extremities

- Red face

- The fingers twist around each other

- Red tongue without coating

- Fine, Weak and Hidden pulse

Key symptoms
Wizened body, wizened limbs and dry gums.

Treatment principle
Rescue *yin* and drain Heat.

Acupuncture points
Choose from: *Jing*-well points, UB 40, Sp 10, LI 11, Kid 1, Kid 3, Kid 6 and Ren 4.

Needle technique
Draining on UB 40, Sp 10 and LI 11. Tonifying on Kid 1, Kid 3, Kid 6 and Ren 4.

Explanation

- *Jing*-well points, UB 40, Sp 10 and LI 11 drain *xue* Heat.

- Kid 1, Kid 3, Kid 6 and Ren 4 rescue *yin*.

Herbal formula

- *Da Bu Yin* (Rescues *yin*)

Relevant advice
The person will probably be in intensive medical care.

Yin expiring and extreme dehydration can be caused by the following patterns of imbalance

- *Qi*-level Heat

- *Ying*-level Heat

Yin expiring and extreme dehydration can result in the following pattern of imbalance

- *Yin* and *xue xu*

Diagnosis according to *San Jiao* theory

Diagnosis according to *san jiao* theory was developed by Wu Ju Tong (1758–1836 CE). Whilst he lived, his home region was affected by many epidemics, including measles, scarlet fever and smallpox. This meant that he focused his energy on the study of infectious diseases and used the Four Level diagnostic model as his starting point. Diagnosis according to *san jiao* theory was not exactly a new theory but more another way of utilising the diagnostic model of the Four Levels. Where the Four Levels analyses the progression of disease in relation to the energetic depth and severity of the symptoms, the *san jiao* model utilises a more two-dimensional analysis of the body. In this model, disease is differentiated from where in the body the disease is located and in which *jiao* the affected organs are located.

- When exogenous *xie qi* is in the upper *jiao*, the *wei qi*, Lung or Pericardium is affected. This is equivalent to the *wei*, *qi* and *ying* levels respectively in the Four Level model.

- The middle *jiao* patterns are seen when exogenous *xie qi* affects the *yangming* organs and the Spleen. This will be similar to *qi*-level Heat in the Four Levels.

- The lower *jiao* patterns are the most serious. In these patterns, the exogenous *xie qi* has affected the Kidneys and Liver. This corresponds to *xue*-level patterns in the Four Levels.

Upper jiao

When there is an invasion of exogenous *xie qi* in the upper *jiao*, it is the Lung and Pericardium that are affected. The Heart is protected by the Pericardium and therefore cannot be attacked by the exogenous *xie qi*.

An invasion of *xie qi* in the upper *jiao* may be relatively superficial, such as when exogenous *xie qi* disrupts the functioning of *wei qi*. This will be similar to the *wei* level in the Four Level model. Upper *jiao* Heat can also be deeper than the *wei* level in the Four Level model, Lung Heat in the *san jiao* model being similar to *qi*-level Heat. If the *xie qi* invades the Pericardium, it is a relatively serious condition and will correspond to *ying*-level Heat.

Xie qi can jump directly from the Lung and *wei qi* aspect to the Pericardium and the *xue* aspect. This is due to the close proximity that these two organs have to each other in the upper *jiao*.

Wind-Heat invasion in the upper *jiao*

For a description of the symptoms and pathomechanisms in this pattern, the reader is referred to the section discussing Wind-Heat in the Four Levels (page 671), as these imbalances are virtually identical.

Aetiology
Exposure to *xie* Heat.

Symptoms and signs

- Acute fever with mild aversion to wind and cold
- No or little sweating
- Throbbing headache
- Thirst
- Sore throat
- Red, swollen throat
- Cough
- Irritability
- Restlessness
- Yellowish or dried mucus in the nose
- The forehead may feel warm to the touch
- The tip of the tongue may be red and there may be a thin, yellowish coating on the front
- Rapid and Superficial pulse

Key symptoms
Fever or feverish sensation and an aversion to cold, Superficial and Rapid pulse.

Treatment principle
Expel Wind-Heat, activate *wei qi*.

Acupuncture points
Choose from: Du 14, LI 4, LI 11, Lu 7, Lu 10, Lu 11, UB 12, UB 13 and GB 20.

Needle technique
Draining. Cupping is recommended.

Explanation

- Du 14 activates *wei qi* and drains Heat.

- LI 4, LI 11, Lu 7, UB 12 and UB 13 expel Wind and Heat.

- Lu 10 and Lu 11 drain Heat from the Lung and throat.

- GB 20 expels Wind and drains *yang* from the head.

Herbal formula

- *Yin Qiao San* (Expels Wind-Heat)

Relevant advice

When there is an invasion of Wind-Heat in the upper *jiao*, it is best not to eat at all or to only eat light food. The person should drink tea that is cooling and spicy in its dynamic, such as elderflower, chrysanthemum or mint.

An invasion of Wind-Heat in the upper *jiao* can be caused by the following pattern of imbalance

- No previous pattern

An invasion of Wind-Heat in the upper *jiao* can result in the following patterns of imbalance

- Middle *jiao* Heat

- Lower *jiao* Heat

- Pericardium Heat

Damp-Heat in the upper *jiao*

This is an early stage of a Damp-Heat invasion; the Lung and the skin are affected.

For a discussion of the symptoms and pathomechanisms, please see the section describing Damp-Heat in diagnosis according to the Four Levels (page 673), as these two imbalances are virtually the same.

Aetiology

Exposure to Damp-Heat *xie qi*.

Symptoms and signs

- Fever that is highest in the afternoon

- Nausea

- Aversion to cold

- Heavy and aching arms and legs

- Poor appetite

- Abdominal bloating

- Heavy headache

- Chest oppression

- Lack of sweating or sticky sweat

- Fatigue

- Diarrhoea or constipation

- Greasy, yellow tongue coating

- Rapid and Slippery pulse

Key symptoms
Heavy headache, heaviness in the limbs, Rapid and Slippery pulse.

Treatment principle
Expel and drain Damp-Heat, activate *wei qi*.

Acupuncture points
Choose from: Du 14, LI 4, LI 11, Lu 7, Sp 3, Sp 9, Ren 12 and Pe 6.

Needle technique
Draining.

Explanation

- Du 14 drains Heat and activates *wei qi*.

- LI 4 and Lu 7 activate *wei qi* and expel *xie qi*.

- LI 11 expels *xie qi* and drains Damp-Heat.

- Sp 3 and Sp 9 drain Damp-Heat.

- Ren 12 and Pe 6 regulate the *qi* mechanism in the middle and upper *jiao*.

Herbal formula

- *Huo Po Xia Ling Tang* (Expels Damp-Heat from the exterior)

Relevant advice
When there is an invasion of Damp-Heat, the person should avoid consuming food and beverages that create Damp-Heat.

An invasion of Damp-Heat can be caused by the following pattern of imbalance

- No previous pattern

An invasion of Damp-Heat can result in the following patterns of imbalance

- Middle *jiao* Heat

- Lower *jiao* Heat

- Pericardium Heat

- Spleen *qi xu*

Lung Heat

This pattern is the same as the one discussed in *qi* level Heat in the Four Level diagnostic model; for a description of the symptoms and pathomechanisms, please see this section (page 676).

Aetiology
Exposure to *xie* Heat.

Symptoms and signs

- Fever or feeling of heat, without aversion to cold

- Cough with yellow, sticky sputum that is difficult to expectorate

- Profuse sweating

- Thirst

- Chest pain

- Dyspnoea

- Red face

- Restlessness

- Restless sleep

- Red tongue with yellow coating

- Rapid pulse

Key symptoms
Fever, cough with sticky sputum, thirst, Rapid pulse.

Treatment principle
Drain Heat from the Lung, regulate Lung *qi*.

Acupuncture points
Choose from: Lu 1, Lu 5, Lu 10, Lu 11, LI 4, Du 14 and UB 13.

Needle technique
Draining. Du 14 can be bled.

Explanation

- Lu 1, Lu 5 and UB 13 drain Heat from the Lung and regulate Lung *qi*.

- Lu 10 and Lu 11 drain Heat from the Lung.

- Du 14 and LI 11 drain *shi* Heat.

Herbal formula

- *Qin Qi Hua Tan Tang* (Drains Phlegm-Heat from the Lung)

- *Xie Bai San* (Drains Lung Heat)

Relevant advice
The person should avoid consuming food and beverages that will create additional heat in the body and avoid the inhalation of tobacco smoke.

Lung Heat can be caused by the following patterns of imbalance

- No previous pattern

- Wind-Heat

Lung Heat can result in the following patterns of imbalance

- Middle *jiao* Heat

- Lower *jiao* Heat

- Phlegm-Heat in the Lung

- Lung *yin xu*

Pericardium Heat
This corresponds to *ying*-level Heat in diagnosis according to the Four Levels; the reader is therefore referred to this section (page 687) for a description of the symptoms and pathomechanisms.

Aetiology
Exposure to *xie* Heat.

Symptoms and signs

- Fever that is worse at night

- Insomnia

- Restlessness

- Dry mouth but no thirst

- Petechiae

- Skin rashes

- Unconsciousness or coma

- Delirium

- Raving

- The skin on the torso can feel hot, but the hands and feet are icy cold

- Dark, red tongue without coating

- Rapid, Fine pulse

Key symptoms
Fever that is worse at night, dry mouth but no thirst, red tongue without coating, Rapid and Fine pulse.

Treatment principle
Drain Heat from the Pericardium and nourish *yin*. Possibly restore consciousness.

Acupuncture points
Choose from: Pe 3, Pe 8, Pe 9, Du 14, Du 26, Kid 6, Sp 10 and UB 40.

Needle technique
Draining. Bleed Pe 9, Du 26 and UB 40.

Explanation

- Pe 3, Pe 8 and Pe 9 drain Heat from the Pericardium.

- Du 26 restores consciousness.

- Du 14 drains Heat.

- UB 40 and Sp 10 drain *xue* Heat.

- Kid 6 nourishes *yin*.

Herbal formula

- *Qing Ying Tang* (Clears *ying* level Heat)

- *An Gong Niu Huang Wan* (Clears *ying* Heat and restores consciousness)

Relevant advice
The patient will probably be in biomedical treatment.

Pericardium Heat can be caused by the following patterns of imbalance

- No previous pattern

- Lung Heat

- Middle *jiao* Heat

Pericardium Heat can result in the following pattern of imbalance

- Lower *jiao* Heat

Middle jiao
The most important differentiation here is whether it is Heat or Damp-Heat that is the dominant *xie qi*. If the *xie qi* has penetrated down to the middle *jiao* and generated Heat, the pattern will correspond to Heat in the Stomach in diagnosis according to the Four Levels or the *yangming* stage in the Six Stages.

If Damp-Heat is the dominant pathogen, this will corresponds to Damp-Heat in diagnosis according to the Four Levels.

Yangming Heat
Xie Heat has directly invaded or penetrated down to the Stomach, which will correspond to the *yangming* stage and *qi*-level Stomach and Large Intestine Heat. The reader is therefore referred to the relevant section in diagnosis according to the Six Stages (page 642) and diagnosis according to the Four Levels (page 669) for a description of the symptoms and pathomechanisms.

Aetiology
Exposure to *xie* Heat.

Symptoms and signs

- Constipation or green watery diarrhoea (false diarrhoea caused by a blockage of compacted faeces in the Intestines)

- Abdominal bloating and distension that feels worse when palpated

- Fever, especially late in the afternoon, but no aversion to cold

- Profuse sweating

- Mental confusion

- Restlessness

- Frontal headache

- Bleeding gums

- Red face

- Red tongue with a dry, yellow coating

- Rapid, Full and Flooding pulse

Key symptoms
Constipation, bloated abdomen, fever, Rapid and Flooding pulse.

Treatment principle
Drain Heat from the Stomach and Large Intestine.

Acupuncture points
Choose from: LI 11, SJ 6, St 25, St 34, St 37, St 44, UB 21, UB 25 and Du 14.

Needle technique
Draining. Du 14 can be bled.

Explanation

- LI 11, SJ 6, St 25, St 37 and UB 25 drain Heat from the Stomach and Large Intestine and move *qi* in the Intestines.

- St 34, St 44 and UB 21 drain Heat from the Stomach.

- Du 14 drains *qi*-level Heat.

Herbal formula

- *Da Cheng Qi Tang* (Purges *yangming* Heat and moves *qi* in the Intestines)

Relevant advice
The patient should eat foods that are cooling and moistening in their dynamic. They should avoid foods and beverages that have a hot energy. Boiled or steamed spinach and cabbage will be beneficial, as will sauerkraut.

Yangming Heat can be caused by the following patterns of imbalance

- No previous pattern

- Upper *jiao* Heat

Yangming **Heat can result in the following pattern of imbalance**

- Lower *jiao* Heat

Spleen Damp-Heat

This pattern corresponds to the *qi*-level Damp-Heat pattern in the Four Levels; for a discussion of the symptoms and signs and their pathomechanisms, please see this section (page 673).

Aetiology
Exposure to *xie* Heat.

Symptoms and signs

- Fever that is reduced by sweating but soon rises again

- Fever that is worse in the afternoon and comes in waves

- Heavy and aching muscles, especially in the limbs

- Nausea

- Poor appetite

- Loose, sticky, odorous stools

- Abdominal distension or bloating

- Heavy and possibly pounding headache

- Difficulty in thinking clearly

- Oily skin

- Yellowish complexion

- Restlessness or irritability

- Red tongue with yellow, sticky coating

- Rapid and Slippery pulse

Key symptoms
Odorous diarrhoea, fever, yellowish, greasy tongue coating, Rapid and Slippery pulse.

Treatment principle
Drain Damp-Heat.

Acupuncture points
Choose from: Du 14, LI 11, St 25, St 44, Sp 9, Sp 6 and Ren 12.

Needle technique
Draining.

Explanation

- Du 14 and LI 11 drain Heat.

- St 25 and St 44 drain Damp-Heat from the Intestines.

- Sp 6 and Sp 9 drain Damp-Heat.

- Ren 12 drains Dampness from the middle *jiao*.

Herbal formula

- *San Ren Tang* (Drains Damp-Heat)

Relevant advice
The person should avoid consuming foods that produce Dampness or Heat.

Spleen Damp-Heat can be caused by the following patterns of imbalance

- No previous pattern

- Upper *jiao* Damp-Heat

Spleen Damp-Heat can result in the following pattern of imbalance

- Lower *jiao* Heat

Lower jiao

Xie Heat has penetrated the lower *jiao*; it will be the Liver or Kidneys that are affected and the imbalances will correspond to *xue*-level Heat in diagnosis according to the Four Levels or the *shaoyin* Heat stage of diagnosis according to the Six Stages.

There can also be a direct invasion of Damp-Heat in the Large Intestine or Urinary Bladder.

Damp-Heat in the lower jiao

It is usually the Urinary Bladder and Large Intestine that are affected in Damp-Heat in the lower *jiao*. This will resemble Damp-Heat in the middle *jiao*, but here there will be signs that the Urinary Bladder's functions are disrupted or that there is Damp-Heat in the Large Intestine.

Aetiology
Exposure to *xie* Damp-Heat.

Symptoms and signs

- Fever that is reduced by sweating but soon rises again

- Fever that is worse in the afternoon and comes in waves

- Heavy and aching muscles, especially in the limbs

- Nausea

- Poor appetite

- Difficult urination

- Painful urination

- Dark, odorous urine

- Cloudy or oily urine

- Burning pain on urination

- Loose, sticky, odorous stools

- Abdominal distension or bloating

- Heavy and possibly pounding headache

- Difficulty thinking clearly

- Oily skin

- Yellowish complexion

- Restlessness or irritability

- Red tongue with yellow, sticky coating

- Fast and Slippery pulse

Key symptoms
Odorous diarrhoea, painful urination, fever, yellowish, greasy tongue coating, Rapid and Slippery pulse.

Treatment principle
Drain Damp-Heat from the lower *jiao*.

Acupuncture points
Choose from: LI 11, St 25, St 44, Sp 9, Sp 6, Ren 3, UB 28, UB 32, UB 40 and UB 53.

Needle technique
Draining.

Explanation

- LI 11, St 25 and St 44 drain Damp-Heat from the Intestines.

- Sp 6 and Sp 9 drain Damp-Heat.

- UB 28, UB 32, UB 40 and Ren 3 drain Damp-Heat from the Urinary Bladder.

- UB 53 opens the water passages and disperses stagnation in the Urinary Bladder.

Herbal formula

- *Bai Tou Weng Tang* (Drains Damp-Heat from the Intestines)

- *Ba Zheng Wan* (Drains Damp-Heat from the Urinary Bladder)

Relevant advice
The person must avoid consuming foods that produce Dampness or Heat.

Damp-Heat in the lower *jiao* can be caused by the following patterns of imbalance

- No previous pattern

- Upper *jiao* Heat

- Middle *jiao* Heat

Damp-Heat in the lower *jiao* can result in the following pattern of imbalance

- Heat in the Liver or Kidneys

Kidney Heat

If *xie* Heat is not expelled or is treated improperly or inadequately, the Heat can damage the Kidney *yin*. This will result in Kidney *yin xu* Heat symptoms and signs.

This level corresponds to the *shaoyin* Heat Stage in diagnosis according to the Six Stages; for an explanation of pathomechanisms behind the symptoms please see this section (page 666).

Aetiology
Exposure to exogenous *xie* Heat that has injured the Kidney *yin*.

Symptoms and signs

- Irritability

- Insomnia

- Night sweats

- Mental restlessness

- Palpitations

- Malar flush

- Evening fever

- Dryness of the mouth, especially at night

- Dark and scanty urine

- Red tongue without coating, the tip of the tongue is the most red

- Rapid and Fine pulse

Key symptoms
Night sweats, insomnia, dry mouth, red tongue without coating.

Treatment principle
Nourish Kidney *yin*.

Acupuncture points
Choose from: Kid 3, Kid 6, Kid 7, Ren 4, Sp 6, UB 23 and UB 52.

Needle technique
Tonifying.

Explanation

- Kid 3, Kid 6, Kid 7, Ren 4, Sp 6, UB 23 and UB 52 nourish Kidney *yin*.

Herbal formula

- *Da Bu Yin* (Nourishes Kidney *yin*)

Relevant advice
The patient must get sufficient sleep, go to bed early and try not to overexert themselves. Coffee and other stimulants or caffeine-rich substances should be avoided because they over-activate the Heart and thereby consume *yin*. Alcohol, hot spices and grilled and fried food will all create Heat, which will further injure the *yin* and should be avoided.

Kidney Heat can be caused by the following patterns of imbalance

- Upper *jiao* Heat

- Middle *jiao* Heat

Kidney Heat can result in the following patterns of imbalance

- Liver Heat generating Wind

Liver Heat generating Wind

In this pattern, exogenous *xie qi* has injured the Liver's *yin* aspect and generated Heat in the Liver. The Heat causes Liver Wind to stir and the deficient *yin* cannot control it. This pattern corresponds to the pattern of *xue* Heat generating Wind in the Four Levels diagnostic model and the reader is referred to this section (page 691) for an explanation of the symptoms and signs and their pathomechanisms.

Aetiology
Exposure to exogenous *xie qi* that has created Heat in the Liver and injured Liver *yin*.

Symptoms and signs

- Seizures and convulsions
- Stiffness of the neck muscles
- Muscle spasms, cramps and tremors
- Grinding of the teeth
- Headache
- Dizziness
- Red eyes
- Upwardly staring eyes
- Irritability
- Mania
- Fever that is worse at night
- Thirst
- Dark, red tongue without coating
- Rapid, Fine pulse or Wiry pulse

Key symptoms
Fever cramps, stiffness of the neck muscles, dark, red tongue and rapid pulse.

Treatment principle
Drain Heat from the Liver, nourish Liver *yin* and calm Wind.

Acupuncture points
Choose from: *Jing*-well points, *shixuan* (Ex-UE 11) points, UB 62, SI 3, Sp 10, LI 4, Liv 2, Liv 3, Liv 8, GB 20, Du 16, Du 20 and Sp 6.

Needle technique
Draining, apart from Sp 6 and Liv 8, which should be tonified. The *jing*-well and *shixuan* points should be bled.

Explanation

- *Jing*-well points, *shixuan* points and LI 11 drain Heat.

- Liv 2 and Liv 3 drain Heat from the Liver and calm Wind.

- GB 20, Du 16 and Du 20 descend *yang* and calm Wind.

- Sp 6 and Liv 8 nourish Liver *yin*.

Herbal formula

- *Da Ding Feng Zhu* (Extinguishes Wind and nourishes *yin* and *xue*)

Relevant advice
The person will probably be in intensive medical care.

Liver Heat generating Wind can be caused by the following patterns of imbalance

- Upper *jiao* Heat

- Middle *jiao* Heat

- Kidney Heat

Liver Heat generating Wind can result in the following pattern of imbalance

- Kidney Heat

DIAGNOSIS ACCORDING TO THE 12 REGULAR CHANNELS

The channels and organs form a holistic structure where changes in one will affect the other. This means that the organ imbalances can manifest with a disruption of the associated channel and vice versa. Although organs and channels are inextricably linked, there can still be, and often are, imbalances in one without this manifesting in the other. Diagnostically and therapeutically, it is therefore most appropriate to diagnose them separately and use diagnosis according to *zangfu* organs to diagnose organ imbalances.

Channel imbalances can arise when a channel is invaded by exogenous *xie qi*, when there is repetitive movement or strain of a limb or joint, when there is physical trauma and when there are imbalances in the channel's related *zangfu* organ.

Diagnosis in relation to the 12 regular channels is most commonly used in the diagnosis of musculosceletal problems and *bi* syndromes.

Diagnosis in relation to the 12 channels focuses on which channels are affected. Channel diagnosis is, by definition, an exterior imbalance in relation to the Eight Principles, but the channel diagnosis can relate to an interior *zangfu* imbalance.

Diagnosis will be based on where in the body changes have manifested themselves. These changes should be seen in relation to the internal and external pathways of the 12 regular channels. It is important to determine whether there is a *xu* or a *shi* condition. Palpation of the channel is indispensable in this process. The muscles and tissue along the path of the channel should be palpated to see if there are any changes in the tissue. Changes in the tissue could be the presence of nodules, graininess in the tissue, sponginess, tightness, hardness, softness or weakness. There can also be changes in the temperature and moistness of the skin along the channel.

The size, depth and hardness of any changes along the path of the channel are also important diagnostic factors.

Tightness, hardness and tension are usually indicative of a *shi* condition in the channel or its associated organ. The more superficial the hardness, the more acute the condition is likely to be.

Softness and weakness in the tissue along the path of the channel is a sign of a *xu* condition in the channel or its associated organ. If there is a *xu* condition, the palpation will feel more pleasant for the patient than if there is a *shi* condition.

Cold and *xue* stagnation can manifest with nodules that are hard with clearly defined edges, whereas Phlegm and Dampness nodules will tend to be smoother and more slippery with less clearly defined edges.

Longer, more stick-like nodules can also be felt along the path of the channel. If the stick-like nodules are very bumpy and lie along the channel, this is a sign that it is a chronic condition that can be difficult to treat. Stick-like nodules that can be felt transverse to the path of the channel are typically acute or are due to stagnations of *qi* and are thereby easier to treat.

If the patient reports sensations of numbness whilst an area is being palpated, this can be due to Phlegm blocking the channel.

Additionally, individual acupuncture points along the channel should be palpated to see whether there is tenderness or pain or whether the patient feels the pressure is pleasurable or gives some form of relief.

There can be changes in the temperature of the skin along the channel when there is Heat or Cold in the channel.

Visual observation of the channel is also important. Heat in the channel can manifest with redness along the channel's path or with spots, pimples or other skin changes.

Observation of the joints is particularly important. This is because it is at the joints that *qi* sinks deeper into the interior or rises up to the surface. This means that it is a place where *xie qi* tend to accumulate.

Problems with sense organs and the body's orifices can often result from imbalances in the channels rather than the *zang* organ that it is controlled by. For example, many problems in the ears are due to imbalances in the Small Intestine, Gall Bladder or *san jiao* channels and not the Kidney organ.

It is important to remember in diagnosis according to the 12 regular channels, that it is not only the channel's main course that is of relevance; the channel's internal pathways, the muscle channels, the *luo*-connecting vessels and the pathways of the divergent channels must also be taken into account, as well as the channel's relationship to its partner channel and its extended channel.

Shi condition in the channel	*Xu* condition in the channel
Tenderness, tightness and tension along the channel	Weakness in the muscles and connective tissues or muscle atrophy along the channel
Tenderness or pain on palpation of the channel	Relief of pain or pleasure in palpation of the channel
Pronounced, cramping or sharp pain in the joints along the channel	Soreness, weakness, numbness or fatigue in the joints along the channel
Red colouration (Heat) or bluish colouration (Cold) along the course of the channel	Pale colour along the channel course
The channel feels warm	The channel feels cold
The relevant pulse position is Full	The relevant pulse position is Weak
Treated with draining needle techniques	Treated with tonifying needle techniques

Heat in the channel	Cold in the channel
The channel feels warm	The channel feels cold
Redness of the skin, pimples, spots or other red colourations along the path of the channel	Bluish or very white skin along the path of the channel
Pimples, spots or other red skin conditions along the path of the channel	Hard, clearly defined nodules in the tissue along the path of the channel
Inflammation, redness, dryness or yellow, sticky exudation from the sense organ or orifice that the channel connects to	Increased, watery discharges from the sense organ or orifice that the channel connects to
Burning, stinging pain in the sense organ or orifice that the channel connects to	Cramping, intense pain in the sense organ or orifice that the channel connects to

Xue stagnation in the channel
Dark or purple discolouration of the skin along the path of the channel
Sharp, stabbing pain along the path of the channel
Inhibited movement of the joint along the path of the channel
Hard, clearly defined nodules in the tissue along the path of the channel

Treatment of channel problems

The treatment of pain conditions in the channel is mainly based on: the use of local points along the course of the channel; the use of points in the local area; distal points at the opposite end of the channel, on the wrist or on the ankle. If there is a long distance between the distal point and local points, the treatment can be supplemented by using a powerful 'supporting point' somewhere on the channel in between them. This is called a 'chain and lock' treatment. For example, if there is pain in the shoulder joint corresponding to the Large Intestine channel, LI 4 can be used as a distal point and LI 15 as a local point, supplemented with the adjacent points LI 14, LI 16 and SJ 14, as well as LI 10 as a supporting point. A-*shi* points are always important in the treatment of pain conditions and blockages of *qi* and *xue* along the path of the channel.

If there is a stagnation in a joint along the course of the channel, the 'cross channel' method can be utilised. This very effective method was developed by Dr Zhou Yu Yan. In 'cross channel' theory, acupuncture points are selected on the opposite side and in the opposite limb according to where the pain is. These acupuncture points must be located either in a similar area, for example if the pain is in the lateral side of the right ankle, you will select an equivalent point on the lateral side of the left wrist, or the cross channel point should be located on the equivalent spot on the same great channel, for example St 36 on the left side to treat the area corresponding to LI 10 on the right side, because they are both *yangming* channel points and are located in similar positions along the channel.

In addition to acupuncture points on the channel and local points, other points that are relevant to the diagnosis can be used. If there is Heat, for example, acupuncture points that drain Heat can be used. If there is a *qi xu* condition in the channel, relevant *qi*-tonifying points can be used. This means that LI 10, for example, would be the relevant point to choose if there is *yangming* channel shoulder pain that is due to a *xu* condition, whereas LI 11 would be chosen if there are signs of Heat in the joint.

Luo-connecting points can also be used to regulate *qi* in the channel. These points can allow *qi* to flow to or from the partner channel. *Luo*-connecting points can also be used to regulate *qi* and *xue* in the small, superficial *luo* vessels. This is especially relevant when there are joint problems along the course of the channel, because the stagnation is often located in these small, superficial *luo* vessels.

Lung channel imbalances
Symptoms and signs

- Tenderness, weakness or pain along the course of the Lung channel

- Skin changes along course of the Lung channel

- Dyspnoea

- Sore throat

- Blocked nose

- Chest oppression

- Tenderness or pain under clavicle

- Shortness of breath

- Pimples around the nose, upper back and chest

Acupuncture treatment
Local, distal and *a-shi* points on the Lung channel, possibly combined with LI 6.

Large Intestine channel imbalances
Symptoms and signs

- Pain, weakness or tenderness along the course of the Large Intestine channel

- Skin and tissue changes along the course of the Large Intestine channel

- Sore, red and swollen throat

- Paradentosis

- Tooth pain

- Bleeding gums

- Red and swollen gums

- Shoulder pain

- Frozen shoulder

- Elbow pain

- Wrist pain

- Facial paralysis

- Nosebleeds

- Runny or blocked nose

- No sense of smell

- Red and swollen eyes

- Borborygmi

- Abdominal pain

- Ulcers, spots, acne, etc. around the mouth, on the cheekbones, upper back and chest

Acupuncture treatment
Local distal and *a-shi* points on the Large Intestine channel, possibly combined with Lu 7.

Stomach channel imbalances
Symptoms and signs

- Pain, weakness or tenderness along the course of the Stomach channel

- Skin and tissue changes along the course of the Stomach channel

- Red eyes

- Stinging or burning pain in the eyes

- Styes

- Paredentosis

- Toothache

- Bleeding gums

- Mouth ulcers

- Red and swollen gums

- Jaw pain and tension

- Nosebleeds

- Tenderness or pain in the breasts

- Sore throat and pain in the oesophagus

- Stomach ache and abdominal pain

- Facial paralysis

- Muscle wasting or muscle weakness in the legs

- Ulcers, spots, acne, etc. around the mouth, on the cheekbones, upper back and chest

Acupuncture treatment
Local distal and *a-shi* points on the Stomach channel, possibly combined with Sp 4.

Spleen channel imbalances
Symptoms and signs

- Pain, weakness or tenderness along the course of the Spleen channel

- Skin and tissue changes along the course of the Spleen channel

- Heavy, cold or weak legs

- Abdominal pain

- Vaginal discharge

Acupuncture treatment
Local distal and *a-shi* points on the Spleen channel, possibly combined with St 40.

Heart channel imbalances
Symptoms and signs

- Pain, weakness or tenderness along the course of the Heart channel

- Skin and tissue changes along the course of the Heart channel

- Chest and cardiac pain

- Pain or other sensations that radiate out from the chest along the arm

- Hot or sweaty palms

Acupuncture treatment
Local distal and *a-shi* points on the Heart channel, possibly combined with LI 7.

Small Intestine channel imbalances

Symptoms and signs

- Pain, weakness or tenderness along the course of the Small Intestine channel
- Skin and tissue changes along the course of the channel
- Ear pain
- Deafness
- Jaw pain or stiffness
- Sore or stiff neck
- Neck and shoulder tension or pain
- Elbow pain
- Fever and aversion to cold

Acupuncture treatment

Local distal and *a-shi* points on the Small Intestine channel, possibly combined with He 5.

Urinary Bladder channel imbalances

Symptoms and signs

- Pain, weakness or tenderness along the course of the Urinary Bladder channel
- Skin and tissue changes along the course of the channel
- Sore eyes
- Sinus pain
- Headache
- Sore or stiffness in the neck
- Back pain
- Sore or stiffness in the lower back or sacrum
- Pain along the back of the legs
- Sciatica
- Blocked nose
- Nosebleeds
- Fever and aversion to cold

Acupuncture treatment
Local distal and *a-shi* points on the Urinary Bladder channel, possibly combined with Kid 4.

Kidney channel imbalances
Symptoms and signs

- Pain, weakness or tenderness along the course of the Kidney channel
- Skin and tissue changes along the course of the channel
- Lumbar soreness
- Sore knees
- Sore ankles
- Sore feet
- Dry throat

Acupuncture treatment
Local distal and *a-shi* points on the Kidney channel, possibly combined with UB 58.

Pericardium channel imbalances
Symptoms and signs

- Pain, weakness or tenderness along the course of the Pericardium channel
- Skin and tissue changes along the course of the channel
- Cardiac pain
- Chest pain

Acupuncture treatment
Local distal and *a-shi* points on the Pericardium channel, possibly combined with SJ 5.

San jiao channel imbalances
Symptoms and signs

- Pain, weakness or tenderness along the course of the *san jiao* channel
- Skin and tissue changes along the course of the *san jiao* channel
- Sore eyes or eye pain

- Red eyes

- Ear pain

- Deafness

- Exudation from the ears

- Sore throat

- Stiffness and pain in the shoulders

- Elbow pain

- Alternating fever and chills

Acupuncture treatment
Local distal and *a-shi* points on the *san jiao* channel, possibly in combination with Pe 6.

Gall Bladder channel imbalances
Symptoms and signs

- Pain, weakness or tenderness along the course of the Gall Bladder channel, especially when there is pain or soreness of the eyes, ears, jaw, the side of the head, the neck, shoulders, hip, the side of the ribs and the side of the legs

- Skin and tissue changes along the course of the channel

- Hemilateral headache

- Red eyes

- Exudation from the ears

- Deafness

- Alternating fever and chills

Acupuncture treatment
Local distal and *a-shi* points on the Gall Bladder channel, possibly combined with Liv 5.

Liver channel imbalances
Symptoms and signs

- Pain, weakness or tenderness along the course of the Liver channel

- Skin and tissue changes along the course of the Liver channel

- Pimples or spots around the mouth up to or during menstruation

- Sores and ulcers around the mouth or the genitals

- Pain or tenderness in the groin

- Incomplete or difficult urination

- Genital pain or tenderness

- Impotence

- Permanent erection

- Abdominal pain

- Painful eyes

- Headache

- Leg cramps

- Lump in the throat

Acupuncture treatment
Local distal and *a-shi* points on the Liver channel, possibly combined with GB 37.

DIAGNOSIS ACCORDING TO THE EIGHT EXTRAORDINARY VESSELS

Diagnosis is based on the observation of changes in the functions or structures that are controlled by the eight extraordinary vessels.

Du mai and *ren mai* have their own channel points, whereas the other extraordinary vessels 'borrow' points from other channels, and the course of these extraordinary vessels partly follows the course of more than one regular channel. This means that they can be treated locally with points that are meeting points, i.e. acupuncture points where two or more channels meet. GB 20 is, for example, an acupuncture point on the Gall Bladder channel, but it is also a point on *yang qiao mai*, *yang wei mai*, as well as an acupuncture point where the *san jiao* channel meets with the Gall Bladder channel. This means that this acupuncture point can treat multiple channels at the same time.

As was seen in Section 10, 'Diagnosis According to the 12 Regular Channels', it is important to remember that the channels have both internal and external pathways and that there can be branches of the channel that separate from the main channel. This means that there can be symptoms and signs in places other than along the path of the external vessel.

Treatment of the extraordinary vessels

The most popular approach to activating the extraordinary vessels is to use combinations of so-called opening points. These acupuncture points, which are not usually located along the course of the extraordinary vessel, can be understood as being a key that activates the *qi* in the extraordinary vessel. In this approach the opening point will either be used alone to activate the vessel or used in combination with acupuncture points along the channel.

The opening points that most people agree upon when activating the extraordinary vessels are as follows.

- *Du mai* – SI 3

- *Ren mai* – Lu 7

- *Chong mai* – Sp 4

- *Dai mai* – GB 41

- *Yang qiao mai* – UB 62

- *Yin qiao mai* – Kid 6

- *Yang wei mai* – SJ 5

- *Yin wei mai* – Pe 6

In addition to using the opening point of an extraordinary vessel, most people recommend coupling the opening point with a so-called partner point. These acupuncture points are also opening points, but for one of the other extraordinary vessels that is believed to have a relationship with the vessel that is to be activated.

The most common approach is to insert the first needle of the treatment in the opening point of the extraordinary vessel that is to be activated. The next acupuncture point that is needled will then be the opening point of the partner vessel. Only after these needles have been inserted, and in this order, will the remaining needles be inserted in the other acupuncture points that are to be utilised in the treatment. At the end of the treatment, the needles will be removed again in reverse order, i.e. the needle inserted in the partner vessel's opening point will be taken out, as the penultimate needle to be removed and vessel's own opening point, last.

Maciocia writes that the opening point should be used on the right-hand side of women and the partner opening point on the left-hand side (Maciocia 2005, p.832). This will be reversed in the treatment of men, with the opening point being activated on the left-hand side and partner opening point on the right-hand side. Personally, I generally use the opening and partner opening points bilaterally, but will still insert the first needle in the opening point of the extraordinary vessel on the left-hand side in men and right-hand side in women, because there is no reason not to do it in that order.

Below is the most common presentation of opening point/partner opening point relations among the extraordinary vessels.

- Lu 7 (*ren mai*)/Kid 6 (*yin qiao mai*)

- SI 3 (*du mai*)/UB 62 (*yang qiao mai*)

- Sp 4 (*chong mai*)/Pe 6 (*yin wei mai*)

- GB 41 (*dai mai*)/SJ 5 (*yang wei mai*)

As was the case with the regular channels, local and distal points can be used along the pathway of the vessel to activate *qi* in the vessel. For example, it is possible to use Du 3 and Du 4 as *du mai* local points and Du 26 as a distal point in the treatment of lower back pain. This can be done both with or without the use of the vessel's opening and partner opening point.

Du mai imbalances
Symptoms and signs

- Aches, pains, weaknesses or problems along the path of the vessel, especially pain in the spine, tail bone, neck

- Imbalances along the spine

- Headache

- Nasal problems

- Seizures, convulsions and tremors

- Haemorrhoids

- Rectal prolapse

- Tinnitus

- Fever and aversion to cold

- Manic behaviour

- Depression

- Superficial and Long pulse in the left-hand pulse positions

Acupuncture treatment
SI 3, UB 62, local, distal and tender points along the course of the *du mai*.

Ren mai imbalances
Symptoms and signs

- Soreness, weakness, pain or problems along the path of the vessel, especially pain in the abdomen, chest and neck

- Infertility

- Irregular menstrual periods

- Amenorrhoea

- Hot flushes

- Night sweats

- Urinary disorders

- Involuntary ejaculation

- Accumulations in the abdominal cavity

- Thin, Tight and Long pulse in both *cun* positions

Acupuncture treatment
Lu 7, Kid 6, local, distal and tender points along the course of the *ren mai*.

Chong mai imbalances

Symptoms and signs

- Aches, pains, weaknesses or problems along the path of the vessel, especially pain in the abdomen, uterus and chest

- Irregular menstrual periods

- Dysmenorrhoea

- Clotted menstrual blood

- PMS

- Purple, painful spots around the mouth during and up to the menstruation

- Restlessness or turmoil rising up from the abdomen to the chest and the neck (running piglet *qi*)[27]

- Anxiety

- Shortness of breath

- Nausea and vomiting

- Infertility

- Palpitations

- Muscular atrophy in the legs

- Warm sensation in the face

- Cold and purple feet

- Hot flushes and night sweats during menopause

- Deep and Confined pulse in both *guan* positions or in all positions on both sides. The pulse may also be Wiry in both *guan* positions

Acupuncture treatment

Sp 4, Pe 6, local, distal and tender points along the path of the *chong mai*.

Dai mai imbalances

Symptoms and signs

- Aches, pains, weaknesses or problems along the path of the vessel, especially pain in the hip and waist region

- Abdominal bloating

- A sensation of sitting in a tub of cold water

- Vaginal discharge
- Irritability
- Lumbar weakness
- Uterine prolapse
- Miscarriages
- Infertility
- Burning and difficult urination
- Cold feet
- Weakness and muscle atrophy in the legs
- Dragging, heavy menstrual pain
- Cold or moist genitals
- Heaviness and fatigue of the whole body
- Wiry pulse in both *guan* positions that vibrates from side to side

Acupuncture treatment
GB 41, SJ 5, local, distal and tender points along the course of the *dai mai*.

Yin qiao mai imbalances
Symptoms and signs

- Aches, pains, weaknesses or problems along the path of the vessel, especially problems with the neck and eyes
- Dry throat
- Dry eyes
- Insomnia
- Constipation
- Urinary problems
- Uterine bleeding
- Irregular menstrual bleeding
- Tightness, weakness or atrophy in the muscles of the inner side of the legs
- The feet point inwards
- Uneven hips or one leg is longer than the other

- Cramps and spasms at night

- Leg cramps

- Wiry pulse in both *chi* positions and the pulse vibrates from side to side

Acupuncture treatment
Kid 6, Lu 7, local, distal and tender points along the course of the *yin qiao mai*.

Yang qiao mai imbalances
Symptoms and signs

- Aches, pains, weaknesses or problems along the path of the vessel, especially problems with the neck, lower back, hips, eyes and head

- Insomnia or narcolepsy

- Cramps and spasms

- Hemilateral paralysis

- Facial paralysis

- Headache

- Dizziness

- Tension, weakness or atrophy of the muscles of the outside of the legs

- Sciatic pain where the pain is along both the back and outer side of the leg

- The feet point outwards

- Structural imbalances between the right and left, e.g. one leg is longer than the other or one shoulder is higher than the other

- Red eyes

- Manic behaviour

- Wiry pulse in both *cun* positions and the pulse can vibrate from side to side

Acupuncture treatment
UB 62, SI 3, local, distal and tender points along the course of the *yang qiao mai*.

Yin wei mai imbalances
Symptoms and signs

- Aches, pains, weaknesses or problems along the path of the vessel, especially in the heart, chest and ribs

- Headache

- Anxiety

- Insomnia

- Mental unrest

- Depression

- Sadness

- Poor memory

- Palpitations

- The pulse in the *chi* position rolls towards the thumb or up to the *cun* position and is deep, wide and *shi*

Acupuncture treatment
Pe 6, Sp 4, local, distal and tender points along the course of the *yin wei mai*.

Yang wei mai imbalances
Symptoms and signs

- Aches, pains, weaknesses or problems along the path of the vessel, especially along the lateral side of the body and leg

- Alternating fever and chills

- Dizziness

- Earache

- Deafness

- Tinnitus

- Stiff neck

- The pulse in the *chi* position rolls towards the little finger or towards the *cun* position and is superficial, broad and *shi*

Acupuncture treatment
SJ 5, GB 41, local, distal and tender points along the course of the *yang wei mai*.

Section 12

DIAGNOSIS ACCORDING TO THE FIVE PHASES

The diagnosis according to the Five Phases is not used much in modern Chinese medicine. It is, however, used more in countries such as Vietnam, Korea and Japan. In the West, this diagnosis model is used mainly by students of the JR Worsley Five Element tradition.

In this diagnostic model, symptoms and signs are differentiated in relation to the *sheng* (creative) cycle and the *ke* (controlling) cycle.

There are three main possibilities for imbalance within this model: a phase not nourishing and tonifying the subsequent phase in the *sheng* cycle, for example Water not nourishing Wood; a phase dominating another phase in the *ke* cycle, for example, Fire dominates Metal; a phase that instead of being controlled by another phase, becomes too strong and 'insults' the phase that should have controlled it, for example Metal 'insulting' Fire.

The imbalances are treated by drawing *qi* via the phase points on the various channels so that the *xu* phase is tonified and the *shi* phase drained.

Sheng phase patterns

In these patterns of imbalance, the mother phase does not nourish the child, i.e. the next phase in the *sheng* cycle. There will be signs and symptoms that the organ of the son phase is *xu*.

The pattern is treated by using the mother point on the deficient organ's channel. For example, if there is a deficiency in the Wood Phase, the mother point of the Liver channel can be tonified. In this example, Liv 8 would be tonified, as it is the Water point on the Liver channel.

Wood not generating Fire

This corresponds to the *zangfu* pattern of Heart and Gall Bladder *qi xu*.

Symptoms and signs

- Being easily startled

- Shyness

- Nervousness

- Lack of courage

- Indecision

- Insomnia, especially waking early in the morning and not being able to fall asleep again

- Difficulty making decisions

- Pale face

- Poor memory

- Palpitations

- Weak pulse in the left *cun* position

Acupuncture treatment
He 9, which is the Heart channel's Wood point, should be tonified.

Fire not generating Earth
This is similar to the *zangfu* pattern of Kidney and Spleen *yang xu*.

Symptoms and signs
- Loose stools

- Poor appetite

- Aversion to cold

- Weakness of the arms and legs

- Cold limbs

- Abdominal bloating

- Oedema

- Pale complexion

- Weak pulse in the right *guan* position

Acupuncture treatment
Sp 2, which is the Spleen channel's Fire point, should be tonified.

Earth not generating Metal
This is similar to the *zangfu* pattern of Lung Phlegm-Dampness caused by Spleen *qi xu*.

Symptoms and signs

- Cough with loose sputum

- Phlegm in the throat

- Fatigue

- Slight breathlessness

- Pale complexion

- Weak pulse in the right *cun* position

Acupuncture treatment
Lu 9, which is the Lung channel's Earth point, should be tonified.

Metal not generating Water

This is similar to the *zangfu* pattern of Kidney and Lung *yin xu* and Kidney *qi* not grasping Lung *qi*.

Symptoms and signs

- Dyspnoea

- Shortness of breath

- Slight breathlessness

- Weak voice

- Sparse and dark urination

- Weak knees

- Lumbar soreness

- Dry, tickling cough

- Dry throat

- Weak pulse in the left *guan* position

Acupuncture treatment
Kid 7, which is the Kidney channel's Metal point, should be tonified.

Water not generating Wood

This is similar to the *zangfu* pattern of Liver and Kidney *yin xu*.

Symptoms and signs

- Dizziness

- Headache

- Difficulty focusing the eyes

- Dry eyes

- Tinnitus

- Lumbar soreness

- Weak knees

- Emaciated body

- Weak pulse in the left *guan* position

Acupuncture treatment
Liv 8, which is the Liver channel's Water point, should be tonified.

Ke phase dominating patterns

In these imbalances the 'controlling' phase dominates the phase that succeeds it in the *ke* cycle. There will be signs and symptoms that the controlling phase is *shi* and that the controlled phase is *xu*.

These patterns will be treated by draining *qi* from the phase that dominates the succeeding phase in the *ke* cycle. For example, if the Metal Phase dominates the Wood Phase, the Metal Phase's son point, which is Lu 5, is drained. The deficient phase can then be tonified via its mother point, in this case Liv 8.

Wood dominates Earth

This pattern corresponds to the *zangfu* imbalance of Liver *qi* invading the Spleen.

Symptoms and signs

- Abdominal bloating

- Hypochondriac pain or distension

- Irritability

- Loose stools

- Poor appetite

- Nausea

- Greenish tinge to the complexion

- Headache

- Flatulence

- Fatigue

- Full pulse in left *guan* position and a Weak pulse in the right *guan* position

Acupuncture treatment
The Liver's Fire point, Liv 2, is drained and the Spleen's Fire point, Sp 2, is tonified.

Earth dominates Water

This pattern is similar to an accumulation of fluids due to Kidney and Spleen *yang xu*.

Symptoms and signs

- Oedema

- Lack of thirst

- Difficult or frequent urination

- Yellowish face

- Cold limbs

- Fatigue

- The right *guan* pulse is Full and right *chi* pulse is Weak

Acupuncture treatment
The Spleen's Metal point, Sp 5, is drained and the Kidney's Metal point, Kid 7, is tonified.

Water dominates Fire

This pattern is similar to the *zangfu* patterns of Heart and Kidney *yang xu*, overflowing water.

Symptoms and signs

- Oedema of the ankles and legs

- Aversion to cold

- Lumbar soreness

- Dizziness

- Palpitations

- Cough with watery sputum

- Slight breathlessness

- Weak pulse in the left *cun* position, Full pulse in the left *chi* position

Acupuncture treatment
The Kidney's Wood point, Kid 1, is drained and the Heart's Wood point, He 9, is tonified.

Fire dominates Metal
This pattern corresponds to the *zangfu* patterns of Lung Heat or Lung Phlegm-Heat.

Symptoms and signs

- Loud cough with yellowish, sticky sputum

- Fever or an aversion to heat

- Thirst

- Red face

- Full pulse in the left *cun* position and a Weak pulse at the right *cun* position

Acupuncture treatment
The Heart's Earth point, He 7, is drained and the Lung's Earth point, Lu 9, is tonified.

Metal dominates Wood
This pattern corresponds to the *zangfu* patterns Lung and Liver *qi* stagnation.

Symptoms and signs

- Fatigue

- Irritability

- Hypochondriac tension or chest oppression

- Dyspnoea

- Cough

- White face

- Weak pulse in the left *guan* position and a Full pulse in the right *cun* position

Acupuncture treatment
The Metal's Water point, Lu 5, is drained and the Liver's Water point, Liv 8, is tonified.

Ke phase 'insulting' patterns

In these imbalances the 'controlling' phase is dominated or 'insulted' by the phase that comes after it in the *ke* cycle. There will be signs and symptoms that the phase that should be controlled by the other phase is *shi*, while the phase that should be the controlling phase in the *ke* cycle will be *xu*.

The imbalance can be treated by draining the son point of the insulting phase's channel. For example, if the Wood Phase insults Metal, the Wood Phase's son point is drained. In this example, Liv 2 would be drained. The deficient phase can then be tonified via its mother point, in this case Lu 9.

Wood insults Metal

This pattern is similar to the *zangfu* pattern of Liver Fire invading the Lung.

Symptoms and signs

- Cough with yellowish or bloody sputum

- Dyspnoea

- Chest oppression and hypochondriac tension

- Irritability

- The left *guan* pulse position is Full

Acupuncture treatment
The Liver's Fire point, Liv 2, is drained and the Lung's Earth point, Lu 9, is tonified.

Metal insults Fire

This pattern corresponds to the *zangfu* patterns of Lung and Heart *qi xu*.

Symptoms and signs

- Palpitations

- Insomnia

- Lack of joy

- Shortness of breath

- The right *cun* pulse is Full

Acupuncture treatment
The Lung's Water point, Lu 5, is drained and the Heart's Wood point, He 9, is tonified.

Fire insults Water

This pattern is similar to the *zangfu* patterns of Kidney and Heart *yin xu* Heat.

Symptoms and signs

- Palpitations

- Insomnia

- Dry mouth at night

- Dry throat

- Lumbar soreness

- Malar flush

- Dizziness

- The left *cun* position is Full and the left *chi* pulse is Weak

Acupuncture treatment
The Heart's Earth point, He 7, is drained and the Kidney's Metal point, Kid 7, is tonified.

Water insults Earth

This pattern corresponds to the *zangfu* pattern of Spleen and Kidney *yang xu*.

Symptoms and signs

- Loose stools

- Oedema

- Aversion to cold

- Fatigue

- Weak limbs

- The left *chi* position is Full and right *guan* position is Weak

Acupuncture treatment
The Kidney's Wood point, Kid 1, is drained and the Spleen's Fire point, Sp 2, is tonified.

Earth insults Wood

This pattern corresponds to the *zangfu* pattern Liver Damp-Heat.

Symptoms and signs

- Jaundice

- Hypochondriac tension or pain

- Nausea

- Loose stools

- The right *guan* position is Full and the left *guan* position is Weak

Acupuncture treatment

The Spleen's Metal point, Sp 5, is drained and the Liver's Water point, Liv 8, is tonified.

Appendix 1

SUPPORTING THE TREATMENT OF
THE PATIENT THROUGH *YANGSHEN*

In Chinese culture, there is a concept called *yangshen* – to nurture life. *Yangshen* includes all the possible physical and spiritual practices that can be utilised to strengthen and nourish not only the physical body, but also the *shen*. *Yangshen* includes everything from dietary principles, various forms of exercise such as qi gong and tai ji, and meditation techniques to diverse sexual practices. *Yangshen* is relevant to us as practitioners of Chinese medicine in the West, as there is a concept in Chinese medicine that is summarised in the saying: 'Seven parts care and three parts treatment.' Care in this context denotes dietary and lifestyle changes. For a patient to get the maximum effect from an acupuncture or a Chinese medicine herbal treatment, it is important that the patient supports their treatment through dietary and lifestyle changes. This is because their patterns of imbalance have not arisen by themselves but are the consequence of various aetiological factors. Many patterns of imbalance emerge directly and indirectly from dietary factors and through either too much, too little or incorrect exercise. Furthermore, although diet and exercise were not directly involved in the creation of the imbalances, they can often be used to influence the body in a positive direction. The best results will be achieved if the patient addresses the factors that are helping to create and/or aggravate their patterns of imbalance. We can treat the patient with as many needles and elegant point combinations as we like, but if the patient does not address the root cause of their imbalances, the imbalances will often just regenerate themselves. It is not uncommon that it is only when a patient begins to comply with the advice that they have been given that there is a significant and lasting change in their condition. Often the greatest help that we can give our patients is to give them the tools to heal themselves. This can be acupuncture points that they can press on or treat themselves with moxa, or it could be advice with regard to diet, exercise, relaxation, meditation or breathing exercises. By giving the right advice to each individual patient, we can give this person the power to take control of their own life, so that they control their patterns of imbalance and their patterns of imbalance do not control them. To some people, this might sound as if we thereby erode our own economic foundation as a therapist. First, our primary motivation as therapists should always be to help others in the most effective way possible and should not be financially determined. Second, you will achieve quicker and better results when the patient cooperates and makes changes in the factors contributing to their problem. Patients who get well, particularly patients who get well quickly, are the best advertising you can get as a therapist.

Cooperating with the patient

Nutrition and lifestyle recommendations are only effective if the patient puts the recommendations into practice. Even the very best advice will have absolutely no effect if the patient does not follow these recommendations. In fact, advice that is not put into practice can quickly turn into a guilty conscience, which can itself become an aetiological factor that creates new, or exacerbates existing, patterns of imbalance in the patient.

There can be many reasons why patients have difficulty complying with the recommendations you give them.

Lack of time and energy

This is especially relevant in relation to things such as exercise, meditation and dietary changes that involve the preparation of food in a different way. Many people ought to be able to find time during the day to meditate for 20 minutes, but the spare time that they do have is often consumed by Facebook, watching television, playing games on their smartphone and so on. However, there are people who literally do not have any free time due to the pressures of work, family and other obligations. This means that you should be realistic in the recommendations that you give to them. At the same time, it is often important that precisely these people do try and create a space for themselves in their lives. This is because you can hear that these people are constantly active, constantly *yang*. These people have an even greater need to have some time while they are awake where they are in a more *yin* state.

When people find it difficult to find time during the day to meditate, practice qi gong or do something similar, you can suggest that they get up 20 minutes earlier each day. Even though they lose a little sleep, the benefit they receive from the meditation, qi gong, etc. will often more than offset the lost sleep.

Exercise can also be integrated into the daily routine of people whose time is limited. You can suggest that they bike to work instead of taking the bus or driving or that they take the stairs instead of using the elevator and so on.

Other people do actually have the time, but they do not use it ideally. These people need to have more self-discipline and this may require stricter words from their therapist.

Finally, you can also remind people who say that they are too busy to meditate, of the Zen proverb: 'Everyone should meditate for 20 minutes each day, except those who are too busy. They should meditate for one hour.'

Difficulty adhering to dietary recommendations

When we start to tinker with people's eating habits, we must be aware that there are many reasons why people eat. They do not eat only to create *qi* (or in Western physiology to ingest nutrients such as carbohydrates, oils, proteins, minerals, vitamins and so on).

We mainly eat for a whole host of other reasons, most of these being psycho-emotional reasons:

- habit
- social interaction with friends and family
- traditions
- culture
- pleasure

- business meetings

- social gatherings

- desire

- cravings

- boredom

- comfort

- security

- reward

- procrastination

- curiosity

- fashion and fads

- beliefs

- therapy

- patterns of imbalance such as Stomach Fire.

Something we should keep in mind when we give people dietary advice is the very first experience this person had when they left the dark, warm, secure and quiet existence of their mother's womb and entered into a noisy, scary world. This experience was to be taken up to their mother's breast, hear her heartbeat, feel her warmth and have something sweet enter into their mouth. When they cried as a baby, whether it was because they were hungry, had pain or were insecure, their mouth and stomach was filled with sweet breast milk or sweet formula from a bottle. In this way a connection was formed between the consumption of something sweet and comfort and security at a time when their psyche was in the process of being formed.

The connection between the consumption of something that tastes good, especially something sweet, and emotional well-being was reinforced for many people when they were given something sweet to eat if they had fallen or hurt themselves as a child. A person may also have been rewarded with something sweet when they had excelled themselves or been good. Christmas, birthdays and other celebrations were often social gatherings that were associated with happy memories, but also subconsciously with the consumption of something sweet.

From a Chinese medicine perspective, not only will the Spleen and thereby *gu qi* have been nourished in these situations, but also the sweet taste will have become inextricably associated with pleasure, comfort and social contact – things that nourish the Heart *qi* and the *shen*. It is therefore no wonder that many people comfort eat, especially cake, sweets and chocolate when they are sad, are insecure, feel challenged or are just bored.

Furthermore, we know that most of the patients we meet in the clinic are Spleen *qi xu* and will therefore also have cravings for the sweet taste. This is because it is the body's signal to the mind that it is time to take action and strengthen the Spleen *qi*.

Furthermore, people with Stomach Fire, who again form a significant proportion of the clients we see, will have an increased or an insatiable appetite.

All these factors can make it difficult for the person to control their dietary intake in a reasonable and appropriate manner.

Conflicting advice

Another problem we have to deal with is that our advice may be in conflict not only with the advice given to the patient by their Western medical doctor, but also with the advice they have received from other practitioners of complementary medicine.

Some clients are used to our perception of what is healthy being at odds with the views of Western medicine, and some even expect this. Unfortunately, it is not rare that other complementary medicine therapists have given them advice that we do not necessarily think is appropriate to their condition or their constitution. Fortunately, there will most often be consistency between our advice and that of others. For example, it is typical that when there is Damp-Heat and Spleen *qi xu*, the patient may have been diagnosed as having a candida imbalance by a naturopath. However, a difference in this situation could be that we may also have diagnosed Liver *qi* stagnation. This means that even though there will be no conflict between the foods we think that they should stay away from and the foods the naturopath has proscribed, we will often be more flexible and less restrictive in our recommendations than the naturopath is. This is because we do not want to create frustration and irritation in the patient by giving them too many rules and restrictions. Furthermore, we may well also have recommended exercise and discussed the effect that frustration and irritation can have on their imbalances.

Where we often come into conflict with the advice and opinions of both Western and complementary medicine practitioners is with regard to how much water a person should drink and the use of ice when there is a physical injury. In these situations, our advice can sometimes seem almost heretical.

The problem is that clients with chronic conditions – i.e. those who make up the bulk of our client base – are often people who see several therapists simultaneously or consecutively. This can result in confusion when they get conflicting advice from the different practitioners.

The only things we can do are to try to:

- find a common denominator in the advice that they have been given and our advice

- be convincing in our explanation of how we comprehend their body's physiology, pathology and aetiological factors.

Lack of familiarity with or access to certain foods

It is important to remember that not everyone is familiar with the foods that we recommend. We may have eaten tofu all our lives, whereas the patient has never even heard of it. Furthermore, a patient living in the countryside will often not have the same access to the variety of foods that are available in a large city. This means that we must be realistic in our dietary advice, tailoring and modifying it so that it is relevant to each individual client.

Their children and partner eat differently

It can be difficult for a person to alter their diet radically when they live and eat with other people, for example a husband and two children. Even though they are willing to change their eating habits, the rest of the family may not have the same motivation.

It can complicate the situation if several members of the same family are being treated and they have patterns of imbalance that require conflicting dietary approaches.

Ethical reasons

Some people find it difficult to change the diet in an appropriate direction due ethical principles. This could be a vegan patient who is extremely *xue xu*. Our job is to educate people about the causes and effects of, as well as the possibilities to positively influence, their imbalances. They can then make their own choices; we should not be the judge of these choices.

Desire, enjoyment

Our advice will often conflict with a person's desires and passions. As I just wrote, I think it is important that we present people with the information that can improve their condition, but from then on it is their own choice. This is especially important when people do things that from a Chinese medicine perspective are detrimental to their health. They often do these things because they give pleasure or because, in fact, they help to ameliorate another pattern of imbalance. Some people, for example, do excessive physical training because it relieves their Liver *qi* stagnation. If they did not exercise as much they do, the symptoms and signs of their Liver *qi* stagnation would be accentuated. This creates a conundrum if they are simultaneously Liver *xue xu*. The excessive physical training relieves their Liver *qi* stagnation but is also an aetiological factor in their Liver *xue xu*.

It is also a complicating factor when inappropriate behaviour or diet are sources of pleasure and enjoyment. By stopping someone from drinking a glass of red wine in the evening or running 20 kilometres in the woods three times a week, we remove something from their life that is nourishing their Heart *qi*. In these cases, it is important to try and find something else that gives them pleasure or something that they are passionate about so that we do not exacerbate or create a new pattern of imbalance in their Heart.

Their patterns of imbalance mean that they have difficulty complying with the recommendations

A person with Spleen *qi xu* will often have a very sweet tooth. Their craving for sweetness will make it difficult for them to avoid eating sugar, sweets, cakes, honey, dried fruit and so on. They could also have a Heart imbalance that means that they comfort eat these sweet things.

It is important that the patient does not feel that we judge them. They are often very good at doing this themselves without our help. It is, of course, a balancing act – trying to be strict enough that they adhere to our recommendations but at the same time not creating feelings of guilt and inadequacy when they don't succeed in doing what is best. We must find a way to support and help them without them feeling judgement on our part.

How do you get people to comply with your advice?

The greatest chance of relieving and preventing the recurrence of a disorder in a patient exists when the person actively participates and cooperates in their treatment by making relevant changes in their diet and lifestyle. In order to get the patient to assist in their treatment, it is important to explain to the patient which patterns of imbalance they have and how these patterns may have arisen; then you can tell them what they can do to help promote the healing process. Most patients are interested in making relevant changes, especially when they can see a logic in the advice they are given. When explaining to patients which patterns of imbalance they have and how these have arisen, it is, of course, important to explain these concepts so they are understandable to a layman who has not had a three-year training as an acupuncturist.

As well as there being differences in what advice you would give to each individual patient, there are also differences in how to present this advice to different people, especially in relation to the amount and the extent of the changes that they should make. All of this will, of course, depend upon the patient's patterns of imbalance. Some clients will get overwhelmed or give up if you give them too much information and too much advice in one go; others can accommodate more and will be more motivated to change their habits and diet. It is often a case of suggesting small, realistic changes. It is difficult enough to change long-term habits in general, but this is even more complicated with regards to the diet. This is because there are so many factors that come into play in relation to why we eat, what we eat and how we eat it. For some, the situation is further complicated by the fact that they are not fully in control of what they eat. This may be because they eat in the canteen at work, share their meals with others or frequently have to eat out.

Implementing 75 per cent changes that are maintained for weeks, months or years is often not only more realistic but also more beneficial than making a 100 per cent change for 14 days or three weeks, only to return to the original diet because the dietary changes were too hard to maintain. It is hoped that when the patient makes relevant changes in their diet, they will experience an improvement in their symptoms. Often they will also experience a deterioration of their symptoms when they at some point do eat what is detrimental for them. This will in itself create a motivation to continue with the dietary changes. It will also result in a completely different *qi* dynamic. They will no longer experience the dietary changes as a set of rules and restrictions dictated by their therapist, something that may cause their Liver *qi* to stagnate and prevent them from consuming things that give them pleasure (i.e. nourishing their Heart). Now they begin to experience motivation. They, for example, no longer want to eat wheat and cheese because this will result in a state of discomfort and they feel better when they don't. This motivation will have a completely different effect on their *qi* to a perceived ban. It may even end up benefiting their Heart because they now feel that they are doing something that is good for them and are taking care of themselves, which makes them happy, thereby nourishing their Heart *qi*. It is enormously important that our advice does not become an aetiological factor in their imbalances. This is especially important when they do not live up to their own expectations and their perceptions of our expectations. This can result in feelings of guilt and a lack of self-esteem, which will have a negative impact on their Liver and Heart *qi*.

Undergoing a course of treatment – any treatment that involves having to make changes in your diet and lifestyle habits – is something all therapists should try. It helps to create a sense of understanding when a client has difficulty conforming to the advice we give them. I sometimes share with my clients my own experiences and failings as a client of others. It can be a relief for them and their conscience to know that I am not different from them. It also helps to bring me down from the pedestal that they often have put me up upon.

There are, though, other types of clients who benefit from a more stern approach where you are more strict and give them little leeway, either because of the severity of their condition or because of the type of person that they are. This means that we must constantly adjust our approach from client to client – sometimes being strict, sometimes being understanding and accommodating, sometimes being humorous and sometimes being stern.

The severity of the patient's condition will usually be a significant factor. A person who has a slight aching in their lower back will probably be less motivated to make major changes in their life, than someone who has just been diagnosed with a serious heart problem.

The verbal strategies you that you utilise in all these situations will depend on your own character and temperament, as well as that of your client. I do not think there are any hard-and-fast rules of how to get clients to comply with therapeutic recommendations and each situation must be tackled individually.

In general, it is best to dose your advice and only give the patient new challenges once they have implemented the previous ones.

Resistance to giving things up

It is typical for most clients to ask: 'What can I eat or what can I take that will be good for me?' Unfortunately, a lot of the dietary advice that I then give tells them what they should avoid in their diet, as well as recommending exercise, rest, meditation and so on. As I list the foods they should avoid, they often exclaim: 'But there must be something that will be good for me to eat, something that is beneficial?' Here we can see a fundamental problem with our Western consumer mentality. We have developed an expectation that we can purchase or consume a solution. Every time that we are dissatisfied or when life does not live up to our expectations, we believe that there must be something we can buy or at least assume that there will be something that will be salutary for us to consume – some sort of magical pill or superfood. In general, we have more difficulty with the more Eastern, esoteric approach that happiness – in this context healing – is a process of letting go of of things. Eastern philosophies have often focused on abandoning the bonds of materialism, letting go of bad habits and ultimately letting go of the ego. Usually, the healing process of the physical body is also about avoiding certain foods and letting go of bad habits. This is because it is these things that have given rise to the problematical condition. Simply consuming something new – something additional – does not remove the causes of the problem. In fact, it increases the risk of creating a new problem. For example, if a person has a Fire condition, it will be beneficial for them not to consume things like chilli, alcohol, pepper, garlic, lamb, cinnamon, chips, crisps, fried food and so on. If they do not drop these things and instead just consume foods that are extremely cold in their energy to counteract the Fire condition, they will risk injuring their Spleen *qi* without necessarily creating an improvement in their symptoms, because they are still ingesting things that aggravate the Fire condition. This is similar to people who believe that by eating some organic carrots, they can continue to eat chips, cakes, cream puddings and chocolate and drink copious amounts of red wine. The organic carrots may well be packed with vitamins and minerals, but they do not counterbalance the other things being consumed. Salutary foods should be instead of, not at the same time as, at least if you want to create long-term harmony in the body.

Another thing we often hear when we start telling people which things they ought to exclude from their diet, is that they exclaim: 'But that's everything that I eat!' Although in reality they probably do eat other things, there is a reason that they have developed certain patterns of imbalance, and this is often due to the excessive consumption of an inappropriate diet that is very one-sided.

The central role of the Stomach and Spleen

Central to all Chinese medicine diet therapy is maintaining the health of the Spleen and Stomach. No matter what imbalances there are, account should always be taken of what affects the suggested changes in the diet will have on the Spleen and Stomach. This is because the Stomach receives all the food that is ingested through the mouth, and the Spleen *yang qi* that must transform this food into *gu qi* and extract the essence out of it. This means that regardless of what other qualities the food has and no matter what organs and channels this food affects, it will always also have an influence and an effect on the Stomach and the Spleen. This therefore means that diet therapy is sometimes a bit of a balancing act in which you try to achieve a therapeutic effect whilst trying not to injure the Spleen and the Stomach.

This relates back to some of the very first classes we had in our acupuncture training. In these classes we learnt about the production of *qi*. We learnt how the Stomach can be envisioned as a cauldron that is filled with the food and liquids that we ingest. The Spleen *qi* is the flames below the cauldron that transform the ingested food and liquids into a soup from which rises an aromatic and nourishing vapour. More precisely, we learnt that the Stomach receives the food and liquids ingested through the mouth and it 'ripens and rots' these, preparing them so that the Spleen can transform the ingested food and liquid into *gu qi* and extract the essences from it. Furthermore, because of their location in the centre of the body and their dynamic of sending *qi* upwards and downwards, the Stomach and Spleen will affect the movement and communication of *qi* in the whole body. It is therefore paramount that we support the Spleen and Stomach as much as possible through the diet. This can be done by following a few basic guidelines. We could call these the ten golden rules of eating in Chinese medicine. Most of the recommendations actually also make good sense from a Western medicine physiological perspective.

The 10 golden rules of eating in Chinese medicine

- **Chew your food well.** This will help the Stomach to mature and rot the ingested food so that the Spleen can transform it. From a Western perspective, the digestive process starts in the mouth. Chewing the food will increase the surface area that the digestive enzymes in the mouth can work on. Chewing will also help to physically break down the cell walls and mix the ingested food with the digestive enzymes. Furthermore, food that is physically cold will also be warmed up before descending into the stomach. This, as we will see in the second golden rule, is something that is important from both Western and Chinese perspectives.

- **Avoid eating cold food, i.e. food that is physically cold, such as raw vegetables, salads, cold beverages and food eaten directly from the refrigerator, as well as food that is energetically cold.** From a Western perspective, physically cold food will negatively affect the digestion, because the gastric enzymes are most efficacious when the temperature in the stomach is between 37 and 42 degrees Celsius. When foods and beverages that are physically cold are consumed, these enzymes will be less effective and the digestion will thereby be weakened. Chinese medicine states that the Spleen fears cold. The consumption of energetically and physically cold foods and beverages burdens the Spleen because the Spleen must expend more *yang qi* to warm and transform the ingested food. In the long run, too many cold foods and beverages can lead to Spleen *qi xu* and Spleen *yang xu.*

- **Eat as much prepared food as possible, especially things like soups and stews.** This is because if the food has been cooked in some way, the transformation process has already been initiated, thereby placing less demand on the resources of the Stomach and Spleen. Even though there are more vitamins and minerals in a raw carrot, the body will not necessarily be able to access, extract and absorb as many nutrients from a raw carrot, as it will from a steamed, stir-fried or boiled carrot. The cooking process helps to break down the cell walls in the food so that nutrients can be more easily released into the digestive system and absorbed through the intestinal wall. If the person insists on eating raw or unprepared food, they should ensure that the food is very finely chopped or grated and that they chew it thoroughly. Drinking some hot ginger tea with the raw food will also help.

- **Do not drink too much water or other beverages, and drink between meals.** Too much liquid will drown the Spleen's 'digestive fire'. A single cup of hot water or tea can, on the other hand, support the process (the Stomach hates dryness). This also makes sense from a Western perspective. Too much fluid will dilute and thereby weaken the acidity in the stomach. This will have a negative impact on the gastric enzymes, which function optimally in an acidic environment.

- **Do not eat too much.** Eat until you are 75 per cent full, otherwise you will overburden the Stomach and Spleen, which could cause food stagnation because the Spleen will not be able to transform so much food in one go and the Stomach will have difficulty rotting and ripening the food, as well as sending it downwards after the Spleen has transformed it. From a Western perspective, it takes a while for the brain to register that the stomach is full. This means that the stomach is full before you are aware that you are full. It also takes time for the food to move down through the oesophagus and into the stomach.

- **Eat your main meal as early as possible and avoid eating in the evening prior to going to bed.** Chinese medicine posits that the *yang* processes of transformation and transportation halt at night and only begin once more in the morning, when *yang* activity in general increases again. This means that if you eat late at night, the food stagnates and remains untransformed in the Stomach, where it will begin to generate Heat. In general, the main meal should be eaten as early in the day as possible. In relation to the Chinese medicine horary clock, the Stomach and Spleen are at their strongest between seven and eleven in the morning and therefore at their weakest between seven and eleven in the evening. In Western medicine physiology, peristalsis and digestion cease at night, so the food remains undigested in the stomach. Many cultures in fact have sayings along the lines of: 'Eat like a king in the morning, a peasant at lunchtime and a beggar in the evening.'

- **Choose foods that have vitality.** This can be seen, for example, when the vegetables are crisp and juicy or when the eyes of a fish are still bright and not dull.[28] In practice, this means as much fresh food as possible. Freshly picked vegetables, for example, contain many more vitamins than vegetables that have been transported and stored. Avoid industrially produced food, such as ready-made meals and canned foods. Not only do they contain very little *qi*, but they also usually contain various chemicals and additives such as preservatives, flavour enhancers, artificial flavourings, emulsifiers and so on, as well as excessive sugar and salt.

- **Enjoy what you eat.** This nourishes the Heart. We eat not only to create *gu qi*, but also for a variety of emotional reasons such as comfort and security, as well as the sheer pleasure obtained from the taste, smell and the sight of good food. This enjoyment is often accentuated by the pleasure of eating with others. Strict, spartan diets will remove this source of nourishment of the Heart. Frustration and irritation over dietary restrictions will also stagnate Liver *qi*. If you are going to eat something that you know is not good for you, do so without guilt. Guilt will only increase the negative effect that this food has on the body. Instead, really enjoy every mouthful, savouring the taste. Even though the food may be creating Dampness or Heat or whatever, it will at least nourish the Heart.

- **Try to eat in as tranquil a state as possible.** It is best to sit down and relax whilst eating and to avoid stress and quarrels. Heated discussions can disrupt the Liver *qi*, which may then invade and disrupt the Stomach and Spleen *qi ji*. Stress can also disrupt the *qi ji* in the middle *jiao*, as will worry and speculation. It is best not to read, watch television or surf the internet whilst eating. *Qi* should be used to digest food and not information during the transformation of the food.

- **Sit upright in a relaxed position and do not twist the trunk or sit in a slumped position.** A twisted or slumped posture will block the free passage of food and *qi* in the middle and lower *jiao*. From a Western medicine perspective, these postures will hamper the peristalsis of the intestines. Gentle stretching exercises or going for a light walk after a meal will help to circulate *qi* in the middle *jiao*, thereby supporting the Stomach and Spleen *qi*, or, in Western terms, it will activate the abdominal muscles, thereby supporting peristalsis. Sun Si Miao recommended that a person walks 100 steps after meals but that they do not count the number of steps.

Dietary recommendations

It is beyond the scope of this book to discuss and analyse the various qualities attributed to various foods. In Appendix 2 and throughout the main text I have superficially discussed certain foods in relation to various types of imbalance. For a more detailed discussion and understanding of the dynamics of food and how this can be utilised in Chinese medicine, the reader is referred to the following books. Some of these books can also be recommended to enthusiastic clients who would like to gain a deeper understanding of Chinese medicine dietetics:

- *Chinese Nutrition Therapy* (Kastner 2009)
- *Helping Ourselves* (Leggett 1994)
- *Recipes for Self Healing* (Leggett 1999)
- *Healing with Whole Foods* (Pitchford 1993)
- *The Tao of Healthy Eating* (Flaws 1995).

Mental and emotional approach to life

Most of us are not trained as psychotherapists. It is therefore important that we are conscious of our limitations, particularly as many of our clients present with imbalances that have their roots in psycho-emotional factors. As practitioners of Chinese medicine, we can try to make people aware of the emotional factors that may be influencing or generating their patterns of imbalance, we can create a space where they can discuss their problems without being judged, but we should also encourage them to seek additional help from relevant professionals when this is relevant.

I often explain clients' Chinese medicine diagnosis to them and tell them which emotional aspects Chinese medicine views as being potential aetiological factors in these patterns of imbalance. Often the client will have already mentioned certain emotional factors in their life, but if they haven't it gives them the opportunity to reflect and possibly recognise emotional factors that could be affecting their physical and emotional health. I do not start advising the client with regards to how they should act in situations that are creating these emotional imbalances, but talking about possible aetiology and the way emotions can affect the dynamic of the body's *qi* can help the client to become conscious of the relevance of these factors. It is then up to the client how they will work with these emotions and situations. Often the emotional baggage has been created at a very early age and is difficult to influence. Acupuncture is very good at changing the way a person and their *qi* reacts to these influences. It is not uncommon that a person who has been to counselling or other forms of psychotherapy for years finds that they have a breakthrough or start reacting differently in situations after they have started acupuncture sessions. This is because acupuncture harmonises the *qi* imbalances that are being affected by, but also manifesting as, emotional distress and detrimental behaviour.

When we are in a state of dissatisfaction or distress, especially emotionally, we should act to rectify the situation in some way and if this is not possible, we should try to reach a state of acceptance. What we should not do is to constantly live in a state of tension between these two poles. This is an area where acupuncture can often be of great help. Harmonising the *qi* means the person can find the strength or the vision to act or they can find the peace of mind that helps them to accept situations that cannot be changed.

It can also be relevant to explain to clients that we always have three possibilities in life when we are not satisfied, whether it is with our present situation or our past. *We can act and try to change the situation.* Sometimes this is a possibility; sometimes it is not. If we have the ability to change anything that we are unhappy with, we should do this. If, for example, we are dissatisfied with the way a person treats us, we can ask or tell the person to act differently. We must not remain in a situation that makes us discontent if we have the possibility or the ability do something about it. Many times, though, it is not possible to change the situation. In this example, it could be that this person cannot or will not change the way that they are behaving. If it is not possible to change the situation itself, you can still act by moving away from the situation or the condition that is making you discontent. *We can get up and leave.* This, though, is also not always an option. There can be many reasons why people have to remain in an unsatisfactory situation – economic reasons, family relationships, the limitations of the physical body, chronic illness, fear or because what is creating the emotional pain happened years ago in childhood. In these and many other situations, changing the situation or leaving it is not a possibility. *This then only leaves the option of acceptance* – to accept things as they are and thereby find peace. This peace of mind will often also mean that it becomes possible to see what other options and possibilities there are in the situation.

We can illustrate this model by using a couple of examples. If we are dissatisfied with something banal such as the colour of our bedroom wall, we can just paint it and then we have rectified the situation that is causing the discontentment. The Danish weather, though, is something that many people constantly complain about but have no influence over. They cannot change the weather. Some people have the possibility to move to another country with a different climate. This means that they can leave the situation that is causing their dissatisfaction. However, most people do not have this possibility due to financial reasons, family ties, employment situation, language difficulties and so on. If they cannot move away from and cannot change the Danish climate, then there is only one option left and that is acceptance: accepting things as they are and then working within the options that are left. Through acceptance we will often not only discover other possibilities, but also recognise what is advantageous or beneficial in the situation. I am lucky: I love all kinds of weather and I love all seasons. Each season and each climate has something special and something beautiful about it. Winter is hard for some people, but the light in the winter in Denmark can be magical and the sensation of the cold biting into my cheeks is something that I love. If I constantly fought against the winter and was dissatisfied until the spring, I would not be able to appreciate this.

Clothing

Discussing clothing is particularly relevant for patients who are *yang xu* and *wei qi xu* and those who have a tendency to be invaded by exogenous *xie qi* in certain areas of the body, for example the knees or the lower back. Being appropriately dressed may sound very trivial and obvious, but unfortunately this is certainly not the case for all clients.

Factors that may be relevant and can be reasons why clients dress inappropriately are:

- fashion

- poverty

- ignorance.

Unfortunately, it is only the latter that we, as therapists, can do anything about. We can inform clients of the consequences that inadequate or inappropriate clothing will have for their patterns of imbalance or their health, for example that exposure to cold and dampness may be a factor in their knee pain and that it is therefore important that they wear clothing that keeps their knees warm and dry. We must also, though, accept that they may prioritise looking smart over keeping their knees warm and dry. What we have given them is relevant knowledge so that they can make a conscious choice.

Exercise and rest

Exercise is good. However, this does not mean that the more you exercise the better it is. It is typical of our Western, linear thinking that when something is good, even more of it will be even better. Unfortunately, many of our clients live by this logic. One can quickly see flaws in this logic if you replace the word 'exercise' with the words 'eating food'. Eating food is vital: if we did not eat food we would die, therefore eating food is good for us. Nobody, though, is of the opinion that constantly eating excessive amounts of food will benefit their health. However, we do see clients who are exercising themselves to death because they believe that the more they train, the healthier they will be. We see women who are extremely *yin xu* and *xue xu* running several kilometres a day, as well as going to the gym, because they are training to do an Ironman event.

What makes things even more complicated is that it is not possible to say how much exercise is too much or how little exercise is too little. The right amount of exercise is completely individual and will depend on the person's constitution, patterns of imbalance, age and gender and the season, time of day and so on. This is something that is hard to accept for many patients who are looking for straight guidelines. A rule of thumb, though, is the more *shi* their imbalances and the more stagnation there is, the more exercise and physical activity will be good for them (within reason). Likewise, the more *xu* that their imbalances are, the less they should train.

Just as exercise is good, so is rest. Rest and relaxation are extremely important for all people. This is something that many people do not consider in their attempt to achieve a healthy lifestyle.

Sleeping, for example, is vital. However, as well as needing sleep, there must be a balance between *yang* activity (both mental and physical) and *yin* rest. How the balance between *yin* rest and *yang* activity should be is dependent on many factors, such as constitution, age, gender, patterns of imbalance, diet and so on. Once again, there are no fixed rules that people can grasp hold of. It is always a question of dosage – both too much and too little rest and relaxation are harmful. Too little rest will initially exhaust *qi* and *yang*, and over time it will exhaust *xue*, *yin* and finally *jing*. Too much rest, on the other hand, and too little activity will stagnate *qi* initially, and with time it may stagnate *xue* and *jinye*.

Sleeping at night should not be the only *yin* state a person experiences during a 24-hour period. People need to create spaces in their day when they consciously gear down, relax and cultivate tranquillity of the mind and body. The more physically and mentally active a person is, i.e. the more *yang* that they are, the more *yin* they need to be to balance this. Sleep and physical relaxation are a good balance to physical activity, whilst meditation, mindfulness, introspection and reflection are a good counterbalance to mental over-stimulation and stress.

Yoga, tai ji and qi gong are physical activities that most people will benefit from. This is because they combine physical movement of the body, and thereby the movement of *qi* and *xue*, with mental relaxation and mindfulness. They are activities that harmonise *yin* and *yang* at the same time. Furthermore, these forms of movement stimulate the internal organs and the channel system, thereby increasing the production of *qi*. A problem, though, is that they can be too slow for people whose *shen* is agitated by Heat, especially when there is Liver *qi* stagnation Heat. These people will often not have enough patience and they will experience these forms of movement as being too slow and boring, which will further stagnate their Liver *qi*.

Following the natural rhythm of life

The invention of electric lighting has given us the possibility to disrupt the natural circadian rhythm, which challenges our physiology. The evening and night are *yin*. These periods of the day are dark and cool, activity decreases and there is tranquillity. Most animals and birds go to rest. This is what most people did before the advent of electric lighting. Now we have the opportunity to be alert and active at night because we have electric lighting and have also acquired computers, smartphones and televisions, which are extremely *shen* stimulating. Televisions, smartphones and computers activate our *shen*, which is the most *yang* aspect of the body and thereby consumes *yin*. These devices are problematical enough during the day if used excessively, but they are especially harmful in the evening and at night, when *shen* should be calm and placid and we should be in a *yin* dormant state.

On the other hand, during the day when we should be *yang* and thereby physically active, many people no longer work manually using their bodies. A great many people now have sedentary daytime jobs that involve very little physical activity.

Unfortunately, it is not only the diurnal cycle we have become out of sync with. December is the darkest and most *yin* time of year. Many animals hibernate or at least significantly reduce their physical activity. Plants draw their sap down into their roots or into a bulb in the ground. Traditionally, people who worked together with nature would have had a high level of activity in the summer. In summer they would have worked hard from when the sun rose at dawn until it set in the evening. In the winter the working day would have been shorter and they would have got up later and gone to bed earlier than they did in the summer. Winter was also characterised by the winter solstice and, later on in history, Christmas. These were festivals of light during the dark days of winter (the *yang* dot of white in the black *yin* of the *taiji* symbol). December was a time for quiet communion and reflection. Now December has become the time of the year when people run around like headless chickens and are constantly stressed for a whole month. They rush around juggling Christmas shopping with office parties, arranging family gatherings and cooking extravagant meals. As soon as Christmas is over, this excessive *yang* activity continues with the New Year's Eve celebrations. All of this is then counterbalanced by people lying around lazing in the sun in a state of *yin* passivity in the *yang* summer, when they should be physically active! Unfortunately, it is unlikely that we as therapists are going to be able to rectify these tendencies in society.

Where we can have an influence is to increase people's awareness of the cycles of *yin* and *yang*. These cycles can be seen throughout life and are something we must accept and adapt our lives to. When we are young, we have an excess of *yang*. This means that it is not only beneficial, but also a necessity, that we are physically quite active. In this period of life, there is also a more natural tendency to be more extrovert and sociable, which is also a *yang* property.

As we age and our *yang* declines, we become less extrovert and seek more peace and quiet. We have less energy available for physical exertion and a greater need to get to bed at a proper time. It is important that we learn to listen to our bodies and our minds and do not vainly try to fight against windmills by living like a 20-year-old when we are 50. This is something we must try and make our clients aware of, especially as the media has a tendency to glorify a *yang*, youthful lifestyle. Many middle-aged and older people end up feeling inadequate or that there is something wrong with them, because they physically cannot maintain, or no longer enjoy, this lifestyle, even though they did when they were younger.

Acupressure

Acupressure is a good way to involve the client in their own healing process, thereby creating quicker results. It also helps to give the client the responsibility and the tools to maintain their own health. We must, however, also remember that most of our clients are not acupuncturists and are not trained in locating acupuncture points. It can be difficult for them to remember how many fingerwidths St 36 is located below the kneecap and how far away from the shin bone. Initially, it can also be difficult to sense where an acupuncture point is with your fingertips until you have trained and practised for a while. This is why I usually choose acupressure points that are easy to locate, even though other points would be more efficacious. So, for example, instead of recommending St 36, I would show them how to locate and stimulate Sp 3, because it is easier to find. It is better that the client stimulates an acupuncture point that is not the most effective than pressing the muscle five centimetres adjacent to a more appropriate point.

Moxa

I sometimes give clients who are *qi xu* and *yang xu* a stick-on mini moxa to take home with them. I give them detailed instruction and training in how to use the stick-on mini moxa and what to be observant of. I also control them on return at the next appointment. Like acupressure, the domestic use of moxa will speed up the healing process and it will involve the client in the treatment. Again, I only give them points that are easy to locate and safe to use, as well as strict instructions not to use the moxa on other places.

Meditation and mindfulness

Meditation is one of the best ways, apart from sleeping, that a client can nourish their *yin*. It is not only patients who are *yin xu*, though, who will benefit from meditation. As stated earlier, most people are too *yang* in their lifestyle and we constantly further activate our *yang* aspects through the use of computers, smartphones, televisions and so on in our leisure time. It is important to balance all this *yang* activity and stimulation with *yin* tranquillity. Meditation is an excellent tool to cultivate quietude and something that I encourage many clients to practise in some form or other.

I'm not an experienced meditation instructor, therefore I usually urge clients to either find a meditation teacher or buy a meditation CD. I do, however, sometimes give clients individual instructions. Again, it is important to be realistic in your expectations and even more important to get the client to be realistic as well. Ten minutes a day, every day, is far better than an hour's session every second week.

I also use myself and my own experience as an example – I can find it difficult to stay focused while I meditate. Sharing this experience is not only a relief, but also an inspiration to many clients. Most people believe that it is only them who have this problem and therefore that they are incapable of meditating. If they find out that others, particularly people they look up to (which people unfortunately tend to do with therapists), they become more willing to try to carry on, even though it is difficult.

Sometimes I do not use the term 'meditation', but instead just call it breathing techniques and relaxation exercises, where they should sit or lie down, focus on their breathing, possibly place a hand on their stomach, which should rise and fall each time they breathe in and out, and relax as much as possible.

THE ENERGETIC PROPERTIES
OF CERTAIN FOODS

Cereals

Most cultures' diet is cereal based. This is also in accordance with Chinese medicine dietetic theories in which cereals such as rice, millet and corn should constitute the greatest portion of food that is consumed.

Most grains are relatively neutral in their temperature and generally strengthen *qi* and *xue*. This means that regularly consuming relatively large amounts of them will generally not create imbalances in the body.

Most cereals also have slight Damp-draining qualities but unfortunately not all. Modern wheat is particularly problematic. This is because as well as having a cooling energy, wheat has also been modified to produce a higher yield and to suit the needs of the baking industry. This has resulted in wheat having a tendency to produce Dampness in the body. This is particularly problematical, given how many people's diet is based on the consumption of bread, pasta and other wheat-based foods.

Barley

Salty, sweet and slightly cooling. Drains Dampness and Heat; Nourishes *yin*.

Maize/corn

Sweet and neutral. Strengthens *qi* and *xue*.

Millet

Sweet, salty and neutral (some sources classify millet as being either slightly warming or slightly cool). Strengthens the Kidney and Spleen *qi*; transforms Dampness and Phlegm.

Oats

Sweet, neutral/warm. Strengthens *qi* and nourishes *xue*.

Quinoa

Sweet, salty and slightly warm. Strengthens Kidney *yang*.

Rice

Neutral and sweet. Strengthens *qi* and *xue*; harmonises the Stomach and strengthens the Spleen.

Rye

Bitter and neutral/slightly cooling. Drains Dampness.

Spelt

Sweet and neutral/slightly cooling. Strengthens *qi* and nourishes *xue*. Less Dampness and Phlegm-creating than modern wheat.

Wheat

Sweet, cool or slightly cold. Drains Heat; nourishes the *qi* and nourishes *xue*. Has a tendency to create Dampness and Phlegm.

Dairy products

Generally sweet and cool or neutral (goat and sheep milk is neutral or slightly warming, which makes it a better option for people who are Spleen *qi xu*). Dairy products are very rich in flavour (*wei*) and therefore can have a tendency to create Dampness.

Fish

Freshwater fish are usually sweet and salty in their flavour, whilst being neutral or slightly warm in their temperature. Saltwater fish usually have a salty flavour and a cool temperature. Trout is slightly hot and salmon is warm. A lot of shellfish are warming.

Fruit

Generally sweet, sour and sometimes bitter. Most fruit is cooling in its thermal dynamic. Exceptions to this are apricot, raspberry and cherry, which are slightly warming. Tropical fruit is generally cold and should preferably be eaten in warm, *yang* climates, not in the autumn and winter in Northern Europe. The sweet and sour taste helps to create fluids, but the sour taste will bind the fluids in the body, which is not good when there is Dampness.

Meat

Meat is generally warm. Meat is good at tonifying *yang*, *qi* and *xue*. Because meat is very rich in its flavour (*wei*), it can be difficult to transform and it can lead to the creation of Phlegm and Heat.

The various kinds of organ meats, such as kidney, liver and so on, will tonify the corresponding *zangfu* organ in the body. It is, however, highly recommended that the liver and kidney are organic, due to the use of growth promoters, antibiotics, medicine and other chemicals used in the production of meat.

Beef

Sweet and neutral or slightly warm.

Chicken

Sweet and warm.

Duck

Sweet, salty and neutral or slightly cooling. Nourishes *yin* and *xue*.

Lamb

Sweet and hot. Strengthens *qi* and *yang*, nourishes *xue*. Can aggravate Heat and Fire conditions.

Pork

Sweet, salty and neutral or slightly cooling. Nourishes *yin* and *xue*. Tendency to create Dampness and Phlegm.

Venison

Spicy, sweet and hot. Strengthens *qi* and *yang*, circulates and invigorates *xue*. May aggravate Heat and Fire conditions.

Nuts and seeds

Generally sweet, neutral or warm. Nuts are rich in flavour (*wei*). This means that they also have a tendency to produce food stagnation, Dampness and Phlegm if too many are eaten at a time.

Seaweed

Salt and cold. Nourishes *yin*; dissolves Phlegm accumulations and drains Heat.

Vegetables

Vegetables are generally neutral or cooling in their dynamic, although there are exceptions (the onion family, for example, is warm). A rule of thumb is that vegetables that grow quickly and contain a lot of water, for example lettuce, tomato, cucumber and so on, are often more cooling. In the past, you could only grow and buy these vegetables in the summer when their cooling energy was more appropriate to the *yang* season. Now people eat them all year round, even in winter and in countries with a very *yin* climate.

Beans

Generally good for the Kidneys. Nourish *xue* and tonify *qi*. Dried beans help to drain Dampness. Tofu is good for the Lung.

Green, leafy vegetables

Generally nourish *xue* and strengthen *qi*. Many of them will also cool the Liver and nourish Liver *yin*. Cabbage is especially beneficial for the Intestines. White cabbage is slightly warming, Chinese cabbage is a little more cooling and drains Damp-Heat. Spinach soothes the walls of the Intestines and is beneficial when there is Heat or *yin xu* in the Stomach and Large Intestine.

Lettuce, tomato, cucumber

Cold in their energy and therefore drain Heat.

Mushrooms

Many mushrooms drain toxins and transform Phlegm.

Onion family

Warm, spicy and sweet. Due to their spicy flavour, plants from the onion family help to disperse stagnations and expel exogenous *xie qi*.

Root vegetables

Generally sweet and generally strengthen the Stomach and Spleen *qi*. Nourish *qi* and *xue*.

Temperature of common foods

Cold	Cool	Neutral	Warm	Hot
Asparagus	Apple	Alfalfa sprouts	Basil	Alcohol
Banana	Aubergine	Almonds	Bell pepper	Chilli
Bean sprouts	Avocado	Beans	Blackcurrant	Chocolate
Celery	Barley	Beef	Butter	Cinnamon
Crab	Beer	Beetroot	Cherry	Curry
Cucumber	Broccoli	Carrot	Chicken	Deep-fried food
Fruit juice	Buckwheat	Cauliflower	Eel	Garlic
Lemon	Courgette	Cheese	Fennel	Lamb
Melon	Marjoram	Corn	Ginger	Paprika
Salt	Mushroom	Cow milk	Goat milk	Pepper
Seaweed	Orange	Duck	Ham	Trout
Tofu	Pea	Egg (chicken)	Leek	Venison
Tomato	Pear	Goose	Lobster	Yogi tea
Watermelon	Rabbit	Grapes	Nutmeg	
Yoghurt	Radishes	Hazelnut	Oats	
	Salad	Herring	Onion	
	Shrimp	Lentil	Oregano	
	Spearmint	Mackerel	Parsley	
	Spinach	Millet[29]	Peach	
	Strawberry	Olive	Rosemary	
	Tea	Plum	Sage	
	Wheat	Pork	Salmon	
		Potatoes	Thyme	
		Rice	Walnut	
		Rye		
		Sardines		
		Sesame		
		Spelt		

HERBAL FORMULAS

An Gong Niu Huang Wan

Niu huang 30g, shui niu jiao 30g, she xiang 7.5g, huang lian 30g, huang qin 30g, zhi zi 30g, xiong huang 30g, bing pian 7.5g, yu jin 30g, zhu sha 30g, zhen zu 15g (to make 90 pills)

Ba Zhen Tang

Ren shen 9g, bai zhu 12g, fu ling 15g, zhi gan cao 3g, dang gui 15g, shu di huang 18g, bai shao 15g, chuan xiong 9g

Ba Zheng San

Mu tong 3g, hua shi 21g, che qian zi 12g, qu mai 9g, bian xu 9g, zhi zi 6g, da huang 6g, deng xin cao 6g, zhi gan cao 3g

Bai He Gu Jin Tang

Bai he 12g, sheng di huang 9g, shu di huang 9g, mai men dong 4.5g, xuan shen 2.4g, chuan bei mu 4.5g, jie geng 2.4g, dang gui 9g, bai shao 3g, gan cao 3g

Bai Hu Jia Gui Zhi Tang

Shi gao 30g, zhi mu 9g, zhi gan cao 3g, geng mi 6g, gui zhi 9g

Bai Hu Tang

Shi gao 30g, zhi mu 9g, zhi gan cao 3g, geng mi 9g

Bai Tou Weng Tang

Bai tou weng 15g, huang bai 12g, huang qin 6g, qin pi 12g

Ban Xia Hou Po Tang

Ban xia 12g, hou po 9g, fu ling 12g, zi su ye 9g, sheng jiang 12g

Bao He Wan

Shan zha 18g, shen qu 6g, lai fu zi 3g, ban xia 9g, fu ling 9g, chen pi 3g, lian qiao 3g

Bei Xie Fen Qing Yin I

Bei xie 9g, yi zhi ren 9g, wu yao 9g, shi chang pu 9g, fu ling 9g

Bei Xie Fen Qing Yin II

Bei xie 10g, huang bai 3g, shi chang pu 3g, fu ling 5g, bai zhu 5g, lian zi xin 4g, dan shen 7g, che qian zi 7g

Bei Xie Shen Shi Tang

Bei xie 9g, yi yi ren 15g, huang bai 9g, fu ling 12g, mu dan pi 9g, ze xie 9g, tong cao 6g, hua shi 15g

Bu Fei Tang

Huang qi 18g, shu di huang 18g, ren shen 9g, zi wan 6g, sang bai pi 9g, wu wei zi 6g

Bu Gan Tang

Shu di huang 15g, dang gui 9g, bai shao 12g, chuan xiong 6g, mu gua 6g, suan zao ren 9g, mai men dong 6g, zhi gan cao 3g

Bu Zhong Yi Qi Tang

Huang qi 15g, ren shen 9g, bai zhu 9g, dang gui 9g, chen pi 6g, chai hu 3g, sheng ma 3g, zhi gan cao 3g

Chai Hu Shu Gan Tang

Chai hu 6g, chuan xiong 4.5g, xiang fu 4.5g, chen pi 6g, zhi ke 4.5g, bai shao 4.5g, zhi gan cao 1.5g

Chuan Xiong Cha Tiao Tang

Chuan xiong 12g, jing jie 12g, bai zhi 6g, qiang huo 6g, xi xin 3g, fang feng 4.5g, bo he 2.4g, gan cao 6g

Da Bu Yin Wan

Shu di huang 18g, zhi mu 12g, huang bai 12g, gui ban 18g

Da Chai Hu Tang

Chai hu 15g, huang qin 9g, bai shao 9g, ban xia 9g, zhi shi 9g, da huang 6g, sheng jiang 15g, da zao 5pcs

Da Cheng Qi Tang

Da huang 12g, mang xiao 9g, zhi shi 12g, hou po 15g

Da Ding Feng Zhu

Bai shao 18g, e jiao 9g, gui ban 12g, sheng di huang 18g, huo ma ren 6g, wu wei zi 6g, mu li 12g, mai men dong 18g, ji zi huang 2pcs, bie jia 12g, zhi gan cao 12g

Da Jian Zhong Tang

Hua jiao 6g, gan jiang 12g, ren shen 6g, yi tang 21g

Dan Shen Yin

Dan shen 30g, sha ren 5g, tan xiang 5g

Dao Chi San

Sheng di huang 9g, mu tong 9g, dan zhu ye 6g, gan cao 6g

Di Tan Tang

Ban xia 7.5g, dan nan xing 7.5g, fu ling 6g, zhi shi 6g, ju hong 4.5g, shi chang pu 3g, ren shen 3g, zhu ru 2.1g, gan cao 2.1g

Ding Chuan Tang

Bai guo 9g, ma huang 9g, zi su zi 6g, kuan dong hua 9g, xing ren 6g, sang bai pi 9g, huang qin 6g, ban xia 9g, gan cao 3g

Ding Zhi Wan

Ren shen 9g, fu ling 9g, yuan zhi 6g, shi chang pu 6g

Du Huo Ji Sheng Tang

Du huo 9g, sang ji sheng 6g, du zhong 6g, niu xi 6g, xi xin 3g, qin jiao 6g, fu ling 6g, rou gui 6g, fang feng 6g, chuan xiong 6g, ren shen 6g, dang gui 6g, bai shao 6g, sheng di huang 6g, gan cao 6g

E Jiao Ji Zi Huang Tang

E jiao 6g, bai shao 9g, shi jue ming 15g, gou teng 6g, sheng di huang 12g, mu li 12g, luo shi teng 9g, fu shen 12g, ji zi huang 2pcs, zhi gan cao 1.8g

Er Chen Tang

Ban xia 15g, chen pi 15g, fu ling 9g, zhi gan cao 5g, sheng jiang 3g, wu mei 1pc

Fang Ji Huang Qi Tang

Fang ji 12g, huang qi 15g, bai zhu 9g, gan cao 6g, sheng jiang 4 slices, da zao 1pc

Fu Zi Li Zhong Tang

Fu zi 6g, ren shen 9g, bai zhu 9g, gan jiang 9g, zhi gan cao 6g

Gan Mai Da Zao Tang

Gan cao 9g, fu xiao mai 15g, da zao 6 pcs

Ge Gan Tang

Ge gen 12g, ma huang 6g, gui zhi 6g, bai shao 6g, sheng jiang 9g, da zao 4pcs, zhi gan cao 6g

Ge Xia Fu Zhu Yu Tang

Dang gui 9g, chuan xiong 6g, tao ren 9g, hong hua 9g, mu dan pi 6g, chi shao 6g, wu ling zhi 9g, yan hu suo 3g, wu yao 6g, xiang fu 4.5g, zhi ke 4.5g, gan cao 9g

Gui Pi Tang

Huang qi 12g, ren shen 6g, dang gui 6g, bai zhu 9g, fu ling 12g, long yan rou 9g, suan zao ren 12g, yuan zhi 6g, mu xiang 4.5g, sheng jiang 6g, da zao 5pcs, zhi gan cao 6g

Gui Zhi Fu Ling Tang

Gui zhi 9g, fu ling 9g, mu dan pi 9g, tao ren 9g, chi shao 9g

Gui Zhi Tang
Gui zhi 9g, bai shao 9g, zhi gan cao 6g, sheng jiang 9g, da zao 3pcs

Hou Po Wen Zhong Tang
Hou po 12g, chen pi 12g, fu ling 9g, cao dou kou 6g, mu xiang 6g, gan jiang 4.5g, zhi gan cao 3g, sheng jiang 3 slices

Huang Lian E Jiao Tang
Huang lian 12g, huang qin 6g, e jiao 9g, bai shao 6g, ji zi huang 2pcs

Huang Lian Jie Du Tang
Huang lian 9g, huang qin 6g, huang bai 6g, zhi zi 9g

Huang Qin Tang
Huang qin 9g, bai shao 9g, zhi gan cao 3g, da zao 4pcs

Huang Tu Tang
Zao xin huang tu 21g, bai zhu 9g, fu zi 9g, sheng di huang 9g, e jiao 9g, huang qin 9g, gan cao 9g

Huo Po Xia Ling Tang
Huo xiang 6g, hou po 3g, ban xia 4.5g, fu ling 9g, xing ren 9g, yi yi ren 15g, bai dou kou 3g, zhu ling 4.5g, dan dou chi 9g, ze xie 4.5g, tong cao 12g

Huo Xiang Zheng Qi Tang
Huo xiang 9g, ban xia 6g, bai zhu 6g, chen pi 6g, hou po 6g, jie geng 6g, da fu pi 3g, bai zhi 3g, zi su ye 3g, fu ling 3g, zhi gan cao 7.5g, sheng jiang 6g, da zao 1pc

Ji Sheng Shen Qi Wan
Shu di huang 6g, shan zhu yu 12g, shan yao 12g, ze xie 12g, fu ling 12g, mu dan pi 12g, fu zi 6g, rou gui 6g, chuan niu xi 6g, che qian zi 12g

Jian Pi Wan
Ren shen 6g, bai zhu 9g, fu ling 6g, chen pi 3g, shen qu 3g, sha ren 3g, mai ya 3g, shan zha 3g, shan yao 3g, rou dou kou 3g, mu xiang 3g, huang lian 1.5g, gan cao 3g

Jin Gui Shen Qi Tang
Shu di huang 24g, shan zhu yu 12g, shan yao 12g, ze xie 9g, fu ling 9g, mu dan pi 9g, fu zi 3g, gui zhi 3g

Ju Pi Zhu Ru Tang
Ju pi 9g, zhu ru 9g, ren shen 3g, sheng jiang 6g, da zao 4pcs, gan cao 3g

Juan Bi Tang
Qiang huo 9g, jiang huang 9g, dang gui 9g, chi shao 9g, fang feng 9g, huang qi 9g, zhi gan cao 3g, sheng jiang 3g

Li Zhong An Hui Tang

Ren shen 2.1g, bai zhu 3g, fu ling 3g, hua jiao 0.9g, wu mei 0.9g, gan jiang 1.5g

Li Zhong Tang

Ren shen 6g, gan jiang 6g, bai zhu 9g, zhi gan cao 6g

Ling Gan Wu Wei Jiang Xin Tang

Fu ling 12g, gan jiang 9g, xi xin 3g, wu wei zi 6g, gan cao 6g

Ling Jiao Gou Teng Yin

Ling yang jiao 4.5g, sang ye 6g, gou teng 9g, ju hua 9g, bai shao 9g, chuan bei mu 12g, sheng di huang 15g, zhu ru 15g, fu shen 9g, gan cao 2.4g

Liu Jun Zi Tang

Ren shen 9g, bai zhu 6g, fu ling 9g, chen pi 6g, ban xia 6g, gan cao 3g

Liu Wei Di Huang Tang

Shu di huang 24g, shan zhu yu 12g, shan yao 12g, fu ling 9g, ze xie 9g, mu dan pi 9g

Long Dan Xie Gan Tang

Long dan cao 6g, huang qin 9g, zhi zi 9g, ze xie 9g, mu tong 9g, che qian zi 9g, dang gui 3g, sheng di huang 9g, chai hu 6g, gan cao 6g

Ma Huang Tang

Ma huang 9g, gui zhi 6g, xing ren 9g, zhi gan cao 3g

Ma Zi Ren Wan

Huo ma ren 12g, bai shao 6g, zhi shi 6g, da huang 12g, hou po 6g, xing ren 6g

Mai Men Dong Tang

Mai men dong 9g, ban xia 6g, ren shen 6g, geng mi 9g, da zao 8 pcs, gan cao 3g

Ping Wei San

Cang zhu 15g, hou po 9g, chen pi 9g, gan cao 4.5g, sheng jiang 2 slices, da zao 2 pcs

Qi Ju Di Huang Tang

Shu di huang 24g, shan zhu yu 12g, shan yao 12g, fu ling 9g, ze xie 9g, mu dan pi 9g, gou qi zi 9g, ju hua 9g

Qiang Huo Sheng Shi Tang

Qiang huo 6g, du huo 6g, gao ben 3g, fang feng 3g, chuan xiong 3g, man jing zi 2g, zhi gan cao 3g

Qing Luo Yin

He ye 6g, jin yin hua 6g, si gua pi 6g, xi gua cui yi 6g, bian dou hua 6g, dan zhu ye 6g

Qing Qi Hua Tan Tang

Gua lou ren 9g, dan nan xing 6g, huang qin 6g, ban xia 9g, chen pi 6g, xing ren 6g, zhi shi 6g, fu ling 6g

Qing Wei San

Sheng di huang 12g, dang gui 6g, huang lian 4.5g, mu dan pi 9g, sheng ma 6g

Qing Ying Tang

Shui niu jiao 60g, xuan shen 9g, sheng di huang 15g, mai men dong 9g, jin yin hua 9g, lian qiao 6g, huang lian 4.5g, dan zhu ye 3g, dan shen 6g

Run Chang Wan

Huo ma ren 15g, tao ren 9g, dang gui 9g, sheng di huang 12g, zhi ke 6g

San Ren Tang

Xing ren 15g, yi yi ren 18g, bai dou kou 6g, hua shi 18g, tong cao 6g, dan zhu ye 6g, ban xia 6g, hou po 6g

San Shi Tang

Hua shi 9g, shi gao 15g, han shui shi 9g, xing ren 9g, zhu ru 6g, jin yin hua 9g, jin zhi 1 glass, tong cao 6g

San Wu Bei Ji Wan

Da huang 30g, gan jiang 30g, ba dou 30g (made into pills)

San Zi Yang Qin Tang

Bai jie zi 6g, zi su zi 9g, lai fu zi 9g

Sang Ju Yin

Sang ye 7.5g, ju hua 3g, xing ren 6g, lian qiao 6g, bo he 2.5g, jie geng 6g, lu gen 6g, gan cao 2.5g

Sang Xing Tang

Sang ye 3g, xing ren 4.5g, sha ren 6g, zhe bei mu 3g, dan dou chi 3g, zhi zi 3g, li pi 3g

Sha Shen Mai Men Dong Tang

Sha shen 9g, mai men dong 9g, yu zhu 6g, sang ye 4.5g, bian dou 4.5g, tian hua fen 4.5g, gan cao 3g

Shao Fu Zhu Yu Tang

Xiao hui xiang 1.5g, gan jiang 2g, yan hu suo 3g, dang gui 9g, chuan xiong 3g, rou gui 3g, mo yao 3g, chi shao yao 6g, pu huang 9g, wu ling zhi 6g

Shao Yao Tang

Bai shao 15g, dang gui 9g, huang lian 9g, bing lang 5g, mu xiang 5g, huang qin 9g, da huang 9g, rou gui 5g, gan cao 5g

Shen Fu Tang

Ren shen 9g, fu zi 6g

Shen Tong Zhu Yu Tang

Qin jiao 3g, chuan xiong 6g, tao ren 9g, hong hua 9g, qiang huo 9g, mo yao 3g, dang gui 9g, wu ling zhi 6g, xiang fu 3g, chuan niu xi 9g, di long 6g, gan cao 6g

Sheng Mai San

Ren shen 9g, mai men dong 15g, wu wei zi 6g

Shi Hui San

Da ji 9g, xiao ji 9g, he ye 9g, ce bai ye 9g, bai mao gen 9g, qian cao gen 9g, zhi zi 9g, da huang 9g, mu dan pi 9g, zong lu pi 9g

Shi Wei San

Shi wei 6g, che qian zi 9g, qu mai 6g, hua shi 9g, dong kui zi 6g, jin qian cao 60g, hai jin sha 30g, ji nei jin 15g

Si Miao San

Huang bai 12g, yi yi ren 12g, cang zhu 6g, huai niu xi 6g

Si Ni Tang

Fu zi 9g, gan jiang 4.5g, zhi gan cao 6g

Si Sheng Wan

He ye 9g, ai ye 9g, ce bai ye 12g, sheng di huang 15g

Si Wu Tang

Dang gui 9g, shu di huang 12g, bai shao 12g, chuan xiong 6g

Su Zi Jiang Qi Tang

Zi su zi 9g, ban xia 9g, dang gui 6g, qian hu 6g, hou po 6g, rou gui 3g, zhi gan cao 6g, zi su ye 2g, sheng jiang 2 slices, da zao 1pc

Suo Quan Wan

Wu yao 12g, yi zhi ren 12g, shan yao 15g

Tao He Cheng Qi Tang

Tao ren 15g, da huang 12g, mang xiao 6g, gui zhi 6g, zhi gan cao 6g

Tao Hong Si Wu Tang

Shu di huang 15g, dang gui 12g, bai shao 9g, chuan xiong 9g, tao ren 6g, hong hua 6g

Tian Ma Gou Teng Yin

Tian ma 9g, gou teng 12g, shi jue ming 18g, zhi zi 9g, huang qin 9g, niu xi 9g, du zhong 12g, yi mu cao 9g, sang ji sheng 9g, ye jiao teng 9g, fu shen 9g

Tian Tai Wu Yao San

Wu yao 12g, mu xiang 6g, xiao hui xiang 6g, qing pi 6g, gao liang jiang 9g, bing lang 9g, chuan lian zi 12g, ba dou 70 pcs

Tian Wang Bu Xin Dan

Sheng di huang 24g, mai men dong 12g, tian men dong 12g, dang gui 12g, dan shen 3g, xuan shen 3g, suan zao ren 12g, bai zi ren 12g, ren shen 3g, fu ling 3g, yuan zhi 3g, wu wei zi 3g, jie geng 3g

Wei Ling Tang

Ze xie 12g, fu ling 9g, zhu ling 9g, bai zhu 9g, gui zhi 9g, cang zhu 6g, hou po 12g, chen pi 9g, gan cao 4.5g, sheng jiang 3 slices, da zao 2 pcs

Wen Dan Tang

Ban xia 6g, zhu ru 6g, zhi shi 6g, chen pi 6g, fu ling 9g, sheng jiang 4.5g, da zao 1pc, zhi gan cao 3g

Wen Jing Tang

Dang gui 9g, wu zhu yu 9g, bai shao 6g, chuan xiong 6g, ren shen 6g, gui zhi 6g, e jiao 6g, mu dan pi 6g, ban xia 6g, mai men dong 9g, sheng jiang 6g, gan cao 6g

Wu Ling San

Fu ling 9g, zhu ling 9g, ze xie 15g, bai zhu 9g, gui zhi 6g

Wu Mei Wan

Wu mei 9g, xi xin 3g, gan jiang 6g, huang lian 9g, dang gui 3g, fu zi 3g, hua jiao 2g, gui zhi 3g, ren shen 3g, huang bai 3g

Wu Pi San

Sheng jiang pi 9g, sheng bai pi 9g, chen pi 9g, da fu pi 9g, fu ling pi 9g

Wu Zhu Yu Tang

Wu zhu yu 12g, ren shen 9g, da zao 12 pcs, sheng jiang 18g

Xi Jiao Di Huang Tang

Xi jiao 3g, sheng di huang 24g, chi shao 12g, mu dan pi 9g

Xiao Chai Hu Tang

Chai hu 12g, huang qin 9g, ren shen 6g, ban xia 6g, zhi gan cao 4.5g, sheng jiang 9g, da zao 4 pcs

Xiao Feng San

Dang gui 3g, sheng di huang 3g, fang feng 3g, chan tui 3g, zhi mu 3g, ku shen 3g, hei zhi ma 3g, jing jie 3g, cang zhu 3g, niu bang zi 3g, shi gao 3g, mu tong 1.5g, gan cao 1.5g

Xiao Qing Long Tang

Ma huang 9g, gui zhi 6g, bai shao 9g, gan jiang 9g, xi xin 3g, wu wei zi 3g, ban xia 9g, zhi gan cao 6g

Xiao Yao San

Chai hu 9g, dang gui 9g, bai shao 12g, bai zhu 12g, fu ling 15g, bo he 3g, wei jiang 6g, zhi gan cao 6g

Xie Bai San

Di gu pi 15g, sang bai pi 15g, zhi gan cao 3g, geng mi 9g

Xie Xin Tang

Huang lian 3g, huang qin 9g, da huang 6g

Xing Su San

Zi su ye 6g, xing ren 6g, ban xia 6g, fu ling 6g, chen pi 6g, qian hu 6g, jie geng 6g, zhi ke 6g, sheng jiang 6g, da zao 2pcs, gan cao 3g

Xue Fu Zhu Yu Tang

Tao ren 12g, hong hua 9g, dang gui 9g, sheng di huang 9g, chuan xiong 4.5g, chi shao 6g, chuan niu xi 9g, jie geng 4.5g, chai hu 3g, zhi ke 6g, gan cao 3g

Yi Pi Tang

Tai zi shen 12g, fu ling 9g, bai zhu 9g, jie geng 3g, shan yao 9g, lian zi rou 9g, yi yi ren 9g, qian shi 6g, bai bian dou 9g, shi hu 12g, gu ya 9g, zhi gan cao 3g

Yin Chen Zhu Fu Yu Tang

Yin chen hao 12g, bai zhu 9g, fu zi 6g, gan jiang 6g, rou gui 3g, zhi gan cao 6g

Yin Qiao San

Jin yin hua 9g, lian qiao 9g, jie geng 6g, bo he 6g, dan zhu ye 4.5g, gan cao 4.5g, jing jie 4.5g, dan dou chi 4.5g, niu bang zi 9g, lu gen 6g

You Gui Wan

Shu di huang 24g, shan zhu yu 9g, shan yao 12g, gou qi zi 12g, tu si zi 12g, lu jiao jiao 12g, du zhong 12g, dang gui 12g, rou gui 9g, fu zi 9g

Zhen Gan Xi Feng Tang

Niu xi 30g, dai zhe shi 30g, long gu 15g, mu li 15g, gui ba 15g, bai shao 15g, xuan shen 15g, tian men dong 15g, chuan lian zi 6g, mai ya 6g, yin chen hao 6g, gan cao 4.5g

Zhen Ren Yang Zang Tang

Ren shen 6g, dang gui 9g, bai zhu 12g, rou dou kou 12g, rou gui 3g, bai shao 15g, mu xiang 9g, he zi 12g, ying su ke 21g, zhi gan cao 6g

Zhen Wu Tang Tang

Fu zi 9g, bai zhu 6g, fu ling 9g, bai shao 9g, sheng jiang 9g

Zhi Bai Di Huang Tang

Shu di huang 24g, shan zhu yu 12g, shan yao 12g, fu ling 9g, ze xie 9g, mu dan pi 9g, zhi mu 6g, huang bai 6g

Zhi Zi Dou Chi Tang

Zhi zi 9g, dan dou chi 9g

Zou Gui Wan

Shu di huang 24g, shan zhu yu 12g, shan yao 12g, gou qi zi 12g, tu si zi 12g, chuan niu xi 9g, lu jiao jiao 12g, gui ban jiao 12g

GLOSSARY

A-*shi* points	Spots on the body that are sore on palpation or are reactive.
Back-*shu* points	Back transport points. Category of acupuncture points, all of which are located on the Urinary Bladder channel. These acupuncture points can transport *qi* directly to their same name internal organ.
Bao	Envelope, wrapping. The Uterus; the place where the semen is stored; the space between the Kidneys.
Bao luo	The channel that connects the Kidneys and the Uterus.
Bao mai	The channel that connects Heart and the Uterus.
Bei	Sorrow, sadness, melancholy.
Ben	Root or cause.
Bi	Painful blockage of channel *qi*.
Biao	Branch or manifestation.
Cou li	The space between the skin and muscles; spaces in the tissue.
Cun	Chinese body measurement unit.
Da qi	'Big' *qi* or air *qi*.
Fu	Hollow organ.
Gao	Fatty tissues.
Gu qi	Food or basis *qi*. *Gu qi* is an antecedent and the foundation of *xue* and *zong qi*.
Huang	Membranes.
Hui-gathering points	*Hui* can be translated as 'meeting', 'collecting' or 'gathering'. It is a place where certain energies gather or meet.
Hun	The ethereal spirit. The *shen* aspect of the Liver.
Jiao	Space or burner. There are three *jiao* – *san jiao*. Some people define the three *jiao* as being the organs that are located in that part of the body. Others define the three *jiao* as being the cavity around these organs. A third definition is that *san jiao* is all the spaces in the body, i.e. that *san jiao* can be defined as being the following: the space between the organs; the spaces between connective tissue and the skin; the spaces in the tissue itself and between the individual cells.
Jin	Tendons.
Jin	Thin, light body fluids.
Jing	Essence or the innate *qi* inherited from the parents. The form of *qi* in the body that is the most *yin*.
Jing	Shock, fright, terror.
Jing luo	Channels and collaterals.
Jinye	Body fluids.
Jueyin	Terminal *yin*. Liver and Pericardium.
Kong	Fear.
Le	Joy.
Luo-connecting points	The place on a channel where the *luo*-connecting vessel branches away from the primary channel.
Mingmen	Gate of fire. The source of all *yang qi* in the body.
Mu-collecting points	Category of acupuncture points that are almost exclusively located on the front of the body. A *mu*-collecting point is the place where an organ's *qi* collects.
Nu	Anger.
Po	Corporeal spirit. *Shen* aspect of the Lung.
Qi	*Qi* is often translated as energy or bio-energy, but this is a very narrow definition of something that is very encompassing and vast. *Qi* is the fundamental substance or energetic matter of the universe. At the same time, *qi* is the energy or the potential that creates all the movement and all change in the universe. In the body *qi* is the sum of all

the vital substances and of all physiological activity in the body. At the same time, there are specific forms of *qi* in the body that are further differentiated from each other.

Qi ji	*Qi* mechanism, *qi* dynamic.
Rou	Muscle, meat, flesh.
Shan	*Shan* can have three definitions. It can be an organ or tissue that protrudes or has sunk from its position, for example a hernia in Western medicine. It can be extreme abdominal pain when there is concurrent urinary difficulty or constipation. Finally, it may be disorders that relate to the external genitalia.
Shaoyang	Lesser *yang*. *San jiao* and Gall Bladder.
Shaoyin	Lesser *yin*. Heart and Kidneys.
Shen	*Shen* encompasses concepts such as mind, awareness, consciousness, vitality and spirit. *Shen* is the sum of all the five organs' *shen* aspects, whilst being the specific *shen* aspect of the Heart. *Shen* is the form of *qi* in the body that is most *yang*.
Shi	Full, excess or surplus.
Shu transport points	Category of five points on each channel. The five *shu*-transport points are *jing*-well, *ying*-spring, *shu*-stream, *jing*-river and *he*-sea.
Si	Worry, speculation, pensiveness.
Taiyang	Greater *yang*. Urinary Bladder and Small Intestine.
Taiyin	Greater *yin*. Spleen and Lung.
TCM	Traditional Chinese Medicine.
Tian gui	Heavenly or celestial water. Menstrual blood; semen. Created when *jing* is transformed by Heart fire.
Wei qi	Defensive or protective *qi*. The aspect of *zhen qi* that flows under the skin. *Wei qi* moistens and warms the skin whilst protecting the body against invasions of *xie qi*.
Wu xing	Five Phases, Five Movements or Five Elements.
Xi	Happiness, joy, ecstasy.
Xi-cleft points	Category of acupuncture points. *Xi*-cleft points are the place where *qi* gathers before plunging deeper into channel.
Xie qi	Evil, perverse or pathogenic *qi*. It is a pathological form of *qi*.
Xu	Emptiness, vacuum, a lack of. Often translated as deficiency.
Xue	Blood. *Xue* is a more physical form of *qi*. *Xue* is more than just blood in Western physiology. *Xue* nourishes and moisturises the body. *Xue* also nourishes and anchors *shen*.
Yang	One of the two opposing but at the same time complementary forces in the universe.
Yangming	*Yang* Brightness. Stomach and Large Intestine.
Ye	The denser and more turbid aspect of the body fluids.
Yi	*Shen* aspect of the Spleen. *Yi* can be defined as our mental faculties, our intellectual focus and intention.
Yin	One of the two opposing but at the same time complementary forces in the universe.
Ying qi	Nourishing *qi*. Nourishes both *zangfu* organs and the whole body. *Ying qi* flows together with *xue* in the channels.
You	Oppression, anguish, restraint.
Yuan qi	Original *qi*. *Jing* that has been transformed into *qi*.
Yuan-source points	The place on a channel where *yuan qi* enters the channel and the place where *yuan qi* can be accessed.
Yun hua	Transportation and transformation.
Zang	Solid organ.
Zangfu	Internal organs.
Zhen qi	True *qi*, formed when *zong qi* is transformed by *yuan qi*. *Zhen qi* has a *yin* and a *yang* aspect that are *wei qi* and *ying qi* respectively.
Zheng qi	Correct, upright or healthy *qi*. The sum of the body's anti-pathogenic *qi*. The term is normally only used as a contrast to *xie qi*.
Zhi	*Shen* aspect of the Kidneys. Determination, will power.
Zong qi	Basis, ancestral, inherited or gathering *qi*. *Zong qi* is generated when air inhaled by the Lung is combined with *gu qi*.

REFERENCES

Ching, N. (2016) *The Fundamentals of Acupuncture*. London: Singing Dragon.

Clavey, S. (1995) 'Spleen and Stomach yin deficiency – Differentiation and treatment.' *Journal of Chinese Medicine 47*, January.

Flaws, B. (1995) *The Tao of Healthy Eating*. Boulder: Blue Poppy Press.

Gascoigne, S. (2001) *The Clinical Medicine Guide: A Holistic Perspective*. Clonakilty: Jigme Press.

Gascoigne, S. (2003) *The Prescribed Drug Guide: A Holistic Perspective*. Clonakilty: Jigme Press.

Hicks, A., Hicks, J. and Mole, P. (2004) *Five Element Constitutional Acupuncture*. Edinburgh: Churchill Livingstone.

Kastner, J. (2009) *Chinese Nutrition Therapy*. Stuttgart: Thieme.

Leggett, D. (1994) *Helping Ourselves*. Totnes: Meridian Press.

Leggett, D. (1999) *Recipes for Self Healing*. Totnes: Meridian Press.

Maciocia, G. (2004) *Diagnosis in Chinese Medicine*: *A Comprehensive Guide*. Edinburgh: Churchill Livingstone.

Maciocia, G. (2005) *The Foundations of Chinese Medicine, Second Edition*. Amsterdam: Elsevier Churchill Livingstone.

Matsumoto, K. and Birch, S. (1983) *Five Elements and Ten Stems*. Brookline: Paradigm.

Oleson, T. (2014) *Auriculotherapy Manual, Fourth Edition*. Edinburgh: Churchill Livingstone.

Pitchford, P. (1993) *Healing with Whole Foods*. Berkeley: North Atlantic Books.

Wang, J. Y. and Robertson, J. (2008) *Applied Channel Theory in Chinese Medicine*. Seattle: Eastland Press.

Worsley, J. R. (1990) *Traditional Acupuncture Volume II – Traditional Diagnosis*. Leamington Spa: The Traditional College of Acupuncture.

Xiao, F. and Liscum, G. (1995) *Chinese Medical Palmistry*. Boulder: Blue Poppy Press.

FURTHER READING

Beinfeld, H. and Korngold, E. (1991) *Between Heaven and Earth*. New York: Ballantine Books.

Buck, C. (2015) *Acupuncture and Chinese Medicine, Roots of Modern Practice*. London: Singing Dragon.

Ching, N. (2016) *The Fundamentals of Acupuncture*. London: Singing Dragon.

Clavey, P. (2003) *Fluid Physiology and Pathology in Traditional Chinese Medicine*. Edinburgh: Churchill Livingstone.

Deadman, P. and Al-Khafaji, M. (1998) *A Manual of Acupuncture*. Hove: Journal of Chinese Medicine Publications.

Deng, T. (1999) *Practical Diagnosis in Chinese Medicine*. Edinburgh: Churchill Livingstone.

Feit, R. and Zmeiwski, P. (1989) *Acumoxa Therapy, Volumes 1 and 2*. Brookline: Paradigm.

Flaws, B. (1995) *The Secrets of Pulse Diagnosis*. Boulder: Blue Poppy Press.

Flaws, B. (1995) *The Tao of Healthy Eating*. Boulder: Blue Poppy Press.

Flaws, B. (1997) *A Handbook of Menstrual Diseases in Chinese Medicine*. Boulder: Blue Poppy Press.

Focks, C. (2008) *Atlas of Acupuncture*. Edinburgh: Churchill Livingstone.

Gascoigne, S. (2001) *The Clinical Medicine Guide: A Holistic Perspective*. Clonakilty: Jigme Press.

Gascoigne, S. (2003) *The Prescribed Drug Guide: A Holistic Perspective*. Clonakilty: Jigme Press.

Hammer, L. (1990) *Dragon Rises, Red Bird Rises*. New York: Station Hill Press.

Hammer, L. (2001) *Chinese Pulse Diagnosis*. Seattle: Eastland Press.

Hammer, L. and Bilton, K. (2012) *Handbook of Contemporary Chinese Pulse Diagnosis*. Seattle: Eastland Press.

Hicks, A., Hicks, J. and Mole, P. (2004) *Five Element Constitutional Acupuncture*. Edinburgh: Churchill Livingstone.

Jiao, S. D. (2005) *Ten Lectures on the use of Formulas from the Personal Experience of Jiao Shu-De*. Taos, New Mexico: Paradigm Publications.

Kaptchuk, T. (1983) *Chinese Medicine. The Web That has No Weaver*. London: Rider.

Kastner, J. (2009) *Chinese Nutrition Therapy*. Stuttgart: Thieme.

Kirschbaum, B. (2000) *Atlas of Chinese Tongue Diagnosis, Volume 1*. Seattle: Eastland Press.

Kirschbaum, B. (2002) *Atlas of Chinese Tongue Diagnosis, Volume 2*. Seattle: Eastland Press.

Larre, C. (1994) *The Way of Heaven*. Cambridge: Monkey Press.

Larre, C. and Rochat de la Vallee, E. (1989) *The Kidneys*. Cambridge: Monkey Press.

Larre, C. and Rochat de la Vallee, E. (1989) *The Lung*. Cambridge: Monkey Press.

Larre, C. and Rochat de la Vallee, E. (1990) *The Spleen and Stomach*. Cambridge: Monkey Press.

Larre, C. and Rochat de la Vallee, E. (1991) *The Heart*. Cambridge: Monkey Press.

Larre, C. and Rochat de la Vallee, E. (1992) *The Heart Master and Triple Heater*. Cambridge: Monkey Press.

Larre, C. and Rochat de la Vallee, E. (1994) *The Liver*. Cambridge: Monkey Press.

Larre, C. and Rochat de la Vallee, E. (1995) *Rooted in Spirit*. Barrytown: Station Hill.

Larre, C. and Rochat de la Vallee, E. (1996) *The Seven Emotions*. Cambridge: Monkey Press.

Larre, C. and Rochat de la Vallee, E. (1997) *The Extraordinary Meridians*. Cambridge: Monkey Press.

Larre, C. and Rochat de la Vallee, E. (1999) *The Essence, Spirit, Blood and Qi*. Cambridge: Monkey Press.

Larre, C. and Rochat de la Vallee, E. (2003) *The Secret Treatise of the Spiritual Orchard*. Cambridge: Monkey Press.

Legge, D. (1997) *Close to the Bone*. Sidney: Sydney College Press.

Leggett, D. (1994) *Helping Ourselves*. Totnes: Meridian Press.

Leggett, D. (1999) *Recipes for Self Healing*. Totnes: Meridian Press.

Li Shi Zhen (1985) *Pulse Diagnosis*. Sydney: Paradigm Publications.

Liu, J. (1995) *Chinese Dietary Therapy*. Edinburgh: Churchill Livingstone.

Lu, H. (1986) *Chinese System of Food Cures*. New York: Sterling.

MacClean, W. and Lyttleton, J. (1998) *Clinical Handbook of Internal Medicine, Volume 1*. Campbeltown: University of Western Sydney.

MacClean, W. and Lyttleton, J. (2000) *Clinical Handbook of Internal Medicine, Volume 2*. Campbeltown: University of Western Sydney.

MacClean, W. and Lyttleton, J. (2010) *Clinical Handbook of Internal Medicine, Volume 3*. Sidney: Pangolin Press.

Maciocia, G. (1987) *Tongue Diagnosis in Chinese Medicine*. Seattle: Eastland Press.

Maciocia, G. (1998) *Obstetrics and Gynaecology in Chinese Medicine*. Edinburgh: Churchill Livingstone.

Maciocia, G. (2004) *Diagnosis in Chinese Medicine: A Comprehensive Guide*. Edinburgh: Churchill Livingstone.

Maciocia, G. (2005) *The Foundations of Chinese Medicine, Second Edition*. Amsterdam: Elsevier Churchill Livingstone.

Maciocia, G. (2006) *The Channels of Acupuncture*. Edinburgh: Churchill Livingstone.

Maoshing N. (1995) *The Yellow Emperor's Classic of Medicine*. Boston: Shambala

Matsumoto, K. and Birch, S. (1983) *Five Elements and Ten Stems*. Brookline: Paradigm.

Matsumoto, K. and Birch, S. (1986) *Extraordinary Vessels*. Brookline: Paradigm.

McCann. H. (2014) *Pricking the Vessels*. London: Singing Dragon.

Montakab, H. (2014) *Acupuncture and Channel Energetics*. Munich: Keiner.

Neeb, G. (2007) *Blood Stasis*. Edinburgh: Elsevier.

Oleson, T. (2014) *Auriculotherapy Manual, Fourth Edition*. Edinburgh: Churchill Livingstone.

Pitchford, P. (1993) *Healing with Whole Foods*. Berkeley: North Atlantic Books.

Rochat de la Vallee, E. (2009) *Wu Xing*. Cambridge: Monkey Press.

Scheid, V., Bensky, D., Ellis, A. and Barolet, R. (2009) *Formulas and Strategies, Second Edition*. Seattle: Eastland Press.

Scott, J. and Barlow, T. (1999) *Acupuncture in the Treatment of Children*. Seattle: Eastland Press.

Shao, N. F. (1990) *Diagnostics of Traditional Chinese Medicine*. Shandong: Shandong Science and Technology Press.

Sionneau, P. and Lü, G. (1996-2000) *The Treatment of Disease in TCM, Volumes 1–7*. Boulder: Blue Poppy Press.

Solos, I. (2013) *Gold Mirrors and Tongue Reflections*. London: Singing Dragon.

Spears, J. (2010) *Meridian Circuit Systems*. Charleston: Integrative Healing Press.

Torsell, P. (2000) *Kinesisk Kostlära*. Stockholm: Akunpunkturakademin.

Unschuld, P. (1986) *Nan-Ching – The Classic of Difficult Issues*. Berkeley: University of California Press.

Unschuld, P. and Tessenow, H. (2011) *Huang Di Nei Jing – Su Wen*. Berkeley: University of California Press.

Wang, J. Y. and Robertson, J. (2008) *Applied Channel Theory in Chinese Medicine*. Seattle: Eastland Press.

Wen, J. M. and Seifert, G. (2000) *Warm Disease Theory, Wen Bing Xue (trans)*. Brookline: Paradigm.

Worsley, J. R. (1990) *Traditional Acupuncture Volume II – Traditional Diagnosis*. Leamington Spa: The Traditional College of Acupuncture.

Wu J. N. (2002) *Ling Shu or The Spiritual Pivot*. Honolulu: University of Hawai Press.

Xiao, F. and Liscum, G. (1995) *Chinese Medical Palmistry*. Boulder: Blue Poppy Press.

Yan, D. X. (2000) *Aging and Blood Stasis*. Boulder: Blue Poppy Press.

Young Jie De, G. and Marchment, R. (2009) *Shang Han Lun Explained*. Chatswood, NSW: Elsevier

Zong, L.X. (2001) *Pocket Handbook of Chinese Herbal Prescriptions*. Miami: Waclion International.

ENDNOTES

Part 1

1. Dao De Jing – Lao Zi.
2. Traditional Chinese Medicine (TCM) is a modern version of acupuncture, created in the second half of the 20th century. It is based on classical Chinese acupuncture but is also heavily influenced by modern Western medicine. TCM is the primary acupuncture style practised in mainland China today.
3. In Chinese medicine physiology, the Lung is a singular organ.
4. *Qing* is a green/blue colour and is described as the colour that a dragon has. A more domestic comparison is the colour of peacock feathers or the colour on the head of a mallard duck.
5. In humans and most other mammals, cutaneous respiration accounts for one to two per cent of respiration.
6. Western medicine differentiates between macules that are larger or smaller than one centimetre in diameter. Chinese medicine does not have this differentiation.
7. ECIWO (Embryo Containing Information of the Whole Organism) is a modern acupuncture system.
8. Pain will always indicate that there is some form off stagnation. This is summarised in the saying '*Bu ze tong tong, tong ze bu tong*' which translates as 'Where there is stagnation, there is pain. Where there is free circulation, there is no pain.'
9. I have capitalised the names of specific Chinese medicine pulse qualities.
10. Older texts refer to only five *zang* organs – the Heart, Lung, Liver, Spleen and Kidneys.
11. For example, the *Shen*/Hammer pulse system,
12. The left side is considered to be *yang*. This is because when the Emperor sat on his throne facing south, the Sun rose on the left side of his body and sank on the right side.
13. This is why it is unfortunate that arthritis patients and others with joint pain are encouraged to swim. Exercise is good to move the stagnant *qi* and thereby relieve pain, but if they have Cold or Damp *bi* syndrome, swimming can aggravate the cause of their *qi* stagnation.

Part 2

14. Although there is *wei qi xu*, it will never be a pure *xu* condition, because the moment the body is invaded by *xie qi* there is a relatively *shi* condition due to the presence of *xie qi* in the body.
15. In 'cross channel' theory, acupuncture points are selected on the opposite side and in the opposite limb to where the pain is. These acupuncture points must be located in a similar area, for example if the pain is in the lateral side of the right ankle, you will select an equivalent point on the lateral side of the left wrist, or on the equivalent spot on the same great channel, such as St 36 on the left side to treat the area corresponding to LI 10 on the right side, because they are both *yangming* channel points.
16. An exception is *shaoyang* patterns. In *shaoyang* patterns *xie qi* is 'locked', the energetic 'hinge' between the interior and the exterior.
17. Often it is only the hands that feel warm. It is rare for Western patients to report that they have a warm sensation in the centre of the chest.
18. It is important that the liver is organic. This is because the Western function of the liver is to clean and break down chemicals and drugs from the blood. This means that there will be a higher concentration of toxins and chemicals in the liver than in other meat.
19. It is important to be aware of the seriousness of this situation, and the patient should be investigated by a Western medicine doctor.
20. It is important to be aware of the seriousness of this situation, and the patient should be investigated by a Western medicine doctor.
21. In Chinese medicine, fever is defined by the patient's subjective sensation of heat in the body or by the practitioner's observation, i.e. palpation of the skin and visual observation, rather than via a thermometer.

22. Another explanation is that Dryness is the climatic influence that resonates with the Metal Phase. The Gobi desert, where the air is extremely dry, is located in the west of China.

23. For a more thorough discussion of Spleen *yin xu*, the reader is referred to Steve Clavey's excellent article on the subject in the *Journal of Chinese Medicine* (Clavey 1995).

24. It is the bitter taste that is traditionally associated with Fire conditions. My own experience is that many of the patients whom I would expect to have a bitter taste in the mouth report that they have a metallic taste instead. I therefore perceive the bitter taste as encompassing the metallic taste.

25. It is important that the liver is organic. This is due to the liver's function of cleansing chemicals and drugs from the blood, which means that there will be a higher concentration of toxins and chemicals in liver than in other meat.

26. It is important that the liver is organic. This is due to the liver's function of cleansing chemicals and drugs from the blood, which means that there will be a higher concentration of toxins and chemicals in liver than in other meat.

27. 'Running piglet qi' is a sensation that arises when rebellious qi ascends uncontrolled up through *chong mai*. It can feel like 'butterflies' in the Stomach and chest, but it can also feel like a panic attack. There are often palpitations, chest oppression, a choking sensation in the throat and an inner turmoil.

Appendices

28. Unfortunately, supermarkets and the food industry are aware that consumers consciously and unconsciously choose such wares. This means that we are often deceived into believing that the products are fresher and more vibrant than they really are. This is done using all sorts of practices and substances that we would probably rather not know too much about.

29. Millet is classified in some texts as being neutral, whilst in others it is either slightly warm or slightly cool.

INDEX